Springer

Tokyo
Berlin
Heidelberg
New York
Barcelona
Budapest
Hong Kong
London
Milan
Paris
SantaClara
Singapore

Heart Replacement

Artificial Heart 6

The 6th International Symposium on
Artificial Heart and Assist Devices, July 30–31, 1996
Tokyo, Japan

Editors:
Tetsuzo Akutsu and Hitoshi Koyanagi

Associate Editors:
Pierre M. Galletti
Robert L. Kormos
Kazutomo Minami
Johannes H. Müller
Victor L. Poirier
Peer M. Portner
Setsuo Takatani
John T. Watson

Mitsuhiro Hachida
Kou Imachi
Kazunori Kataoka
Yoshinori Mitamura
Takeshi Nakatani
Hiroshi Nishida
Shin-ichi Nitta
Chisato Nojiri
Hiroyuki Suga
Yoshiyuki Taenaka
Mitsuo Umezu
Ryohei Yozu

With 380 Illustrations, Including 6 in Color

 Springer

Tetsuzo Akutsu, M.D., Ph.D.
Chairman, Terumo Corporation, Shonan Center, 1500 Inokuchi, Nakai-machi, Ashigarakami-gun, Kanagawa 259-01, Japan

Hitoshi Koyanagi, M.D.
Chairman and Professor, Department of Cardiovascular Surgery, The Heart Institute of Japan, Tokyo Women's Medical College, 8-1 Kawada-cho, Shinjuku-ku, Tokyo 162, Japan

Library of Congress Cataloging-in-Publication Data

International Symposium on Artificial Heart and Assist Devices (6th: 1996: Tokyo, Japan)
    Heart replacement: artificial heart 6 / the 6th International Symposium on Artificial Heart and Assist Devices, July 30–31, 1996, Tokyo, Japan; editors, Tetsuzo Akutsu and Hitoshi Koyanagi; associate editors, Pierre M. Galletti . . . [et al.].
        p. cm.
    Includes bibliographical references and index.
    ISBN 4-431-70209-1 (hardcover: alk. paper)
    1. Heart, Artificial—Congresses. 2. Heart—Transplantation—Congresses. I. Akutsu, Tetsuz-o, 1922– . II. Koyanagi, Hitoshi, 1936– . III. Title.
    [DNLM: 1. Heart, Artificial—congresses. 2. Heart Transplantation—congresses. 3. Assisted Circulation—congresses. 4. Biocompatible Materials—congresses. WG 169.5 I608h 1998]
    RD598.35.A78I57   1996
    617.4′120592—dc21
    DNLM/DLC
    for Library of Congress   97-41992
                                                                                                CIP

ISBN 4-431-70209-1 Springer-Verlag Tokyo Berlin Heidelberg New York

Printed on acid-free paper

© Springer-Verlag Tokyo 1998
Printed in Japan

Typesetting: Best-set Typesetter Ltd., Hong Kong
Printing & binding: Sanshodo, Tokyo
SPIN: 10646549

Preface

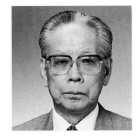

It has been just 40 years since total artificial heart (TAH) and ventricular assist devices (VAS) projects both started at the same time at two different laboratories in the United States in 1957. The number of clinical uses of TAH and VAS has now exceeded 2000 — mainly for temporary use in severe heart failure related or unrelated to heart surgery, and the rest as a bridge to heart transplantation.

Our International Symposium on Artificial Heart and Assist Devices has now entered the second decade and has been well recognized worldwide. *Artificial Heart 6* (with heart replacement as the main theme), which we present here with great pleasure, is the proceedings of the 6th meeting, which took place July 30–31, 1996, in Tokyo.

The proceedings consists of nine sessions: TAH, Heart Transplantation, Biomaterials, VAS, Clinical Application, Pathophysiology, Engineering, New Approaches, and Special Session. Session V, Clinical Application, has three sections: 1, 2, and Muscle Pumps. Excluding the last two invited special lectures, Session IX (Special Session) has three selected papers under the category of "From Pulsatile to Nonpulsatile." In the Fifth Symposium, three subjects — nonpulsatile pumps, muscle-powered pumps, and control physiology — were presented in three independent sessions as New Approaches 1, 2, and 3. I hope some topics in Session VII (Engineering) and Session VIII (New Approaches) of the present proceedings will also develop further and will comprise a major session someday.

The scientific exhibition which started in the 2nd symposium has become completely established as a regular event, and reports on approximately 20 displays have also been included in this volume. I am sure that all of you will find the proceedings interesting as well as instructive.

The 7th symposium has tentatively been scheduled to take place in the summer of 1999. I hope to meet with all of you again here in Tokyo.

Tetsuzo Akutsu
Vice President

Congratulatory Addresses

Dr. Akutsu, Vice President of the Organizing Committee; Mr. Fujiki, Director of the Life Science Division, Science and Technology Agency; Dr. Morioka, Vice President of the Japan Medical Association; Dr. Koyanagi, Secretary General of the Organizing Committee; Distinguished Guests; Ladies and Gentlemen:

It is my great pleasure and privilege to be given an opportunity to say a few words at the opening ceremony of the 6th International Symposium on Artificial Heart and Assist Devices. On behalf of the Ministry of Health and Welfare, I should like to extend my warmest welcome to all the participants, especially those who are from abroad.

Development of artificial organs which will take over the function of a part of the human body will certainly improve the quality of health care. Some remarkable progress in this field, such as the pacemaker, has been saving many patients from serious diseases. We believe that further development of artificial organs will give us great benefits and play a greater role in solving various health problems.

The government of Japan also participates with the health-care industry in joint research and development efforts for artificial organs, including the artificial heart. In overseas countries, responding to various demands and based upon new technology, new products are being developed. I believe that international cooperation in this field should be furthered, utilizing such opportunities as this symposium. Development of medical products including the artificial heart is what medical professionals are looking forward to as one of the most important vehicles to improve the quality of health care. We are now trying to increase our efforts; however, at the same time, we also recognize that it is very important for us to guarantee safety and effectiveness.

Research and development in this field necessitates a huge amount of time and financial costs and, needless to say, continuous efforts by all of you. We depend greatly on your work, and we would appreciate it if you, in the process of developing such devices, will be aware of the needs of suffering patients and of medical staff working in the clinical fields.

Finally, we believe that this symposium will surely contribute to the provision of better and efficient health-care services.

May your discussions be fruitful and productive in better understanding the complex problems in the study of the artificial heart.

Thank you.

Shuichi Tani
Director-General
Health Policy Bureau
Ministry of Health and Welfare

Ladies and Gentlemen:

I would like, first of all, to congratulate the Japan Research Promotion Society for Cardiovascular Diseases and all those who have made efforts to convene this 6th International Symposium on Artificial Heart and Assist Devices. It is a great honor for me to have an opportunity to speak at this important symposium.

As the Director of the Life Sciences Division of the Science and Technology Agency, I am in charge of promotion of life sciences, which aims first at elucidating the complex sophisticated mechanisms of life, and then at utilizing the result of research, including research on artificial organs, to find solutions to various problems in human life.

The research on artificial organs, which we are about to discuss today, is, in my view, of great importance in Japan, where the number of elderly people is rapidly increasing. Also in other countries, where organ-replacement technology is rather widely applied, the development of artificial organs is eagerly awaited as well, due to an insufficient supply of natural organs. Recognizing this importance, the Council for Science and Technology, which is a supreme advisory body for science and technology policy in Japan, chaired by the prime minister, pointed out in its 1980 report, among others, the need for introducing engineering techniques into the medical field, in particular, the necessity and importance of the development of artificial organs in such areas as circulatory and metabolic systems, as an important measure for improving human health.

In response to this report and following reports of the Council for Science and Technology, my agency has been making efforts to promote research on artificial organs, in particular, circulatory and metabolic artificial organs. For example, we have been promoting research for the development of the artificial heart by using a mechanical technique simulating the human circulatory system since FY 1991.

It goes without saying that research on artificial organs requires extensive cooperation and coordination among research institutions and researchers in such fields as medicine, biology, and engineering. In this sense, I believe, this symposium could provide participants with an extremely useful opportunity to exchange the most up-to-date research information, which, I am sure, will greatly contribute to significant progress in this field.

Thank you very much for your attention.

Kanji Fujiki
Director for the Life Sciences Division
Research and Development Bureau
Science and Technology Agency

Mr. President, Ladies and Gentlemen:

On behalf of the Japan Medical Association, I would like to congratulate you on holding the 6th International Symposium on Artificial Heart and Assist Devices.

Recent progress in science and technology has been remarkable, and in the field of medicine, the introduction of medical engineering has enabled us to achieve further development of new medical treatments. Particularly, the development of artificial organs has made steady progress.

Unfortunately, heart transplants have not yet been performed in Japan. Some Japanese surgeons, however, have actually made great contributions to the development of the artificial heart. I think, therefore, it is very significant for us to have this symposium here in Japan this year.

Nature stands firmly in front of us like a thick wall against our further progress in science. We must make every effort to break down this wall in order to continue to make further advances.

I hope that this symposium will contribute to the substantial development and practical use of the artificial heart.

Thank you.

Yasuhiko Morioka
Japan Medical Association

Past and Future Perspectives of the Symposium

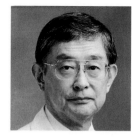

Twelve years have passed since the first symposium was held in 1985. The International Symposium on Artificial Heart and Assist Devices has been held in Tokyo, usually biennially, in the midsummer of 1985, 1987, 1990, 1992, 1995, and 1996.

Dedicated and enthusiastic investigators from the world's major artificial heart research laboratories were invited to participate at all six symposia.

A dream I had years ago, that basic scientists and clinical surgeons would get together, even if only in a small conference room, and discuss and rebuild a new concept of the artificial heart and heart replacement, came true in 1985. Since then, the symposium has been growing in size from 150 participants in 1985 to over 500 members in 1996.

The 4th, 5th, and 6th symposia differed in various important respects from the previous three. First, they featured presentations limited to the subject of heart replacement, with specific in-depth descriptions of selected techniques. Since so many more abstracts were received from abroad than had been expected, we could accept only those that were very strictly selected by the program committee.

Five hundred cardiovascular surgeons and engineers from all over the world, including 13 invited speakers, joined us in the 6th symposium. We were particularly delighted and honored that Dr. Michael E. DeBakey from Houston, who has been active for a long time as leader of the cardiovascular surgical field in the United States, addressed us with the impressive story of this exciting field.

The symposium program has been directly influenced by dramatic advances in artificial heart and heart transplantation. We are planning the 7th symposium to be held in the summer of 1999. I am looking forward to seeing all of you in 1999, here in Tokyo.

In closing, I would like to thank all the individuals and organizations who made this symposium possible. Their support was indispensable for holding the 6th symposium, and we hope for their continued support.

Hitoshi Koyanagi
Secretary General

The Yoshioka Memorial Prize, the Akutsu Prize, and the Koyanagi Scientific Exhibition Prize

The Yoshioka Memorial Prize

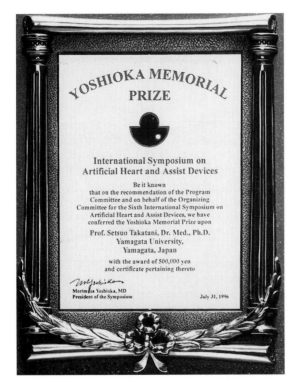

The International Symposium on Artificial Heart and Assist Devices is a biennial event that has been held six times since the 1st symposium in 1985. The president of the 6th symposium, Morimasa Yoshioka, was the third generation of the Yoshioka family to hold the position. Hiroto Yoshioka was president of the 1st, 2nd, and 3rd symposia; Hiromitsu Yoshioka, the 4th symposium; and Morimasa Yoshioka, the 5th and 6th. Just before 6th symposium we heard with profound sorrow the sudden news that Morimasa Yoshioka had died of prostatic carcinoma on July 8. All were descendents of Professor Yayoi Yoshioka, M.D., the founder of Tokyo Women's Medical College, who was especially noted for her accomplishments and devotion to the education of women in the field of medicine. Tokyo Women's Medical College opened the first heart institute in Japan in 1954 under the auspices of the late Professor Shigeru Sakakibara, an internationally recognized pioneer in cardiovascular surgery in Japan, to conduct comprehensive studies, both in research and in clinical cardiovascular diseases. During the 40 years since the institution was established, the Yoshiokas have been tireless in their efforts to financially support the development of clinical and research work for patients with heart disease. To promote research in this field, they have also sponsored the International Symposium on Artificial Heart and Assist Devices and assumed responsibility as its president. The Heart Institute of Japan has played a leading role in the field of cardiovascular surgery, cardiology, and pediatric cardiology not only in Japan but also worldwide. The Yoshioka Memorial Prize was established to honor the contributions of the late Hiroto Yoshioka, M.D., who served as president of the international symposium for the six years following its inception in 1985. The prize is presented to the author of the best clinical paper contributed to the symposium and includes an award of 500000 yen.

First Laureate, 1992: Kenji Yamazaki, M.D.
The Heart Institute of Japan, Tokyo Women's Medical College
Second Laureate, 1995: Ryohei Yozu, M.D.
Department of Surgery, Keio University
Third Laureate, 1996: Setsuo Takatani, Ph.D.
Faculty of Engineering, Yamagata University

The Akutsu Prize

The Akutsu Artificial Heart Prize was created to honor contributions to the development of the artificial heart and to celebrate the 10th anniversary of the symposium. The prize carries an award of 300000 yen. Dr. Tetsuzo Akutsu's contribution to development of the artificial heart, with Dr. Kolff, is well known worldwide. From the early stages of the development of the artificial heart up to the present, his tireless efforts manifest his courage and dignity as a researcher. The prize is awarded for the best paper contributed in the area of basic research of the artificial heart. It is hoped that many young researchers, inspired by the discipline shown by Dr. Akutsu, will devote their efforts to development of the artificial heart and that the results they achieve will be for the benefit of mankind.

First Laureate, 1995: J. Vašků, M.D.
Vacord Bioengineering Research Company
Second Laureate, 1996: Hiroaki Harasaki, M.D.
Cleveland Clinic Foundation

Koyanagi Scientific Exhibition Prize

Professor Hitoshi Koyanagi is a cardiovascular surgeon in the Department of Cardiovascular Surgery, the Heart Institute of Japan, Tokyo Women's Medical College, and studied under Professor Shigeru Sakakibara with Professor Soji Konno at the dawn of the era of cardiovascular surgery. Professor Konno, who succeeded to Professor Sakakibara's position, died at the young age of 43 years. However, all cardiovascular surgeons must remember his name in the Konno-Rastan procedure for aortic stenosis with patch grafts and a prosthetic bileaflet valve, and in the Konno-Sakakibara bioptome. The Heart Institute of Japan has contributed greatly to the development of cardiovascular surgery in Japan, and Professor Koyanagi has borne important responsibilities since his appointment to his present position in 1980. He believes his mission is to promote heart replacement treatments such as transplantation and artificial hearts for many patients suffering from severe intractable heart failure since those treatments are performed daily in the Western world. As Secretary General, Professor Koyanagi has served the international symposium five times with Dr. Akutsu acting as vice-president since 1985, his aim being the realization of treatment by heart replacement. In commemoration of the 10th anniversary of the symposium and as an expression of their gratitude to Professor Koyanagi for his efforts in handling the symposium's general affairs, the program committee members established the Koyanagi Scientific Exhibition Prize. The prize carries an award of 100000 yen.

First Laureates 1995: Tokyo University Group,
Tohoku University Group
Second Laureates 1996: Kenji Yamazaki, M.D.
The Heart Institute of Japan, Tokyo Women's Medical College;
University of Pittsburgh; Waseda University;
Sun Medical Technology Research Corporation

Toyoko Komatsu, Symposium Secretary

Contributors

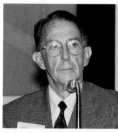

J.T. Watson

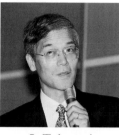

S. Takatani

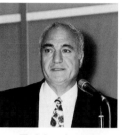

T. Mussivand

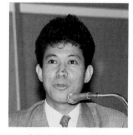

M. Kobayashi

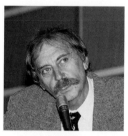

H.M. Reul for
R. Kaufmann

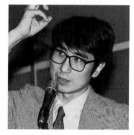

Y. Abe

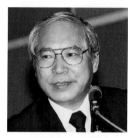

H. Harasaki

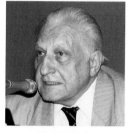

J. Vašků

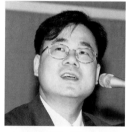

W.W. Choi

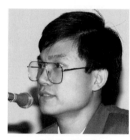

M.J. Choi

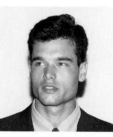

C.B. Howarth

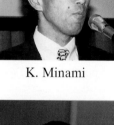

K. Minami

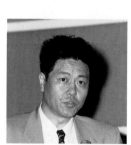

M. Hachida

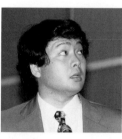

O. Tagusari

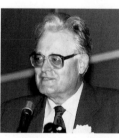

P.M. Galletti

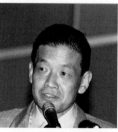

K. Imachi

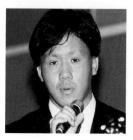

M. Waki

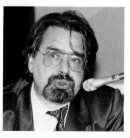

V.V. Nikolaychik

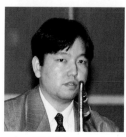

Y. Takewa

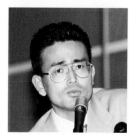

Y. Takami

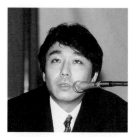

H. Ito

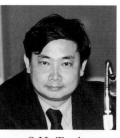

S.H. Teoh

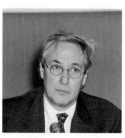

T. Okoshi

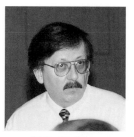

V.L. Poirier

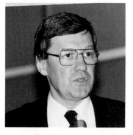

S. Westaby

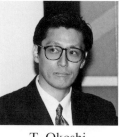

O.H. Frazier

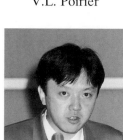

R.J. Mullaly

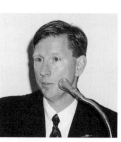

M. Nonoyama

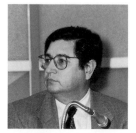

R.M. Adamson

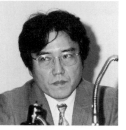

T. Masai

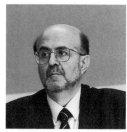

E. Castells

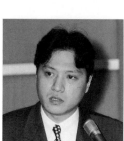

H. Niinami

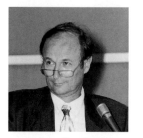

A. Pavie

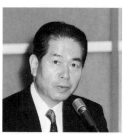

M. Okada

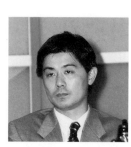

S. Isoda

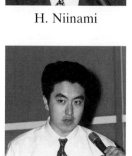

M. Nogawa

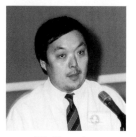

Y. Kaneko

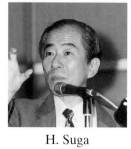

H. Suga

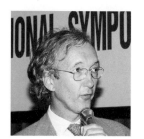

J. Müller

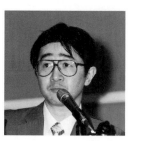

E. Tatsumi

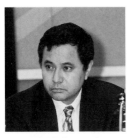 T. Nakatani

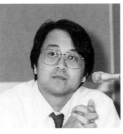 T. Yambe

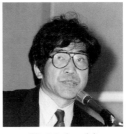 K. Mabuchi

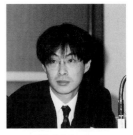 K. Nakata

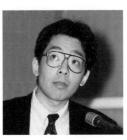 H. Konishi

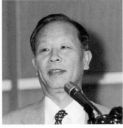 B.G. Min

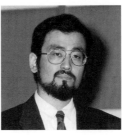 K. Yamazaki

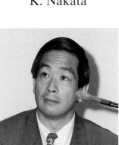 M. Umezu

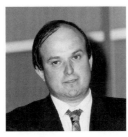 H. Schima

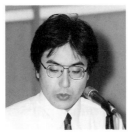 S. Nanka

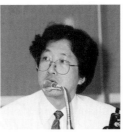 M. Yoshizawa

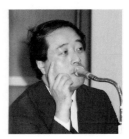 H. Nishida

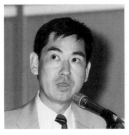 K. Nishimura

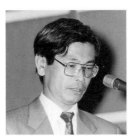 T. Yamane

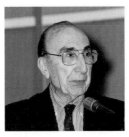 M.E. DeBakey

Table of Contents

Part I   Total Artificial Heart

— Implantable Devices

— Basic Research

Part I
Total Artificial Heart

Implantable Devices
Basic Research

Prospects for Implantable Circulatory Support

John T. Watson

Summary. The National Heart, Lung, and Blood Institute (NHLBI) recognizes that heart failure death and morbidity are a significant burden to society. During the period 1977–1992 the Institute supported the development of implantable ventricular assist devices designed for a 2-year lifetime. These devices have proven to be safe and clinically useful in over 1200 patients, the longest implantation exceeding 2 years. Patient quality of life seems relatively normal, requiring special attention to the implanted device but allowing complete freedom for most activities, including moderate exercise. The prospect of using implantable mechanical circulatory support (MCS) to treat heart failure is quite promising. The results with vented, implanted ventricular assist devices suggest that for some patients they may prove a long-term treatment for end-stage disease. For other patients, extended use of MCS may lead to reversal of the maladaptive remodeling processes and the restoration of normal function. Interestingly, clinical reports indicate that MCS systems may also be useful in conducting heart failure research. Towards its vision, the NHLBI is supporting programs for the implantable total artificial heart and for second-generation, innovative ventricular assist systems (IVAS) designed for a 5-year lifetime. The total artificial heart (TAH) program is beginning its final phase and the innovative ventricular assist systems (IVAS) program is nearing the end of its first year of design efforts. These results and the prospects for implantable circulatory support bespeak the talent, persistence, and continuing dedication of the worldwide pool of researchers, clinicians, and industrialists working in this field.

Key words: Artificial heart — Implantable circulatory support — Ventricular assist device

Introduction

The National Heart, Lung, and Blood Institute (NHLBI) is emphasizing research on heart failure. Research advances on several fronts have yet to improve the prospects for patients once diagnosed with heart failure. Cardiac transplant remains the only treatment for end-stage disease but is limited in application due to the storage of donors' organs. To meet this societal need, the NHLBI is continuing research and development of implantable ventricular and artificial heart systems as a possible alternative treatment for patients with debilitating heart failure.

Vision

The Institute's vision is for implantable mechanical circulatory support (MCS) systems that will function safely for 5 years and provide a good quality of life at an affordable cost. Two programs are funded to fulfill this vision:

1. The *implantable artificial heart* program is entering the phase of demanding laboratory tests of system reliability, and animal tests of performance, biocompatibility, and adverse events, before the initiation of human clinical trials. The total artificial heart (TAH) program is undergoing peer-review.

2. A new program for developing second-generation *implantable ventricular assist systems* is building upon the MCS experience and research supported by the NHLBI over the past 20 years. Support is provided to six investigative teams to study rotary, centrifugal, muscle-powered, pulsatile, and non-blood-contacting approaches.

This communication discusses the status of and prospects for implantable circulatory support system research, development, and clinical use.

Need and Clinical Options

The prevalence and incidence of heart failure continues to trend upwards in the United States. Heart failure affects more than 4.7 million patients in the USA and the death rate is over 47000 patients per year [1]. The condition afflicts both women and men. It is the largest diagnosis-related group of US hospitalized patients over 65 years of age [2].

Treatment options remain limited. Beta-blockers and the angiotensim-converting enzyme inhibitors seem to unload the ventricles and decrease wall tension [3]. These therapies modestly enhance survival and quality of life. Investigators are also studying

National Heart, Lung, and Blood Institute, National Institutes of Health, Bethesda, Maryland 20892-9050, USA

other experimental heart failure therapies, including new drugs, cardiomyoplasty, surgical ventricular remodeling, xenotransplantation, and Food and Drug Administration (FDA)-approved mechanical circulatory support systems.

Estimates based on current and projected mortality rates suggest that 35000–70000 patients annually would benefit from long-term mechanical circulatory support in the year 2010. The extremes of the candidate pool correspond to an upper age limit of 75 of 85 years of age for both men and women [4].

Clinical Use

Two implantable, vented ventricular assist systems (VAS) are in worldwide clinical use: the Novacor N100 left ventricular assist system (LVAS) Novacor-Baxter, Oakland, CA, USA, and the Thermo Cardiosystems (TCI; Woburn, MA, USA) Heartmate. These systems are disigned for 2-year, high-reliability use. The US FDA has approved these devices as a bridge to cardiac transplantation. In Europe, these systems are additionally approved for the long-term treatment of end-stage heart failure. Over 1200 patients have received treatment with these two devices, half pneumatically and half electrically activated (P. Portner, V. Poirier, 1996, personal communications). A few dozen of these patients have what are considered "permanent" implants. The longest TCI implant was for 1.4 years, and an ongoing Novacor implant has been operating for over 2 years.

Other than daily changing of the batteries supplying primary power to the implanted device, patients lead relatively normal lives. They must also take special precautions with their percutaneous electrical lead and vent to prevent mechanical trauma or the introduction of fluids and other contaminants. These patients have been seen playing volleyball, basketball, and tennis. Some have returned to daily work. Adverse event rates are low and should decrease with clinical experience and design improvements.

This early clinical experience suggests that MCS provides clinical benefit, is relatively safe, and provides a good quality of life. However, this has not been shown in a formal clinical trial. The question is no longer "Will MCS perform as designed?" Rather, the question is now "What are the prospects for MCS?" The status of the Institute's MCS research and development programs follows.

Innovative Ventricular Assist Systems

The aim of the new innovative ventricular assist systems (IVAS) program is to design a new generation of devices which are fully implantable, permanent, and suitable for the general worldwide population of male and female patients, with a highly reliable operating lifetime of 5 years [5]. Because of the risks of infection associated with long-term implanted devices, these systems will require no venting to atmosphere or patient percutaneous access. Each project is completing the first year of research and experimentation:

Nimbus (Rancho Cordova, CA, USA) and the University of Pittsburgh are collaborating on an axial flow rotary blood pump system for supporting the left or right ventricle. Primary electrical power is transmitted inductively across the intact skin to a controller near the blood pump located in a left subcostal space under the rectus abdominis muscle. The controller energizes the motor and maintains rotation speed to meet physiologic needs. Another implanted module provides secondary power for periods up to 45 min. The blood pump has a volume of 62 cm^3 and weighs 166 g. The blood pump has undergone 6-month animal and laboratory tests.

The Cleveland Clinic Foundation (CCF) IVAS uses a radial flow impeller as its primary element. Collaborating with the CCF are Ohio State University, Smith and Nephew Richards (Memphis, TN, USA), Mechanical Technology (Latham, NY, USA), and the NASA-Lewis Research Center (Cleveland, OH, USA). The blood pump rotating assembly is supported on a hydrodynamic, fluid film bearing and powered by an inverted, brushless d.c. motor. Demand-responsive pacemaker technology will set the running speed of the system to existing physiologic conditions. It is designed for a left hemithorax location. Prototype testing in a mock loop with a blood analog at body temperature has exceeded 500 days.

Transicoil (Trooper, PA, USA) is developing an intraventricular axial blood flow pump system. The system consists of a small axial flow blood pump (25 cm^3, 85 g) which resides in the left ventricle, dual internal control electronics and transcutaneous energy transfer, and shapeable lithium-ion batteries for internal and external power. The system is implanted in the left ventricular apex. The pump radial and thrust bearings are immersed in blood. Six-month laboratory and animal tests with the blood pump demonstrate resting cardiac output and pressure with an acceptable host response.

Pennsylvania State University at the Hershey Medical Center is working to develop a pulsatile, ventless, totally implantable ventricular assist system. It employs electromechanical actuation which mimics natural blood flow and pressure pulse. The focus of this activity is the proof-of-the-concept for totally implanting a pulsatile ventricular assist device. The blood pump and energy converter are being redesigned utilizing a comprehensive system model. New materials, bearings, and geometries are under consideration. Improvements in energy efficiency, size, manufacturability, and patient management are expected.

- Abiomed (Danvers, MA, USA) and the Columbia Presbyterian Medical Center are working together to develop an artificial myocardium (AM) to mimic the contraction–relaxation of the natural myocardium. The AM wraps the natural heart and the contractile action is performed by inflating balloon-like tubes conforming to the epicardium, which decreases the circumference of the device. This motion causes blood to be ejected from the natural ventricles. The tube design allows for hydraulic amplification using a single- or double-layer configuration. The design model is complete and fabrication prototyping studies are underway.
- A skeletal-muscle-powered left ventricular assist system is being developed by Whalen Biomedical (Cambridge, MA, USA) and the University of Utah. A uniaxial blood pump is hydraulically coupled to a separate drive bladder. Contraction of the latissimus dorsi muscle, wrapping the drive bladder, displaces hydraulic fluid into the blood pump housing. This fluid transfer causes the collapse of the uniaxial blood pump and ejection of blood into the thoracic aorta. The "dynamic conditioning" model of Guldner et al [6] is used to transform the skeletal muscle to perform like cardiac muscle. Commercially available myostimulators powered by internal batteries will control the impulses to activate this biologically powered device. Counterpulsation is the primary mode of operation. If successful, this system has the potential to provide a quality of life that may be superior to that provided by systems powered by external electric batteries.

These investigative teams collectively bring a critical mix of innovative science and technology to bear to this important public health problem. Obstacles such as thrombogenicity, infection, reliability, size, and efficiency are challenging, and the research and development required through this program requires intensive efforts and collaboration by all the investigative teams.

Prospects for Clinical (Therapeutic) Use

Implantable VADs have proved safe and beneficial for patients as a bridge to cardiac transplant. Observation of these patients suggests that following cardiac transplantation, they are discharged from hospital more rapidly than conventional cardiac transplant patients. The vented, electrically powered, implantable VADs are being investigated in a few European centers as an experimental alternative to cardiac transplantation (P. Portner, V. Poirier, 1996, personal communications).

The ability of left ventricular assist devices to support the circulation is undisputed [7]. Chronic, sustained ventricular unloading is associated with improved native ventricular function [8]. Reports show a reversal of maladaptive remodeling, an example being the reversal of chronic ventricular dilatation in patients with end-stage cardiomyopathy and the restoration of normal structure and biology. Another report indicates that mechanical support produced a reduction in anti-β_1 adrenoceptor autoantibodies and an improvement in cardiac function for nonischemic cardiomyopathy patients. One patient, with significant improvement, was explanted and is doing well with normal native cardiac function [9].

These findings suggest three therapeutic roles for VAD: (1) temporary support for "bridging" patients to a second procedure, (2) permanent support for end-stage heart failure, and (3) chronically unloading the heart, which promotes reversal of the maladaptive structural, hormonal, and biological processes that occur as heart failure progresses. Role 3 also implies that circulatory support could serve as a basis for staging other interventions to promote angiogenesis, regulate gene expression and products, and perhaps implant functional myocytes [10].

Research

Mechanical support is becoming useful as a research tool in the study of heart failure pathophysiology. In practice, patients with severe left ventricular failure who are administered nitric oxide to decrease pulmonary vascular resistance have an increased left ventricular filling pressure. To understand the mechanism of the increased filling pressure, circulatory support was used as a research methodology [11]. Patients inhaled nitric oxide while the device was operated in either a fixed or variable cardiac output mode. Filling pressure increased with the device in the fixed mode, suggesting that if cardiac output cannot increase in heart failure, then nitric oxide may decrease pulmonary vascular resistance while increasing venous return, leading to an elevated left ventricular filling pressure. Further studies may implicate nitric oxide in the pathophysiology of heart failure.

Total Artificial Heart (TAH)

The NHLBI is supporting three TAH teams: Nimbus/ Cleveland Clinic Foundation, Penn State/3M Corporation, and Abiomed/Texas Heart Institute. These programs are completing the first of two phases for the "Readiness-Testing of Implantable total Artificial Hearts." The objectives of this program are to complete the development of electrically powered, totally implantable TAH systems and to use common protocols to establish the reliability, performance, and quality of these TAH systems as a prerequisite to consideration for clinical trial [12]. At the present time the Institute is using peer-review and monitoring visits to evaluate the design of these TAH systems, documentation of quality control and manufacturability, and performance in animals, before deciding which of the three teams will proceed into Phase II device readiness testing.

This readiness-testing program is patterned after the left ventricular assist device (LVAD) readiness-testing program of the 1980s. In 1984, for the first time, four teams began a program to fabricate and test four different LVAD systems [13]. The outcome of the 1984 program is the core technologies for three therapeutic devices in use worldwide for the treatment of acute and chronic heart failure: the Abiomed BVS 5000, the ThermoCardiosystems Heartmate, and the Novacor N100 LVAS. A similar outcome is anticipated for the new TAH readiness-testing regimen.

In 1997, the first of the TAH systems will undergo formal reliability testing, submerged in body-temperature saline and attached to a mock loop. A minimum of eight systems will undergo a weekly duty cycle and be required to operate continuously for two years without failure or significant degradation in performance. This provides a reliability of 0.80 at a confidence level of 80%. Additionally, failure-free TAH operation with acceptable adverse event rates for infection, thromboembolism, bleeding, and intimal hyperplasia is required in a minimum of 24 months of testing in animals.

A Data Review Roard will provide independent oversight of the readiness-testing results, and advice to the NHLBI. The FDA and other interested federal agencies will participate in the program. The Phased Readiness Testing of TAH program is scheduled for completion at the turn of the century. With Institutional Review Board and FDA approval, these devices will enter clinical trial. General use of the implantable artificial heart should begin in 2010.

References

1. Braunwald E, Katz AM, Abboud FM, Cohn JN (1994) Proceedings of the National Heart, Lung, and Blood Institute Task Force on Heart Failure, Bethesda, MD
2. Kannel WB, Ho K, Thom T (1994) Changing epidemiological features of cardiac failure. Br Heart J 72 (2 Suppl):53–59
3. The SOLVD Investigators (1991) Effect of enalapril on survival in patients with reduced left ventricular ejection fractions and congestive heart failure. N Engl J Med 325:293–302
4. Hogness JR, VanAntwerp M (eds) (1991) The artificial heart: prototypes, policies, and patients. National Academy Press, Washington, DC
5. Castle JR (1994) Request for proposals (RFP) NHLBI-HV-94-25: innovative ventricular assist system (IVAS). National Heart, Lung, and Blood Institute, Bethesda, MD
6. Guldner NW, Eichstaedt HC, Klapproth P, Tilmans MHI, Thaudet S, Umbrain V, Ruck K, Wyffels E, Bruyland M, Sigmund M, Messmer BJ, Bardos P (1994) Dynamic training of skeletal muscle ventricles: a method to increase muscular power for cardiac assistance. Circulation 89:1032–1040
7. McCarthy PM (1995) HeartMate implantable left ventricular assist device: bridge to transplantation and other applications. Ann Thorac Surg 59:S46–S51
8. Levin HR, Oz MC, Chen JM, Packer M, Rose EA, Burkhoff D (1995) Reversal of chronic ventricular dilatation in patients with end-stage cardiomyopathy by prolonged mechanical unloading. Circulation 91:2717–2720
9. Mueller J, Wallukat G, Weng Y, Luther H-P, Siniawski H, Ziegler U, Hetzer R (1995) Simultaneous reduction in anti-β1 adrenoceptor antibodies and an improvement in cardiac function during mechanical support. An indication for weaning from assist device? Circulation (abstract): 92:I–378
10. Koh GY, Soonpa MH, Klug MG, Pride HP, Cooper BJ, Zipes DP, Field LJ (1995) Stable fetal cardiomyocyte grafts in the hearts of dystrophic mice and dogs. J Clin Invest 96:2034–2042
11. Hare JM, Sherman S, Body S, Graydon E, Colucci WS, Couper G (1995) Beneficial hemodynamic effects of inhaled nitric oxide in patients on the HeartMate left-ventricular assist device. Circulation 92:I–378
12. Frye DW (1992) Request for proposals (RFP) NHLBI-HV-92-28: phased readiness testing of implantable total artificial hearts. National Heart, Lung, and Blood Institute, Bethesda, MD
13. Castle JR (1983) Request for proposals (RFP) NHLBI-84-1: device readiness testing of implantable ventricular assist systems. National Heart, Lung, and Blood Institute, Bethesda, MD

Discussion

Dr. Nosé:
One of the major problems of improving the efficiency of your electrohydraulic system is the length of the actuator conduit. I though you shortened it, but in the picture you showed today it's still long. Why did you extend it again to a long one?

Dr. Taenaka:
That was an old picture. Right now it is about 20 cm.

Dr. Nosé:
Still long. You should shorten it.

Dr. Taenaka:
Yes, we know. The important thing is that in the chronic animal experiment, as you know, the placement of the actuator is limited. In the clinical case, the length from the pump to the actuator could be very small, so I don't think that is a big problem; but, still, we need to improve.

Dr. Portner:
Yes, I'd like to follow up on that question because I'm also concerned about the long drive lines. Have you examined the limitation on responsiveness in terms of rate and possible gravitational effects on the system?

Dr. Taenaka:
I don't think the gravitation is a big problem because the characteristic of that regenerative pump is that the afterload, or the head, is not a big problem. Do you understand "head"?

Dr. Portner:
I understand "head," but that's precisely my concern. You have to create the momentum of the column of blood in the conduit for each pumping cycle. I would have thought that would limit rate responsiveness and would also affect pump performance with positional change from lying down to standing up.

Dr. Taenaka:
Yes, the rate limitation — we know that that is a big problem, so we increased the stroke volume at the pump to compensate to overcome the problem.

Dr. Jarvik:
The use of the magnetic holding device for your transducer or sensor, do you have information on what the amount of magnetic force you can apply without causing tissue necrosis is, that would be a quantitative value of how tightly we can hold magnetically to the skin?

Dr. Taenaka:
Actually we have not evaluated how strong a magnet should be used. We don't have any information about that.

Dr. Watson:
I have a quick question before you leave. On the lithium ion battery, are they flexible?

Dr. Taenaka:
Oh, yes.

Dr. Watson:
And are they safe to use? I mean you can implant them? They are implantable! Very very good. Thank you.

Ultracompact, High-Performance, Completely Implantable Permanent Electromechanical Total Artificial Heart

Setsuo Takatani[1], Hitoshi Koyanagi[2], Masamichi Nogawa[1], Taro Inamoto[1], and Hiroshi Nishida[2]

Summary. An ultracompact, high-performance, completely implantable permanent electromechanical total artificial heart (TAH) intended for physically smaller populations like the Japanese has been designed, utilizing the desirable features of the TAHs that are already being developed elsewhere. The design specifications include: (1) it should fit in 60–65 kg adults, (2) it should have 4–5 l/min average pump output with a maximum flow of 8 l/min, (3) system efficiency should be 15%–20%, and (4) durability should be 3–5 years. The TAH is a one-piece design with left and right pusher-plate type blood pumps (55 cm^3 stroke volume) sandwiching a miniature electromechanical actuator consisting of a smaller-size planetary roller screw in combination with a d.c. brushless motor. The blood-contacting surfaces, including the inner surface of the pump housing, flexing diaphragm, and inflow/outflow valves, were fabricated with polyurethane, Bio-Span. The pump housings were fabricated with carbon fiber. Two sets of 16-bit microprocessors were incorporated to operate the TAH in the left and right alternately ejecting mode, based on the commutation sensor pulses and pusher-plate position signals. Energy is transmitted inside the body using a transcutaneous energy transmission system. The left and right flow difference is compensated for by the implantable compliance chamber. The diameter of the pumping unit is 88–90 mm with the thickness being 73 mm. The overall fabrication cost has also been reduced through incorporation of built-in polyurethane valves. This ultracompact, high-performance, completely implantable TAH is expected to be suitable for permanent replacement of the failing heart of end-stage cardiac patients.

Key words: Electromechanical total artificial heart — Planetary roller screw — Polyurethane valves — Pusher-plate blood pumps — Alternate ejection

Introduction

Artificial heart research, started in 1957 by Akutsu and Kolff [1], has made remarkable progress in the 1980s and 1990s. Patients implanted with portable ventricular assist devices (VAD) can be sent home while waiting for heart transplantation. This significantly reduces the cost involved with the patients' hospital stays. Currently, there are two devices, Novacor and TCI systems [2,3], available for bridge-to-transplantation use and also for permanent support of the heart. The permanent application of the TCI device was initiated in 1996 with older patients who may have difficulty in undergoing heart transplantation.

Since 1988, development of completely implantable permanent total artificial heart (TAH) systems has been ongoing under government contracts in the United States. Although the program was stopped temporarily in 1988, it was reinstituted later that year, confirming the usefulness of the VAD and TAH to salvage end-stage cardiac patients. It was estimated that in the United States alone from 30000 to 50000 people will benefit from such permanent systems. Currently, there are three systems being developed and tested in animals [4–6]; they are (1) an electromechanical system, by the Pennsylvania State University with Sarns 3M Inc. (Ann Arbor, MI, USA); (2) an electrohydraulic (high-pressure) system, by the Cleveland Clinic with Nimbus Inc. (Rancho Cordova, CA, USA); and (3) a low-pressure electrohydraulic system, by Abiomed Inc. (Danvers, MA, USA) with the Texas Heart Institute. The common features among these three groups include (1) a one-piece pumping system, with the left and right hearts alternately ejecting; (2) either electromechanical or electrohydraulic conversion of the electrical energy; (3) energy transmission inside the body relying on the transcutaneous energy transmission (TET) system; (4) an internal battery, which should be able to support pumping for 30–40 min in case of disconnection or failure in the external power system; and (5) an internal volume compensator (compliance chamber) to adjust for the left and right pump output difference. System reliability for 5 years, with a reliability factor of 90% or greater, is required for a permanent device. Currently, animal survival for close to 6 months has been reported with the energy transmitted with the TET system [7]. The development program will finish in the year 2000, when clinical trials will start.

Although both VAD and TAH systems developed in the United States have advanced to clinical trial

[1] Biomedical Systems Engineering, Yamagata University, 4-3-16 Joh-nan, Yonezawa, Yamagata 992, Japan
[2] Tokyo Women's Medical College, Cardiovascular Surgery, 8-1 Kawada-cho, Shinjuku-ku, Tokyo 162, Japan

stages, mainly for bridging to heart transplantation, from anatomical and systems points of view they may not be suitable for smaller-size people like the Japanese. Downsizing of the pumping chamber and an improvement in system performance are required. In Japan, since heart transplantation has not yet been reinstituted, mechanical circulatory assist devices for permanent use will be particularly important. The development of such devices will stimulate the need for heart transplantation in Japan. This study aims at the development of an ultracompact, high-performance, completely implantable, permanent, electromechanical TAH that will be applicable to smaller-size people such as the Japanese. In this paper, the design concept of the ultracompact TAH system will be described.

Design Specifications

Following the guidelines established by the NIH, the following specifications were included in the pump design:

1. The TAH should fit in 60–65-kg adults; Japanese are 10%–15% smaller than Americans and Europeans.

2. The average pump output should be 4–5 l/min with a preload of 10 mmHg, and a maximum output of 8 l/min with a preload of 15 mmHg, against a 100-mmHg afterload.

3. The system efficiency should be 15%–20%. This will allow a power requirement of 5–8 W to provide a pump output of 4–5 l/min against a 100-mmHg afterload.

4. The durability should be at least 3–5 years. Exchange of the device can be considered after 3–5 years, if necessary. At that time, heart transplantation can be considered if a donor heart is available and if the patient's condition allows the operation.

5. A TET system should be used for energy transmission. The external power source should last 7–8 h or longer before needing recharging.

6. The compliance chamber will be implanted to compensate for the left and right pump flow differences.

7. Cost performance should be justifiable. The major drawback of the artificial heart or assist device is its high cost. The overall cost needs to be reduced for wide usage.

Figure 1 shows the anatomical layout of the completely implantable TAH. A one-piece pumping unit will be implanted orthotopically in the space resulting from the removal of the natural heart. The hybrid motor controller package will be placed inside the internal battery pack. The internal battery pack should be able to supply power to the motor for at least 30–40 min in case the external power is accidentally disconnected. The energy will be transmitted inside the body utilizing the TET system.

Ultracompact TAH

To achieve the specified design requirements, either a pulsatile or a nonpulsatile device can be considered. Although it has been demonstrated up to 100 days in calves that pulsatility is not essential for the survival of

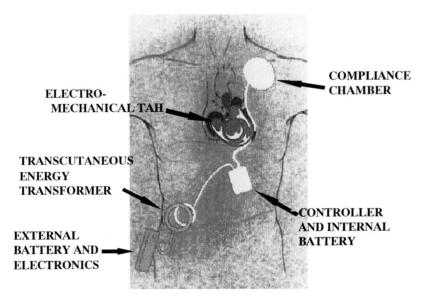

Fig. 1. Anatomical layout of the completely implantable permanent electromechanical total artificial heart (*TAH*)

the biological system [8], long-term nonpulsatile total perfusion and its control is still in question from the physiological and device points of view. In this research, therefore, we chose a pulsatile system, into which the following features have been incorporated. Figure 2 shows a schematic diagram of the pumping unit. The prototype TAH pumping unit together with a miniature roller screw and brush-less motor are shown in Fig. 3. First, the pumping unit was designed as a one-piece unit with the left and right blood pumps sandwiching a miniature electromechanical actuator in between. As for the blood pump, a pusher-plate pump with a nominal stroke volume of 55 cm^3 was designed. The pump fills passively without requiring active filling; the left and right flow difference will be automatically compensated for by the compliance chamber. This pump capacity will allow a pump output of 4–5 l/min at a pump rate of 80 bpm and 8 l/min at

140 bpm. The conical flexing diaphragm will be made from polyurethane through a dip-coating technique. An electromechanical actuator, consisting of a miniature d.c. brushless motor and a planetary roller screw, will be placed in the space available behind the two conical pusher-plates. The rotational motion of the motor will be converted to a rectilinear motion of the roller screw to actuate the left and right blood pumps alternately. A miniature-size planetary roller screw (Fig. 3) obtained from SKF (Chambery Cedex, France) together with a specially designed bruch-less DC motor from Kollmorgen Inland Motor will be used to reduce the size of the pumping unit. As for the material for the pumping unit, the pump housing will be made from carbon fiber reinforced with epoxy resin, forming a strong, light, biocompatible material. The blood-contacting surface will be covered with a seamless polyurethane. The inflow and outflow ports

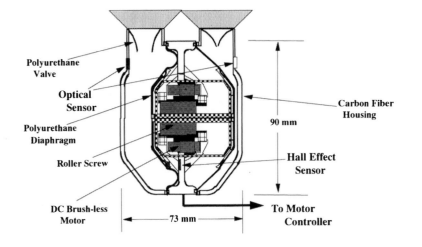
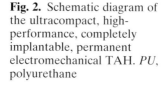

Fig. 2. Schematic diagram of the ultracompact, high-performance, completely implantable, permanent electromechanical TAH. *PU,* polyurethane

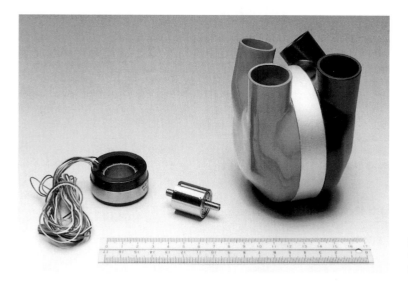

Fig. 3. A prototype TAH pumping unit with a miniature roller screw and brush-less motor

will house built-in polyurethane trileaflet valves (diameters: inflow 25 mm, outflow 21 mm) that will be developed together with the Helmholtz Institute [9,10] (Fig. 4). The longest dimension of the pumping unit is approximately 90 mm with the thickness being 73 mm.

Figure 5 shows a schematic diagram of the controller. The commutation sensor signals, 3 Hall sensors, and pusher-plate position signal will be used to control the motor speed, stroke length, and motor rotation direction. Two sets of dedicated 16-bit microprocessors will be used to monitor and control the motor speed as well as its direction. The position signal from the left pump will be used to trigger ejection of the left pump, followed by the right ejection. The left and right pump ejection motor speed will be regulated to minimize the time between the right end-ejection and left pump filling time. This will optimize the pump performance in response to the left atrial pressure as well as changes in the venous return. The commutation sensor signals will be counted to obtain the desired

stroke length, since each rotation will result in a specified number of commutation pulses. In addition, an optical sensor will be mounted in each pump housing to monitor blood hemoglobin content and oxygen saturation, from which pump output can be controlled to meet oxygen demand in peripheral tissues.

Discussion

An ultracompact, high-performance, completely implantable, permanent, electromechanical TAH has been designed to meet the anatomic requirements of physically smaller people such as the Japanese. Although VAD and TAH that have been developed in the United States are now in clinical use, their size seems to be too large for Japanese. A 10%–15% reduction in size would be advantageous for implantation inside 60–65-kg adults.

To attain ultracompactness, the electromechanical driving concept, as implemented in the Penn State and Baylor TAH, in combination with the Cleveland Clinic conical pusher-plate, has been adopted. The Penn State group has demonstrated continuous pumping in calves for over a year with the roller screw electromechanical design. The Baylor TAH, which adopted the concept of the Penn State electromechanical design and the Cleveland Clinic conical pusher-plate design, showed excellent fit in 77-kg heart transplant recipients [11,12]. The conical design reduces the distance between the left and right pump housing so as to obtain better anatomical fit. However, its size seems to be still too large for 60–65-kg adults, who require a reduction in the overall size by another 10%–15%. To attain this goal, a smaller-size roller screw and motor were employed, which reduced the

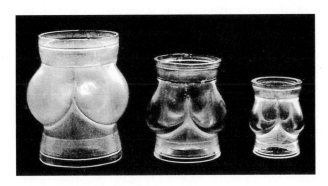

Fig. 4. Polyurethane trileaflet valves

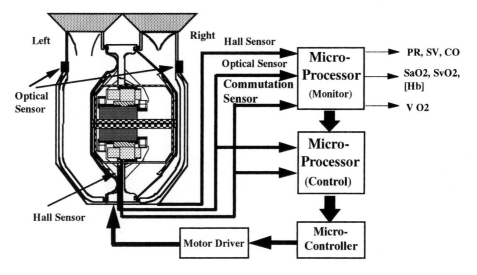

Fig. 5. Schematic diagram of the control drive system. *MCU*, Micro-Control Unit

diameter as well as the thickness of the pumping unit by approximately 10mm from the previous Baylor design. Also, carbon fiber was employed to fabricate the pump housing. This allowed a reduction in the pump housing thickness and also the total weight.

High performance can be obtained through efficient and durable performance of the planetary roller screw. The mechanical durability of the d.c. motor in combination with the roller screw has been demonstrated over a year of performance in calves. Theoretical calculation indicates that the period giving a 10% probability of failure of the roller screw in revolution in a blood pump may be greater than 10 years, and its mechanical efficiency over 95%, provided the force applied is only in the axial direction[1] [13]. The roller screw can withstand longer-term durability, provided the axial load design meets the specifications.

To achieve long-term antithrombogenesis, a flexing diaphragm was fabricated from polyurethane (Biospan-SPU, Polymer Technology Group, Emeryville, CA, USA), through a dip-coating technique. The Bio-Span, which is similar to Biomer, has a flexing life of over 200 million cycles which is close to 4–5 years [14]. The blood-contacting surface of the pump housing was also coated with the seamless polyurethane. In addition to these features, polyurethane trileaflet valves were incorporated in the inflow and outflow ports with built-in small sinuses. This eliminates the abrupt junction that usually exists when mechanical or tissue valves are incorporated in the respective ports. Thus, the internal blood-contacting surface consists of all seamless polyurethane material to allow better antithrombogenic performance.

For efficient control, commutation sensor pulses were counted to control precisely the stroke length as well as the motor speed. To attain this goal, two sets of microprocessors were employed, one for the monitor and the other for the control, to regulate precisely the motor speed in response to the changes in the left and right atrial pressures. The left pump pusher-plate position signal can be used to initiate left pump ejection, followed by right ejection. The time between the right end-ejection and left pump end-fill can be regulated to within preset levels through adjustment of the motor speed to balance the left and right atrial pressure changes. Also, the left pump ejection time control through regulation of the motor speed allowed pump-output changes in response to the left and right atrial pressure changes. Control of the left pump ejection time through regulation of the motor speed allowed pump output changes in response to the afterload changes. In addition, the optical sensor mounted on each housing should help to evaluate oxygenation in the lungs as well as to evaluate adequacy of oxygen delivery to peripheral tissues.

The built-in polyurethane valves will reduce the major cost, since four valves are necessary for each TAH. Each valve will cost US$7000–$8000, so a total of $28000–$32000 will be necessary for each TAH. Also, the use of commercially available components such as the d.c. brushless motor and the planetary roller screw can cut down the development cost. Thus, the overall cost per device is effectively reduced.

In conclusion, an ultracompact, high-performance, completely implantable permanent electromechanical TAH has been designed using the best features of the existing TAHs and components. The extra smaller-size planetary roller screw, in combination with the d.c. brushless motor, use of carbon fiber reinforced with epoxy resin for the pump housing, and use of polyurethane material for the blood-contacting surface and the inflow and outflow valves, all contributed to achieving the desired design features. The ultracompact TAH should satisfy the requirement for a permanent TAH for physically smaller people such as the Japanese. It should provide a means of supporting failing hearts for bridging to heart transplantation or as a permanent circulatory support. The fabrication, bench testing and animal study of the prototype TAH will follow in the immediate future.

References

1. Akutsu T, Kolff WJ (1958) Permanent substitutes for valves and hearts. ASAIO Trans 4:230–232
2. Prista JM, Stephen W, Nastala CJ, Gifford J, Conner EA, Brovets HS, Griffith BP, Portner PN, Kormos RL (1995) Protocol for releasing Novacor left ventricular assist system patients out-of-hospital. ASAIO J 41(3):M539–543
3. Cloy MJ, Myers TJ, Stutts LA, Macris MP, Frazier OH (1995) Hospital charges for conventional therapy vs left ventricular assist system therapy in heart transplant patients. ASAIO J 41(3):M535–538
4. Kung RT, Yu LS, Ochs RD, Parnis SM, Macris MP, Frazier OH (1995) Progress in the development of the Abiomed total artificial heart. ASAIO J 41:M245–M248
5. Snyder AJ, Rosenberg G, Weiss W, Pierce WS, Pae WE, Prophet GA, Dailey W, Kawaguchi O, Nazarian RA, Ford SK, Marlotte JA (1993) Completely implantable total artificial heart and heart assist systems: Initial in vivo testing. In: Akutsu T, Koyanagi H (eds) Heart re-

[1]Ten percent probability of failure of the roller screw in revolution was calculated from $L_{10} = (C/F_m)^3 \times 10^6$ revolutions, where L_{10} = life corresponding to a 10% probability of failure, C = dynamic nut capacity, and F_m = sum of the load N during left and right ejection. When $C = 2000\,N$, $F_m = 127\,N$, then $L_{10} = 3904 \times 10^6$ revolutions. Since the screw makes 3 revolutions per stroke, it will make 6 revolutions for the left and right ejection. For a 100-bpm pulse rate, it will make 8.64×10^5 revolutions per day. Thus, L_{10} becomes 4519 days, which is 12 years.

placement. Artificial heart 4. Springer, Tokyo, pp 117–126

6. Harasaki H, Fukamachi K, Massiello A, Fukumura F, Muramoto K, Chen J-F, Himley S, Kiraly R, Golding L, McCarthy P, Thomas D, Rintoul T, Carriker W, Butler K (1993) Development of an implantable total artificial heart: Initial animal experiments. In: Akutsu T, Koyanagi H (eds) Heart replacement. Artificial heart 4. Springer, Tokyo, pp 173–184

7. Fukamachi K, Benavides ME, Wika KE, Manos JA, Massiello AL, Harasaki H (1995) Assessment of circulating blood volume in calves with a total artificial heart. ASAIO J 41:M262–M265

8. Golding L, Murakami G, Harasaki H, Takatani S, Jacobs G, Yada I, Tomita K, Yozu R, Valdes F, Fujimoto L, Koike S, Nosé Y (1982) Chronic nonpulsatile blood flow. ASAIO Trans 28:81–85

9. Knierbein B, Rosaius N, Unger A, Reul H, Rau G (1992) CAD-design, stress analysis and in vitro evaluation of three leaflet blood-pump valves. J Biomed Eng, pp 275–283

10. Eilers R, Harbott P, Reul H, Rakhorst G, Rau G (1994) Design improvements of the HIA-VAD based on animal experiments. Artif Organs 18:473–478

11. Takatani S, Shiono M, Sasaki T, Glueck J, Noon GP, Nosé Y, DeBakey ME (1992) Development of a totally implantable electromechanical total artificial heart. Artif Organs 16:398–406

12. Takatani S, Orime Y, Tasai K, Ohra Y, Naito K, Mizuguchi K, Ling J, Noon GP, Nosé Y (1994) Totally implantable TAH and VAD with multipurpose miniature electromechanical energy system. Artif Organs 18(1):80–92

13. Lemor PC (1988) Planetary roller screws; expanding the limits of linear actuators. Machine Des

14. Ward RW, White KA (1994) Development of a new family of polyurethane urea biomaterials. Proceedings from the 8th CIMTEC — forum on new materials. Topical symposium VIII, materials in clinical applications, Florence, Italy, July 1994

Discussion

Dr. Nosé:
Dr. Takatani, I really would like to congratulate you on what you have done in such a short period of time. I think it is only 12 months. One question. Baylor TH's stroke volume is in the range of 55cc and cardiac output of 8 liters, and you reduce the original Baylor design to the 90-mm diameter and also the width. However, its cardiac output remains in the same range. What is your secret, if you can tell us.

Dr. Takatani:
Just simply that, as I indicated, this smaller-size roller screw actually has a diameter and also the length, and also leads are reduced. That allows the incorporation or one smaller-size motor, so that we can actually downsize as far as the diameter of the pump and also the stroke length. This may be the same but actually the thickness of the pump can be also reduced. Thus, I think this is the only thing. Also, incorporation of this further built-in valve may actually reduce the size of the inflow and outflow area.

Dr. Puran:
Thank you very much. I just want to know what would be the estimated cost, the price?

Dr. Takatani:
Estimated cost? I haven't done any calculations yet, so how much do you pay?

Dr. Puran:
I am from Nepal and I just wanted to know.

Dr. Takatani:
I don't know. It all depends on the components and also development costs. Maybe I can give you a figure later, but I don't have a figure now.

Dr. Watson:
Thank you, Dr. Takatani. In addition to those costs, there is also the cost of regulation and potential liability. Now I will turn the session over to my colleague, Dr. Imachi, to introduce the remaining speakers.

Development of a Totally Implantable Intrathoracic Ventricular Assist Device

Tofy Mussivand, Paul J. Hendry, Roy G. Masters, and Wilbert J. Keon

Summary. A compact, totally implantable electrohydraulic ventricular assist device (Unified System) has been developed. The device utilizes transcutaneous energy and information transfer systems to eliminate the need for percutaneous connections. Designed for intrathoracic implantation (pleural space), the Unified System has an overall volume of 480 ml. The intrathoracic implant location provides for more direct cannulation to the natural heart, and allows for a less extensive surgical implantation procedure. Long-term in vitro durability testing has been conducted, and several systems have run failure-free for 1–3.75 years. Eleven in vivo evaluations (bovine) of the complete system have been conducted. Perioperative and postoperative powering and monitoring/control of the Unified System was successfully demonstrated utilizing the developed transcutaneous energy and information transfer systems. The sustained circulation duration ranged from 1.5–96 hours with no deaths due to device failure. The in vitro and preliminary in vivo assessment has demonstrated that the Unified System can function effectively as a totally implantable assist device (i.e., without percutaneous connections). Chronic in vivo evaluation is planned in preparation for clinical trials.

Key words: Ventricular assist device — Durability testing — In vivo assessment — Transcutaneous energy transfer — Totally implantable

Introduction

A totally implantable intrathoracic ventricular assist device, which has been designed for long-term or permanent use outside of the hospital setting, is under development. The design configuration is intended to allow for left, right, or bi-ventricular mechanical circulatory support.

The most common complications with mechanical circulatory support are bleeding, thrombus/embolus, and infection [1]. Reduction in the incidence of bleeding through the use of aprotinin during the implantation of these devices has been observed [1]. Recently, improvements in thrombus/embolus-related events have been attributed to both medical therapy and im-

proved device design [1]. However, infection remains a serious complication leading to morbidity and even mortality [2]. Infection affects around 25% of mechanical circulatory support patients, and is both costly and difficult to treat [3]. To reduce the incidence of infection, the totally implantable system was designed with no percutaneous leads or vents. This approach has the potential to have a significant impact in reducing the incidence of infection [2,3]. Furthermore, an effective totally implantable device will enable patients to return to relatively normal day-to-day activities outside of the hospital, which is critical for long-term or permanent implants.

The device development program has focused on two major tasks: (1) the development of the main blood pumping unit (the Unified System), and (2) the development of associated subsystems which allow for transcutaneous powering, monitoring, and control of the implanted device.

Methods

Design Constraints

Early versions of the device focused on the feasibility of the concept and development of appropriate subsystem technologies. More recently, the design and development efforts have focused on optimization of the intrathoracic fit (i.e., volume reduction) and integration of the developed subsystems. Evaluation of the device through in vitro and in vivo testing of the complete system has also been conducted on an ongoing basis to assess the design for function and fitness for purpose.

Durability Testing

System level in vitro testing has been conducted on mock circulation loops to assess device function. In addition, several systems have been run nonstop (24 h a day) for extended periods of time to assess the long-term performance of critical components. Logs of accumulated run time on the mock circulation loops have been maintained to aid in design analysis and reliability determinations.

Cardiovascular Devices Division, University of Ottawa Heart Institute, 1053 Carling Avenue, Room H560B, Ottawa, Ontario, K1Y 4E9, Canada

Bovine (In Vivo) Evaluation

A series of bovine experiments utilizing the complete system have been conducted to assess implantability and functionality of the developed device in a physiological system [4]. The bovine experiments provided valuable input for design optimization of various components (connectors, controller, cannulae), specifically in regard to ease of use in the surgical setting.

Device and Subsystem Development

Unified System

The Unified System (version 5.0) is shown in Fig. 1; it combines the blood pump, volume displacement chamber (VDC), energy converter, and internal controller electronics into a single unit. The Unified System is designed for implantation in the left hemithorax, adjacent to the natural heart. The use of an intrathoracic implant site provides several important benefits: (1) the connecting cannulae can be short, with minimal hydraulic losses, and a reduced risk of thromboembolic incidents, due to the short blood flow pathway; (2) the implantation procedure is much less intrusive than abdominal implantation, since the need to extend the sternotomy incision to the umbilicus and to perforate the diaphragm will be eliminated; and (3) the chest wall can provide an anchoring base for the system, to prevent device migration.

Anatomical dimensions for intrathoracic implantation of the Unified System have been assessed using fit trials in cadavers and intraoperatively in patients as small as 64 kg, using a 630-ml model of the Unified

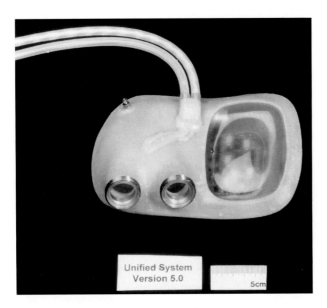

Fig. 1. Unified System (Version 5.0)

System [5]. Using these results, and those from other anatomical studies [6,7], along with fluid dynamics analysis, the overall size and geometrical constraints for the Unified System were determined. Recent optimization progress has significantly reduced the volume of the device (version 5.0) to ~480 ml. This volume reduction is expected to provide acceptable fit in a wider range of patients, specifically smaller individuals who have previously been precluded from this type of device.

To support the operation of the Unified System, several subsystems have been developed: (1) Energy Systems to provide operating power to the Unified System, and (2) Information Systems to allow the Unified System to be controlled and monitored, both locally and remotely.

Energy Systems

Power to operate the Unified System comes either from an external source through the transcutaneous energy transfer system or from the internal battery pack. The transcutaneous energy transfer system was developed to power the Unified System without the need for percutaneous connections [8]. The system consists of an internal and an external coil along with associated electronics located inside the Unified System and also on a wearable external controller. The internal coil is implanted subcutaneously in the upper clavicle region (or other suitable location) and connected to the Unified System via a hermetically sealed electrical connector. The external coil is located directly over the top of the implanted coil, at the outside of the body and connected to the external controller. Power delivered from the external battery, a wall socket, or an automobile cigarette lighter, drives an oscillator which energizes the external coil. Energy is electromagnetically coupled across the skin and tissue to the implanted internal coil. The induced voltage in the internal coil is then converted from an alternating current (a.c.) to a direct current (d.c.) by the control electronics mounted inside the Unified System. The 10–25-V output from the a.c. to d.c. conversion is used to power the Unified System and simultaneously recharge the internal battery pack when required. Autotuning circuitry reduces the impact of variations in coil separation and coil misalignment by tracking the natural resonant frequency of the transformer and providing feedback control to the oscillator.

An internal battery pack has been designed for subcutaneous implantation and is rechargeable via the transcutaneous energy transfer system [4]. The 12-V battery pack serves as an interim power reserve when exchanging external batteries, in the case of emergencies, and also allows the patient to be disconnected from an external power source for limited periods of time, such as to bathe or to shower. Currently, nickel-cadmium (Ni/Cd) battery cells have been selected [9]; however, lithium ion cells are also being investigated, because of their increased energy density. As battery technologies advance, it is anticipated that the Ni/Cd cells will be replaced with newer battery chemistries which provide improved performance and longer operating times.

Information System

A transcutaneous biotelemetry system has been developed to allow control and monitoring of the implanted Unified System [10]. The biotelemetry system utilizes infrared transmitter/receiver modules mounted in each of the energy transfer coils to establish an infrared communications link between the implanted Unified System and the outside of the body. The wearable external controller provides the ability to monitor the Unified System using a liquid crystal display (LCD) to display the system status (i.e., operating mode, the beat rate, systolic fraction, internal operating voltage, warning messages, etc.). The LCD also displays a waveform representing the movement of the blood pump diaphragm, to allow filling and ejection of the blood pump to be monitored and tailored to specific requirements (Fig. 2). Additionally, the wearable external controller provides an interface to a personal computer, for controlling various Unified System operating parameters during implantation and postoperative recovery.

Recent efforts have also focused on implementing modifications to allow secure control and monitoring of the implanted Unified System from remote locations using various public communication systems (phone lines, asynchronous transfer mode systems [ATM], cellular networks, etc.). Using this technology, health-care professionals will be able to control and/or monitor the function of the Unified System in discharged patients periodically, without the need to

have patients return to the hospital. To facilitate this home monitoring, patients would connect the wearable external controller to a phone jack (or other public communication system) and the clinician would have secure access to the implanted Unified System for control and monitoring purposes. This capability has been recently demonstrated successfully with ATM systems, public telephone lines, and cellular networks [11].

Results

A totally implantable ventricular assist system (called the Unified System) has been designed, fabricated, and evaluated. The overall size and geometry of the Unified System is compatible with intrathoracic implantation in the pleural space as determined through cadaver and intraoperative fit trials. The recent design optimization efforts have resulted in significant reductions to the overall volume (Table 1). This volume reduction is expected to provide acceptable fit in a greater number of patients, specifically those smaller patients who have previously been denied this type of device because of anatomical limitations. Optimization is ongoing and the preliminary design for the next iteration has shown that the overall volume can be further reduced to approximately 420ml.

System-level in vitro testing on mock circulation loops has been conducted to assess device function. Figure 3 shows the accumulated run time for each of the systems under test. The longest running prototype,

Table 1. Volume reduction of the Unified System

Unifed System version	Device volume (ml)	Size reduction (%)
Version 4.0 — prototype	630	—
Version 5.0 — prototype	480	24
Version 6.0 — design	420	12

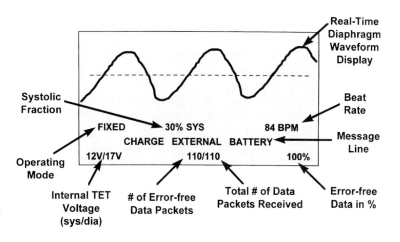

Fig. 2. Liquid crystal display screen providing the operating status of the Unified System

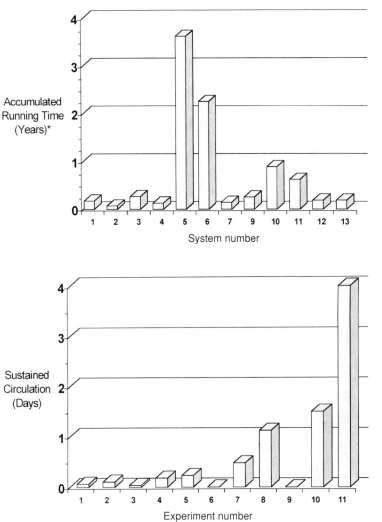

Fig. 3. In vitro durability testing: duration on mock circulation loops. *, as of May 30, 1996

Fig. 4. In vivo evaluation: duration of sustained circulation

an early prototype, has now functioned for over 3.75 years without failure, which is equivalent to over 100 million cycles.

In vivo studies to assess individual components, as well as the entire system, have been conducted to assess the implantability and functionality of the developed device. Eleven implants (bovine) utilizing the complete system have been conducted. The sustained circulation on the Unified System ranged from 1.5–96h as shown in Fig. 4. Further in vivo evaluation is planned: specifically, chronic evaluation to further assess the blood chamber design.

Discussion

As the use of mechanical circulatory support devices moves from the experimental to a mainstream therapy, the need for devices which are truly suitable for use outside of the hospital increases. Therefore, future devices must not only provide safe and effective cardiac support, but must also be designed for the patient, such that they provide minimal limitations and offer a relatively normal day-to-day lifestyle for the recipient. It is believed that a totally implantable system such as the Unified System that has no percutaneous connections and can be controlled and monitored remotely, will help to meet those criteria.

An important issue facing all developers of mechanical circulatory support devices is anatomical fit. Currently, certain patients (smaller individuals, children, teenagers) are precluded from existing devices due to the size of available devices. This situation has driven the Unified System development team to strive for continual reduction in the overall size of the implantable components of the device. It is hoped that this approach will ensure fewer patients are denied this type of lifesaving technology solely because of their body size. To further address this situation, perhaps a family of devices of different sizes and outputs, may be required to address specific patient populations.

It is hoped that in the not too distant future, patients who are functionally and physiologically able to leave the hospital, but are confined in hospital rooms tethered to the very systems which have saved their lives, will be but a memory. Only then will the many scientists involved in artificial heart technology be able to say with a clear conscience that we have truly succeeded in this field.

References

1. Mehta SM, Aufiero TX, Pae WE, Miller CA, Pierce WS (1995) Combined registry for the clinical use of mechanical ventricular assist pumps and the total artificial heart in conjunction with heart transplantation: Sixth official report — 1994. J Heart Lung Transplant 14:585–593

2. Holman WL, Murrah CP, Ferguson ER, Bourge RC, McGiffin DC, Kirklin JK (1996) Infections during extended circulatory support: University of Alabama at Birmingham experience 1989 to 1994. Ann Thorac Surg 61:366–371

3. McCarthy PM, Schmitt SK, Vargo RL, Gordon S, Keys TF, Hobbs RE (1996) Implantable LVAD infections: Implications for permanent use of the device. Ann Thorac Surg 61:359–365

4. Mussivand T, Masters RG, Hendry PJ, Keon WJ (1996) Totally implantable intrathoracic ventricular assist device. Ann Thorac Surg 61:444–447

5. Mussivand T, Masters RG, Hendry PJ, Rajagopalan K, Walley VM, Nahon D, Hicks A, Keon WJ (1992) Critical anatomic dimensions for intrathoracic circulatory assist devices. Artif Organs 16:281–285

6. Fujimoto K, Smith W, Jacobs G, Pazirandeh P, Kramer J, Kiraly R, Golding L, Matsushita S, Nosé Y (1985) Anatomical considerations in the design of a long-term implantable human left ventricle assist system. Artif Organs 9:361–374

7. Fujimoto K, Jacobs G, Pazirandeh P, Collins S, Meaney T, Smith W, Kiraly R, Nosé Y (1984) Human thoracic anatomy based on computed tomography for development of a totally implantable left ventricular assist systme. Artif Organs 8:436–444

8. Miller JA, Belanger G, Mussivand T (1993) Development of an auto-tuned transcutaneous energy transfer system. ASAIO J 39:M706–M710

9. MacLean GK, Aiken PA, Adams WA (1995) Evaluation of nickel-cadmium battery packs for mechanical circulatory support devices. ASAIO J 39:M423–M426

10. Mussivand T, Hum A, Diguer M, Holmes KS, Vecchio G, Masters RG, Hendry PJ, Keon WJ (1995) A transcutaneous energy and information transfer system for implanted medical devices. ASAIO J 41:M253–M258

11. Mussivand T, Hendry PJ, Masters RG, Holmes KS, Hum A, Keon WJ (1996) A remotely controlled and powered artificial heart pump. Artif Organs 20:1314–1319

Discussion

Dr. Harasaki:
I congratulate you for your success. I have two questions. What kind of valve do you use, and, secondly, possibly you could tell us what has been the main failure mode in your in vitro tests?

Dr. Mussivand:
I'll start with the last question. We had no failure in vitro. We have had failure in vivo and the failure in vivo was a surgical failure, not the device's. For example, bleeding was one of the major failures. The other issue was pulmonary edema and nondetected disease of the lung. Basically, in the last one, it showed at the 96th hour we had a lung which already had pneumonia before we opened the chest. Going back to the valve, at this time we use the Medtronic Hall valve. As you know, you need anticoagulation with the mechanical valves. We are planning to use tissue valves. We are looking for good tissue valves, and I am very much interested to hear from the presenters to see what you are using, and hopefully we will switch.

Dr. Wolner:
Do you have any concerns about the space and the size of your device in the left chest? I suspect when you do chronic implantations in animals or in humans that you have a compression of the left lower lobe and this is the source for infection, pneumonia, and so on. Have you any idea to remove one lobe of the lung, or what are your ideas for this?

Dr. Mussivand:
This is a very important question. We have done two things. First, in animals, we have no problem. The major problem has been to make sure the short cannulation is not pulling on the natural heart. In human beings, this design was based on many anatomical studies, both the ones that we did at Cleveland Clinic under the direction of Dr. Nosé and subsequent to that we had 29 cadavers and what we called intraoperative patients for anatomical study; and we have put this device in patients of 64 kg with no observable compression of the lungs. The main reason is that it is very flat and it goes in the pleural cavity rather than being bulky in front. We are hoping — of course we have not yet tested it in a living patient — we are hoping that it is no problem. At this time we have not seen any problem. The total volume is less than 500 ml.

Dr. Takatani:
What is the volume of the internal compliance?

Dr. Mussivand:
The stroke volume at this time is 68 ml. I believe the compliance is slightly larger than that.

Dr. Takatani:
You said bleeding is one of the causes of termination in the animal experiment. From where?

Dr. Mussivand:
Yes, we call this bleeding "diffuse" bleeding. Those of you who are familiar with bleeding both in humans and in animals, when you anticoagulate the patient you have lots of bleeding. Unfortunately it is not one place so that you go and suture it. Basically I think it was caused by heavy anticoagulation.

Use of an Improved Linear Motor-Driven Total Artificial Heart in an Acute Animal Experiment

Manabu Kobayashi[1], Hajime Yamada[1], Tsutomu Mizuno[1], Hiroshi Mizuno[1], Mitsuji Karita[2], Minoru Maeda[2], Yuichiro Matsuura[3], and Shintaro Fukunaga[3]

Summary. Linear motor-driven total artificial hearts (linear TAH) have been developed and evaluated by our group. A linear motor is capable of directly driving the reciprocating motion of pusher plates in a pulsatile artificial heart. A linear TAH has the advantages of a simpler transmission mechanism and fewer components in comparison with a rotary motor-driven TAH. The improved linear TAH was developed with a view to high thrust generation and low flow resistance. The total volume of the linear TAH is 580 mL. The linear TAH provided a maximum left pump flow rate of 5.9 L/min at a pumping rate of 113 bpm in a mock circulatory system. An acute animal experiment using a sheep was conducted to evaluate the hemodynamic performance. The maximum flow rate of the left pump was 4.2 L/min at 85 bpm in this animal experiment.

Key words: Total artificial heart — Linear motor — Linear pulse motor — Mock test — Acute animal experiment

Introduction

A linear motor-driven total artificial heart (linear TAH) is a pulsatile artificial heart driven by a linear motor [1–4]. The linear TAH has the advantages of a simpler transmission mechanism and fewer components in comparison with a rotary motor-driven TAH, because the linear motor is capable of directly driving the reciprocating pusher plates.

This paper deals with the following aspects of the newly developed linear TAH:

1. Basic structure of the improved linear TAH.
2. Flow rate characteristics in a mock test.
3. Hemodynamic performance in an acute animal experiment.

Linear TAH

Figure 1 shows the structure of the linear TAH [5]. The linear TAH has a linear pulse motor (LPM) for an

[1] Shinshu University, Faculty of Engineering, 500 Wakasato, Nagano 380, Japan
[2] Shinko Electric Co., Ltd., Development Laboratory New Products, 100 Takegahana, Ise, Mie 516, Japan
[3] Hiroshima University School of Medicine, 1-2-3 Kasumi, Minami-ku, Hiroshima 734, Japan

actuator, two pusher plates, two sac-type blood pumps, and four Jellyfish valves. The total volume of the TAH is 580 mL and the total mass is 1.9 kg. The linear TAH pumps the blood by expanding and compressing the sacs according to the reciprocating motion of the pusher plates attached to the mover in the LPM.

The LPM consists of a pair of stators, a flat mover, and two linear ball bearings for maintaining the width of the air gaps at 40 μm between the stators and the mover. The mover reciprocates with a stroke length of 17.6 mm using electromagnetic force generated from the excitation coils and permanent magnets in the stators. The LPM generates a maximum static thrust of 155 N with a 2-phase excitation current of 1.4 A, rms.

The blood pumps are made of segmented polyether polyurethane. Part of the blood flowing through the aorta branches to the bronchial artery and returns to the pulmonary vein without passing through the right ventricle in an organism. Therefore, it is necessary to have the left pump (aortic) flow rate in the TAH higher than the right pump (pulmonary arterial) flow rate for appropriate organic evaluation [6]. The difference in flow rates was set by adjusting the sizes of the blood pumps and the pusher plates. The stroke volumes of the left and right blood pumps are 60 mL and 54 mL, respectively. The diameters of the left and right pusher plates are 58 mm and 55 mm, respectively. These blood pumps are designed so that the flow resistance in the inflow and outflow ports is as low as possible. The blood pumps were covered with acrylic housings. These housings are not hermetic. Both sides of the sacs were bonded to the pusher plates and the housings using adhesive tape.

Four Jellyfish valves were used in the improved linear TAH. A Jellyfish valve consists of a valve membrane and a valve seat [7]. The valve membrane is made of blood-compatible polyurethane. The valve seat is made of polyurethane and is coated with the same material as is the valve membrane. The inner diameter of the Jellyfish valve on the inflow side is 25 mm and that on the outflow side is 18 mm.

A microstep driver and a pulse controller are used as the driving circuit of the LPM. The driving velocity

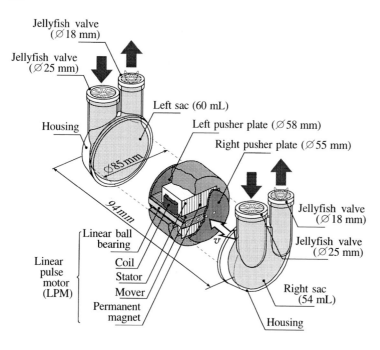

Fig. 1. Structure of the linear total artificial heart (TAH). φ, diameter

pattern of the pusher plate is an acceleration–deceleration control with a triangular wave form.

Mock Test

An overflow-type mock circulatory system was used to measure the flow rate characteristics of the linear TAH. A physiological saline solution was used in this system. The afterloads of the left and right pumps were 104.5 mmHg, and 34.21 mmHg, respectively. The preloads of the left and right pumps were both 10 mmHg. The left and the right flow rates were measured by electromagnetic flowmeters.

The flow rate characteristics in the mock test are shown in Fig. 2. The mean flow rate of the left and right pump, q_L and q_R, were increased in proportion to the pumping rate, f_P, approximately. The left pump flow rate q_L is expressed by the following function, $q(f_P)$:

$$q(f_P) = kV_s f_P \ (L/min) \qquad (1)$$

where k fillness factor = 0.83
$\quad V_s$ (stroke volume of the left pump) = 0.06 (L)
$\quad f_P$ (pumping rate) = 60–113 (bpm)

The maximum flow rate of the left pump was 5.9 L/min at a pumping rate of 113 bpm. Beyond the pumping rate of 113 bpm, the linear TAH could not work because of a step-out of the LPM. The difference in flow rates, γ, calculated by Eq. 2 was in the range of 3.2%–16.9% in this mock test.

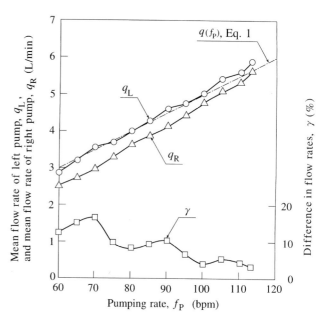

Fig. 2. Flow rate characteristics of the linear TAH in the overflow-type mock circulation test. q_L, q_R, mean flow rate of left (*circles*) and right (*triangles*) pump, respectively; $q(f_P)$, left pump flow rate expressed by Eq. 1; (*broken line*) γ, difference in flow rate between left and right pump (*squares*). Both sides of the sacs were bonded to the pusher plates and housings, respectively

$$\gamma = \frac{q_L - q_R}{q_L} \qquad (2)$$

where q_L is the mean flow rate of the left pump and q_R is the mean flow rate of the right pump.

Acute Animal Experiment

The experimental protocol described here was approved by Research Facilities for Laboratory Animal Science, Hiroshima University School of Medicine, and met the standards outlined in the "Guide for the Care and Use of Laboratory Animals" (NIH publication no. 85-23, revised 1985).

An adult sheep of weight 58 kg was used in this acute animal experiment. The descending aortic flow rate of the natural heart was 2.6 L/min at a heart rate of 111 bpm. The linear TAH was not implanted into the pleural cavity of the sheep as shown in Fig. 3 because the anatomical suitability and the compliance chamber of the linear TAH could not be considered sufficiently. The artificial circulation was maintained for two hours.

Figure 4 shows the hemodynamic performance of the linear TAH at a pumping rate of 90 bpm in the acute animal experiment. The aortic pressure, p_a, was between 170 and 100 mmHg, the central venous pressure, p_{cv}, was 13 mmHg, the pulmonary arterial pressure, p_p, was between 34 and 22 mmHg, and the left atrial pressure, p_{la}, was 20 mmHg. The mean flow rate in the descending aorta, q_{ad}, was 3.4 L/min, and the mean flow rate of the left pump, q_L, and that of the right pump, q_R, were 4.2 and 3.9 L/min, respectively.

The mean flow rate of the left pump versus the pumping rate characteristics is shown in Fig. 5. The mean flow rate in the acute animal experiment, q_L, is expressed by $q_L = q(f_P) - \Delta q_L$. $q(f_P)$ is a function given by Eq. 1 and Δq_L is the difference between the flow rates in the mock test and the acute animal experiment.

When pumping rates were between 70 and 80 bpm, the mean flow rate, q_L, decreased by $\Delta q_L'$, caused by a fall in the maximum filling of the pump. The left atrial pressure, p_{la}, was between 8.5 and 9 mmHg at this time.

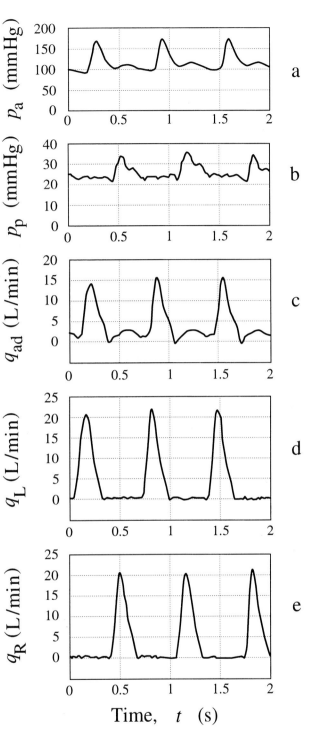

Fig. 4. Hemodynamic performance of the linear TAH in an acute animal experiment. **a** Aortic pressure p_a; **b** pulmonary arterial pressure p_p; **c** descending aortic flow rate q_{ad}; **d** left pump flow rate (aortic flow rate) q_L; **e** right pump flow rate (pulmonary artery flow rate) q_R. The pumping rate, f_P, was 90 bpm

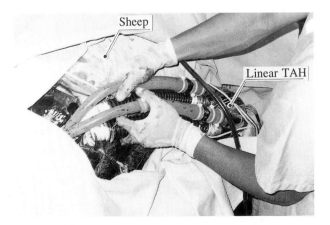

Fig. 3. In vivo evaluation of the linear TAH using a sheep

The left atrial pressure, p_{la}, was increased to 20 mmHg by a transfusion at a pumping rate of 85 bpm. The mean flow rate, q_L, was 4.2 L/min in this condition. This value was similar to that obtained from the mock testing. At pumping rates between 90 and 100 bpm, the mean flow rate, q_L, decreased by $\Delta q_L''$, the cause being a step-out of the LPM. The linear TAH was completely prevented from working by the step-out of the LPM beyond 100 bpm. The difference in flow rates, γ, calculated by Eq. 2, was in the range of 0% to 9.1% in this experiment. It was difficult to adjust the difference in flow rates, γ, by the volume difference between the left and right pumps.

Figure 6 shows the temperature characteristics on the surface of the linear TAH during the acute animal experiment. The ambient temperature, T_a, at the start of the experiment was 31.3°C. The room temperature was 23°C. The temperature of the linear TAH reached 48°C an hour after the start of the experiment, and then the temperature remained between 48°C and 50°C. The temperature rise, ΔT, can be approximately expressed by Eq. 3. The thermal time constant, λ, and saturation temperature, T_s, depend upon the iron loss, the copper loss, and the thermal conductivity of the linear TAH.

$$\Delta T = \left\{ 1 - \exp\left(-\frac{t}{\lambda} \right) \right\} (T_s - T_a)(°C) \qquad (3)$$

where t is the driving time (min)
  λ (thermal time constant) = 33 (min)
  T_s (saturation temperature) = 50 (°C)
    (the value of the temperature in the saturation state)
  T_a (ambient temperature) = 31.3 (°C)

Discussion

The mean flow rate of the left pump, q_L, ranged from 2.9 to 5.9 L/min at pumping rates, f_P, of 60–113 bpm in the mock test. The flow rate, q_L, in the acute animal experiment was 3–4.2 L/min at pump rates, f_P, of 60–85 bpm, but at higher pump rates, insufficient flow was obtained because of the lack of thrust of the linear TAH.

The desired value of the difference in flow rates between the left and right pumps, γ, was 10%–15%. However, the values of γ obtained in the animal experiment were in the range 0%–9.1%. It is necessary to improve the mechanism controlling this difference in flow rates in the future.

The temperature rise, ΔT, on the surface of the linear TAH was 18.3°C, and the temperature, T, reached 49.6°C 2 h after the beginning of the animal experiment. The main cause of this temperature rise was the iron loss in the linear motor. The linear motor needs to be redesigned to reduce the iron loss.

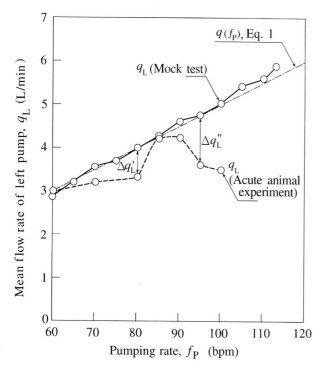

Fig. 5. Mean flow rate of left pump q_L at various pumping rates f_P. *Dashed line* joins q_L values obtained in the acute animal experiment; *solid line*, q_L from the mock circulation experiment (Fig. 2). The differences $\Delta q_L'$, $\Delta q_L''$ are shown with *double-arrowed lines*

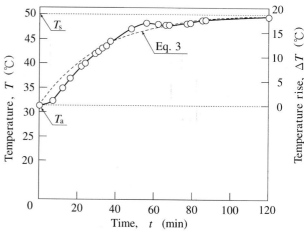

Fig. 6. Temperature change on the surface of the linear motor during the 2-h animal experiment. T_a, starting temperature (31.3°C); T_s, saturation temperature (50°C)

Conclusions

A new, linear motor-driven total artificial heart (linear TAH) was developed and evaluated in a mock circulatory system and an acute animal experiment. In conclusion:

1. The total volume of the linear TAH is 580 mL. The maximum static thrust is 155 N at an excitation current of 1.4 A, rms.

2. The maximum flow rate was 5.9 L/min at a pumping rate of 113 bpm against a 104.5-mmHg afterload in the overflow-type mock circulatory system.

3. In the acute animal experiment using a sheep, the maximum flow rate was 4.2 L/min at 85 bpm. The flow rate was not sufficient at pumping rates greater than 86 bpm because of the short thrust of the linear motor. The difference in flow rates between the left and right pumps was 0%–9.1%. It is necessary to improve the control mechanism so that the difference in flow rates ranges from 10% to 15%.

4. The temperature on the surface of the linear TAH rose to plateau at between 48°C and 50°C after an hour from the start of the experiment. The linear motor needs to be redesigned to reduce the iron loss which was the main cause of the temperature rise.

Acknowledgments. The authors wish to thank Taijiro Sueda, Yoshihiko Koura, Satoru Morita, Hiroshi Hotei, Shinji Hirai, Masafumi Sueshiro, and Kazunori Iwase of Hiroshima University School of Medicine for their helpful discussions. The authors also would like to thank Professor Kou Imachi, the University of Tokyo, for preparing Jellyfish valves, and Tetsumasa Konishi, Shinshu University, for preparing a driving circuit for the linear TAH.

References

1. Yamada H, Yamaguchi M, Karita M, Matsuura Y, Fukunaga S (1994) Acute animal experiment using a linear motor-driven total artificial heart. J Magn Soc Jpn 18:519–524
2. Yamada H, Yamaguchi M, Kobayashi K, Matsuura Y, Takano H (1995) Development and test of a linear motor-driven total artifical heart. IEEE Eng Med Biol 14:84–90
3. Yamada H, Kobayashi M, Watanabe M, Yamaguchi M, Karita M, Matsuura Y, Fukunaga S (1995) Performance evaluation of a linear motor-driven total artificial heart in an acute animal experiment. Jpn J Artif Organs 24:858–863
4. Yamada H, Kobayashi M, Watanabe M, Wakiwaka H, Karita M, Maeda M, Matsuura Y, Fukunaga S, Hotei H (1996) Second type of linear motor-driven total artificial heart. In: Akutsu T, Koyanagi H (eds) Heart replacement. Artificial heart 5. Springer, Tokyo, pp 121–124
5. Yamada H, Kobayashi M, Watanabe M, Yamaguchi M, Karita M, Maeda M, Fukunaga S (1995) Performance characteristics of a linear motor-driven total artificial heart for the second step. In: Proceedings of the first international symposium on linear drives for industry applications (IEEJ), 31 May–2 June, 1995, Nagasaki, pp 453–456
6. Taenaka Y, Kinoshita M, Masuzawa T, Nakatani T, Akagi H, Sakaki M, Matsuo Y, Inoue K, Baba Y, Anai H, Araki K, Takano H, Fujita T (1993) In vivo performance of an electrohydraulic total artificial heart toward the development of a totally implantable system. Jpn J Artif Organs 22:674–678
7. Imachi K, Mabuchi K, Chinzei T, Abe Y, Imanishi K, Yonezawa T, Kouno A, Ono T, Nozawa H, Isoyama T, Atsumi K, Fujimasa I (1992) Fabrication of a Jellyfish valve for use in an artificial heart. ASAIO Trans 38:237–242

Artificial Heart with a Highly Efficient and Sensorless Fuzzy-Controlled Energy Converter

Ralf Kaufmann, Christoph Nix, Helmut Reul, and Günter Rau

Summary. An anatomically integrated, electromechanical total artificial heart (HIA-TAH I), driven by a uniformly and unidirectionally rotating actuator with a patented hypocycloidic pusher plate displacement gear unit, has been developed. The elimination of any sliding guide mechanisms leads to a 98% mechanical efficiency of the gear unit and considerably increases the long-term reliability. Depending on the finally chosen eccentricity value of the pusher plate displacement gear, both of the free-filling pump chambers (stroke volume 65 ml) simultaneously provide a 2:3 ejection: filling-time relation. This measure increases the specific pump chamber efficiency to 65%–75%. In addition, a novel internal gas volume compliance system called the mean pressure compensator–pulsatile pressure compensator (MPC–PPC) is presented. It strongly supports the left–right output flow balance by dynamic variation of the output difference between 5% and 20% as a function of different left and right preloads. The uniform motor rotation facilitates simple sensorless preload and afterload detection by motor current analysis. After preprocessing of the current curve characteristics, a fuzzy control module, as part of the control loop, evaluates the actual pump status and generates a decision for beat rate adaptation by changing motor speed. The current HIA-TAH I device with its Labtype MPC–PPC system and perfusion controller is presented as well as some relevant in vitro test results.

Key words: Total artificial heart — Efficiency — Compliance — Sensorless preload and afterload detection — Fuzzy control

Introduction

Worldwide, a handful of research groups are involved in the development of orthotopic pulsatile total artificial hearts. The final goal is a device for use as a long-term bridge to heart transplantation and finally for use as a permanent heart-replacement system [1]. The common features of all concepts are double pump chambers with diaphragms or with geometrically adapted blood sacs within rigid housings, and inflow and outflow ports with different types of artificial valves. The different energy converter principles for supplying hydraulic energy to the circulatory system (pulsatile flow and pressure) can be divided into four categories:

1. Electropneumatic
2. Electrohydraulic
3. Electrohydraulic-mechanical
4. Electromechanical

While electropneumatic total artificial hearts (TAHs) cannot be fully implanted, because of their relatively heavy and large gas compressors, the other TAH-driving concepts open the door to fully implantable and anatomically adapted tether-free heart replacement. The main advantages of electrohydraulic energy converters are the elimination of compliance chambers and an easy anatomical adaptation of pump chambers, since they are geometrically more variable. However, many problems occur in balancing right and left output (e.g., interatrial shunts or atrial hydraulic fluid reservoirs are necessary) as well as in the limiting of negative filling pressures or venous suction at high rates of pumping. The electric motors which drive small rotary pumps for hydraulic fluid movement and pressure generation have to be reversed for each stroke [2]. Otherwise, they have to be equipped with technically expenditive flow direction switch valves [3]. Finally, the hydraulic fluid itself is an additional factor which may complicate pump development. The well-known electrohydraulic-mechanical E4T-TAH [4] regains the advantages of free pump chamber filling and right–left balance by stroke volume variation. Its pusher plate actuator is driven by high hydraulic pressure which requires the aforementioned flow-switching technology, and it has to deal with hydraulic fluid related problems. The path of energy conversion within these actuators is rathr long and has limited efficiency. Improved efficiency can be obtained with electromechanically driven TAHs. This is due to a shortened energy conversion path without the hydraulic stage. Electrical input energy is directly converted into mechanical energy of the pusher plate. Within an electromechanical TAH, there are three design areas which can be separately considered for further improvement of overall efficiency:

Helmholtz Institute for Biomedical Engineering, Pauwelsstrasse 20, D-52074 Aachen, Germany

Fig. 1. Helmholtz Institute Aachen total artificial heart (HIA-TAH I) and its anatomical fitting study model (*left side*)

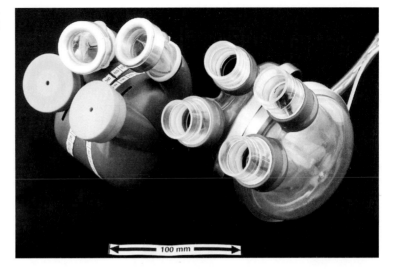

1. Electrical actuator (mostly a brushless d.c. motor)
2. Mechanical displacement gear unit
3. Internal pump chamber geometry and valves

Most of the currently developed electromechanical TAHs use highly integrated gear technologies of the 1970s and 1980s, such as ball or roller screws, and camshafts with hollow wheel motors, d.c.-motors within a moving actuator, or simple linear motors [5–8]. Each of these technologies needs reversing motors. With the technical progress of the 1990s, smaller and stronger d.c.-motors became available. More efficiently actuated TAHs with uniformly and unidirectionally rotating motors, smaller gear units without sliding guides, and easier sensorless preload and afterload detection are now possible. The Helmholtz Total Artificial Heart (HIA-TAH) belongs to this novel category. The development of this TAH was initiated in 1990. Figure 1 shows the system (HIA-TAH I) together with the anatomical fitting model. Both represent the current state of development. The presented version also permits integration of the complete motor commutation and power electronics into the pump housing. This model was derived from the HIA-TAH Labtype [9].

Current Helmholtz Total Artificial Heart

Figure 2 gives a schematic impression of the most characteristic components of the HIA-TAH. The close arrangement of the inlet and outlet ports of the pump chambers supports the proper fitting of all components, considering the anatomical constraints. The overall volume of the current pump unit is 550 ml. Within the housing, two spherical pusher plates en-

close the motor and gear unit in the end-diastolic position. They are linked by simple hinge joints to the piston rods which are supported by a planetary wheel where eccentric bearings generate the special hypocycloid (Fig. 3). Polyurethane membranes which are glued to the pusher plate work as a reliable axial guiding element (see Fig. 2, no. 4). The orientation of the pusher plates during ejection is supported by the rolling fold of the guiding membrane. Because of the spherical pusher plate surface, the membrane deforms in a circular rolling fold which expands in a concentric way during the ejection phase. The guiding membrane is perforated for free venting of the gas behind the actual diaphragm of the pump chamber.

Hypocycloidic Pusher Plate Displacement Gear

The displacement gear transforms the unidirectional constant rotational movement of a sensorless commutated brushless d.c. motor with internal rotor (Etel SA, Môtiers, Switzerland) [1] into translatory pusher plate movements (Fig. 3). This feature permits the elimination of rotor position sensors and rotational switches which decrease the general reliability. The mean efficiency of this motor (mechanical work per cycle divided by electrical work per cycle) is between 60% and 70%. The displacement curves of the pusher plates provide flow output curves similar to those of the natural heart. This leads to a left systolic duration of 40% of the cycle time and a prolonged passsive filling time of 60%. The unidirectionally rotating motor drives the toothed sun wheel (Fig. 3, no. I). This again drives a planetary wheel of the same diameter (Fig. 3, no. II). Due to the fixed hollow wheel (Fig. 3, no. III) which

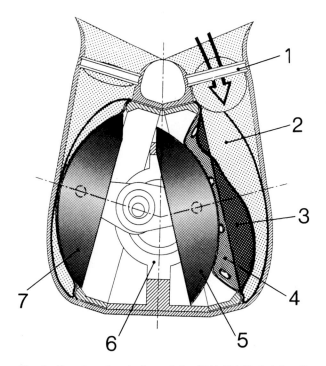

Fig. 2. Cross-sectional view of the HIA-TAH: *1*, inlet disc valve; *2*, pump chamber; *3*, double-layered diaphragm; *4*, pusher plate guiding membrane; *5*, right pusher plate in end-diastolic position; *6*, motor-gear unit; *7*, left pusher plate in end-systolic position

supports the planetary wheel, an eccentric bearing on the planetary wheel (Fig. 3, point E) describes a three-edged hypocycloid. One of the corners of the hypocycloid has to be orientated into the axial dis-

placement direction. The chosen eccentricity provides a mean radius of about 25 mm of the long edges of the hypocycloid (Fig. 3, curve L) which is identical with the left piston rod length (Fig. 3, no. IV) [10]. The mean mechanical efficiency of this continously operating gear unit is 98% [11]. Despite identical chamber and pusher plate design, the right pump chamber has a higher specific hydraulic efficiency than the left one [1]. This is due to the smaller pressure difference between the right atrium and the pulmonary artery. However, three methods can be used to reduce the right pump output:

1. With a right bearing eccentricity of zero, a sinoidal displacement curve (Fig. 3, right side) is obtained, which provides a 1:1 systolic–diastolic time relation. This causes a 10% reduction in filling time associated with a slight decrease of stroke volume.

2. A positive side effect of the novel compliance system (see Fig. 4) can also be used. It generates a dynamic pump balance by a certain filling delay (FD) at the right pump chamber (Fig. 3, curve part FD).

3. An outward shift of the right pump chamber of only 2 mm along the displacement axis causes a fixed stroke volume reduction of about 7% realative to the left pump chamber. This effect is due to the nonlinear displacement length–stroke volume relationship. The right displacement length is not affected. To keep the overall volume of the TAH constant, it is necessary to reduce the right pump chamber height by the same amount, 2 mm.

In vitro results (see Fig. 8) show that for right–left output balance a combination of methods 1 and 2 is

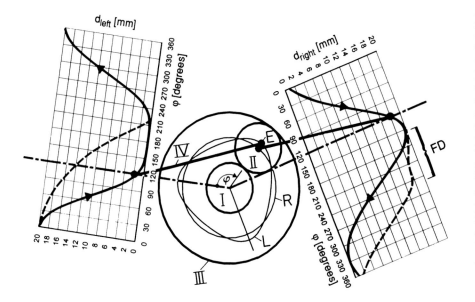

Fig. 3. Kinematic principle of left and right pusher plate displacement curve generation (*continuous curves*). The displacement axes are marked by dot-dash lines. The diaphragm displacement is marked by *dashed curves*: φ, cycle angle counted from left end-systolic position; *I*, uniform unidirectionally rotating sun-wheel; *II*, planetary wheel; *III*, hollow wheel; *IV*, piston rod (*left*); *E*, eccentric bearing of the left piston rod; *L*, hypocycloidic movement curve of point E; *R*, circular movement curve of the bearing of the right piston rod; *FD*, right filling delay

sufficient to achieve physiological conditions. Depending on preload and afterload, mean pump chamber efficiencies (arterial hydraulic work per cycle divided by mechanical pusher plate work per cycle) between 65% and 75% for the left pump chamber and between 50% and 65% for the right pump chamber can be achieved. The overall efficiency of the HIA-TAH (complete arterial hydraulic work per cycle divided by electrical input work per cycle) is between 30% and 51% [11].

MPC–PPC Compliance Concept

The pressure difference across the diaphragm between the venous system and the gas within the housing of the energy converter has to provide a nearly undisturbed filling of the pump chamber without suction effects. Due to this requirement, the relative gas pressure within the pump housing has to change in a special manner with a small amplitude (±15mmHg) around a mean value of –4mmHg which represents the intrathoracic pressure (see Fig. 7). Limitation of gas pressure oscillations is the task of the intrathoracically placed MPC–PPC compliance system [12]. This system has a substantially rigid housing which exerts only low strains on the surrounding lung tissue because of its very small pulsating volume of 30ml only. It consist of two parts (Fig. 4):

1. A semi-rigid mean pressure compensator (MPC) which contains 70ml of a hydraulic fluid (e.g., silicone oil)
2. A small compliance chamber (PPC) with a volume of 30ml

Both parts are conected via a throttle through which fluid can pass from one compartment to the other (Fig. 4, no. 6). The MPC compensates long-term changes of internal gas pressure which may be due to atmospheric pressure changes or other environmental pressure effects. The PPC compensates short-term changes of gas volume caused by pump action.

Sensorless Load Detection and Fuzzy Control Concept

The main task of a TAH control system is to achieve sufficient organ perfusion at different load conditions due to changes in physiological exercise. Some general restrictions have to be observed. It is not possible to increase cardiac output (CO) if the available amount of blood at the pump inlet is too low. Aortic pressure has to be in a range which maintains a pressure gradient high enough for diffusion on one side, and low enough to prevent any high-pressure damage on the other. Full–empty pumping has to be ensured for both pump chambers. Our concept follows the Frank-Starling law: "High venous return causes an increase of cardiac output." An increase of CO is achieved by increasing the pump rate. Active adaptation to organ perfusion demand is achieved by controlling the rotational speed of the motor (Fig. 5) within a range of 1000–2700rpm. The control circuit (Fig. 5) consists of two parts: first, the HIA-TAH itself, with its inner control circle for the adjustment of motor speed to the guiding input voltage U_{k+1}; and second, the control unit which contains a fuzzy module for adaptation decisions to body perfusion demands. The fuzzy control unit was first implemented on a PC platform and has now been ransferred to a Siemens 80C166 microcontroller (Siemens, Munich, Germany) which combines all necessary features such as analog–digital (A/D) converters, pulse width modulation (PWM) output signals, and software tools (fuzzy TECH 3.1, Inform GmbH, Aachen, Germany) for the fuzzy control concept [13].

Fig. 4. Design study of the MPC–PPC system with mean pressure compensator (MPC) and pulsatile pressure compensator (PPC). **a** PPC actuation at high relative environmental pressures. **b** PPC actuation at low relative environmental pressures. *1*, tube to internal gas space of the TAH; *2*, circular gas distribution tube; *3*, PPC diaphragm; *4*, diaphragm stop mesh; *5*, internal MPC-diaphragm; *6*, fluid throttle; *7*, rigid compliance frame; *8*, external MPC-diaphragm

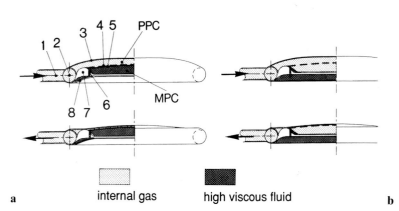

internal gas   high viscous fluid

Because of the unidirectional motor movement and the highly efficient gear unit, there is a high affinity between the motor current curve $I_{k(t)}$ and preload and afterload conditions. Several pieces of information can be derived from the time course of the motor current curve $I_{k(t)}$ (Fig. 6). The current maximum ($I_{k_{max}}$) is nearly a linear function of the afterload at the left pump outlet. Points A and B represent the start of the pump chamber ejection phase. It is expected that due to atrial inflow, the diaphragm contacts the resting pusher plate a few milliseconds before displacement begins. An estimation of the preload on the left side is possible by a mathematical algorithm which is based on an analysis of the shaded area of the current curves [14]. Filling information can also be inferred from the course of the current curve.

Results and Discussion

The in vitro test results presented here were obtained from studies with the HIA-TAH Labtype [9]. Despite its larger stroke volume of 73 ml compared to the current HIA-TAH I version with 65 ml, the results give a good representation of the principal features of the overall concept. The compliance chamber function of the HIA-TAH I will be even better because of the smaller displaced chamber volumes. Figure 7 shows the internal gas pressure pG over normalized cycle time with and without the MPC–PPC system. Without the compliance system, pump rates above 100/min generated dangerous negative pressures (Fig. 7, upper panels). Suction and excess pressure of the internal gas alternated at twice the pump frequency. With the compliance system the internal gas pressure was well controlled. The MPC kept the mean internal gas pressure

at the intrathoracic environmental pressure for the TAH (–4 mmHg) due to passive shifting of the fluid volume via a throttle (Fig. 4, no. 6). For in vitro testing, this situation was simulated by increasing the atrial and arterial pressures by about 4 mmHg relative to their nominal values. This "trick" facilitates the simulation of a mean intrathoracic hypopressure. With the volume compensator, small excess pressures at pump rates above 140/min can be observed (Fig. 7, lower panels). These positive gas pressure peaks are respon-

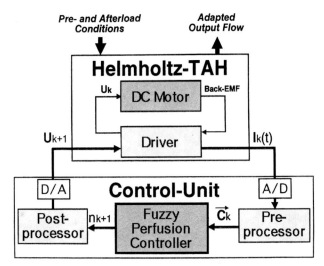

Fig. 5. Schematic diagram of the perfusion control circuit for the HIA-TAH. $I_{k(t)}$, motor current of the actual cycle; $\vec{C}_k$, motor current related characteristic load vector; n_{k+1}, adapted rotational speed of the next cycle; U_{k+1}, target voltage of the next cycle; U_k, voltage of the actual cycle; *Back-EMF*, rotor induced voltage: *A/D*, analog/digital converter; *D/A*, digital/analog converter

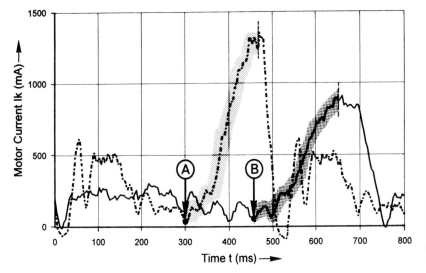

Fig. 6. Left–right preload and afterload related motor current curves $I_{k(t)}$ at 80 bpm (*solid trace*) and 120 bpm (*dashed trace*). *A, B*, start of pump chamber ejection phase

sible for decreased right filling times (Fig. 3, curve part FD). All of these results are nearly invariant with various right atrial pressures between 0 and 12 mmHg. Figure 8 shows the compiled results of fuzzy-controlled pumping at left preload dependent pump rates n (Fig. 8a), mean left and right pump outputs $Q_{l,r}$ (Fig. 8b), as well as the resulting relative shunt flows (Fig. 8c). In contrast to the present motor current analysis, optimal left chamber filling was directly detected by means of an infrared switch sensor within the pusher plate of the HIA-TAH Labtype. Physiological aortic pressures of $P_{ao} = 120/80$ mmHg and pulmonary artery pressures of $P_{pa} = 25/10$ mmHg were simulated. The afore-mentioned right-side filling decrease was additionally supported by the special right displacement kinematics which finally led to a reduced right

pump flow and established the pump volume balance. The achieved balance was optimal at 5%–12% reduced right pump flow at right atrial pressures of about 6 mmHg (Fig. 8c).

Conclusions

The gear unit transforms a uniform unidirectional rotational motor movement into translatory pusher plate movements without sliding guides and with a prolonged left filling time. This highly efficient operation has the following consequences:

— low heat generation by motor and gear unit (the maximum value is 4 W), and therefore reduced need for heat dissipation
— low friction and wear as well as low stress and strain on functional parts, which generally improves lifetime and system reliability
— better detection of load effects (e.g., preload and afterload detection for pump output control)
— low inertia effects, vibration, and noise

The in vitro tests confirm that the very small volume of the small compliance chamber (PPC), about 30 ml, is able to limit efficiently the gas pressure oscillations to ±15 mmHg around a mean pressure compensator (MPC)-controlled value within the pump housing. The separation of the MPC and PPC results in a safer and more stable volume compensation for an implantable artificial heart. Because of the incompressibility of the fluid and the damping effect of the throttle, this volume compensator is less sensitive to external shocks and compression than common completely gas-filled chamber compensators. The successful application of sensorless preload and afterload data acquisition in combination with a control unit which contains fuzzy-based decision-making modules is one of the benefits of this approach. A technically improved version, called HIA-TAH II, is under development and will be used for initial animal testing. In this context our contribution should be regarded as part of an evolutionary

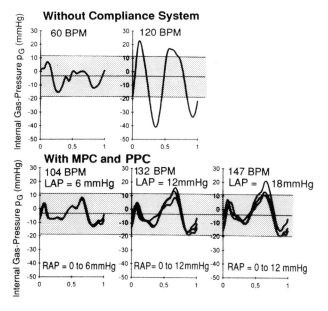

Fig. 7. Internal gas pressure (ρ_G) effects versus normalized cycle time with and without the MPC–PPC system. *LAP*, left atrial pressure; *RAP*, right atrial pressure

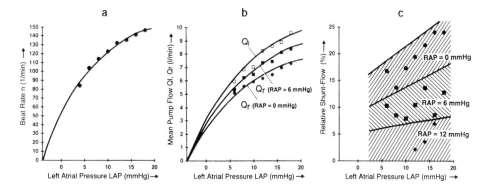

Fig. 8. Left preload controlled beat rates (**a**), mean left and right pump performances for different right atrial pressures (RAP) (**b**), and dynamic flow balances for different RAP (**c**). Q_l, Q_r, mean pump flow (left, right)

process which may hopefully lead to improved patient care and patient survival.

References

1. Kaufmann R, Reul H, Rau G (1995) Total artificial heart with high-efficiency motor-gear unit. In: Unger F (ed) Assisted circulation 4. Springer New York, pp 249–263
2. Olsen DB, White KR, Long JW, Khanwilkar PS (1991) Right–left ventricular output balance in the totally impantable artificial heart. Int J Artif Organs 6:359–364
3. Yu LS, Finnegan M, Vaughan S, Ochs B, Parnis S, Frazier OH, Kung RTV (1993) A compact and noise free electrohydraulic total artificial heart. ASAIO J 39:386–391
4. Rintoul TC, Butler KC, Thomas DC, Carriker JW, Maher TR, Kiraly RJ, Massiello A, Himley SC, Chen J, Fukamachi K, Harasaki H, Savage R, McCarthy P (1993) Continuing development of the Cleveland Clinic — Nimbus total artificial heart. ASAIO J 39:168–171
5. Snyder AJ, Rosenberg G, Weiss W, Pae WE, Prophet GA, Dailey W, Kawaguchi O, Nazarian RA, Ford SK, Marlotte JA, Pierce WS (1993) Completely implantable total artificial heart and heart assist systems: Initial in vivo testing. In: Akutsu T, Koyanagi H (eds) Artificial heart 4, heart replacement. Springer, Tokyo, pp 117–123
6. Shiono M, Takatani S, Sasaki T, Minato N, Orime Y, Swenson Ca, Noon GP, Nosé Y (1993) Baylor multipurpose one-piece total artificial heart (TAH) system for short-term to long-term use. In: Akutsu T, Koyanagi H (eds) Artificial heart 4, heart replacement. Springer, Tokyo, pp 153–156
7. Min BG, Kim HC, Lee SH, Chang JK, Choi JW, Kim JW, Seo KP, Rho JR, Ahn H, Kim SW, Olsen DB (1991) Design of moving-actuator total artificial heart (Korean Heart). In: Akutsu T, Koyanagi H (eds) Artificial heart 3. Springer, Tokyo, pp 229–233
8. Yamaguchi M, Yamada H, Wakiwaka H, Karita M (1993) System estimation of linear pulse motor-driven artificial heart. In: Akutsu T, Koyanagi H (eds) Artificial heart 4, heart replacement. Springer, Tokyo, pp 127–132
9. Kaufmann R, Reul H, Rau G (1994) The Helmholtz total artificial heart labtype. Artif Organs 7:537–542
10. Kaufmann R, Reul H, Rau G, Bitdinger R (1993) United States Patent 5 263 978. Blood pump for pulsating operation
11. Kaufmann R (1996) Entwurf eines vollimplantierbaren elektromechanischen Künstlichen Herzens. VDI, Düsseldorf, pp 1–238
12. Kaufmann R, Nix C, Reul H, Rau G (1995) A new compliance chamber concept for fully implantable bloodpumps. Research Report 1993/94 of the Helmholtz Institute for Biomedical Engineering, Aachen, pp 61–70
13. Kaufmann R, Becker K, Nix C, Reul H, Rau G (1995) Fuzzy control concept for a total artificial heart. Artif Organs 4:355–361
14. Kaufmann R, Nix C, Klein M, Reul H, Rau G (1997) The implantable fuzzy controlled Helmholtz-left ventricular assist device — first in vitro testing. Artif Organs 2:131–137

Discussion

Dr. Minami:
Thank you very much, Dr. Reul. I enjoyed your paper. How do you deside to use two different types of valves? One is a mechanical one for the outflow cannula, and a jellyfish or polyurethane valve for the inlet.

Dr. Reul:
Yes, that is our first idea because we would like to use mechanical vales at the inlet in order to save some space. You know, the outlet valve has a certain length, which is about the diameter of the valve, a little more, and you use the natural atria because you would like to have the inlet as short as possible and use a flat valve. That is the first concept. Maybe we will change that again but it looks like from an anatomical point of view for the inlet valve you have to be as flat as possible.

Dr. Minami:
Do you have to use anticoagulation with the two valves?

Dr. Reul:
Yes.

Dr. Jarvik:
Dr. Reul, that's a very impressive system. How do you deal with the right-left balance situation?

Dr. Reul:
We have changed the kinematics of the right side pusher plate a little bit, so on the right side we have a 50-to-50 fill-empty time ratio. On the left side we have 60% filling, 40% ejection, and on the right we have 50–50.

Dr. Jarvik:
You have independent motors for the right and left, or does one motor drive them both?

Dr. Reul:
No, no. It's the same motor, but the pusher plate of the right side is coupled to the gear at a different location and that changes the kinematics a little bit.

Dr. Jarvik:
Thank you.

Dr. Nosé:
Mr. Kobayashi, probably I missed the point: What is the maximum afterload your system can pump at this time?

Mr. Kobayashi:
In a mock test or animal test?

Dr. Nosé:
It doesn't matter.

Mr. Kobayashi:
104.5 mmHg.

Dr. Nosé:
So how about 150 mmHg or 180 mmHg? Can your system pump it?

Mr. Kobayashi:
Now, I am afraid I cannot do that, at 180 mmHg.

Dr. Watson:
Mr. Kobayashi, what are your plans to make the system implantable? You mentioned that it was too long, I think. What are your plans to reduce the size?

Mr. Kobayashi:
For implantable — hermetic structures, compliance chamber and the mass of the linear motor.

Dr. Watson:
I see, the mass of the linear motor.

Mr. Kobayashi:
Yes.

Dr. Watson:
Thank you.

Over 500 Days' Survival of a Goat with a Total Artificial Heart with 1/R Control

Y. Abe[1], T. Chinzei[1], K. Mabuchi[2], T. Isoyama[3], K. Baba[1], H. Matsuura[2], A. Kouno[1], T. Ono[1], S. Mochizuki[1], Y. Sun[1], K. Imanishi[4], K. Atsumi[1], I. Fujimasa[2], and K. Imachi[1]

Summary. The 1/R control was developed to provide control over the output of a total artificial heart (TAH) by the central nervous system by using the peripheral vascular conductance (1/R) the vasodilatation in for the control signal. The physiologic stability of the 1/R control algorithm was tested by using goats with TAH. To apply the 1/R control equation to TAH in goats, real-time and continuous measurements of cardiac output, aortic pressure, and right atrial pressure were performed throughout the survival period. Left atrial pressure was also measured, to prevent lung edema. Under the 1/R control, 532 days' survival was obtained in a goat with a TAH. Findings over the course of the experiment showed no hemodynamic or metabolic abnormality. Autopsy findings showed macroscopically no congestion in the liver. The experiment demonstrated the physiologic stability of the 1/R control algorithm for an extended period. Improvement of methods for measurement, such as the development of feasible techniques for the noninvasive measurement of the required hemodynamic parameters, will make it possible to use 1/R control in practice, especially for a totally implantable TAH system.

Key words: Total artificial heart — Control — Central nervous system — Conductance — 1/R

Introduction

In the Institute of Medical Electronics, University of Tokyo, research aimed at total replacement with an artificial heart (AH) began in 1981. By using the paracorporeal total artificial heat (TAH) system, in 1984, 344 days of long-term survival were obtained in a goat using the fixed cardiac output method [1], in which the drive parameters of the TAH were fixed to maintain the TAH output within the range of physi-ological normal values. However, the long-surviving goats with TAH gradually began to suffer from hemodynamic abnormalities including systemic venous hypertension sufficient to cause marked hepatic congestion, and slight arterial hypertension. To overcome these problems, development of a new automatic control method (1/R control) was begun in 1991 [2]. After various developments and improvements, 360 days' survival of a goat with a TAH with 1/R control was obtained in 1993 [3]. Survival for 532 days was achieved in 1995.

Materials and Methods

Implantation

An adult female goat weighting 47.6 kg was used. Heparin (5000 IU/kg) was given before the implantation. During surgery with 72 min of extracorporal circulation, the natural heart was resected at the atrioventricular groove. Pump inflow cannulae were attached via atrial cuffs sutured to the remnant atria. The pulmonary outflow cannula was inserted into the pulmonary artery and ligated. The systemic outflow cannula was anastomosed end-to-side with descending aorta; the ascending aorta was closed using an arterial clamp. Pneumatically driven blood pumps [4] with a sac volume of 60 ml (Nihon Zeon, Tokyo, Japan) were connected to the cannulae and set outside the body on the chest wall. A computer controllable artificial heart drive unit (Corart 103C; Aisin Seiki, Aichi, Japan) was used. Protamine sulfate (30 mg) was given for neutralization of heparin at the time when TAH pumping started.

Measurements

The cardiac output (CO) was measured at the outlet cannula of the left pump using an electromagnetic flow meter (Nihon Koden, Tokyo, Japan). The aortic and left and right atrial pressures (AoP, LAP, RAP) were measured using pressure transducers (Nihon Koden) through fluid-filled side catheters built into the outlet port of the left pump and the atrial cuffs. Pressure

[1] Institute of Medical Electronics, Faculty of Medicine, University of Tokyo, 7-3-1 Hongo, Bunkyo-ku, Tokyo 113, Japan
[2] Research Center for Science and Technology, University of Tokyo, Tokyo 153, Japan
[3] Aisin Research and Development Company, Ltd., Aichi 448, Japan
[4] Division of Cardiovascular Surgery, Daini Hospital of Tokyo Women's Medical College, Tokyo 116, Japan

transducers were affixed externally to the chest wall so that they remained near the level of the heart as the animal moved about. Pressure transducers were calibrated every 1–2 weeks. All pressure lines received slow, continuous infusions of heparinized saline to prevent clotting, using infusion bags. Infusion bags were exchanged every 3–5 days. Infusion lines were exchanged every 2–3 months.

Hemodynamic data were low-pass filtered (time constant = 3 s) to cancel the vibration caused by the movement of the animal or water-hammer effects from the mechanical valves. The signals were then collected through an analog/digital (A/D) converter into the microcomputer (PC9801VM2; NEC, Tokyo, Japan), and an average of each was computed for each beat period. The averaged data were sampled every 2 s for the automatic control.

Blood chemical and hormonal data were analyzed every 1–2 months. Hematocrit and total protein were measured every 1–2 weeks.

1/R Control Protocol

The 1/R control was constructed to provide control over the output of the TAH by the body, specifically the cardiovascular center, by using the autonomic plasticity. As an alternative to direct access to nerve signals, we selected the peripheral vascular conductance (1/R), the reciprocal of the resistance (R), modified to select out vasodilatation, as the signal for controlling TAH where the natural heart was not present. The practical control equation for 1/R control is composed of a conductance based main term and arterial pressure based correction, as is shown in Eq. 1:

$$CO_{TAH} = \left(AoP_{SET} - RAP_{SET}\right) \cdot \frac{CO}{AoP - RAP}$$
$$+ CP \cdot BW \cdot \left(AoP - AoP_{SET}\right) \quad (1)$$

$$AoP_{SET}(t) = e^{-T/\tau} \cdot AoP_{SET}(t - T)$$
$$+ \left(1 - e^{-T/\tau}\right) \cdot AoP(t) \quad (2)$$

where CO_{TAH} is the target cardiac output required for the TAH; AoP_{SET} is the set point for the aortic pressure determined according to Eq. 2; RAP_{SET} is the set point for the right atrial pressure; BW is body weight; CP is the gain of the correction; and τ is the time constant, set to 12 h to capture the circadian rhythm in arterial pressure changes. In the experiment, CP was set to 0.6 and RAP_{SET} was set to 6.

The left blood pump was maintained at a constant stroke volume, SV_{SET}, which was set to 46. Active control over left–right balance was enforced by the manipulation of the right pump stroke volume to maintain a fixed relationship between the atrial pressures:

$$LAP = a \cdot RAP + b \quad (3)$$

In the experiment, a was set to one and b was set to 3 according to the difference in the height of the two atria, to keep the filling pressures of the left and right pumps equal. Both enforcement of the constant left pump stroke volume and control of the right pump stroke volume to maintain the left–right balance relationship of Eq. 3 were achieved automatically. The balance and stroke volume control algorithm was executed every two seconds.

With the left pump stroke volume kept constant at SV_{SET}, the cardiac output was set by calculating the required cardiac output according to Eq. 1 and setting the pulse rate to

$$PR = \frac{CO_{TAH}}{SV_{SET}} \quad (4)$$

A new cardiac output value was calculated and a new pulse rate was set in the artificial heart drive unit every 6 s.

Postoperative Management

The goat with the TAH rested for 1 h after surgery and was then extubated. She was provided with nasal oxygen at rate of 5 l/min initially, then this was reduced as required to maintain pO_2 above 80 mmHg, until the chest tubes were removed on the third postoperative day (POD).

Antibiotics (ampicillin sodium 1 g/day and cefotaxime sodium 1 g/day) were given by doping them into the heparinized saline which was infusing the fluid-filled catheters for pressure measurements. The total dosage of heparin in the slow infusion was below 1000 IU/day. Other maintenance medication was not given. No water restriction was imposed.

Results

Postoperative Course

Until POD 5, the TAH was driven at a fixed rate to maintain the right flow around 100 ml·kg^{-1}·min^{-1}. The 1/R automatic control was started on POD 6, and was continued until the final day, maintaining the TAH in a completely stable condition. From POD 43 to 56 and from 64 to 88, a trial to achieve the optimal operating points of both left and right blood pumps was performed by the Tohoku University group [5]: the optimal operating point for 1/R control was used to control automatically the drive conditions of the left and right AHs. Because of thrombus formation inside the blood pumps, the left blood pump was exchanged on POD 312, and the right blood pump was exchanged on POD 414. Bleeding from the chest pressure necrotic wound occurred on POD 372, and produced anemia, but the goat recovered after one month. She suddenly died on POD 532 with acute lung edema caused by the misbalancing of left and right AH flows with the obstruction of the left atrial pressure line caused by infusion line trouble. The total survival period with the TAH was 12760.5 h.

Figure 1 shows the goat with the TAH under 1/R control on POD 507. She was active and alert and appeared to be free of discomfort until the last day. Figure 2 shows the long-term hemodynamic changes. RAP was low and completely stable from the beginning to the end. Figure 3 shows the postoperative blood count data. The temporary decrease in hematocrit on POD 372 was due to bleeding. Figure 4 shows the data from postoperative blood chemical measurements. There were no abnormal findings for liver or kidney function. Figure 5 shows the data from postoperative measurements of five hormones. There were no abnormal findings in hormonal function.

Autopsy Findings

The goat's chest was filled with about 300 ml of serous effusion. The lungs were heavily congested. Infections were found locally in a portion of the inflow cannulae. These sites of infection were surrounded by a heavy tissue capsule. The liver was macroscopically normal. Serious infarctions were found in the kidneys. No ascites was found. The other organs (stomach, intestines, spleen, bladder, great vessels, and uterus) were found to be macroscopically intact.

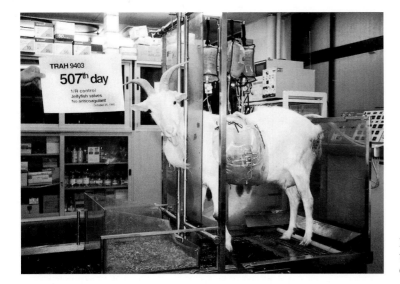

Fig. 1. The goat that survived 532 days with a total artificial heart under 1/R control (postoperative day 507)

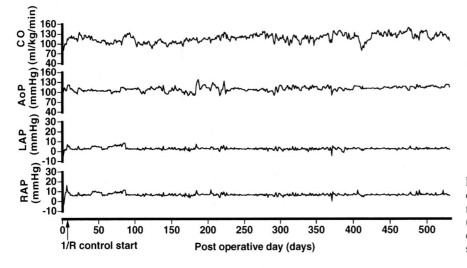

Fig. 2. Hemodynamic changes over the course of the experiment. Right atrial pressure (*RAP*) was low and stable. *CO*, cardiac output; *AoP*, aortic pressure; *LAP*, left atrial pressure

Fig. 3. Blood counts over the course of the experiment. *RBC*, red blood cells; *WBC*, white blood cells; Hb, hemoglobin; Ht, hematocrit

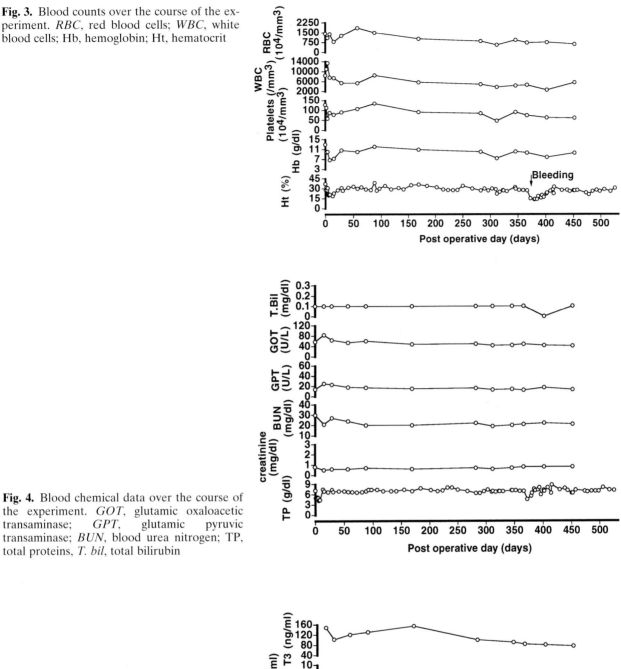

Fig. 4. Blood chemical data over the course of the experiment. *GOT*, glutamic oxaloacetic transaminase; *GPT*, glutamic pyruvic transaminase; *BUN*, blood urea nitrogen; TP, total proteins, *T. bil*, total bilirubin

Fig. 5. Hormonal data over the course of the experiment. T_3, Triiodothyronine; T_4, Thyroxin; ADH, antidiuretic hormone

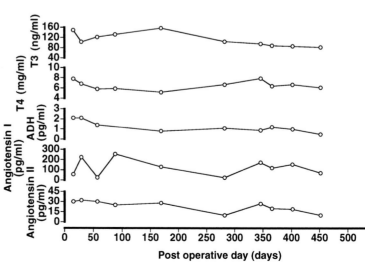

Discussion

To use R or 1/R: that was the first question in constructing the new control method. The goal of the new control method was to provide central nervous system control over the output of the TAH by using the autonomic plasticity, but the problem was to select a control signal. If we were to relate cardiac output control to R, a feedback loop actively using the baroreflex could be constructed. In contrast, using 1/R to control cardiac output, a feedback loop simulating the beta adrenergic system could be constructed. We selected 1/R for the main input parameter because beta adrenergic efferents affect heart rate in the natural system. After several basic animal experiments, we found that 1/R-related control had the potential to realize such a control method, because the control did not fail unless vasoconstriction occurred. Then, we attempted to isolate the vasodilatation by using an arterial pressure based correction, and the 1/R algorithm (conductance and arterial pressure based method) was completed.

To apply the 1/R algorithm to TAH in animals, real-time and continuous measurements of CO, AoP, and RAP are necessary. Measurement of LAP is also necessary, to prevent lung edema. Although physiologic stability depends on the control algorithm, the feasibility of the control system depends on those measurements and instruments. Therefore, for testing the long-term physiologic stability of the 1/R algoirthm in animal experiments, many developments were required, including an automatic system for pressure and flow measurements, computer programs, a remote monitoring system, and a backup system in case of an unexpected power cut. To ensure the continuity of long-term measurements, ceaseless effort to prevent the obstruction of pressure lines by clotting was necessary. Calibrations of instruments were required periodically. The pressure transducers and wiring were exchanged several times in the event of unexpected disorder or snapping.

Finally, we obtained over 500 days' survival of a goat with a TAH with 1/R control. Findings over the course of the experiment showed no hemodynamic or metabolic abnormality. Autopsy findings showed macroscopically no congestion in the liver. Thus, the experiment demonstrated the physiologic stability of the 1/R control algorithm for an extended period. How-ever, the feasibility of performing hemodynamic measurements was the terminal problem. The fatal infarction with thrombus formation in the blood pumps could be avoided by exchanging blood pumps, but it will be also the terminal problem when the 1/R control is applied to an implantable TAH. Further improvement of the anti-thrombogenicity of the blood pump is necessary to achieve survival with a TAH for more than one year.

As the 1/R control equation is written with hemodynamic parameters, it is applicable to any TAH system if the required hemodynamic parameters can be measured. Therefore, the improvement of methods for measurement, such as the development of feasible techniques for the noninvasive measurement of the required hemodynamic parameters, will make it possible to use 1/R control in a totally implantable TAH system.

References

1. Fujimasa I, Imachi K, Nakajima M, Mabuchi K, Tsukagoshi S, Kouno A, Ono T, Takido N, Motomura K, Chinzei T, Abe Y, Atsumi K (1986) Pathophysiological study of a total artificial heart in a goat that survived for 344 days. In: Nosé Y, Kjellstrand C, Ivanovich P (eds) Progress in artificial organs — 1985 ISAO, Cleveland, pp 345–353
2. Abe Y, Imachi K, Chinzei T, Mabuchi K, Imanishi K, Isoyama T, Yonezawa T, Kouno A, Ono T, Atsumi K, Fujimasa I (1993) Reciprocal of peripheral vascular resistance (1/R) control method for total artificial heart. In: Akutsu T, Koyanagi H (eds) Artificial heart 4. Springer, Tokyo, pp 349–351
3. Abe Y, Chinzei T, Imachi K, Mabuchi K, Imanishi K, Isoyama T, Matsuura H, Senih G, Nozawa H, Kouno A, Ono T, Atsumi K, Fujimasa I (1994) Can total artificial heart animals control their TAH by themselves? One year survival of a TAH goat using a new automatic control method (1/R control). ASAIO J 40:M506–M509
4. Atsumi K, Fujimasa I, Imachi K, Nakajima M, Tsukagoshi S, Mabuchi K, Motomura K, Kohno A, Ono T, Miyamoto A, Takido N, Inou N (1985) Long-term heart substitution with an artificial heart in goats. ASAIO J 8:155–165
5. Yoshizawa M, Takeda H, Yambe Y, Nitta S, Abe Y, Isoyama T, Imachi K, Chinzei T, Fujimasa I (1994) Development of optimal operating point controller for implantable total artificial heart. Jpn J Artif Organs 23:551–558

Discussion

Dr. Suga:
Suga from Okayama. I am a physiologist. I have a question about the 1/R control. Very interesting, and I am wondering what the essential difference is between the 1/R control and constant mean arterial pressure control. In the result you showed that aortic pressure is fairly normal, although there are some jagged lines, but it was fairly constant. So, if you try to fix the arterial pressure and to control the arterial pressure, what happens? What's the difference?

Dr. Abe:
By using fixed aortic pressure control, the control of the right atrial pressure is impossible. And the increase of cardiac output during exercise is also impossible. In this system we use the activity of the cardiovascular center. The cardiac output changes according to the beta adrenergic system in the peripheral conductance. Because there was no heart, we could not detect the signal from the cardiovascular center to the heart. Instead of this we detected the signal from the cardiovascular center by using the change of peripheral conductance.

Dr. Suga:
I see. So, because of that, the arterial pressure actually changed a little bit?

Dr. Abe:
Yes.

Dr. Suga:
I see. O.K. Thank you.

Mr. Siess:
Mr. Siess from the Helmholtz Institute. I think it was very impressive to see that you could keep control for about 500 days in the animal, and, in fact, I wanted to ask you if the kind of pressure sensors that you used were stable for that long period. Could you possibly talk on that?

Dr. Abe:
I think there are no stable pressure transducers available now.

Mr. Siess:
Well, that was my idea. That's why I asked.

Dr. Abe:
I must change them maybe in 3 months or 4 months because the pressure transducers were out of order, and I must do calibration once a week. So, I want a stable pressure sensor — it is a key point to realize a practical control method of this 1/R algorithm.

Professor Wolner:
Wolner, Vienna. I want to congratulate you for these excellent results of 500 days. For many years your group reports first with this goat model. First, 30 days, then 60 days, then 200 days. Over the years, Dr. Atsumi and all his co-workers. I have a question in regard to your *period* perspectives. In my opinion, you can never offer to a patient such a paracorporal system. *Longer than short-term bridging* — that's the maximum. Let's say, one week, two weeks, three weeks, maximum, six weeks. What is the rationale behind your now using such a paracorporal system for such a long term? That's very difficult, I know, to get such results. What is your perspective in regard to clinical use of such systems?

Dr. Abe:
I think the durability of this pump is up to 300 days. Because the blood pump is set outside the body, we can exchange the blood pumps when a thrombus formation is found inside the pump. In this case, the blood pumps were also exchanged in order to obtain longer survival.

Professor Wolner:
What is the prospect in terms of usage of this pump for clinical purposes? I think that was the main question.

Dr. Imachi:
Maybe your question is how to prevent infection when it is used for clinical purposes? Is that so?

Professor Wolner:
My question is very simple: What is the practicability for clinical use of a paracorporal system for, let's say,

longer than 1 month? I think it is a senseless approach when you have a patient in cardiac failure with all these problems with infection, so you can never use a paracorporal system longer than a few weeks.

Dr. Abe:
I think this is pure scientific research for the control of other total implantable systems. I think the paracorporal system is not practical for permanent use.

Professor Wolner:
So actually you want to make this one completely implantable in the future?

Dr. Abe:
Yes.

Heat Dissipation from Artificial Hearts: Characterizing Tissue Responses and Defining Safe Levels

Hiroaki Harasaki, Charles R. Davies, Tetsuji Matsuyoshi, Yukio Okazaki, Kent Wika, and Kiyotaka Fukamachi

Summary. Mechanical artificial hearts generate heat, imposing unprecedented biomedical problems. Experiments were conducted in calves to study the effects of chronic heating and the mechanisms of the adaptation response, and to determine the safe levels for device–tissue interfacial temperatures. Electric heat sources which dissipated three different levels of constant heat flux (0.04, 0.06, or 0.08 W/cm^2) were implanted adjacent to lung and muscle for up to seven weeks. The tissue temperatures were continuously monitored at the heater surface and 1, 3, and 7 mm from the surface. Correlating the local tissue temperatures with histologic features, the safe upper limit was identified to be 43°C, or 4°C above the body temperature. There were significant differences in tissue temperatures between the lung and muscle at all distances and with all three fluxes ($P = 0.0001$), reflecting a higher blood perfusion in the lung tissue. With the highest heat flux of 0.08 W/cm^2, and the resultant initial surface temperature of 42.8°C ± 0.9°C, the lung showed no sign of tissue damage or necrosis, while the muscle, with a surface temperature of 45.3°C ± 2.2°C, was necrotic to a distance of 18.1 mm and 3.0 mm from the surface at 2 and 4 weeks, respectively. By the seventh week this muscle necrosis was totally replaced by fibrosis. Gradual decreases in the surface temperatures with the two higher heat fluxes and enhanced angiogenesis have suggested that the tissues adapt to chronic heating by increased perfusion. The expression of heat shock proteins by the tissue repair cells in the tissue capsule also suggests that cellular adaptation to heating is occurring.

Key words: Implantable artificial hearts — Waste heat dissipation — Chronic heating — Device surface temperature — Heat-induced angiogenesis

Introduction

The need for a fully implantable mechanical circulatory assist system (MCS) and total artifical heart (TAH) is widely recognized [1,2]. Any energy source for these devices generates waste heat. The prototype of the Cleveland Clinic–Nimbus total artifical heart, for example, operated at an energy efficiency of 15%–20%. Accordingly, the majority of the input energy was lost as heat with resultant maximum device surface

Department of Biomedical Engineering, Cleveland Clinic Foundation, 9500 Euclid Avenue, Cleveland, OH 44195, USA

temperatures ranging from 43.9°C to 46.2°C, which produced tissue necrosis and significant hyperemia [3]. The existing knowledge in the area of hyperthermia treatment in relation to the heat sensitivity of normal and tumor cells has been of limited value for determining the effects of chronic heating and establishing the safe maximum temperature or thermal dosage, because in hyperthermia, the heat exposure is limited to a few hours' duration [4]. Studies on the effects of chronic heating on device–tissue interactions, including a knowledge of the spatial and temporal distribution of heat and the response of tissues to heat, have not been performed. Consequently, there is no theoretical basis or in vivo data with which we can predict the results of chronic in vivo heating by blood pumps. The feasibility of using implantable artifical hearts depends heavily on their ability to dissipate excess heat into the body without causing any adverse local or systemic effects. Thus, an understanding of the tissue response to chronic heating and of the body's adaptive mechanisms is critically important to identify the safe maximum temperature for chronic heating and to establish a guideline for thermal management of fully implantable mechanical artifical hearts.

To address these questions, a series of calf experiments were conducted by implanting a specially designed heating device that was equipped with multiple thermistors for continuous temperature distribution measurements. Three different levels of constant heat fluxes (0.08, 0.06, and 0.04 W/cm^2) were chosen from our preliminary studies to generate the desired temperature range [3]. The results showed a time-dependent decrease of temperatures, indicating the occurrence of an adaptive response which allowed for increased heat transfer. This decline appeared to have stabilized by the seventh week. It was also shown that the muscle temperatures were higher than the lung temperatures at all heat fluxes tested and for a given distance from the heater, probably reflecting the lower tissue blood flow to the latissimus dorsi muscle than to the lung. In the present study, the tissue response to three different levels of constant heat fluxes was analyzed by a computer-aided morphometry system to identify the maximum safe temperature limit. The time course of heat effects on tissue was also studied.

Immunohistochemical staining was used to identify the cell types and to demonstrate the expression of a heat shock protein and proliferative cell nuclear antigens (PCNA) by the cells adjacent to the heat source. These histological occurrences were correlated with the local tissue temperature. The results have indicated that the safe maximum heat flux is $0.08\,W/cm^2$ for lung and $0.06\,W/cm^2$ for muscle. A tissue temperature of $43°C$, $4°C$ above the body temperature (ΔT), appears to be well tolerated, with an active inflammatory response, collagenization, and angiogenesis.

Materials and Methods

To study the effects of chronic heating on tissues in vivo, we performed experiments in which heated disks were implanted into a total of 25 calves. The tissues against which the heated disks were placed represent a highly vascularized tissue (lung) and a tissue with a rather low resting blood flow rate (latissimus dorsi muscle, LDM). As a practical matter, these are the tissues that must adapt to an implanted artificial heart and its ancillary components. Based upon our preliminary study [5], the required implant duration was determined to be 7 weeks. After this duration, the responses at the three different heat fluxes (0.04, 0.06, and $0.08\,W/cm^2$, 5 calves each) were compared. Also, to study the chronological changes of tissue in response to continuous heating, additional studies were performed at $0.08\,W/cm^2$ by killing 6 animals at 2 weeks and 4 animals at 4 weeks each after implantation. The details of the implantable heater disk have been described elsewhere [5]. In brief, the implantable heater and control disks consist of a 6.35-cm epoxy housing into which conditioning electronics and heating elements were packaged behind a 304 stainless steel heat-conducting surface. A double insulation packaging of Sylgard gel encapsulated the circuit along with epoxy adhesive sealing of the metal face to prevent leakage. The feedthrough included polyvinyl chloride tubing backfilled with silicone to provide strain relief and sealing. A highly stranded, flexible 12 conductor wire (Cooner, Chatsworth, CA, USA) was used in combination with a multiplexor in the heated disks to provide data transfer with a minimum of wires leading through the skin of the calves. The metal face was a 5.1-cm-diameter copper-clad disk which was composed of copper, aluminum, and 304 stainless steel. The copper provided uniform heat transfer while the stainless steel provided a minimally reactive surface contacting the tissues. In order to measure tissue temperatures chronically, two 0.36-mm thermistors (Thermometrics, Edison, NJ, USA) were embedded at the heater surface. Thermistors were also embedded in 21-gauge needles at 1, 3, and 7mm from the heater surface (three at each distance). Control disks had two

surface thermistors and one thermistor each at 3 and 7mm. Prior to final implant preparation, the sealed disks were leak-tested and calibrated. Temperature was monitored using a Curtin Matheson Scientific thermometer (Fisher Scientific, Pittsburgh, PA, USA) with $0.1°C$ increments. The thermistors provided continuous temperature measurements at the tissue interface and in the tissue at distances of 1, 3, and 7mm from the interface. The local tissue temperatures between the measured points were estimated from a mathematical model of dynamic heat transfer, which has been formulated to analyze chronic heating of tissues and is described elsewhere [6].

After killing and gross examination, serial cross-sectional specimens were obtained from the tissue capsule and adjacent lung and muscle, fixed with HistoChoice fixative (Amresco, Solon, OH, USA), paraffinembedded, sectioned, and stained with hematoxylin and eosin, trichrome, von Kossa, and, when indicated, with Gram stain for bacteria and Grocott's methenamine silver nitrate (GMS) for fungi. Immunohistochemical staining was performed using a Jung Histostainer automatic processor (Leica, W. Nushbaum, McHenry, IL, USA). Hydrogen peroxide (0.6%) in methanol was used to remove any endogenous peroxidase present in the tissue. A blocking solution composed of a 1:10 dilution of normal swine serum in phosphate buffered saline was then added before application of the appropriate antibody, which was labeled with an Elite avidin/biotin/peroxidase complex (Vector Laboratories, Burlingame, CA, USA). A chromogen, 3,3-diaminobenzidine, was then used. Polyclonal rabbit antibodies for von Willebrand factor for endothelial cells (EC), heat shock protein (HSP)70, and a monoclonal mouse anti-PCNA (DAKO, Carpinteria, CA, USA) have also been shown to be usable in the calf model in our previous studies to document the in vivo occurrence of heat-induced angiogenesis, cell proliferation, and thermotolerance in inflammatory cells, EC, and fibroblasts. Sections of human tonsil were included with each staining procedure to act as positive controls. The image analysis system that was used in conjunction with the immunostaining technique for the quantification of the tissue response was a Bioquant BQ Meg IV (R&M Biometrics, Nashville, TN, USA). The tissue layer thickness, cell populations, and density of angiogenesis were measured in a quantitative manner. The values for heated disks were compared to the values for nonheated disks in the same animal and heated disks at other heat fluxes, using analysis of variance (ANOVA). In addition, the values of each parameter for different durations of heating were tested for statistical significance. Also, the parameter values for tissue at different distances from the heater were statistically tested.

Results

Systemic Effects of Chronic Local Heating

The systemic effects of chronic heat dissipation were assessed by monitoring vital signs (respiration rate, heart rate, rectal temperature), major organ functions, hematology, and platelet and leukocyte functions. Since one heated disk has a surface area of $20.3\,cm^2$, the total amount of heat that was dissipated to the animals was 1.62 W for the $0.04\,W/cm^2$, 2.44 W for the $0.06\,W/cm^2$, and 3.25 W for the $0.08\,W/cm^2$ heat flux group. With this range of relatively small heat dosage, there were no significant changes observed in the afore-mentioned parameters. Phagocytic function, chemotaxis, and superoxide anion production of leukocytes, and platelet aggregation and ATP release were not affected. Prothrombin time (PT) and activated prothrombin time (APTT) remained normal throughout the experiments. Autopsy disclosed no systemic pathologic finding in the major internal organs attributable to heat dissipation.

Tissue Temperature Distribution and Time Course

The time courses of the temperature profile in the lung and muscle for the three heat fluxes are shown in Fig. 1. For the lung, there was no statistically significant difference observed with time at a given distance from the heater surface. The surface temperature (0 mm) remained unchanged at around 42.8°C–42.5°C. For muscle, there was a distinct time-dependent decline in temperatures with $0.08\,W/cm^2$ from postoperative day (POD) 1 through POD 28 ($P < 0.01$). Initially, at POD 1, the average surface temperature was 45.3°C ± 2.2°C, which was 6.8°C ± 1.0°C above the core temperature (ΔT). As the POD increased, the muscle tissue temperature at all distances dropped, indicating a time-dependent increase in the heat transfer by the tissue. It is evident that the driving force for this adaptation is local, chronically elevated temperature. Even at the furthest distance measured (7 mm), the muscle temperature was still 3.8°C ± 0.9°C above the core temperature on POD 1, suggesting that the heat effects could extend far beyond this distance. The extent of the temperature decline over 7 weeks depended on the distance from the heat source: 2.2°C, 2.8°C, and 1.9°C for 1 mm, 3 mm, and 7 mm, respectively. The larger relative decline seen at 3 mm may be due to increased local blood flow with angiogenesis occurring in the tissue layer at a distance between 1 and 3 mm from the heat source. For the lower heat flux of $0.06\,W/cm^2$, the surface temperature increased less for lung and muscle tissue, to 41.7°C ± 0.7°C and 44.5°C ± 0.7°C respectively, with the corresponding ΔT of 2.6°C and 5.5°C. For the lung, again, there were no statistically

significant changes in temperatures with time. In contrast, the time-dependent decreases in temperatures at the given distance were significant for the muscle between POD 1 and the other three time points ($P < 0.01$). No significant change was noted thereafter. The surface temperature decline for the muscle over the 7-week period was 1.1°C, being smaller than that with $0.08\,W/cm^2$ flux. This decline was seen up to 3 mm, but not at 7 mm. These findings suggest that with this level of heat flux, adaptation as evidenced by an increased heat transfer, may have occurred within 14 days of exposure and with the local temperature above 43°C. For $0.04\,W/cm^2$, the temperature elevation was of the order of 1°C for lung and was near 3.5°C for muscle. The temperature decline over 7 weeks was negligible at all distances.

Local Tissue Response to Chronic Heating

The thickness of the entire tissue capsule and of its constituent tissue layers for the three fluxes for seven weeks are shown in Table 1. The time-dependent changes in tissue capsule thickness and composition with a $0.08\,W/cm^2$ flux are shown in Table 2. The tissue capsule that formed adjacent to the control nonheating discs did not differ between the lung and muscle locations (Table 1) or among the three durations (Table 2). In the lung, thin subpleural atelectasis was a frequent finding underneath the implants. There was mild thinning in the muscle layer underneath the implant, and the thickness was 77.8%, 73.5%, and 70.8% of the adjacent normal muscle thickness at 2, 4, and 7 weeks of implantation, respectively. This thinning was much less than that seen in the heater side as described later. By two weeks of implantation the majority of the tissue capsules appeared whitish and fibrous with an accumulation of only a small amount of tissue fluid and fibrinous material at the interface. Accumulation of calcified deposits, as revealed by von Kossa staining and energy-dispersive X-ray microanalysis, was observed on both the control and heater surfaces, with a tendency towards a greater amount with higher fluxes. The tissue capsule surface was finely granular in appearance and mottled by varying sizes of petechial changes and dark-brown discolorations, being more prominent with higher fluxes. The most distinctive finding in the muscular implants with a $0.08\,W/cm^2$ heat flux was heat-induced necrosis in the muscle layer, extending from the heated interface into the muscle layer, approximately 2 mm in depth at 2 weeks and 3 mm at 4 weeks (Table 2). The presence of a hyperemic and hemorrhagic layer between this necrotic layer and the normal muscle layers suggested enhanced angiogenesis in this area. It was of particular interest to note that this muscle necrosis was com-

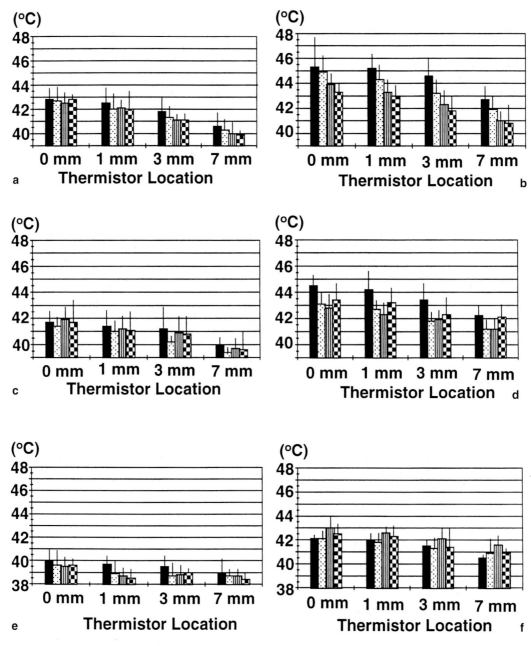

Fig. 1. Tissue temperature profiles as measured at the heater surface (0 mm), and 1, 3, and 7 mm from the surface for 0.08 W/cm^2 (**a,b**), 0.06 W/cm^2 (**c,d**) and 0.04 W/cm^2 (**e,f**) heat fluxes. **a,c,e** Lung; **b,d,f** muscle tissue temperature. Although the temperatures were measured at 20-min intervals throughout the entire experimental period, only selected data from postoperative days (POD) 1 (*black bars*), 14 (*dotted bars*), 28 (*striped bars*), and 48 (*checked bars*) are presented here. The *bar graph* represents the mean and the *error bar*, the standard deviation, from five cases for each heat flux

pletely replaced by fibrosis by the seventh postoperative week. In contrast, no sign of tissue necrosis was observed in the lung adjacent to the heater even with the highest flux (0.08 W/cm^2), regardless of exposure duration.

In Table 1, it is shown that the entire capsule thickness of the lung and muscle heaters does not differ among the control (0.00 W/cm^2) and the three heat fluxes at seven weeks ($P = 0.39$ for muscle, and $P = 0.65$ for lung, one-way factorial ANOVA). Microscopically, the tissue capsule was composed of three layers, in the following order from the heater interface to the normal adjacent tissue: (1) the acellular, fibrinous layer at the interface; (2) the inflammatory cell layer

Table 1. Thickness of tissue layers adjacent to heater disks (7 weeks; unit, mm)

	0.00 W/cm² (n = 15)	0.04 W/cm² (n = 5)	0.06 W/cm² (n = 5)	0.08 W/cm² (n = 5)
Muscle				
Tissue capsule	1.39 ± 1.10	1.87 ± 0.92	1.87 ± 0.49	0.86 ± 0.54
Acellular	0.01 ± 0.02	0.04 ± 0.06	0.03 ± 0.02	0.26 ± 0.31
Inflammatory	0.06 ± 0.03	0.15 ± 0.12	0.08 ± 0.04	0.20 ± 0.34
Collagenous	1.24 ± 1.11	1.66 ± 0.79	1.74 ± 0.46	0.54 ± 0.63
Necrotic	0 ± 0	0 ± 0	0 ± 0	0 ± 0
Fibrosis	0 ± 0	0 ± 0	0 ± 0	1.95 ± 1.26
Lung				
Tissue capsule	1.59 ± 0.44	1.50 ± 0.38	1.76 ± 0.12	1.37 ± 0.49
Acellular	0.02 ± 0.02	0.02 ± 0.03	0.11 ± 0.19	0.03 ± 0.04
Inflammatory	0.06 ± 0.08	0.02 ± 0.02	0.09 ± 0.10	0.12 ± 0.06
Collagenous	1.49 ± 0.45	1.45 ± 0.38	1.68 ± 0.08	1.23 ± 0.47
Necrotic	0 ± 0	0 ± 0	0 ± 0	0 ± 0
Fibrosis	0 ± 0	0 ± 0	0.10 ± 0.18	0.18 ± 0.35

Table 2. Thickness of tissue layers adjacent to heater disks (0.08 W/cm²; unit, mm)

	2 weeks (n = 6)		4 weeks (n = 4)		7 weeks (n = 5)	
	Control	Heat	Control	Heat	Control	Heat
Muscle						
Tissue capsule	1.30 ± 0.55	0.17 ± 0.09	1.38 ± 0.67	0.23 ± 0.05	1.50 ± 1.16	0.86 ± 0.54
Acellular	0.01 ± 0.02	0.23 ± 0.12	0.02 ± 0.02	0.23 ± 0.04	0.03 ± 0.04	0.26 ± 0.31
Inflammatory	0.05 ± 0.02	0 ± 0	0.06 ± 0.02	0 ± 0	0.07 ± 0.04	0.20 ± 0.34
Collagenous	1.25 ± 0.54	0 ± 0	1.29 ± 0.68	0 ± 0	1.26 ± 1.25	0.54 ± 0.63
Necrotic	0 ± 0	1.57 ± 0.82	0 ± 0	2.77 ± 0.83	0 ± 0	0 ± 0
Fibrosis	0 ± 0	1.42 ± 0.74	0 ± 0	1.80 ± 0.76	0 ± 0	1.95 ± 1.26
Lung						
Tissue capsule	1.18 ± 0.76	1.14 ± 0.72	1.62 ± 0.33	0.68 ± 0.40	1.59 ± 0.41	1.37 ± 0.49
Acellular	0.13 ± 0.27	0.07 ± 0.15	0.02 ± 0.02	0.03 ± 0.04	0.01 ± 0.01	0.03 ± 0.04
Inflammatory	0.09 ± 0.11	0.04 ± 0.02	0.04 ± 0	0.01 ± 0.01	0.13 ± 0.12	0.12 ± 0.06
Collagenous	1.04 ± 0.61	1.02 ± 0.81	1.54 ± 0.35	0.64 ± 0.44	1.39 ± 0.40	1.23 ± 0.47
Necrotic	0 ± 0	0 ± 0	0 ± 0	0 ± 0	0 ± 0	0 ± 0
Fibrosis	0 ± 0	0 ± 0	0 ± 0	0 ± 0	0 ± 0	0.18 ± 0.35

with capillary formation (angiogenesis front); and (3) the collagenous layer formed on the visceral pleura or fascia. The thickness of these layers appeared to be affected by the heat dosage only in the muscle site. The acellular layer for muscle with 0.08 W/cm² flux is significantly thicker (0.26 ± 0.31 mm) than with the other heat fluxes ($P = 0.01$). In contrast, the acellular layer for lung is thinner with the same heat flux (0.03 ± 0.04 mm) and shows no difference from other heat fluxes. The thickness of the other layers in the tissue capsule did not show any significant difference in either the muscle or the lung implantation sites. Heat-induced necrosis was not observed either in the muscle or lung by the seventh week. The presence of fibrosis in the muscle layer with 0.08 W/cm² represents replacement of necrotic muscle by fibrosis. Fibrosis seen in the lung parenchyma was due to fibrosis of the atelectatic lesions caused by compression of the tissue by the implants.

When the three exposure durations were compared at a flux of 0.08 W/cm² (Table 2), the capsule thickness for the muscle heater was significantly thinner than the control ($P = 0.001$) and was different for the 2-week (0.17 ± 0.09 mm), 4-week (0.23 ± 0.09 mm), and 7-week (0.86 ± 0.54 mm) durations, gradually increasing in thickness ($P = 0.01$, two-way factorial ANOVA). This difference was mainly caused by the lack of collagenization with this heat flux at the heater–muscle interface. The tissue observed between the heater surface and the fascia at 2 and 4 weeks is composed only of an acellular, fibrin-like material without any inflammatory cells, angiogenesis, or collagen formation. Necrosis of the fascia and muscle, 1.57 ± 0.82 mm and 2.77 ± 0.83 mm at 2 and 4 weeks, respectively, indicates clearly that the tissue temperature in this area was too high for cell survival. Replacement of the necrotic muscle by fibrosis was observed microscopically as early as two weeks after heat exposure and was

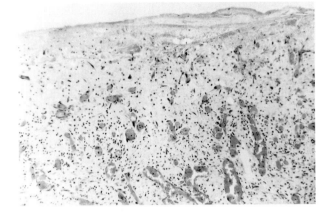

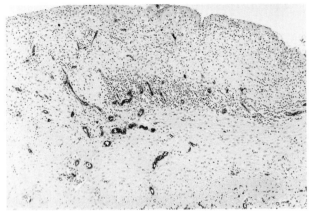

Fig. 2. The tissue capsule formed at the heater–muscle interface after seven weeks of 0.08 W/cm² dissipation. Capillaries are dilated and dense in this area close to the heater–tissue interface, where a layer of fibrin-like substances is observed without involvement of nucleated cells (*top of panel*) (original magnification 10.6×)

Fig. 3. Immunohistochemical staining for heat-shock protein 70 of the tissue capsule formed at the heater–lung interface with 0.08 W/cm² flux for seven weeks. Chronic inflammatory cells and endothelial cells of the capillaries are stained strongly positive. Fibroblasts are also positive (original magnification 10.6×)

complete by the seventh week. No significant change in the thickness of this fibrosis layer was noted with time thereafter ($P = 0.65$). For lung implantation sites, there was no significant difference in the thickness of the entire tissue capsule ($P = 0.47$, two-way factorial ANOVA) of each layer for the three durations, coinciding with the constant local tissue temperatures at the given distance (Fig. 1). No sign of thermal damage was seen histologically in the tissue capsule or in the lung parenchyma, regardless of the heat fluxes and exposure durations. It was shown that a heat flux of 0.08 W/cm² was well tolerated in the highly vascularized tissue such as the lung with the resulting surface temperature of 42.8°C ± 0.9°C, or ΔT of 3.9°C ± 1.0°C.

The major inflammatory cells in the inflammatory cell layer were macrophages and lymphocytes, and this was the layer where neoangiogenesis and interstitial extravasation of blood components took place (Fig. 2). The newly formed blood vessels were frequently dilated, up to 40 μm in diameter. When stained for HSP 70, inflammatory cells, endothelial cells of capillaries, and fibroblasts were shown to express this protein (Fig. 3). These cells also expressed PCNA, suggesting actual proliferation of these cells under elevated temperature.

Discussion

Studies on the feasibility of chronic heat dissipation in animals have been conducted by Norman's group and others [7–14]. In dogs, they showed that 4–23 W delivered to blood over 86 days did not lead to animal death. In calves, the same power levels did not lead to death when tested for up to 2 months. Grillis and Walkup [15] also showed that miniature swine with implanted thoracic aorta heat exchangers did not die as a result of power inputs up to 60 W (4.7 W/cm² flux, 1.1 W/kg body weight) for periods in excess of 12 months. These studies implied that such levels of heat may be safely dissipated in humans. However, the details of tissue-heated surface interactions have not been reported, while the occurrence of suspected heat-induced tissue damage has been reported [7–9]. Our preliminary data from chronic heater implantation in calves showed that a heat flux of 0.12 W/cm² (only 1/40th of that applied by Grills and Walkup) elevated the temperatures at the heater–muscle and heater–lung interfaces by 13°C and 7°C, respectively. These adjacent tissues showed necrosis, calcification, and persistent acute inflammatory reactions. These results motivated the current study which focused on the local tissue effects of chronic heating, and was designed to investigate the spatial and temporal temperature distribution in these two different tissues, to examine the macroscopic and microscopic tissue responses against three different levels of heat levels, and to document the in vivo occurrence of thermotolerance, if any, at both tissue and cell levels. The ultimate goal of this study was to identify the safe maximum temperature for the tissue in order to establish thermal management guidelines for designing implantable devices with an energy source, such as a total artificial heart or a circulatory assist device.

In the present study it was suggested, by measuring the temporal and spatial tissue temperature distributions and corresponding histological features in the adjacent tissue and in the evolving tissue capsules, that the safe maximum temperature at the tissue–device interface was 43°C, which is produced by fluxes of $0.08\,W/cm^2$ for the lung and $0.06\,W/cm^2$ for the muscle. These values have been adopted by other groups as well as our own group in the thermal management of our electrohydraulic total artificial heart (TAH) [16]. Our most recent design channels a substantial portion of the heat that is generated by the electric motor and gear pump into the blood from the blood-pump housing via a thermal conductive graphite heat path and a titanium plate installed in the left pump housing. With this design, the highest device surface–tissue interfacial temperature of the most recent TAH animal experiment was shown to have been maintained below 42°C. Prominent angiogenesis and vasodilation were observed in the tissue capsule adjacent to the "hot" spot, but no sign of thermal damage was noted in the tissue capsule, in the pericardium, or in the adjacent lung.

In the present study we demonstrated the occurrence of tissue adaptation to chronic heating as evidenced by a gradual decline of interfacial temperatures with time when the tissue was heated with constant levels of heat dosage. This decline was clearly demonstrated with the two higher heat fluxes and in the muscle, but not with the lowest flux tested ($0.04\,W/cm^2$) or in the lung. It is of interest to note that the temperature decline is seen when the surface temperature is higher than 43°C, or when the ΔT is more than 4°C, as suggested from the surface temperature data shown in Fig. 1. In the lung, where the temperature did not exceed 43°C even with the highest heat flux of $0.08\,W/cm^2$, no appreciable temperature decline was observed. Furthermore, with $0.06\,W/cm^2$ flux in the muscle, the surface temperature decrease leveled off at 43°C after two weeks to the end of the 7-week experiment. At the lung–heater interface, the temperature elevation was initially 3.9°C with $0.08\,W/cm^2$, and this did not decline appreciably. This observation was thought to be explained by the higher perfusion of lung tissue, allowing for greater convective heat transfer.

From the histologic evaluation of the adjacent tissue, enhanced angiogenesis and a resultant increase in local tissue perfusion were thought to explain the observed temperature changes. In 1967 Rawson et al. [11] also reported on such an adaptation phenomenon, involving vascularization in the tissue encapsulating the heating elements implanted in the abdominal cavity of sheep. The shortest distances from the interface to the capillaries (angiogenesis front) and the topology of capillary density distribution in the tissue capsule are being analyzed using von Willebrand factor (vWF) immunostaining for EC. The preliminary data show that the local tissue temperature of this

capillary front is approximately 42.1°C at the 7th week regardless of the heat fluxes used. The mechanisms of this chronic heat-induced angiogenesis, vasodilation, and increase in blood flow rates are not known. It is postulated that heat stimulates EC directly, with resultant angiogenesis and vasculogenesis, or indirectly by increased production of various growth factors by mononuclear leukocytes (MN).

Immunologic staining of the tissue revealed sustained heat-shock protein (HSP) expression by fibroblasts, endothelial cells, and chronic inflammatory cells involved in the tissue capsule. The ability of both eukaryote and prokaryote cells to withstand heat in culture is known to be influenced by their previous thermal history. A brief exposure to heat induces a transitory resistance to subsequent challenges at higher temperatures, i.e., thermotolerance. Within a few minutes of this exposure, the cell rapidly synthesizes a group of proteins known as HSP. HSP are evolutionarily highly conserved proteins that form in response to various stresses such as heat, ischemia, anoxia, UV radiation, drug (amphetamine)-induced hyperthermia, and oxidative stress [17,18]. The observations of heat-induced HSP production in this study may indicate the occurrence of thermotolerance in vivo in tissue under chronic heating as an adaptation response.

In our previous series of animal experiments with thermally powered left ventricular assist devices with 20-W total heat dissipation, no significant systemic adverse effects were noted [19], coinciding with the results of the present study. In these assist systems, heat was mainly dissipated into blood through the blood pump. The neointima formed on the flocked blood-contacting surface was thinner with heat when compared with the one on the nonheated surface [19]. The results of our previous in vitro studies on the effects of heat on blood components have indicated that a significant effect is exerted by a relatively short-term exposure to a moderate degree of supranormal temperature (>42°C). Blood becomes less coagulable with suppression of both the extrinsic and intrinsic pathways of coagulation [20]. Aggregation, retention, and release functions of platelets are also significantly suppressed [20], due to the heat-induced changes in surface glycoproteins [21]. Heat-induced alterations of surface receptors were also noted in lymphocytes and monocytes [22]. Leukocyte phagocytic function was totally lost with 30 min of exposure to 46°C [23]. The osmotic fragility of erythrocytes was found to be increased with a temperature range lower than the level previously recognized, and significant hemolysis was induced with 42°C when the exposure time was prolonged to more than 24 h [24]. Thus, heat appears to have significant effects on the blood–surface interaction, and further study is warranted.

Acknowledgments. The authors are very grateful to Professor Gerald Saidel of the Department of Biomedical Engineering of the Case Western Reserve University for his participation in mathematical modeling of dynamic heat transfer in tissues which has been helpful in estimation of tissue temperature. We would like to express sincere thanks to Dr. Fumio Fukumura of the Kyushu University School of Medicine, Dr. Kunio Nakamura of the Miyazaki University School of Medicine, and Dr. Ryuji Kunitomo of the Kumanoto University School of Medicine for their participation in animal experiments and data collection. We also thank Ms. Maria Benavides, Ms. Kathy Bucknell, Ms. Shailaja Mude, and Mr. John Manos for their invaluable technical assistance. This work has been supported by NIH Grant 1RO1 HL43127 and NIH Contract NO1-HV-38129.

References

1. Altieri FD, Watson JT (1987) Implantable ventricular assist systems. Artif Organs 11:237–246
2. Hogness JR, Van Antwerp M (eds) (1991) The artificial heart: prototypes, policies, and patients. Committee to Evaluate the Artificial Heart Program of the National Heart, Lung, and Blood Institute. Division of Health Care Service, Institute of Medicine, National Academy Press, Washington, DC
3. Harasaki H, Fukamachi K, Massiello A, Fukumura F, Muramoto K, Chen JF, Himley S, Kiraly R, Golding L, McCarthy P, Thomas D, Rintoul T, Carriker W, Butler K (1994) Development of an implantable total artificial heart: initial animal experiments. In: Akutsu T, Koyanagi H (eds) Heart replacement. Artificial heart 4. Springer, Tokyo, pp 173–179
4. Hahn GM (1982) Hyperthermia and cancer. Plenum, New York
5. Davies CR, Fukumura F, Fukamachi K, Muramoto K, Himley SC, Massiello A, Chen JF, Harasaki H (1994) Adaptation of tissue to a chronic heat load. ASAIO J 40:M514–M517
6. Davies CR, Saidel GM, Harasaki H (1997) Sensitivity analysis of one-dimensional heat transfer in tissue with temperature dependent perfusion. J Biomech Eng 119:77–80
7. Norman JC, Molokhia FA, Asimacopoulos PJ, Liss RH, Huffman FN (1971) Heat-induced myocardial angiogenesis, I. ASAIO Trans 17:213–218
8. Huffman FN, Norman JC (1973) Annual progress report to NHLBI. PH43-66-982-6, Study of the effects of additional endogenous heat
9. Norman JC, LaFarge G, Harvey R, Robinson T, Van Someren L, Bernhard WF (1966) Experimental model for inducing acute and chronic hyperthermia. ASAIO Trans 12:282–287
10. Huffman FN, Bernhard WF, Norman JC (1970) Thrombogenic experience with intravascular heat exchangers. Chest 58:590–597
11. Rawson RO, Hardy JD, Vasko KA (1967) Visceral tissue vascularization: an adaptive response to high temperature. Science 158:1203–1204
12. Liss RH, Huffman FN, Warren S, Norman JC (1971) Electron microscopy and thermal analysis of neointima heated and irradiated in vivo for two years. Ann Thorac Surg 12:251–261
13. Whalen RL, Molokhia FA, Jeffery DL, Huffman FN, Norman JC (1972) Current studies with simulated nuclear-powered left ventricular assist devices. ASAIO Trans 18:146–151
14. Whalen RL, Jeffery DL, Asimacopoulos PJ, Norman JC (1974) Chronic intracorporeal heat studies in calves. ASAIO Trans 20B:509–515
15. Grillis MF, Walkup PC (1968) Annual progress report to NIH. PH-43-66-1130. A study on effects of additional endogenous heat relating to the artificial heart
16. Kung RTV, Yu LS, Ochs BD, Parnis SM, Macris MP, Frazier OH (1995) Progress in the development of the ABIOMED total artificial heart. ASAIO J 41:M245–M248
17. Mytin EV (1995) Heat shock proteins and molecular chaperones: Implications for adaptive responses in the skin. J Invest Dermatol 104:448–455
18. Maulik N, Engelman RM, Wei Z, Liu X, Rousou JA, Flack JE, Deaton DW, Das DK (1995) Drug-induced heat-shock preconditioning improves postischemic ventricular recovery after cardiopulmonary bypass. Circulation 92[Suppl II]:II-381–II-388
19. Emoto H, Harasaki H, Fujimoto LK, Navaro RR, White M, Whale R, Kiraly RJ, Nosé Y (1988) Systemic and local effects of heat dissipation in the thermally powered LVAS. ASAIO Trans 34:361–366
20. Nasu M, Matsushita S, Murabayashi S, Lucus F, Oku T, Kambic H, Nosé Y, Harasaki H (1986) A systemic evaluation of heat on coagulation factors and platelet function. ASAIO Abstract 15:28
21. Pasha R, Benavides M, Kottke-Marchant K, Harasaki H (1995) Reduced expression of platelet surface glycoprotein receptor IIb/IIIa at hyperthermic temperatures. Lab Invest 73:403–408
22. Miller ML, Naganuma S, Utoh J, Harasaki H (1990) In vitro modulation of mononuclear cell ultrastructure and differentiation antigens by thermal exposure. Lab Invest 62:67A
23. Utoh J, Harasaki H (1992) Effects of temperature on phagocytosis of human and calf polymorphonuclear leukocytes. Artif Organs 16:377–381
24. Utoh J, Harasaki H (1992) Damage to erythrocytes from long-term heat stress. Clin Sci 82:9–11

Discussion

Dr. Imachi:
Thank you very much for your very important basic research. I have a question. I think heat tolerance depends on the patient's circulatory state. In your experiment, it's maybe a healthy calf, but how about the patient who is operated on after chronic heart failure? Is it tolerated for the same heat flux?

Dr. Harasaki:
Well, it is a very difficult question to answer. I do not know how the cells behave against the extra heat in cardiac failure states. Certainly this is a very important question. I have to keep studying, but my guess is that there won't be any significant difference. I suppose that there is enough tissue blood flow in the organs or tissue that we are discussing now. My guess is based upon our extensive in vitro studies of the heat effect on the various cells, including the endothelial cells, muscle cells, and the fibroblasts, which show a very consistent response to the given heat load.

Dr. Tatsumi:
Could you make any comment on the device's surface materials in terms of microscopic structure or material itself for heat conductivity, because I think such things may influence cell migration or angiogenesis or heat dissipation itself.

Dr. Harasaki:
Certainly. That is, again, a very important issue. First of all, so far, we may have forgotten to study the effect of heat on the tissue response to the foreign materials. We are very careful in selecting the material for the artificial heart or implantable devices, selecting the most inert materials. But extra heat certainly causes noxious effects. In answering your questions, because of that issue in our minds, we implanted the same device, of the same configuration and same volume on the control side without heat, to isolate only the effect of the temperatures. I don't know what happens if the surface is made of titanium, carbon fibers, or other materials, but my guess is that there won't be any significant difference among these different biomaterials.

Brain and Spinal Cord Lesions with Long-Term Total Artificial Heart Pumping

Jaromír Vašků

Summary. Animals surviving for extended periods with a total artificial heart (TAH) device sometimes experience central nervous system (CNS) complications. These are caused by the hypoperfusion of the CNS for various reasons; by microthromboembolization, which is manifested either by the emboli from a primary thrombotic formation or by calcified emboli; or by central nervous hemorrhages, owing to various causes. The central nervous system can be threatened by hypoperfusion, which may be caused particularly by a mechanical obstruction in the input or output tract of the pump, or by inadequate pumping. Clinically, peripheral spinal paralysis with a histological picture of tigrolysis of the ganglionic cells in the brain and spinal cord and encephalomalacia are frequent findings in these cases. Prevention in these cases can partially depend on proper TAH construction and adequate control and driving. Thromboembolic complications affecting the central nervous system can cause immediate termination of an experiment, if the thromboemboli affect the brain-stem centers. If other parts of the brain are impaired, then for some time this situation can be compatible with life; the animal is mostly hemiplegic before it expires after a few days. From the point of pathogenesis we can differentiate the thrombi caused directly by noncompatible thrombogenic material from those caused by incompatible pump construction resulting in "dead areas" where the bloodstream stagnates and thrombi are formed, or from septic thrombi caused by infection in the animal. On the other hand, the thrombus may be calcified (so-called secondary dystrophic calcification) or the driving diaphragm may be affected by "primary calcification." The prevention of simple thromboembolism may be achieved by adequate TAH construction, by the use of nonthrombogenic material, and by avoiding infection, whereas the prevention of primary calcification may be attained by a special anticalcification treatment. Hemorrhagic lesions affecting the CNS are caused by inadequate anticoagulation and antiaggregation therapy, or by idiopathic endogenous disturbances of coagulation based on septic states or hepatic disturbances caused mostly by an increase in central venous pressure. A solution to the prevention of all possible causes of central nervous disturbance in TAH patients is necessary before its use becomes a clinical reality.

Key words: Total artificial heart — Brain and spinal cord lesions — Hypoperfusion — Thromboembolism — Calcified emboli

VACORD Bioengineering Research Company Ltd., BRNO 614 OO-Husovice, Cacovická 53, Czech Republic

Introduction

The artificial heart is a device urgently needed to solve the problem of final heart failure [1–3]. The systems used currently are pneumatic or electromechanical, and they allow only limited comfort for the patient. Therefore, they have been used for short-term application as so-called bridge systems designed for the period preceding heart transplantation. Artificial heart or mechanical heart support systems should be available for these situations. If they are antithrombogenic owing to their construction and mechanical properties, then the patient's central nervous system (CNS) is not so threatened by thromboembolic complications, unless there is infection, which can be the cause of septic thrombi. Even though the Czech artificial heart, TNS-BRNO, is optimal in this respect, in experiments lasting for months, microembolization affecting the CNS, either by primary thrombi or by thromboemboli from the calcified diaphragm, sometimes threatened the duration of survival [4–8]. This danger can be limited by optimal construction of the pump, by a proper antithrombotic treatment, by the prevention of infection, and finally, by affecting the calcification mechanisms biologically or by suitable processing of the diaphragm material to prevent calcifying nucleation. Optimal technology in the production of artificial hearts should entail the complete elimination of potential air embolism into the central nervous system. Therefore, the aim of further research ought to be to design an absolutely defect-free artificial heart which would eliminate any damage to the central nervous system during permanent long-lasting application, owing either to cerebral embolism of any origin, or to CNS hypoperfusion caused by limitations on the pumping capability of the artificial heart.

Materials and Methods

The materials and methods concerning surgery on calves and postoperative care used both in 66 long-term and in short-lasting experiments were published elsewhere [4–6,9–10].

In 62 experiments, a total artificial heart (TAH) TNS-BRNO (model II, III, VII, or VIII) was implanted; in 4 experiments, the ROSTOCK TAH was used [6]. In the short-duration experiments, a TAH TNS-BRNO II or VII was implanted.

The methods for evaluating calcification of the driving diaphragm and the procedure for possible prevention were described elsewhere [4–6].

To assess possible central nervous complications, at the termination of each experiment, a careful autopsy of the central nervous system (brain and spinal cord) was performed and any macroscopic lesions were evaluated. Very important was the evaluation of microscopic sections from all parts of the brain: cortex cerebri, occipital lobe, frontal lobe, parietal lobe, diencephalon, temporal lobe, amygdala region, hippocampus, mesencephalon, brain stem, cerebellum, pons, and medulla oblongata. Several further sections taken from the upper, middle, and lower spinal cord were evaluated. Histological staining methods were: hematoxylin-eosin, methylene blue, von Kóssa, Bielschowsky, van Gieson, and Masson's trichrome. The pathological macro- and microscopic findings in the central nervous system were compared to the clinical symptoms which accompanied death.

Results

In 56 out of 66 animals, the termination of the experiments involved CNS damage from various causes. Tables 1–4 show the four main groups of causes of death where the deleterious effect on the central nervous system was either decisive (the main cause of death) or was at least a serious, accompanying complication. For example, right circulatory insufficiency killed the experimental subject owing to a serious respiratory complication; however, in various parts of brain, serious pathological changes were found. In two calves, observed signs of brain edema, acidotic coloration of the brain tissue, the formation of pseudocysts, dilatation of perivascular spaces in the pons, and dispersed hemorrhages in the thalamus (calves no. 134, "Pluto," which survived 170 days; and no. 121, "Artur," which survived 293 days). Table 5 summarizes the CNS lesions observed.

On the other hand, hypoperfusion, due to serious dislocation of the device, and thrombi, located in the output tracts, led to definite clinical signs of CNS impairment; e.g., cramps immediately before death (calf no. 122, "Richard," which survived 166 days of pumping). A similar situation was encountered with the formation of pannus, which markedly decreased the output and caused serious brain damage. Sometimes this situation was enhanced by the dislocation of the pump (calf no. 144, "Arvid," which survived 190 days)

(Fig. 1). In this case, edema with the degeneration of ganglionic cells, red encephalomalacia, and occasional tigrolysis in all parts of the brain were typical of the findings in such a state of hypoperfusion.

Pannus in the left inflow tract with an extreme blockade of the venae pulmonales with accompanying bronchopneumonia was another main cause of inadequate blood supply into the brain (calf no. 116, "Alarich," which survived 104 days).

Technical failure due to disconnection of the quick connector from the left inflow tract caused massive blood effusion into the space between the pump and the pseudopericardium. Brain death due to multiple foci of local cerebral dystrophy was evident (calf no. 59, "Omar," which survived 173 days [10]).

Another cause of cerebral death was massive cerebral thromboembolism owing to the formation of septic thrombi as a sequel of massive infection. Polynuclear cells and occasionally small glial knots were observed (calf no. 136, "Nero," which survived 142 days; calf no. 133, "Hugo," which survived 110 days; and 16 other cases (Fig. 2).

Successive multiple thromboemboli of calcified material which had broken away from calcified driving diaphragms and migrated into the brain, and marked tigrolysis of cells with encephalomalacia and extensive brain edema, were the causes of death in calf no. 125, "Prokop" (survival 270 days) and no. 123, "Norman" (survival 231 days). However special anticalcification treatment substantially limited the lethal microembolization in the brain and spinal cord by calcified particles in a number of calves

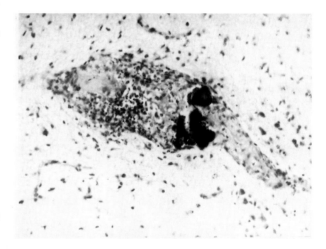

Fig. 1. Calf no. 144, "Arvid." Survived 190 days of pumping. Cause of death: right circulatory insufficiency. *Hippocampus*, focus of the red encephalomalacia with the calcified septic microthromboembolus. Magnification 384×; von Kóssa stain

Table 1. Causes of death in the total artificial heart (TAH) experiments in calves: Group 1

No.	Name	Survival (days)	HP	CHP	LEC	LID	LP LRP	LOTB	RCI
113	Hanibal	184	+						
139	Alfons	83	+						
85	Cesar	98		+					
122	Richard	166		+					
89	Mechmed	97			+				
59	Omar	173				+			
116	Alarich	104					+		
117	Měšek	147					+		
149	Uran	129						+	
142	Juan	314						+	
64	Roman	163							+
66	Roland	133							+
67	Jakub	127							+
100	Armand	153							+
106	Leon	127							+
111	Lena	137							+
114	Arvid	190							+
129	Alfred	196							+
134	Pluto	179							+

HP, Hypoperfusion; *CHP*, cerebral hypoperfusion; *LEC*, lung edema of cerebral origin; *LID*, left inflow tract disconnection; *LP*, left pannus; *LRP*, left, right pannus; *LOTB*, left outflow thrombotic block; *RCI*, right circulatory insufficiency.

Table 2. Causes of death in the TAH experiments in calves: Group 2

No.	Name	Survival (days)	TE	SETE	CATE
53	Florian	155			+
54	Waldemar	31	+		
65	Achmed	175			+
76	Kazan	123			+
79	Ramses	42		+	
82	Perun	39		+	
86	Aram	46		+	
88	Kara mustafa	139		+	
90	Armin	99		+	
93	Hakim	147		+	
94	Kasim	95		+	
95	Rašid	61		+	
97	Gaston	66		+	
102	Pascal	78		+	
120	Amur	97		+	
121	Artur	293		+	
123	Norman	231			+
125	Prokop	270			+
127	Adam	44		+	
130	Ramón	130		+	
133	Hugo	110		+	
136	Nero	142		+	
146	Samuel	147	+		

TE, thromboembolism; *SETE*, septic thromboembolism; *CATE*, calcified thromboembolism.

Table 3. Causes of death in the TAH experiments in calves: Group 3

No.	Name	Survival (days)	HE
50	Hassan	150	+
56	Kamil	35	+
61	Curro	75	+
70	Michal	32	+
74	Girej	71	+
101	Gerard	39	+

HE, hemorrhage.

Table 4. Causes of death in the TAH experiments in calves: Group 4

No.	Name	Survival (days)	DL	AL
52	Samson	104	+	
60	Fatima	75	+	
69	Martin	42	+	
72	Čingiz	100	+	
99	Roger	64	+	
103	Marcel	51		+
107	Harald	226	+	
110	Haakon	218		+

DL, diaphargm leakage; *AL*, air leakage.

Table 5. A survey of the autopsy and histological changes in the various parts of the brain of long surviving calves with a TAH

Group A
Brain edema
Acidotic coloration of the brain tissue
Red encephalomalacia
Dystrophic foci
Necrotic foci
Capillary dilatation
Perivascular edema
Formation of pseudocysts
Tigrolysis of the ganglionic cells
Glial stimulation with the reactive formation of glial knots

Group B
Microthromboemboli
Septic microthromboemboli
Calcified microthromboemboli
Platelet thrombi
Hyaline thrombi
Microemboli in the pial vessels
Dilatation of the pial vessels
Glial stimulation with the reactive formation of glial knots

Group C
Massive hemorrhage in various parts of brain and spinal cord
Hemorrhagic foci
Glial stimulation with the formation of glial knots

The pathohistological findings listed in group A predominantly occurred in cause-of-death groups 1 and 4 of Tables 1 and 4. The findings listed in group B predominantly occurred in group 2, and those listed in group C predominantly occurred in group 3.

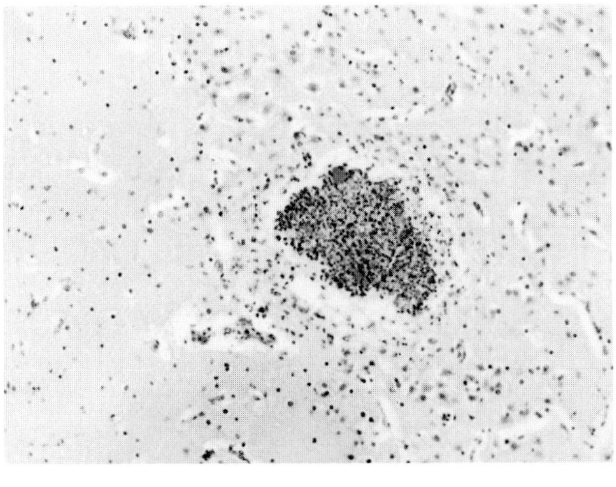

Fig. 2. Calf no. 133, "Hugo." Survived 110 days of pumping. Cause of death: septic thromboembolization. *Right occipital lobe*, septic microthromboembolus. Magnification 302×, hematoxylin-eosin stain

(Figs. 3–5) [4–7]. An interesting observation was a case of hepatocerebral syndrome (calf no. 87 "Mechmed," which survived 97 days) which died of respiratory insufficiency with the formation of pseudocysts in the pons close to the nucleus of the vagus nerve [11,12].

In another calf, we encountered the unusual situation where cerebral ischemia was caused by pathologically low output. This was a unique case, involving pathologically low central venous pressure (CVP) with general vasodilatation in the peripheral circulation. This was a sequel of an anomaly involving the pressoreceptors in the right atrium. The experiment with this particular calf was terminated upon signs of peripheral motor quadriplegia. In the brain and spinal cord tissue, marked disappearance of Nissl bodies from the ganglionic cells (tigrolysis) was evident. Throughout the brain tissue, glial activation was evident, expressed by the occurrence of small dispersed glial knots (calf no. 85, "Cezar," which survived 98 days of pumping [11] (Fig. 7).

Tables 1–4 show that in the majority of experiments, even if the main cause of death did not concern the brain tissue directly, a certain degree of brain lesion was always evident. Table 5 shows the most frequent microscopic lesions observed in the central nervous system of the experimental animals (Figs. 1–12).

In cases of septic microemboli, the microorganisms found most frequently were: *Staphylococcus epidermidis*, *Pseudomonas aeruginosa*, *Escherichia coli*, and *Streptococcus beta-hemolyticus*.

Discussion

In these experiments with total artificial hearts, aimed at long survival, a spectrum of complications influenced the outcome. When the function of the pneumatic pumping system failed and a marked organ hypoperfusion occurred, owing either to technical failure or to pathophysiological disorders such as pannus and thrombotic occlusion at the input or output ports, the general oxygen supply to the internal organs was markedly decreased. First of all, the central nervous tissue was affected due to high sensitivity of the ganglionic cells to the oxygen insufficiency. This situation is typified by group 1 in Table 1 (causes of death). If disturbance of the oxygen supply occurred suddenly (disconnection of the pumping system, dislocation of the device, etc.), then death also came suddenly, and the pathological picture in the brain tissue was typically characterized by acute changes — brain edema, dystrophic and necrotic foci, and encephalomalacia. In cases where the disturbance to the oxygen supply gradually increased, such as gradual growth of pannus or of a thrombotic occlusion in the left or right side, the tissue damage was not so uniform, but somewhat variable. The characteristic changes reflected the gradual impairment of the oxygen supply. In this case, we observed capillary dilatation, perivascular edema,

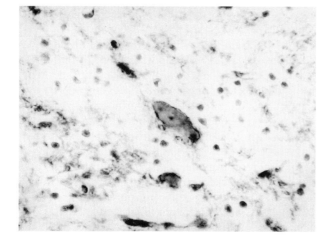

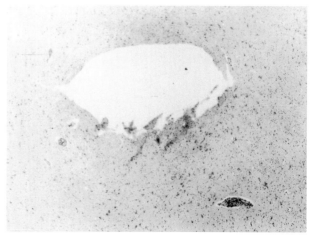

Fig. 3. Calf no. 125, "Prokop." Survived 270 days of pumping. Cause of death: calcified thromboembolism. *Pons*, massive tigrolysis of the ganglionic cells in the left part of pons. Magnification 986× using oil immersion. Hematoxylin-eosin stain

Fig. 5. Calf no. 125, "Prokop." Survived 270 days of pumping. Cause of death: calcified thromboembolism. *Diencephalon*, large pseudocyst, originating from serious metabolic disturbance as a sequel of massive microthromboembolization. In the small arteries, the occurrence of thrombi is clearly visible. Magnification 76×. Hematoxylin-eosin stain

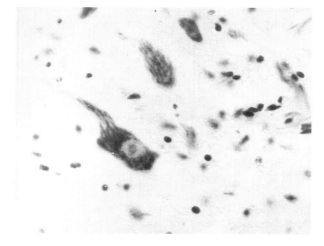

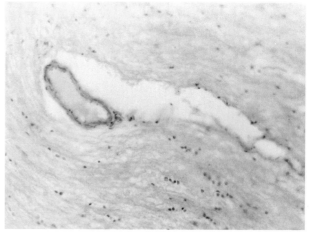

Fig. 4. Calf no. 125, "Prokop." Survived 270 days. Cause of death: calcified thromboembolism. *Pons*, area from the right part of the pons. Here the tigroid structure in the ganglionic cells is well preserved. Magnification 986× using oil immersion. Hematoxylin-eosin stain

Fig. 6. Calf no. 130, "Ramón." Survived 130 days of pumping. Cause of death: septic thromboemolism. *Pons*, in the artery, platelet thrombus with massively edematous dilated perivascular space. Magnificantion 302×. Hematoxylin — eosin stain

tigrolysis of the ganglionic cells, formation of pseudocysts, and also the activation of the glia. As a rule, all connective tissues, including glia, are stimulated by oxygen insufficiency to intense growth. The expression of this state is the occurrence of dispersed glial knots throughout the brain tissue (Figs. 10, 11).

Also, technical failure involving diaphragm air leakage sometimes developed gradually, and the duration of this kind of disorder was sometimes several days.

During this time, the tissue changes included not only the acute, but also the chronic signs of damage which were typical of group 1 in Table 1 and manifested by the pathohistological changes found in group A in Table 5.

A peculiar situation concerning the hypoperfusion of the central nervous system was observed in calf no. 85, "Cezar." Pathological venous hypotension was observed from the beginning of the experiment. This

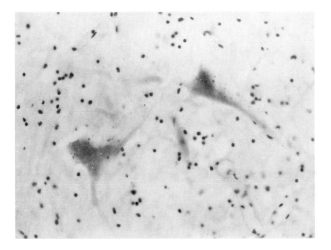

Fig. 7. Calf no. 85, "Cezar." Survived 98 days of pumping. Cause of death: hypoperfusion of the central nervous system. *Lower part of the spinal cord*, tigrolysis of the ganglionic cells in the anterior horns of the spinal cord, with the tissue cleaning reaction (increased activity of cells to remove cellular debris). Magnification 480×. Hematoxylin — eosin stain

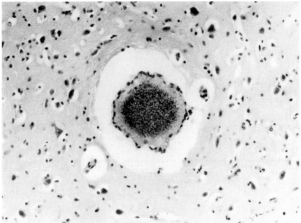

Fig. 9. Calf no. 123, "Norman." Survived 231 days of pumping. Cause of death: calcified thromboembolism. *Left lobus occipitalis*, thrombus with perivascular edema. Magnification 302×. Hematoxylin — eosin stain

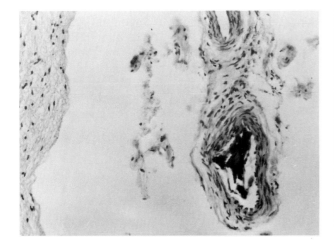

Fig. 8. Calf no. 123, "Norman." Survived 231 days of pumping. Cause of death: calcified thromboembolism. *Medulla oblongata*, calcified microthromboembolus in the pial vessel. Magnification 302×; von Kóssa stain

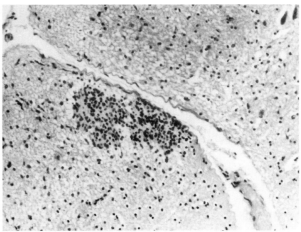

Fig. 10. Calf no. 123, "Norman". Survived 231 days of pumping. Cause of death: calcified thromboembolism. *MESENCEPHALON*, glial knot, formed due to massive oxygen insufficiency. Magnification 302×. Hematoxylin — eosin stain

state was caused evidently by an anomaly in vasomotor regulation with abnormal reactivity of the baroreceptors, which was evidently conditioned by the inborn disturbance of vasomotor regulation. In this animal, the mild hypoperfusion lasted for nearly three months, and increasing ischemia of the neural structures led to peripheral paralysis in the end-stage of the experiment. A conspicuous change, aside from other typical signs of hypoperfusion, was a marked diffuse disappearance of the Nissl bodies from the ganglionic

cells (tigrolysis) in the brain and spinal cord, cellular dystrophy, and dispersed glial knots. The calf died after 98 days of pumping [11].

In another calf (no. 89, "Mechmed") a state of hepatic blockade on the basis of pathological hemolysis developed due to an inborn defect in the osmotic red cell resistance. The hepatic detoxification process was compromised by the products of the RBC destruction. In the human clinic, similar states are known as hepatic cerebropathies [11,12]. The calf finally died from

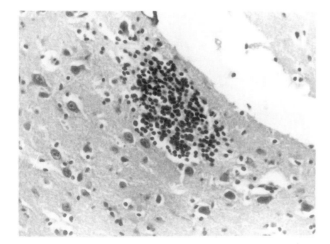

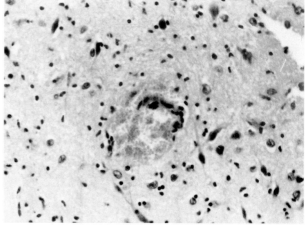

Fig. 11. Calf no. 103, "Marcel." Survived 51 days of pumping. Qause of death: diaphragm leakage. *Hippocampus*, glial knot formed due to oxygen insufficiency. Magnification 484×. Hematoxylin-eosin stain

Fig. 12. Calf no. 103, "Marcel." Survived 51 days of pumping. Cause of death: diaphragm leakage. *Thalamus*, hemorrhagic focus. Magnification 484×. Hematoxylin — eosin stain

abrupt intractable respiratory distress with lung edema due to autotoxic damage to the respiratory center. The experiment was terminated after 97 days of pumping. No thrombi were found in the lungs at autopsy. A marked hemosiderin storage in the renal tubular cells confirmed pathological hemolysis. In the brain (pons) we found pseudocysts in the vicinity of the nucleus of the left vagus nerve, which was markedly damaged [11]. This was also the real cause of death.

In a relatively large group of animals, we encountered cerebral microembolization which originated from thrombi formation due to infection. In 16 calves, the septic microthromboemboli attacked the brain tissue. In 5 cases, we confirmed the presence of calcified microthromboemboli. Unless the embolization affected the vital centers in the brain stem, the state was compatible with further survival, even if signs of cerebral stroke were often clinically evident [10,13]. Concerning the calcified microthromboemboli, compared to the septic embolization, we could decrease the calcifying embolization by a special anticalcification treatment based on the stimulation of endogenous calcifying inhibitors [4–6]. The problem of calcification of the diaphragm was analyzed in detail in [4–7].

Everybody who is familiar with total artificial heart research knows very well how dangerous for the outcome is infection, which endangers the experiment in many ways. In particular, *Staphylococcus epidermidis* and *Pseudomonas aeruginosa* infections are a constant threat in these experiments [14–19]. One important aspect is definitely the formation of septic thrombi. This complication, especially, is an ever-present danger in all long-term clinical applications. Here, in addi-

tion to antibiotic treatment, prevention, based initially on the stimulation of the endogenous defensive reactions (immunomodulation) is important [8].

Thrombosis in the TAH device without the participation of infection still remains a big problem. This problem can be addressed at either the local or general level [8–10,13]. Even if the animal survives for hundreds of days, the danger of a thromoembolic complication accompanies the whole course of the experiment in spite of the anticoagulation and antiaggregation therapy [20]. This danger is also present in clinical applications [21,22]. Vital is the development of totally antithrombogenic surfaces in the blood pumps.

Cerebral hemorrhage was determined as the cause of death in eight calves; sometimes it was accompanied by the leakage of the left driving diaphragm, while in other cases inadequate anticoagulation and antiaggregation therapy could have caused the cerebral hemorrhage. Septic states were often accompanied by cerebral hemorrhages, which were also observed in the case of the hepatocerebral syndrome (Fig. 12) [11].

The blood clotting pathway is very vulnerable, prone either to increased clotting or to increased bleeding wing to abnormal activity of clotting factors [23–25]. The effects on the liver caused by the increased CVP during TAH experiments are very dangerous because this organ has an important impact on the systems which stabilize blood clotting [6,26,27]. Infection and sepsis are inevitably accompanied either by thrombus formation or hemorrhage. From the standpoint of hemostasis, the TAH experiments are balancing on the "edge of a knife".

Conclusions

1. The main aim of this study was to investigate the etiopathogenesis of the brain lesions incurred during TAH pumping.

2. Brain and spinal cord tissues were endangered by technical failures, hypoperfusion, driving diaphragm leakage, defects in the driving tract, etc, resulting in the typical signs of brain and spinal cord damage (Tables 1, 4).

3. Another cause of CNS damage was thromboembolism, which was primary, of septic origin, or caused by calcified microparticles (Table 2).

4. Disturbances in the blood clotting mechanism leading to hemorrhagic states can seriously affect the central nervous system (Table 3).

5. Anomalies in the TAH recipients themselves, such as extremely low blood and venous pressure, hepatic cerebropathy, etc., were accompanied by typical changes in the brain and spinal cord tissue.

6. At present, any blood pump, especially when used for long-term pumping, is not absolutely safe from the stand-point of possible damage to the central nervous system. In some situations, even if the blood pump has excellent attributes, a deficiency in the physiology of the TAH recipient can be a source of certain central nervous complications. This was confirmed by experimental and clinical experience.

Acknowledgments. The author thanks Miss Viola Krejčí for her excellent technical cooperation.

References

1. Olsen DB, Murray KD (1984) The total artificial heart. In: Unger F (ed) Assisted circulation. Springer, Berlin, pp 197–228
2. De Vries WC (1988) The permanent artificial heart. JAMA 259:849–859
3. Pierce WS (1986) The artificial heart 1986: Partial fullfillment of a promise. ASAIO Trans 32:5–10
4. Vašků J, Urbánek P (1995) Electron-microscopic study of driving diaphragms in the long term survival with a total artificial heart. Artif Organs 19:344–354
5. Vašků J (1996) The changes of the TAH driving diaphragms after a long term pumping. Heart replacement. Artificial heart 5, Springer, Tokyo, pp 53–64
6. Vašků J (1993) Perspectives of total artificial heart research as a valuable modelling system for general physiology and pathophysiology. In: Akutsu T, Koyanagi H (eds) Heart replacement. Artificial heart 4. Springer, Tokyo, pp 161–171
7. Vašků J (1992) Pathophysiological assessment of a total artificial heart (TAH) in experimental and clinical work. In: Sezai Y (ed) Artificial heart — the development of biomation in the twenty-first century. Nihon University International Symposium, Saunders, Tokyo, pp 232–239
8. Vašků J (1993) The impact of total artificial heart research on the progress in basic medical sciences. In: Sezai Y (ed) Artificial heart — the development of biomation in the twenty-first century. Nihon University International Symposium, Harwood, Chur, Switzerland, pp 9–21
9. Vašků J (1982) Artificial heart. Pathophysiology of the total artificial heart and of cardiac assist devices. Acta Fac Med Univ Brunensis J E Purkyně, Brno, 397
10. Vašků (1984) Brno experiments in long term survival with total artificial heart. Acta Fac Med Univ Brunensis JE Purkyně, Brno, 622
11. Vašků J (1986) Total artificial heart research in Czechoslovakia. Pathophysiological evaluation of long term experiments performed from 1979–1985. In: Akutsu T (ed) Artificial heart 1. Springer, Tokyo, pp 161–179
12. Bernardini P, Fischer JE (1982) Amino acid imbalance and hepatic encephalopathy. Annu Rev Nutr 2:419–454
13. Vašků J (1990) Central nervous complications in subjects with artificial heart. Bratisl Lk Listy 91:5–20
14. Richards GK, Gagnon RF (1993) The continuing enigma of implant associated infections. Int J Artif Organs 16:747–748
15. Dickinson GM, Bisno AL (1993) Infections associated with prosthetic devices: clinical considerations. Int J Artif Organs 16:749–754
16. Gristina AG, Giridhar G, Gabriel BL, Naylor PT, Myrvik QN (1993) Cell biology and molecular mechanisms in artificial device infections. Int J Artif Organs 16:755–764
17. Costerton JW, Khoury AE, Ward KH, Anwar H (1993) Practical measures to control device-related bacterial infections. Int J Artif Organs 16:765–770
18. Burns GL (1993) Infections associated with implanted blood pumps. Int J Artif Organs 16:771–776
19. Richards GK, Gagnon RF (1993) An assay of *Staphylococcus epidermidis* biofilm responses to therapeutic agents. Int J Artif Organs 16:777–787
20. Fujimasa I, Imachi K, Nakajima M, Mabuchi K, Tsukagoshi S, Kouno A, Ono T, Takido N, Motomura K, Chinzei T, Abe Y, Atsumi K (1986) Pathophysiological sutdy of a total artificial heart in a goat that survived for 344 days. In: Nosé Y, Kjellstrand C, Ivanovich P (eds) Progress in artificial organs — 1985. ISAO Press, Cleveland, pp 345–353
21. Magovern JA, Rosenberg G, Pierce W (1986) Development and current status of a total artificial heart. Artif Organs 10:357–363
22. Sakamoto T, Arai H, Akamatsu H, Suzuki A (1993) Clinical results in postcardiotomy circulatory support. In: Sezai Y (ed) Artificial heart — the development of biomation in the twenty-first century. Nihon University International Symposium, Harwood, Chur, Switzerland, pp 177–181
23. Imachi K (1986) Long term use of artificial heart without anticoagulant. In: Nosé Y, Kjellstrand C, Ivanovich P (eds) Progress in artificial organs — 1985. ISAO Press, Cleveland, pp 319–326
24. Yada J, Onoda K, Shimono T, Tanaka K, Shimpo H, Kusagawa M (1993) Blood coagulation properties and anticoagulant therapy in assisted circulation. In: Sezai Y (ed) Artificial heart — the devlopment of biomation in the twenty-first century. Nihon University

International Symposium, Harwood, Chur, Switzerland, pp 163–165

25. Kagawa Y, Hongo T, Sato N, Uchida N, Miura M, Nitta S, Horiuchi T, Atsumi K, Fujimasa I, Imachi K, Nakajima M (1986) Clinical application of partial artificial heart. In: Nosé Y, Kjellstrand C, Ivanovich P (eds) Progress in artificial organs — 1985. ISAO Press, Cleveland, pp 436–440

26. Vašků J, Vašků J, Dostál M, Guba P, Gregor Z, Vašků A, Urbánek P, Černý J, Doležel S, Cídl K, Pavlíček V, Bednařík B (1990) Evaluation study of calves with total artificial heart (TAH) surviving for 218–293 days of pumping. Int J Artif Organs 13:830–836

27. Vašků J (1996) Actual pathophysiological problems in the contemporary research on the TAH. Ann Thor Cardiovasc Surg 2:315–330

An Adaptive Cardiac Output Control for the Total Artificial Heart Using a Self-Tuning Proportional-Integral-Derivative (PID) Controller

Won Woo Choi[1], Byoung Goo Min[2], Hee Chan Kim[2], Won Kon Kim[3], Yong Soon Won[4], Joon Ryang Rho[3], Young Ho Jo[2], Seong Keun Park[2], Jae Mok Ahn[2], and Jong Jin Lee[1]

Summary. The development of a control method for the totally implantable artificial heart (TAH) to regulate cardiac output according to the change in physiological demand was the goal of this study. The conventional proportional-integral-derivative (PID) controller was used for the automatic regulation of the cardiac output. Furthermore, using a fuzzy gain-tuning algorithm, the PID controller parameters were adaptively tuned to the optimal operating point of the process, which varied with hemodynamic disturbances. To determine the physiological demand, the interventricular pressure (IVP) inside the TAH was used to estimate inflow conditions. The negative peak value of the IVP at each diastolic period has a linear relation to the corresponding atrial pressure. Based on the relationship of atrial pressure to the IVP, the automatic control algorithm proposed regulates the optimal pump rate in terms of sufficient cardiac output delivery under a given venous return. To maintain a well-balanced left and right pump output from the volumetrically coupled, circular moving actuator type TAH, the automatic control also adjusts an asymmetric amount of the moving actuator stroke angle, which provides a different net output of the ventricles. The in vitro performance of the newly developed automatic control method was assessed using a mock circulatory system. Over a physiological range of preload, −3–15 mmHg of right atrial pressure (RAP) and 80–120 mmHg of aortic pressure (AoP), the cardiac output varied from 4.2 to 6.3 l/min with the left atrial pressure (LAP) maintained below 15 mmHg.

Key words: Moving actuator type total artificial heart — Adaptive self-tuning proportional-integral-derivative (PID) controller — Interventricular pressure

Introduction

We have been developing an electromechanical total artificial heart (TAH) since 1983. As several cardiac output control methods have been developed in various parts of the world for long-term use in totally implantable artificial hearts, we have also updated automatic control algorithms to achieve more physiological performance and better stability [1,2]. In this paper, we propose a new adaptive cardiac output control algorithm, using a self-tuning proportional-integral-derivative (PID) controller.

The use of a PID controller does not require an exact process model, hence it is effective for processes for which the derivation of models poses considerable difficulty. Optimal settings for the PID parameters are important to accomplish good performance and stability. Ziegler and Nichols [3] proposed a tuning method based on step response data, and Takahashi and Chan [4] introduced a tuning method for discrete-time PID controllers. However, in spite of the advantages of the PID controllers, there remain several drawbacks. For example, if the operating point of the process is varied due to disturbances, the controller parameters need to be adjusted empirically by a skilled operator to obtain new optimal settings. For systems with interacting loops, this process could be difficult and time-consuming.

Besides, for systems such as the TAH including a circulatory system with variable time-delay, varying plant parameters, large nonlinearities, and significant process noise, the self-adaptation of the PID controller parameters according to fluctuations in the system's operating point overcomes the loss of optimality of the controller parameters. Zhao et al. [5] introduced a scheme for fuzzy gain scheduling of the PID controllers for process control. Fuzzy rules and reasoning were utilized on-line to determine the controller parameters based on the error signal, defined as the difference between the reference signal and the currently measured signal, and its first differential.

For the regulation of cardiac output from the TAH according to the physiological demand, we adopted three basic control requirements: preload sensitivity, moderate afterload sensitivity, and a well-balanced ventricular output. A full-to-empty mode of operation was adopted to utilize maximally the full capacity of the blood pump, and heart rate control was found to be the best way to implement the preload-sensitive response. To obtain information on the preload, we

[1] Department of Biomedical Engineering, College of Engineering, Seoul National University, 28 Youngun-Dong, Chongno-Ku, Seoul 110-744, Korea
[2] Department of Biomedical Engineering and [3] Department of Thoracic Surgery, College of Medicine, Seoul National University, 28 Youngun-Dong, Chongno-Ku, Seoul 110-744, Korea
[4] Department of Thoracic Surgery, College of Medicine, Ehwa Women's University, 11-1 Daehyun-Dong, Seodaemun-Ku, Seoul 120-750, Korea

used the negative peak value of the interventricular spatial pressure (IVP) generated between two blood sacs enclosed by a rigid pump housing. Also, we determined normal peak value when the preload was maintained within the physiological range, even though the heart rate was varying.

An error, defined as the difference between the normal value and the currently measured peak value of these two parameters, forms one input to the self-tuning PID controller. Then the PID controller generates a heart rate appropriate to regulate the error within the acceptable preset range, and in consequence, to maintain the hemodynamics within the physiological range. The adaptive PID controller was robust to the variation of unknown hemodynamics in the circulatory system. The proposed control scheme was evaluated through a series of mock-circulatory experiments.

Materials and Methods

Blood Pump and Electronic Control System

The blood pump is composed of a moving actuator as an energy converter, a right and left ventricle, and the interventricular volume space enclosed by a rigid polyurethane housing. Figure 1 shows a schematic diagram of the moving-actuator type blood pump.

A brushless d.c. motor (S/M 566-18, Sierracin/Magnedyne, Carlsbad, CA, USA) and a three-stage gear train were assembled in the moving actuator. The actuator pumps out blood alternately from each side with the circular motion of an epicyclical gear train.

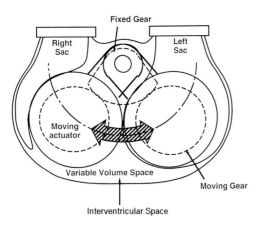

Fig. 1. Schematic diagram of the moving actuator type blood pump. A brushless d.c. motor integrated inside the actuator generates a pendulous motion using an epicyclic gear train. Each ventricle has a double-sac structure, and the interventricular space is filled with air, lubricating oil, and sacs, forming a variable-volume space

Because the TAH is a volumetrically coupled type, a left systolic phase corresponds to a right diastolic period and vice versa. The maximal static stroke volumes of the left and right sacs are $50\,cm^3$ and $45\,cm^3$, respectively. The interventricular space between the two sacs and the moving actuator acts as a variable volume space.

The electronic control system consists of a microcontroller-based implantable internal controller and a human-interfaced external controller. With a control program in the on-chip erasable and programmable read-only memory (EPROM) of the 16-bit microcontroller, 87C196KD (Intel, Folsom, CA, USA), the internal controller performs: (1) brushless d.c. motor commutation using three Hall-effect sensors; (2) position and speed control of the actuator in terms of the physiological control algorithm, analog-to-digital (A/D) conversion of the analog motor-current signal at each 0.17 ms of sampling time; and (4) communication with the external controller, an IBM PC, through an RS-232C serial protocol.

The external controller, in which the proposed automatic control algorithm was implanted, monitors the status of the implanted system, including motor current information, commands the operational mode or control variables, and stores all data.

Balancing Atrial Pressures Without an Extra Compliance Chamber

The imbalance in atrial pressures due to the bronchial circulation and valvular regurgitation has to be circumvented by providing greater output from the left pump than from the right. This larger left stroke volume was achieved by making the left sac larger than the right one, and by setting the control to give a larger left-side stroke angle, defined as *asymmetry* in this paper. Figure 2 depicts the mechanism for setting the asymmetry stroke angle. With an the increase in the left asymmetry value, the left stroke volume increases and the left atrial pressure (LAP) is almost linearly diminished.

Analysis of the Relationship Between the Preload and the Interventricular Pressure

Because the two blood sacs are enclosed by a rigid pump housing, the pressure in the air-filled interventricular space, containing $100\,cm^3$ of lubrication oil, directly reflects the atrial pressure in each diastolic period, with the assumption that all the blood volume at each diastolic phase is fully ejected at the systolic phase. In other words, the negative pressure generated in the interventricular space by ejecting the left ventricular blood, actively drives the right atrial inflow, and vice versa. Therefore, if the inflow volume

Fig. 2. Mechanism of generation of the asymmetric stroke angle. *RV*, right ventricle; *LV*, left ventricle; θL, left stroke angle; θR, right stroke angle

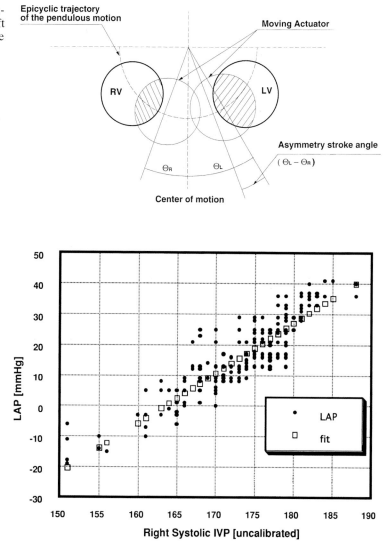

Fig. 3. In vitro relationship between the negative peak of the interventricular pressure (*IVP*) and the left atrial pressure (*LAP*). Linear regression of LAP to right systolic IVP was performed (*squares*): $y = -267.5 + 1.6362x$; $r = 0.88096$

is deficient, the occurrence of a negative pressure in the interventricular space becomes more serious.

In particular, the amplitude of the negative peak of the IVP waveform was adopted as an important information source on the preload. The pressure signal was measured by a pressure transducer (Mpx7200AP, Motorola, Phoenix, AZ, USA) and converted to a digital signal by a commercial A/D converter (AD7870, Analog Device, Norwood, MA, USA). Converted discrete values from 0 to 255 map actual pressure magnitudes from −150mmHg to 30mmHg. Figure 3 shows the in vitro relationship between the negative peak value of the IVP and the left atrial pressure.

Automatic Cardiac Output Control Algorithm

The goal of the automatic cardiac output control is to provide a suitable cardiac output according to the preload while maintaining a well-balanced ventricular output. Cardiac output is regulated by five control variables to control the actuator's speed and moving angle: right systolic speed (RS) and right end-systolic brake time (RBRK), left systolic speed (LS) and left end-systolic brake time (LBRK), and left asymmetry (LAsy). A combination of these five control variables is determined at each stroke termination through the PID controller, adequate to regulate the negative peak of the IVP (mIVP) at the preset reference level (rIVP).

Figure 4 depicts the whole closed-loop control system. The reference level, rIVP, at each diastolic phase was set so that right atrial pressure (RAP) and the LAP were maintained at around −3mmHg and 10mmHg, respectively, in order to provide sufficient cardiac output with balanced atrial pressures. For the adaptation of the PID controller according to parameters, we utilized an on-line gain scheduling scheme based on fuzzy rules proposed by Zhao et al. [5]. In the fuzzification of the error (rIVP minus mIVP) and the

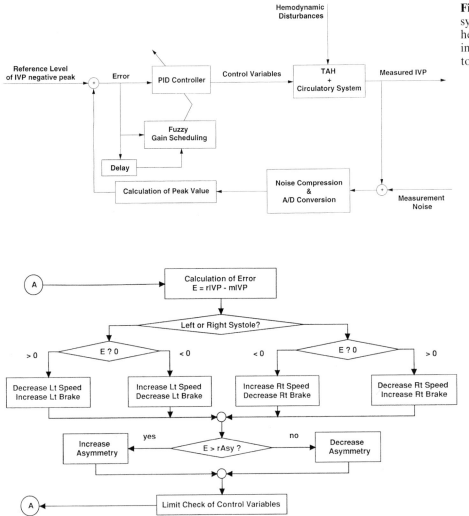

Fig. 4. The closed-loop control system. *TAH*, total artificial heart; *PID*, proportional-integral-derivative; *A/D*, analog to digital

Fig. 5. A flow chart of the automatic cardiac output control algorithm. *E*, error; *rIVP*, preset reference level of interventricular pressure; *mIVP*, negative peak value of interventricular pressure; *A*, loop mark; *Lt*, left; *Rt*, right; *rAsy*, limit level of the error to prevent an increase in left atrial pressure

first differential of the error, triangular membership functions were adopted. The distribution of the membership functions and fuzzy rule bases was based on in vitro experimental results with good step responses. At the defuzzification stage, exponentially curved membership functions were used.

When the left systolic mIVP decreases below the left reference level because the venous return would be decreased, the PID controller increases the LBRK to prevent a succeeding decrease in the right diastolic blood filling rate by waiting for a while, and decreases the LS from the coming stroke to avert a right atrial collapse. The same rule was adapted for the right systolic phase.

If the right systolic mIVP, owing to an increase of the LAP, would be increased over the right reference level, the PID controller increases the LAsy to decrease the increasing LAP. The whole control mechanism is described in the flow chart of Fig. 5.

Mock Circulatory System

A Donovan-type mock circulatory system was used to evaluate the performance and stability of the proposed adaptive control algorithm. Four chamber pressures corresponding to the aortic pressure (AoP), pulmonary arterial pressure (PAP), and the left (LAP) and right atrial pressure (RAP) were monitored by pressure transducers (Cobe, Denver, CO, USA). Also, the systemic flow rate was measured by an ultrasonic flowmeter (T-201, Transonic Systems, USA) at the aortic port of the TAH.

To simulate a limited volume of atrial reservoir, 150-cm³ flexible polymer chambers were connected between the inflow ports of the blood pump and the circulatory system. Also, to simulate the bronchial circulation of the human circulatory system, the left atrial chamber was bypassed through a variable resistance to the aortic chamber.

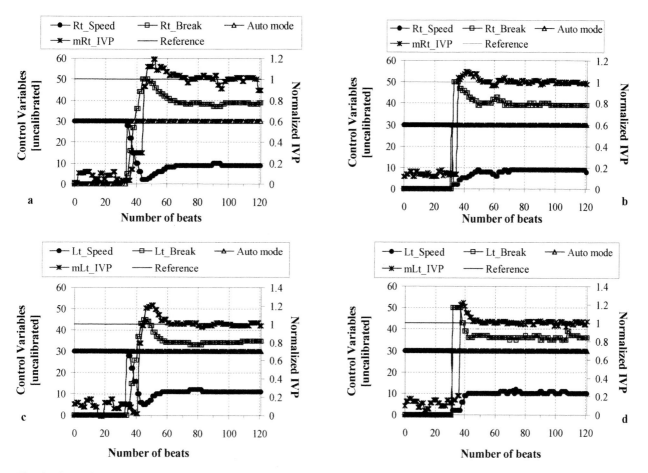

Fig. 6a–d. In vitro step responses of the automatic control system. **a** $K_p = 0.01$, $K_i = 0.2$ at right systole; **b** auto tuned at right systole; **c** $K_p = 0.01$, $K_i = 0.2$ at left systole; **d** auto tuned at left systole. *IVP*, interventricular pressure

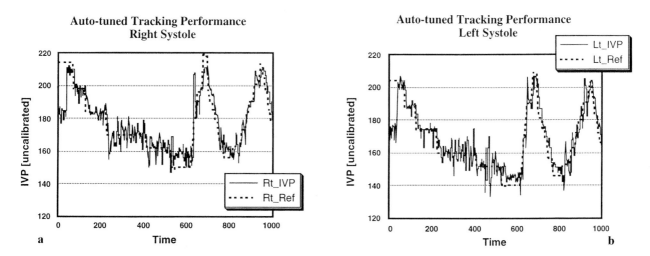

Fig. 7. In vitro tracking performance of the automatic control system. **a** right systole; *solid line*, right interventricular pressure; *dotted line*, its reference level; **b** left systole; *solid line*, left interventricular pressure; *dotted line*, its reference level

Results and Discussion

Prior to in vivo application, the performance of the newly developed automatic control algorithm was assessed through a series of in vitro experiments in a mock circulation system. Input variables to the mock circulatory system were: right atrial pressure within a range of −20–20 mmHg; and the amount of the bypass from the aortic chamber to the left ventricle, up to 630 ml/min, or about 8% of normal cardiac output. The outputs were cardiac output and left atrial pressure.

Figure 6 shows step responses of the measured IVP regulated at the normalized reference level at each systolic phase. The normalized IVP means the ratio of the mIVP to the rIVP. In comparison with the fixed-gain responses, auto-tuned responses have a faster rising time and convergence to a steady state, but bigger overshoots. Therefore, we are trying to diminish the overshoot as much as possible through adjustments of the fuzzy tuning rule and membership function distributions. The performance of the controlled mIVP, which is keeping track of the varying rIVP, is depicted in Fig. 7.

With the proposed control method, the in vitro cardiac output response to the preload changes from −3 to 15 mmHg, as shown in Fig. 8. The cardiac output sensitively increases in response to an increase in RAP from −3 to 6 mmHg, and the resultant response is similar to Starling's curve. Furthermore, the preload sensitivity can be enhanced or diminished by adjustments of the rIVP level. Now, we are trying to find the opti-

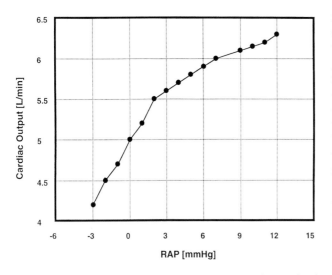

Fig. 8. In vitro cardiac output response to the preload changes. *RAP*, right atrial pressure

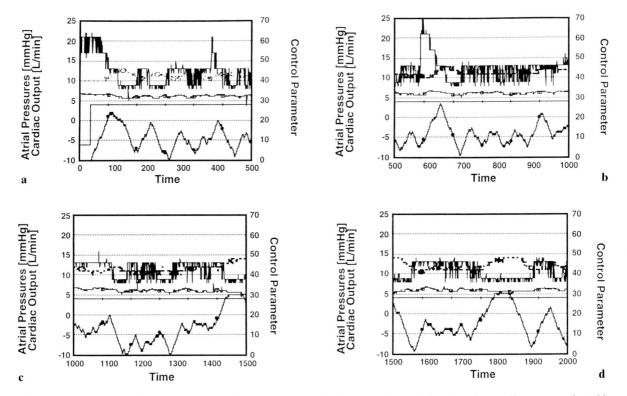

Fig. 9. In vitro atrial balancing performance of the automatic control system. *Line with rectangles*, cardiac output; *dotted line*, right atrial pressure; *line*, left atrial pressure; *line with circles*, imbalance; *line with tickmarks*, control mode. **a–d** show sequential time periods

mal rIVP level to guarantee a given desired preload sensitivity.

Finally, atrial balancing performance is depicted in Fig. 9. The LAP was maintained below 15 mmHg even though there was increased bronchial circulation. When the LAP ascended over 15 mmHg, the automatic control increased the LAsy factor to regulate the right systolic mIVP at the reference level, and from then on, maintain the LAP below 15 mmHg.

Conclusion

In this paper, an adaptive automatic cardiac output control algorithm for a totally implantable electromechanical TAH, using interventricular pressure, was proposed. Based on the appropriate negative peak level of the IVP, the automatic control algorithm provided maximal cardiac output at a given venous return. Also, it maintained a well-balanced left atrial pressure in response to changes in the right atrial pressure and bronchial circulation.

Cardiac output was increased from 4.2 to 6.3 l/min with 80–120 mmHg of aortic pressure according to the increase of preload, and left atrial pressure was maintained at under 15 mmHg at right atrial pressures within the physiological range.

References

1. Kim HC, Lee SH, Kim IY, Min BG, Kim JW, Choi JW, Kim JT, Jung DY (1990) Optimal and physiological control for the new moving-actuator type electromechanical total artificial heart. Artif Organs 14:103–105
2. Choi WW, Kim HC, Min BG (1996) A new automatic cardiac output control algorithm for moving actuator total artificial heart by motor current waveform analysis. Int J Artif Organs 19:189–196
3. Ziegler JG, Nichols NB (1942) Optimum settings for automatic controllers. Trans ASME 15:827–834
4. Takahashi Y, Chan CS (1971) Parametereinstellung bei linearen DDC-algorithmen. Regelungstechnik Prozess-Datenverar-beitung 19:237–244
5. Zhao ZY, Tomizuka M, Isaka S (1993) Fuzzy gain scheduling of the PID controllers. IEEE Trans Systems Man Cybern 23(5):1392–1398

Acoustical Characteristics of a Moving Actuator Type Total Artificial Heart

M.J. Choi[1], B.G. Min[1], S.K. Park[2], S.J. Kim[3], J.W. Choi[2], and S.H. Lee[4]

Summary. The study attempts to characterize the acoustic emission from a moving actuator type, totally implantable, electromechanical, artificial heart. In vitro measurements were made on the acoustic emission from the artificial heart using a highly sensitive measuring microphone, under various operating conditions. Time–frequency spectral analysis, based on the reduced interference distribution kernel, was employed to identify the effects of control parameters of the artificial heart on the acoustic emission. The control parameters considered in this study were the electric current supplied to the d.c. motor of the artificial heart, stroke angle, and the initial interventricular space pressure. The measured acoustic signals were seen to be nonstationary even if a beat cycle yields the periodical repetition by the heart rate. It was shown that the primary spectral peak occurred at 370 Hz under normal operating conditions: stroke angle 140°, initial interventricular space pressure 0 mmHg, and current level 15. The current level used here has no unit and is not directly related to the actual current but controls the motor speed. The primary peak frequency linearly increased with the current level, but was insensitive to the initial interventricular space pressure. When the current level was high, several secondary peaks appeared above 1100 Hz which did not exist at low current levels. The time–frequency energy distribution revealed that the primary frequency, representing the rotational velocity of the motor, was apparent around the middle of both systolic and diastolic periods, and reached its maximum. In contrast, the secondary high-pitched sounds appeared as the cycle approached the end of the systolic period of the left ventricle. It seems that these high-frequency spectral peaks resulted from sac folding and gear sliding. The influence of the motor current on acoustic spectra becomes more significant if the stroke angle of the actuator is increased.

Key words: Acoustic characterization — Total artificial heart — Time–frequency distribution — Sound — Microphone

Introduction

As the clinical implantation of a total artificial heart (TAH) has become a more realistic goal, more attention has been drawn to the evaluation of the reliability of the TAH after implantation. An acoustic technique is considered one of the most promising methods for screening patients with a TAH [1]. Sounds resulting from the dynamic action of the mechanical components of a TAH propagate outwards through the skin. The acoustic emission contains rich information about the condition of each mechanical component of the TAH. The best-known example of acoustic diagnosis is probably auscultation using a stethoscope, a technique which has been in clinical use for a long time. In relatively recent years, the acoustic technique has been proven to provide important information for examining the state of implanted artificial valves [2]. The acoustic technique was not applied to a TAH until the late 1980s, and so far only a few studies have been reported. Sheng et al. [3] investigated the acoustical properties of a pneumatic TAH, and proved the acoustical method to be of use in detecting failures in the blood pump. Lee and Min [4] made acoustic measurements on an electromechanical total artificial heart and were able to observe significant differences between sounds from the TAH with and without damage in the gears, in the frequency ranges around 1300 Hz. Hinrichs [1] proved that the acoustic method can be used to monitor noninvasively the potential wear in bearings of an electrohydraulic TAH. Recently, Kim et al. [5] developed a neural network algorithm to classify automatically the acoustic waveform from the electrohydraulic TAH and to differentiate its mechanical states.

Most of the previous work has focused on examining whether the mechanical parts of the TAH are in order or not. Characteristic patterns of the acoustic emissions from the TAH under the different operating conditions have not yet been thoroughly studied. In this study we have attempted to characterize the sound pitches emitted from an electromechanically driven, moving actuator type TAH under various operating conditions regulated by key control parameters.

---

[1] Institute of Biomedical Engineering, College of Medicine, Seoul National University, 28 Youngun-Dong, Chongno-Ku, Seoul 110-744, Korea
[2] Department of Biomedical Engineering, College of Medicine (or, [3] College of Engineering), Seoul National University
[4] Department of Biomedical Engineering, College of Medicine, Danguk University, Chunahn 330-714, Korea

Materials and Methods

Acoustic measurements were made using a highly sensitive measuring microphone on an electromechanically driven, moving actuator type, total artificial heart which has been developed in our laboratory during the last few years. The TAH employs a pendulous or circular motion of the actuator. The actuator moves back and forth for the alternating ejection of the left and right ventricles. Figure 1 shows a photograph of the TAH (Fig. 1a) and its schematic diagram in a cross-sectional view, together with the position of the measuring microphone (Fig. 1b). The abbreviated terms, RV and LV, represent the right and left ventricles, respectively, and IVS is the interventricular space. A brushless d.c. motor placed inside the actuator generates a pendulous motion by an epicyclic gear train. Each ventricle has a double sac structure. The interventricular space is filled up with air and lubricating oil. The TAH is connected with a mock circulation system (the whole mock system is not shown in the figure) through the inlet and outlet valves in such a way that the TAH experiences preload and afterload. Each mechanical part of a TAH can be a source of sound and, in our TAH, the possible sound sources include gear trains, bearings, blood sacs, fluid flow, and valves. A detailed description of the TAH and the mock circulation system can be found in Min et al. [6].

The microphone used here is a condenser type (no. 4165 Bruel and Kjaer) with a flat frequency response up to 20000 Hz for zero-degree sound incidence. Microphone output was amplified and then sampled at a rate of 50000 Hz for digital signal processing. The sound produced inside the TAH is relatively easily transmitted through the polyurethane window because the acoustic impedance of the polyurethane is low compared with that of the rigid housing steel. For this reason, the sound was picked up by the microphone in front of the flexible polyurethane compliance window. In order to reduce near-field effects [7], the microphone was placed at a distance about 7 cm from the window surface. The detected acoustic signals were stored on an IBM PC together with the synchronized brake and direction signals from the motor, so that the temporal identification of the acoustic signal could be obtained.

The key control parameters considered to alter the operation conditions of the TAH include the initial interventricular space pressure (IIVSP), the electric current supplied to the motor, and the stroke angle. Other conditions such as heart rate, preload, and afterload were adjusted to normal physiological values. The IIVSP enables the TAH to be an actively

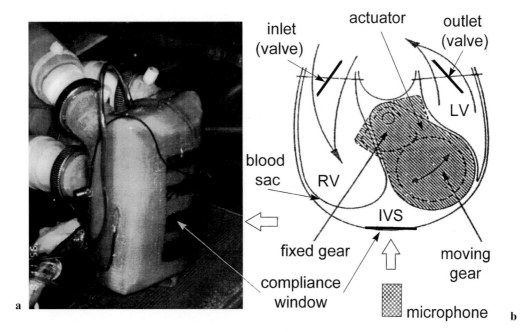

Fig. 1. An electromechanically driven, moving actuator type, totally implantable, artificial heart. **a** Photograph of the artificial heart connected to a mock circulation system. **b** Schematic diagram in a cross-sectional view as indicated by the arrow in **a**. *LV*, left ventricle; *RV*, right ventricle; *IVS*, interventricular space. The measuring microphone (*checks*) was placed in front of the polyurethane compliance window at a distance of 7 cm in order to pick up sounds generated inside the artificial heart and emitted through the window

filling heart during the diastolic period. Although cardiac output goes up with a reduction in IIVSP, the value of IIVSP is required to be maintained so as not to induce negative pressures in the atria. Motor current here represents the pulse width modulation which is used to control the electric current to the 12-V d.c. motor employed in the TAH, and therefore it changes the motor speed. The control algorithm for the TAH recognizes 32 different levels, from 0 to 31 increments of 1, in the pulse width modulation. In the no-load condition, level 1 sets the motor current at 300 mA and level 31 sets it at 1 A. The real electric current supplied to the motor is allowed to change on variation of the actuator load by the control algorithm, even if the value of the current level remains the same. The stroke angle is the total angle that the actuator has moved through its circular track on completion of one cycle of the systolic and diastolic phase.

For the precise analysis of the acoustic signals from the TAH, a time–frequency spectrogram was employed in addition to a conventional averaged frequency spectrum obtained by fast Fourier transformation, since sounds from the TAH are nonstationary. A way is to obtain the energy density in frequency at a time from Cohen's generalized formula [8]:

$$\rho(t,f) = \int \int \int e^{j2\pi\upsilon(u-t)} g(\upsilon,\tau) s*\left(u - \frac{1}{2}\tau\right) s\left(u + \frac{1}{2}\tau\right) e^{-j2\pi ft}$$
$$d\upsilon du d\tau \qquad (1)$$

where $g(\upsilon,\tau)$ is an arbitrary function called the kernel. The detailed description of this equation is omitted here but can be found in [8]. This study employs the reduced interference distribution kernel designed by Williams and Jeong [9,10]. Use of the kernel enables the suppression of the cross-term formulation, providing more interpretable results from multicomponent signals. This equation has been numerically implemented on an IBM PC using a mathematical programming tool called Matlab.

Results

Depicted in Fig. 2 is a typical acoustic signal from the TAH both in the time and frequency domains together with the brake signal and direction signal. The operation conditions were: IIVSP 0 mmHg, motor current level 15, stroke angle 140°, heart rate 70 beats/min, and no preload or afterload. When the brake signal (Fig. 2b) was on just before the end of both the systolic and diastolic period, no electric current was supplied to the motor. The direction signal (Fig. 2c) indicates whether the heart was in the systolic or diastolic period. The ground level, labeled "off" in Fig. 2c, represents the systolic period of the left ventricle; in other words,

the diastolic period of the right ventricle. Unless stated otherwise, references to the systolic and diastolic periods from here on are for the left ventricle. As expected, the acoustic signal in the time domain (Fig. 2a) was seen to be nonstationary even if the beat cycle yields periodical repetition by the heart rate. During the systolic period, the acoustic emission was more significant and this reflects an increased resistance in the TAH due to a greater mechanical load, including afterload. Fourier amplitude variation of the acoustic signal against frequency is shown in Fig. 2e; a primary peak is seen at 370 Hz and several secondary local peaks at frequencies higher than 1300 Hz. The temporal structure of the spectral sound energy is effectively illustrated by Fig. 2d, with the sound energy level contours plotted on the (vertical) frequency axis and the (horizontal) time axis. This figure was obtained using the formula given in Materials and Methods. The primary spectral peak corresponds to the highest level in the contours and is significant around the middle of both the systolic and diastolic periods. In contrast, the secondary peaks appear only in the systolic period; more precisely, after the second half of the systolic period.

The plots shown in Fig. 3 demonstrate the influence of the motor current on the acoustic emission from the TAH. Microphone measurements were carried out at three values of the motor current while keeping the other conditions unchanged: the initial interventricular space pressure 0 mmHg, stroke angle 140°, imbalance 30, preload 10 mmHg, and afterload 100 mmHg. The frequency distribution of the detected acoustic signals is shown in the upper panels (Fig. 3a,c,e), and the changes in frequency with time are depicted in forms of the time-frequency domain sound level contours in the lower panels (Figs. 3b,d,f). For the panels on the left, the motor current level was 10; the middle panels were at 15, and the right most panels were at 26. As seen in the upper panels, the position of the primary peak was shifted to higher frequencies and the secondary high peaks grew greatly as the current level was increased to 26. This shift in the primary peak is more clearly identified in the corresponding time–frequency distributions, shown in the lower panels, by looking at the highest level in the spectral energy contour, marked by the arrows. The time–frequency energy distributions also demonstrate that the secondary peaks are more significant at higher motor current levels and occur during the systolic period only. Figure 4 illustrates that there is a linear relationship between the motor current level and the primary spectral peak frequency.

Plots similar to Figs. 3 and 4 are presented in Figs. 5 and 6, which examine the influence of the initial interventricular space pressure (IIVSP) on the acoustic emission. Acoustic signals were measured when

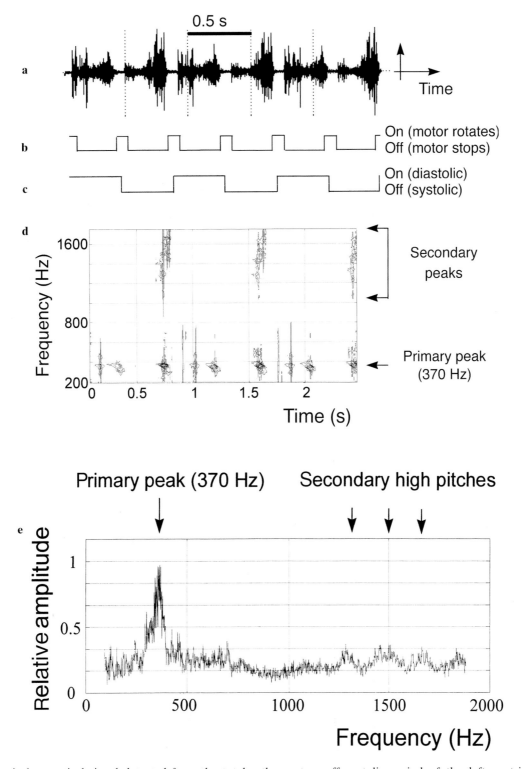

Fig. 2. A typical acoustical signal detected from the total artificial heart under conditions of no preload or afterload. **a** Acoustic amplitude against time. **b** Brake signal to the motor: *on*, motor rotates; *off*, motor stops. **c** Direction signal of the motor: *off*, systolic period of the left ventricle; *on*, diastolic period of the left ventricle. **d** Time–frequency spectral energy distribution. **e** Averaged spectral amplitude against frequency

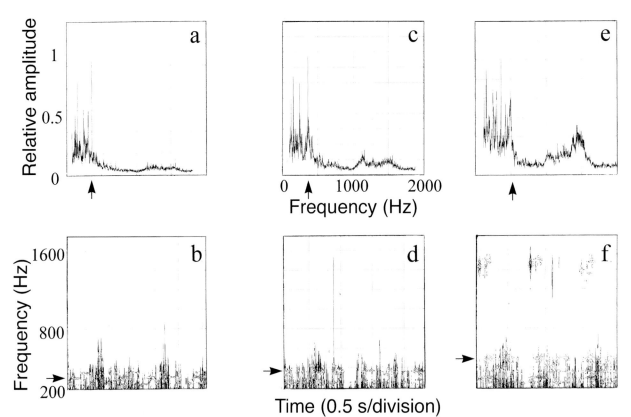

Fig. 3. The influence of the motor current level on the acoustic emission from the total artificial heart. The *upper* panels are the averaged spectral amplitude variations with frequency at the motor current levels of 10 (**a**), 15 (**c**), and 26 (**e**). *Arrows,* position of primary peak. The *lower panels* are the temporal variations of spectral energy at the motor current levels of 10 (**b**), 15 (**d**), and 26 (**f**). The value of the initial interventricular space pressure, IIVSP, was 0 mmHg throughout

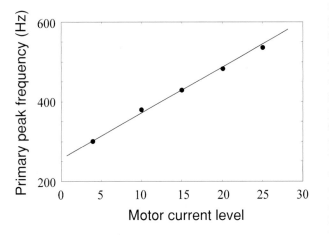

Fig. 4. A plot of the primary peak frequency against the electric current level supplied to the d.c. motor of the total artificial heart. The *solid line* was fitted to the measured data points

altering the value of IIVSP but keeping the other parameters unchanged: the motor current level 15, stroke angle 140°, imbalance 30, preload 10 mmHg, and afterload 100 mmHg. Figure 5a,c,e shows the frequency distribution of the detected acoustic signals (upper panels), while the lower panels (Fig. 5b,d,f) show the changes in frequency with time. The left panels were at the IIVSP of −12 mmHg; the IIVSP was 0 mmHg for the middle panels and 9 mmHg for the panels on the right. It was shown that, unlike the motor current, the initial interventricular space pressure did not influence the acoustic emission. The position of the primary peak remained almost the same regardless of IIVSP, and there were no significant changes in the amplitude of the secondary peak bands even when the value of the IIVSP was altered. Values of the primary peak frequency against IIVSP are plotted in Fig. 6, and it is seen that the primary peak frequency was insensitive to the value of the IIVSP.

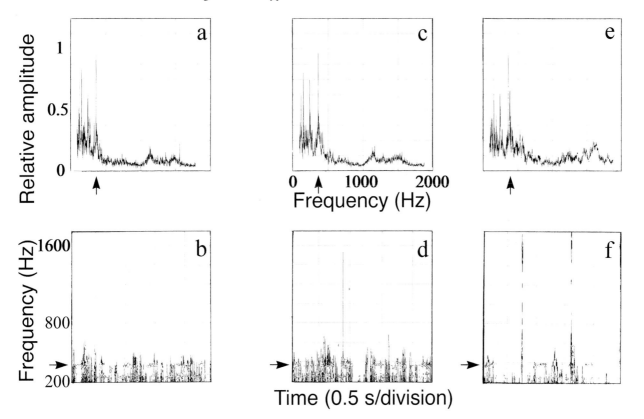

Fig. 5. The influence of the initial interventricular space pressure, IIVSP, on the acoustic emission from the total artificial heart. The *upper panels* are the averaged spectral amplitude variations with frequency at the IIVSP values of − 12 mmHg (**a**), 0 mmHg (**c**), and 9 mmHg (**e**). *Arrows*, posi- tion of primary peak. The *lower panels* are the temporal variations of spectral energy at the IIVSP values of − 12 mmHg (**b**), 0 mmHg (**d**), and 9 mmHg (**f**). The value of the motor current level was 15 throughout

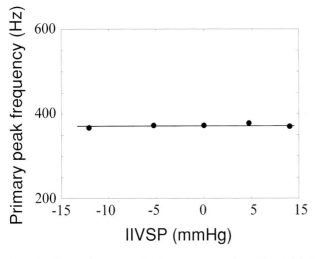

Fig. 6. The primary peak frequency against the initial interventricular space pressure, *IIVSP*. The *solid line* was fitted to the measured data points

Discussion

Microphone measurements were performed in an or- dinary TAH laboratory against a background of un- wanted noises from various sources such as an air conditioning fan and a computer cooling fan. Accord- ingly, the recorded acoustic signals were contaminated by surrounding noises. Nevertheless, this is not a criti- cal problem in our study because the noise is probably insensitive to changes in the operating conditions of the TAH and the noise effects would have been signifi- cantly eliminated when the acoustic signals obtained under the different operating conditions were com- pared. For cases that require noise-free acoustic sig- nals, there may be three possible ways to increase the signal-to-noise ratio. First, as used by Lee and Min [4], an adaptive noise canceller may be employed and, in this case, an extra microphone is required to capture environmental noise signals. Second, noises can be effectively excluded using a contact-type microphone, or a conventional microphone coupled with an acoustic waveguide. This type of microphone can also reduce greatly the near-field effects which cause rapid spatial variations in acoustic amplitudes. Finally, underwater measurements by a hydrophone, detecting sounds from a TAH submerged in a water bath, provide, free of environmental noise, an acoustic signal which may be regarded as a gold standard. It may be worth noting that the vibration signal measured on the surface of a TAH by an accelerometer is free from surrounding acoustic noises. Since the acoustic signal detected at a distance from the TAH represents the oscillation of air molecules induced by the vibrating surface of the TAH, the accelerometer measurement may provide a valuable reference for the detected acoustic signal. As reported in Choi et al. [11], the spectra of the vibrational and acoustic signals are similar to each other, especially for frequencies higher than the heart rate. For clinical use, it may be attractive to use a microphone with a waveguide or a contact-type microphone combined with an adaptive noise canceller.

Two types of spectral peaks were identified from the frequency domain representation of the recorded acoustical signal: the primary and several secondary high-pitch peaks. The primary peak occurred between 300 Hz and 500 Hz and was always seen, regardless of the operating conditions of the TAH. In contrast, the secondary spectral peaks appeared above 1100 Hz and became significant as the motor current level was raised. The primary peak occurred at 370 Hz at the motor current level of 15, and was found to increase linearly with the current level (Fig. 4), but was insensitive to the initial interventricular space pressure (Fig. 6). A more detailed interpretation can be obtained from the time–frequency energy distribution of the detected acoustic signal. As seen in Fig. 2d, the primary peak was apparent around the middle of both the systolic and diastolic periods when the rotational velocity of the motor reached its maximum value. This may be evidence that the primary peak is associated with the electric current which determines the rotational speed of the motor. From the linear relationship between the primary peak frequency and the motor current level (Fig. 4) and the fact that the rotational velocity of the motor highly influences the spectral properties of vibrations in gear trains, the primary peak may be attributed to the mechanical vibrations excited by the first sun and planetary gears, and the spectral bands lower than the primary peak frequency may be related to the mechanical actions of the subsequent gear trains with a high reduction ratio. The time–frequency representation also reveals that the secondary spectral peaks appeared as the cycle approached the end of the systolic period. As seen in

Fig. 3, the secondary peaks almost did not exist at lower current levels, but became apparent as the current level increased. This indicates that such high-pitch noises are likely to emanate from sound sources such as gear sliding and sac folding, which are expected to happen at the end of systolic period, especially when the motor current level is high. Previously, Lee and Min [4] indicated that spectral components around 1400 Hz may be associated with high-pitched sounds due to gear sliding.

The acoustic signals detected include sounds produced by the different mechanical components of the TAH such as bearings, gears, valves, and sac folding, as well as those resulting from accompanying fluid flow. Since the most common problem leading to the failure of our TAH is blood-sac wear and tear, it is appropriate to pay more attention to the acoustic emission associated with the sac. The blood sac is made of polyurethane and has two layers. Once a tear takes place in either side of the sac, surrounding fluid enters into the gap between the two layers. The sac then becomes gradually swollen and this results in the reduction of cardiac output. As the tear progresses further, the complete failure of the TAH eventually occurs. Mechanical stresses causing the sac tear may be due to the folding of the sac, which is likely to happen when the actuator squeezes the sac to its maximum at the end of each systolic period, in particular, in the case that the motor current is high and the stoke angle is large. Sac folding is normally accompanied by high-pitched sounds above 1100 Hz which an experienced operator can easily hear and identify. The appearance of the high-pitched sound around the end of systolic periods at a high motor current level, as shown in Fig. 3e,f, supports the explanation that sac folding is in part associated with the secondary spectral peaks. Accordingly, the spectral structure as the cycle approaches the end of a systolic period can provide an important clue for detecting changes in the mechanical state of the sac exposed to alternating mechanical stresses.

Conclusion

Acoustic signals from the TAH are nonstationary, and therefore the temporal structure of their spectral components is required for precise analysis. The frequency spectrum of the detected acoustic signal was characterized by a primary spectral peak between 300 and 500 Hz and several secondary peaks above 1100 Hz. Time–frequency sound energy level contours, calculated using the reduced interference distribution kernel, clearly illustrate that the primary spectral peaks correspond to the highest levels in the contours and are apparent around the middle of both the systolic and diastolic periods. In contrast, the secondary high-pitched sounds appeared as the cycle approached the end of the systolic period. From spectral analysis on the detected acoustic signals under the various operating conditions of the TAH, it was found that the primary spectral peak frequency was proportional to the motor current level, but insensitive to the initial interventricular space pressure. Continued investigation is suggested into the temporal structure of the sound pitches emitted from the TAH which will enable us to evaluate precisely the mechanical states of the blood sacs and the performance of the TAH. A successful outcome from this study will advance the development of a noninvasive clinical procedure for assessing the physiological condition of the implanted TAH.

References

1. Hinrichs HL (1994) Acoustical analysis of the bearings in the Utah electrohydraulic total artificial heart. MSc thesis, University of Utah, Salt Lake City, UT 84103, USA
2. Anderson FL, Pantalos GM (1986) Phonocardiographic evaluation of total artificial heart valve movement: correlation with pressure waveforms. Artif Organs 10:65–68
3. Sheng YL, Rossi DD, Dario P, Galletti PM (1986) Indwelling acoustic sensor for early detection of total artificial heart failures. In: Abstracts of the international symposium on artificial organs, Biomedical Engineering and Transplantation, 16 January 1986
4. Lee SH, Min BG (1994) Performance evaluation of implantable artificial organ by sound spectrum analysis. ASAIO J 40:M762–M766
5. Kim HC, Hindrich HL, Khanwilkar PS, Bearnson GB, Olsen DB (1994) Non-invasive diagnosis of mechanical failure of the implanted total artificial heart using neural network analysis on acoustical signal. In: Abstracts of the 41st ASAIO annual meeting, Chicago, Illinois, 4–6 May 1995
6. Min BG, Kim HC, Lee SH, Kim JW, Kim JT, Kim IY, Kim SW, Diegel PD, Olsen DB (1990) A moving actuator type electromechanical total artificial heart — Part I: Linear type and mock circulation experiments. IEEE Trans Biomed Eng 37(12):1186–1190
7. Kinsler LE, Frey AR, Coppens AB, Sanders JV (1983) Fundamentals of acoustics. Wiley, New York, pp 176–197
8. Cohen L (1992) Introduction: primer on time–frequency analysis. In: Bashash B (ed) Time–frequency signal analysis: method and application. Longman Cheshire, Melbourne, Chap. 1
9. Jeong J, Williams WJ (1992) Kernel design for reduced interference distributions. IEEE Trans Acoust Speech Signal Processing 40:402–412
10. Williams WJ, Jeong J (1992) Reduced interference time–frequency distributions. In: Bashash B (ed) Time–frequency signal analysis: method and application. Longman Cheshire, Melbourne, Chap. 3
11. Choi MJ, Min BG, Park SK, Park HJ, Lee DJ, Chung WS (1995) Spectral analysis of the acoustic output from a moving actuator type total artificial heart. In: Abstracts of the 5th Korea–Japan Joint Conference, Yong Pyeong, Korea, 13–15 December 1995

Vortex Blood Pump

Charles B. Howarth, John J. De Marco, and John R. Shanebrook

Summary. A new type of blood pump has been designed that utilizes a hemofoil inlet valve to establish a strong vortical motion within a cylindrical pumping chamber. Flow visualization results present clear evidence that the hemofoil occluder generates a starting vortex at the beginning of diastole. This vortex rapidly evolves into a full chamber vortical flow pattern before the end of diastole. Velocity measurements indicate tracer particles vary in speed from about 0.22 m/s to 1.20 m/s. It is concluded that the vortical flow patterns established with this pump design could be beneficial in preventing thromboembolic complications associated with total artificial hearts.

Key words: Thromboembolic complications — Inlet valve vortex generator

Introduction

As discussed by Lelkes and Samet [1], end-stage heart disease affects about 50000 patients annually in the United States alone. These patients could benefit from a total artificial heart (TAH), but successful clinical performance of these devices continues to be hampered by thrombembolic complications.

Attempts to reduce thrombogenic responses to incompatible synthetic materials in TAHs have achieved minimal success, despite the use of anticoagulant drugs. Kolff [2] states that ". . . they introduce about as many problems as they resolve," and Moritz et al. [3] remark on the continued persistence of thrombogenicity being the most destructive complication for recipients of artificial pumping devices.

According to Nosé [4] and Peskin [5], the following factors encourage thrombus formation within circulatory assist devices:

1. The junction of two blood-contacting components
2. The interface of two different biomaterials
3. Undesirable flow patterns within the pumping chamber
4. Poor blood biocompatibility at the surface of the synthetic material

5. Poor performance of some heart valves and their adaptation inside the cardiac prosthesis

Thrombogenicity will be reduced by improving all of these factors. The purpose of this communication is to improve the third and fifth factors by presenting a new type of blood pump design that has exhibited desirable flow patterns within a model pumping chamber. This has been accomplished by employing an airfoil-shaped occluder (hemofoil), for the inlet valve, that additionally serves as a vortex generator during diastolic filling of the pumping chamber.

Materials and Methods

Lugt [6] has presented an extensive account of vortex applications in nature and technology. Included is a description of Leonardo da Vinci's early theory that vortices, generated by the leaflets of the human aortic valve, are beneficial for the efficient functioning of this valve. More recently, Taylor and Wade [7] observed in vivo diastolic flow patterns within dog and sheep ventricles. It was concluded that "The major flow patterns are expanding vortex systems behind the cusps of the mitral and tricuspid valves. These vortex systems appear important in normal valve dynamics." These examples illustrate that the movable portions of human aortic and mitral valves serve not only as occluders but also as vortex generators. Moreover, the resulting expanding vortex systems serve many important hemodynamic functions including a natural cleansing action. These advantages can also be achieved by designing prosthetic valves to be effective vortex generators.

Shanebrook and Bussolari [8] presented in vitro flow visualization results for a hemofoil prosthetic mitral valve that functions much like the anterior leaflet of the human mitral valve. It was demonstrated that the hemofoil occluder generates a large ventricular vortex that has many advantageous characteristics including a natural cleansing action each cycle. This latter characteristic can also be used to advantage in the design of inlet valves for pulsatile blood pumps.

Department of Mechanical Engineering, Union College, Schenectady, NY 12308-3147, USA

Figure 1 presents a hemofoil inlet valve for a pusher-plate blood pump. The hemofoil occluder has a 1.65-mm leading edge thickness, a trailing edge thickness of 0.89 mm, and a trailing edge gap width of 9.02 mm. For in vitro testing, a Plexiglas pump model was constructed with this inlet valve and a 29-mm Björk-Shiley tilting-disk valve at the outlet [9]. The valve ports were tangentially located at the top of the curved boundary of the cylindrical pumping chamber. Pumping action was provided by a cylindrical pusher plate.

Pulsatile flow conditions were established with a mock circulatory system that included an atrial reservoir, two flow capacitors, and three resistance clamps. The capacitors and resistors were arranged in accordance with the findings of Westerhof, who concluded that a sequence of these devices could simulate the elastic response of the human circulatory system [10]. The system was driven by a motor-cam assembly that provided appropriate flow-time characteristics [11].

With water as the test fluid, Pliolite VT particles (Goodyear Chemicals, Goodyear Tire and Rubber, Akron, OH, USA), ground to an approximate mesh size of 80, were used as tracer particles. With a specific gravity of 1.026, these particles can be considered neutrally buoyant in water. Flow patterns within the pump chamber were visualized using a video system. A fiberoptic lamp 3100 (Dolan-Jenner Industries, Woburn, MA, USA), placed normal to the motion of the pusher-plate and flow ports, reflected light from the tracer particles. After carefully positioning the light and utilizing a slit-lighting mechanism to direct the light beam, a video camera VL-L50U (Sharp Electronics, Mahwah, NJ, USA) recorded the fluid motions within the chamber. These results were examined frame-by-frame with the use of a FOR·A video measuring gauge IV-560 (FOR·A, Newton, MA, USA). The video measuring gauge allows the viewer to ascribe (x,y) coordinates to the tracer particle as the particle changes its position from one frame to the next. The Panasonic video cassette recorder Ag-7355 (Matsushita Industrial, Franklin Park, IL, USA) used for this experiment allowed the video tape to be ad-

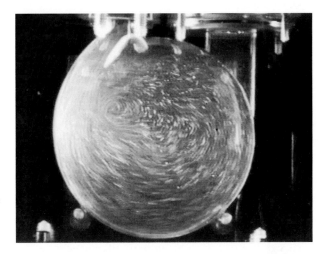

Fig. 2. Photograph of vortex blood pump flow pattern (early diastole). The core of the shed vortex is visible about 1.8 cm directly below the trailing edge of the hemofoil occluder

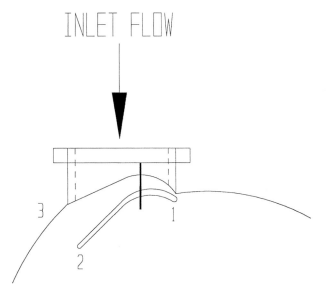

Fig. 1. Sketch of hemofoil inlet valve where (1) denotes the leading edge location, (2) is the trailing edge location, and (3) lies on the chamber surface. The distance from (2) to (3) is the trailing edge gap width

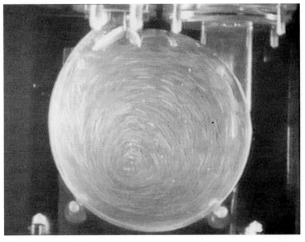

Fig. 3. Photograph of vortex blood pump flow pattern (near end-diastole). The center of the vortical motion is now about 5.5 cm directly below the valve retention strut

vanced field-by-field, resulting in a change in time of $\frac{1}{60}$ second for each displacement reading. Average linear velocities were calculated by measuring the straight line displacement of the particle from one field to the next and dividing the displacement by $\frac{1}{60}$ second.

Results

Figures 2 and 3 are photographs of the flow patterns during diastolic filling of the pumping chamber at 70 beats per minute, and a flow rate of 4.8 l/min. Figure 2 corresponds to an early stage of diastole with the inlet valve (upper left corner) fully open and a starting vortex shed from the trailing edge of the hemofoil occluder. Relatively high wall velocities are visible immediately downstream of the inlet valve as this initially compact vortex begins its expansion process. Figure 3 shows the flow pattern near end-diastole with the hemofoil occluder moving towards closure. The counterclockwise shed vortex has expanded and combined with counterclockwise residual vorticity (from the previous cycle) to form a full chamber vortex motion. The center of the vortical motion has now shifted downwards and to the right; this trend continues during systole with the highest wall velocities moving towards the outlet valve.

The results of particle velocity measurements indicate velocities ranging from 0.22 m/s to 1.20 m/s. The highest velocities occurred immediately downstream from the open inlet valve and the lowest near the vortex center of Fig. 3. From here, the particles accelerated towards the outlet valve where they had velocities between 0.40 and 0.75 m/s. These results are consistent with those reported in [12] for a spiral vortex pump.

Discussion

The results presented here offer a new approach to blood pump design that potentially alleviates thromboembolic complications that currently hinder the long-term performance of TAHs. The hemofoil inlet valve has been shown to be an effective vortex generator that can be used to advantage in providing strong vortical flow patterns throughout the pumping cycle.

Acknowledgments. The authors thank J. Baldwin and W.B. Eulau for their help with the design of the experimental apparatus and Mr. R.A. Smith for providing research fellowships.

References

1. Lelkes PI, Samet MM (1991) Endothelialization of the luminal sac in artificial cardiac prostheses: a challenge for both biologists and engineers. J Biomech Eng 113: 132–142
2. Kolff WJ (1988) Experiences and practical considerations for the future of artificial hearts and of mankind. Artif Organs 12:89–111
3. Moritz A, Wolner E, Nosé Y (1988) Clinical use of the artificial heart, indications, and results. Wien Klin Wochenschr 18:161–167
4. Nosé Y (1990) My life with the National Institutes of Health Artificial Heart Program. Artif Organs 14:174–190
5. Peskin CS (1982) The fluid dynamics of heart valves: experimental, theoretical, and computational methods. Annu Rev Fluid Mechanics 14:235–259
6. Lugt HJ (1983) Vortex flow in nature and technology. Wiley, New York, pp 10–11
7. Taylor DEM, Wade JD (1973) Pattern of blood flow within the heart: a stable system. Cardiovasc Res 7:14–21
8. Shanebrook JR, Bussolari JL (1979) Flow visualization experiments with a hemofoil mitral valve. In: Wells MK (ed) 1979 Advances in bioengineering. ASME, New York, pp 113–116
9. De Marco JJ (1994) The Union College vortex blood pump. Honors thesis, Union College, Schenectady, New York
10. Plant RE (1976) Simple model for the crustacean cardiac pacemaker control system. Math Biosci 32:275–290
11. Howarth CB (1996) In vitro flow experiments with the Union College vortex blood pump. Honors thesis, Union College, Schenectady, New York
12. Nugent AH, Bertram CD (1995) Laser doppler velocimetry of the spiral vortex ventricular assist device. In: Akutsu T, Koyanagi H (eds) Heart replacement: artificial heart 5: Springer, Tokyo, pp 357–360

Discussion

Mr. Mullaly:
Richard Mullaly, from the Children's Hospital in Melbourne. Mr. Howarth, nice presentation. What's the lowest stroke-volume of the device at the present time?

Mr. Howarth:
Right now we can test at a stroke volume or stroke length. I don't know the lowest stroke volume but I know we can minimize the stroke length down to about 26 mm.

Dr. Mullaly:
26 cc?

Mr. Howarth:
Twenty-six-millimeter stroke length, so I don't know what the actual stroke volume would be. The pusher plate can move that a little, but I don't know. Sorry.

Dr. Masuzawa:
Masuzawa, National Cardiovascular Center of Japan. I have one question to Mr. [WW] Choi from Seoul National University. I think the key point of adaptive control is how to eliminate the noise signal or how to eliminate the misidentification or miscalculation of the control parameters. Then, do you have any preventative way to avoid the miscalculation of the adaptive control algorithm parameters?

Mr. WW Choi:
I can't understand miscalculation of the parameters.

Dr. Masuzawa:
If you have some noisy data, then your system will calculate some wrong control gain. Then I think you should have some special detection way for the noise signal to realize some reliable control.

Mr. WW Choi:
Presently we have a big problem with the point you noted, so we are trying to overcome the noise problem but we haven't yet found a good solution to filtering the noise of the signal. The processing is very high-speed real-time processing so we have to find a very fast real-time noise-filtering algorithm. So that is a big problem now.

Dr. Masuzawa:
Also, do you think only noise filtering is enough to prevent data miscalculation?

Mr. WW Choi:
Not an optimal filter, but we use low-pass filtering. So with the low-pass filtering, we didn't have a big noise signal, and there's no significant problem in the control system. We have to find a control system and prepare the control system, but now, presently, we don't have a serious problem with signal noise.

Dr. Antaki:
Jim Antaki, University of Pittsburgh. My question also is for Mr. Choi. You addressed the problem of plant nonlinearity very well with fuzzy-based gain scheduling, but an equally vexing problem which your controller is predicated upon is the selection of the set point. You spoke of a range of intraventricular pressure, I believe minus 3 to 10. How do you plan to address the specification of that set point?

Mr. WW Choi:
We did an estimate of the operating point. I referred to the fuzzy gain scheduling algorithm from Dr. Zhao. If you want information on it, I will give you the reference.

Dr. Harasaki:
Yes, Dr. Vasku, your message that detailed histological examination of the brain and spinal cord is important is well taken. We also take 20 or more histologic sections from the central nervous system to find out if there is any ill effect of the total artificial heart implantation. And it is rather rare to find any pathology. I just wonder, Dr. Vasku, in what percentage did you find this complication in your cases? For instance, the disappearance of the cells, the ganglion cells and hemorrhage, and possibly infarction.

Dr. Vasku:

I think we cannot do a very exact differentiation because sometimes in cerebral hemorrhages you can find even calcified microemboli, if the membrane, the diaphragm, was calcified. In other cases you can observe the typical signs of hypoperfusion because even if hypoperfusion lasts a very short time then Nissl bodies in the ganglionic cells, which are the expression of the metabolic state of the cell, and this is very sensitive to oxygen decrease, immediately disappear. Tigrolysis, the so-called tigrolysis, i.e., disappearance of the Nissl bodies, is a very typical sign of damage of the central nervous system, of ganglionic cells of the central nervous system. On the other hand, glial cells react as connective tissue and in the decrease of oxygen they grow, so sometimes you can find growing knots of glial cells. It is very tedious work because you must cut off several hundred slices of the whole brain if you want to be very exactly informed. So, we had a group which especially dealt with the brain problem.

Dr Reul:

Just a comment to the last speaker. You showed this nice vortex formation in the blood sac. I want to point out that this behavior is not only dependent on the valve you use; it is also dependent on the location of the inflow channel. If you have it very nicely tangential, you can achieve the same thing with the tilting disc valve or with a three-leaflet valve as well.

Mr. Howarth:

But a starting vortex or shed vortex is a very special vortex. It's formed as soon as the flow travels basically the length of the valve occluder and it will form counterclockwise.

Dr. Reul:

But the main thing is that you have a nice washout in the whole territory of the ventricle and you cannot achieve that by other means or by combined means.

Professor Wolner:

I have a comment on Mr. Choi's study on noise and artificial heart. The problem of all these studies is what you measure has nothing to do with what the patient feels. Some years ago we had done a study on noise with different artificial valves. We found, objectively, different noise levels; however, when you ask the patient — that is published in the British Heart Journal — when you ask the patient how you are disturbed by your valve or, when you ask his wife or people around him, how you are disturbed, this has nothing to do with the objective measurements of noise which you measure, let's say, in skin level and 1 meter away. I know that you can measure noise in a mock circulation system, but I warn you to make a conclusion from the noise which you measure here in your model and which will be perhaps in the future the problems for the patient.

Mr. WW Choi:

Thank you for your comment.

Dr. MJ Choi:

Let me have a chance to comment additionally regarding my presentation of acoustics in the total artificial heart. The total artificial heart we are dealing with is a sort of mechanical device and produces sounds when it is in operation. We believe that the sound contains rich information about the mechanical states of the total artificial heart. We try to relate the characteristics of sound to the condition of a mechanical part of the artificial heart. When the implantation of the total artificial heart becomes clinically successful in the future, it will be fun to hear the sound from the implanted artificial heart at the different moods of patients.

Dr. Takatani:

Before closing, I have a simple question for Dr. Ohashi. It is very difficult to simulate the respiratory effect in vitro. Can you tell us just how to simulate that respiratory effect to test the control system?

Dr. Ohashi:

We use left and right, alternative changing mode. That is the same as was developed from in vivo tests, and the changing volume of right side and left side is set in the physiological range.

Dr. Taenaka:

I have a quick question to Dr. Andrade. You measured the flow, but on the outflow part. The important point in this kind of device is the analysis of the flow around the inflow, so did you measure the inflow with this experimental condition?

Dr. Andrade:

Yes, both inflow and outflow.

Dr. Taenaka:

What was the difference?

Dr. Andrade:

For the outflow, we just observed changes in the particle velocities using the motor speeds 720, 900, and 1200 rpm. For the inflow, since the motor speed just changed the ejection time, there was almost no difference; the particle velocity is almost the same; no significant difference was found. And the flow behavior for both sides shows no changing comparing the three motor speeds.

Part II
Heart Transplantation

Bridging for Heart Transplantation by Different Types of Ventricular Assist Device

K. Minami, L. Arusoglu, A. El-Banayosy, N. Mirow, M. Morshuis, N. Reiß, G. Tenderich, M.M. Körner, and R. Körfer

Summary. From the beginning of our heart transplant program in March 1989 until June 1996, 767 orthotopic heart transplantations (HTx) have been performed. The mean age of the patients was 51 years (range: 3 days to 73 years). Almost half (49.1%) of the patients had dilatative cardiomyopathy (DCM); 39.4% had ishemic heart disease (IHD); 5.9%, valvular disease (VD); 3.4%, congenital heart disease (CHD); and 0.4%, acute myocarditis. In 11 patients, re-HTx was necessary. Corresponding to the international experience with restricted number of donor organs, the average waiting time in our patients increased markedly, from 37.6 days in 1989 to 232.5 days in 1995. A total of 448 patients were given transplants between March 1989 and March 1993 (group 1) and 313 patients between March 1993 and June 1996 (group 2). A mechanical assist device (VAD) was used for bridging to HTx in 33 patients (7.3%) in group 1; the VAD types used were Bio-Medicus ($n = 7$), Abiomed ($n = 11$), Thoratec ($n = 15$), and Novacor ($n = 2$). In Group 2, 68 patients (21.7%) were bridged by VAD using Thoratec ($n = 40$), Novacor ($n = 15$), HeartHate ($n = 9$), and Medos ($n = 1$). The early mortality in patients bridged to HTx was 8.7% in group 1 and 5.2% in group 2 ($P < 0.01$). The actuarial survival rate of the patients who were bridged prior to transplantation was 86% in electively bridged patients and 67% in postcardiotomy patients. We conclude that application of VAD in severely ill patients prior to HTx leads to reduction of the early hospital morbidity and mortality due to improvement of hemodynamic and general physical condition.

Key words: Heart transplantation — Mechanical assist device — Bridge to transplantation

Introduction

Norman and co-workers [1] reported in 1978 the first use of a ventricular assist device (VAD) as a bridging to heart transplantation. The first successful application of a VAD as a bridging was performed by DeBakey [2] in 1967 using a centrifugal pump. In 1969 Cooley and co-workers [3] used an artificial heart for a two-stage cardiac replacement. Since then, several types of the mechanical devices have been developed and clinically used [4–7]. Due to increasing waiting

Department of Thoracic and Cardiovascular Surgery, Heart Center North Rhine-Westphalia, University of Bochum, Georgstrasse 11, 32545 Bad Oeynhausen, Germany

time for transplantation — averaging 320 days in the UNOS and 250 days in the Eurotransplant data — having a mechanical assist device is mandatory for a successful heart transplant program.

Patients and Methods

Since starting the heart transplant program in the Heart Center, North Rhine-Westphalia, in March 1989, 767 heart and heart-lung transplantations have been performed up to June 1996. There were 6 heart-lung transplantations and 65 pediatric heart transplantations (Fig. 1).

Nearly half of the recipients suffered from dilatative cardiomyopathy, 39% from end-stage ischemic heart disease, 6% from valvular heart disease, 3.4% from congenital heart disease, and three patients from acute myocarditis. In 13 patients, re-HTx was performed (Table 1). Of the total 761 heart transplant recipients, 643 were male and 118 female. The mean age was 51 years, ranging from 3 days to 73 years. The mean donor age was 38 years, ranging from 3 days to 66 years. The mean ischemic time of the donor hearts was 210 min (Table 2). The majority of the donor hearts had a ischemic time of 2–4 h. In 73 cases, the ischemic time was 4–5 h and in 16 cases, 5–6 h (Fig. 2).

The numbers of waiting patients, transplantations performed, and patients who died on our waiting list are listed in Fig. 3. One sixth of the patients on the waiting list died before a donor heart became available. Due to the increasing shortage of donor organs, the waiting time for transplantation has become dramatically longer in recent years. In our recipients, the waiting time was 37 days in 1989 and 232 days in 1995 (Fig. 4).

Figure 5 indicates the numbers of patients who died while on the waiting list, and of patients who were bridged for HTx. This demonstrates that the increasing use of mechanical ventricular support has had a positive influence in decreasing the number of deaths on the waiting list.

The numbers of HTx and bridging by VAD are given in Fig. 6. It is clearly demonstrated that the bridging rate prior to transplantation markedly in-

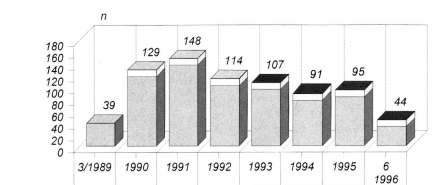

Fig. 1. Number of heart and heart-lung transplantations (March 1989–June 1996) There were 767 transplantations including 6 heart-lung transplantations (*HLTx, dark hatch*) and 65 pediatric (<16 years) heart transplantations (*HTx, light hatch*). The remainder were heart transplantations in adults (*medium hatch*)

	3/1989	1990	1991	1992	1993	1994	1995	6 1996
HLTx ■					1	3	1	1
HTx Children □	1	8	11	11	9	9	11	5
HTx Adults ▨	38	121	137	103	97	79	83	38

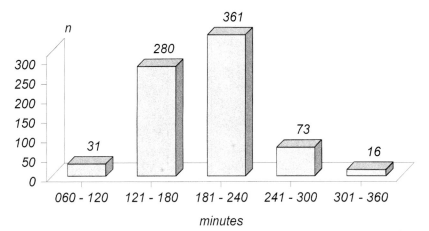

Fig. 2. Ischemic time of donor hearts (*n* = 761): the majority of the hearts had 2–4 h ischemic time; times were 4–5 h for 73 hearts and 5–6 h for 16

Table 1. Indication for heart transplantation

Indication for heart transplantation	*n*	%
Cardiomyopathy	374	49.1
End-stage ischemic heart disease	300	39.4
Valvular heart disease	45	5.9
Complex congenital heart disease	26	3.4
Retransplantation	13	1.7
Acute myocarditis	3	0.4
Total	761	100.0

Table 2. Characteristics of heart transplant recipients and donors, and ischemic time of donor hearts (March 1989–June 1996)

Recipient	*n* = 761 (643 men/118 women)
	Age: 3 days–73 years (mean: 51 years)
Donor	Age: 3 days–66 years (mean: 38 years)
	Ischemic time: 210 minutes (mean)

creased year by year: most recently, 25%–27% of the recipients underwent bridging during the waiting time.

Results

Between March 1989 and June 1996, 761 transplantations, including 13 re-HTx, were performed in our

hospital. In 133 patients, bridging for transplantation was carried out in the same period. The VAD was used in 118 patients electively and in 15 patients with postcardiotomy cardiac failure. Of 133 patients, 101 (76%) were able to be given transplants (Table 3).

Between beginning our transplant program in March 1989 and March 1993 448 patients (group 1)

Fig. 3. The numbers of waiting patients (*light hatch*), transplantations performed (*Tx, medium hatch*), and patients who died on our waiting list (*died on W list, dark hatch*) are shown. One sixth of the patients on the waiting list die before a donor heart is available

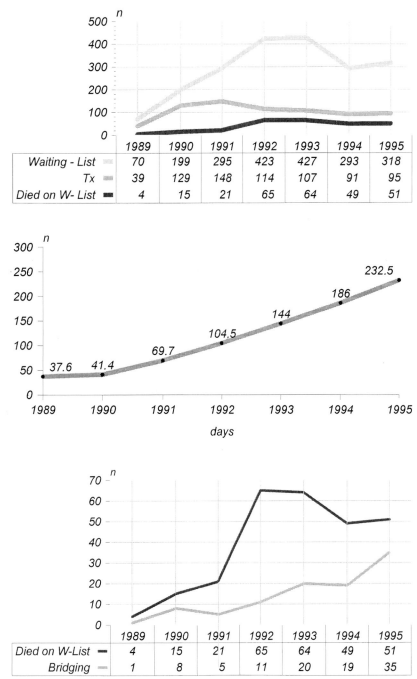

	1989	1990	1991	1992	1993	1994	1995
Waiting - List	70	199	295	423	427	293	318
Tx	39	129	148	114	107	91	95
Died on W- List	4	15	21	65	64	49	51

Fig. 4. Mean waiting time for heart transplantation (Mar 1989–Dec 1995): due to increasing shortage of the donor organs, the waiting time for transplantation became dramatically longer in recent years (37 days in 1989 and 232 days in 1995)

Fig. 5. Numbers of patients who died on waiting list (*dark line*) and the bridged patients (*light line*). Increasing use of mechanical ventricular support has had a positive influence in decreasing the number of deaths on the waiting list

	1989	1990	1991	1992	1993	1994	1995
Died on W-List	4	15	21	65	64	49	51
Bridging	1	8	5	11	20	19	35

Table 3. Numbers of patients given heart transplants, bridging, and both

Total patients for heart transplantation	$n = 761$
retransplantation	($n = 13$)
Bridging for heart transplantation	$n = 133$
Elective	($n = 118$)
Postcardiotomy cardiac failure	($n = 15$)
Bridged patients who received transplants	$n = 101$ (76% of bridged patients)

were given transplants, and between March 1993 and June 1996 transplantation was performed on 313 patients (group 2). In 33 of 448 patients (7.3%), bridging by VAD was performed prior to transplantation, compared with 68 of 313 patients (21.7%) in group 2.

The indications for transplantation in the two groups are shown in Fig. 7. The distribution of the different diagnoses was almost the same in both

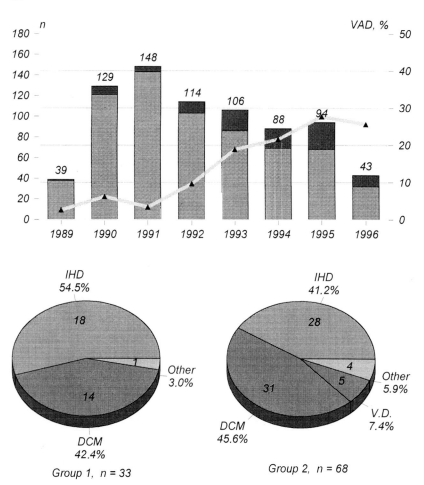

Fig. 6. Number of heart transplantations (*bars*) and bridgings with a ventricular assist device (VAD) (*triangles*). In the last two years, 25%–27% of the recipients underwent bridging during waiting time. *Bars: dark hatch,* children <16 years old; *light hatch,* adults

Fig. 7. Indications for transplantation in the two groups. *Group 1,* Mar 1989–Mar 1993; *Group 2,* Mar 1993–Jun 1996. *IHD,* ischemic heart disease; *DCM,* dilatative cardiomyopathy; *V.D.,* valvular disease

groups: ischemic heart disease (IHD) 54.5%, dilatative cardiomyopathy (DCM) 42.4%, and other causes 3.0%, in group 1; IHD 41.2%, DCM 45.6%, valvular disease (VD) 7.4%, and other causes 5.9%, in group 2. The age distribution of the patients was also similar in the two groups: 50–60 years was the most frequent age group (Fig. 8). There was no difference regarding gender in the two groups: 88% in group 1 and 85% in group 2 were male.

On the left hand side of Fig. 9, the application rate of VAD in both groups is shown. The rate was significantly higher in group 2 (21.7%) than in group 1 (7.3%; $P < 0.001$). The right hand side of Fig. 9 shows the early mortality of all the recipients who underwent heart transplantation during the two time-intervals. The mortality rate in the second time-interval was 5.2%, significantly lower than that in the first interval (8.7%; $P < 0.01$).

In Table 4, the different types of VAD used in 101 patients are listed. During our early experience (group 1). BioMedicus and Abiomed were often used for bridging, whereas later (group 2) in the majority of the patients, more sophisticated devices such as the Thoratec, Novacor, or HeartMate were used. In 2 patients following Novacor implantation as a left ventricular assist device (LVAD), additional use of a right ventricular assist device (RVAD) was necessary: one with Thoratec and one with Medos.

The different types of VAD were used as a LVAD, a biventricular assist device (BVAD), or a RVAD (Table 5). Novacor ($n = 17$) and HeartMate ($n = 9$) pumps were used exclusively as LVAD. For BVAD, BioMedicus ($n = 2$), Abiomed ($n = 6$), and Thoratec ($n = 24$) devices were used. In cases of RVAD, Thoratec ($n = 1$) and Medos pumps ($n = 1$) were used.

In Fig. 10, the outcome for the recipients who had received VAD support is shown. The survival rate of the transplant recipients who were bridged electively was quite high in both groups: 88% in group 1 and 87% in group 2. In cases of postcardiotomy cardiac failure, the survival rate in group 1 was much lower (43%), whereas the survival rate in group 2 was as high as in the elective bridging group (88%). However, the

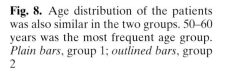

Fig. 8. Age distribution of the patients was also similar in the two groups. 50–60 years was the most frequent age group. *Plain bars*, group 1; *outlined bars*, group 2

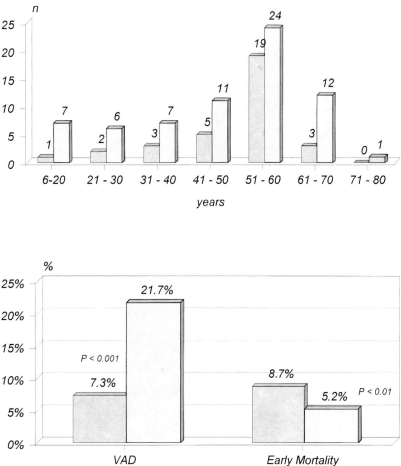

Fig. 9. On the *left-hand side*, the application rate of VAD in each group is shown (7.3% in group 1 vs 21.7% in group 2, *P* < 0.001). The *right-hand side* shows early mortality among the recipients who underwent heart transplantation during the two time-intervals (8.7% in group 1 vs 5.2% in group 2, *P* < 0.01). *Plain bars*, group 1; *outlined bars*, group 2

Table 4. Type of ventricular assist device usd in 101 patients who subsequently received a heart transplant

	BioMedicus	Abiomed	Thoratec	Novacor	HeartMate	Medos
Group 1	7	11	15	2	—	—
Group 2	1	2	40	15	9	1
Total (103)	8	13	55	17	9	1

Two patients received two devices each.
Group 1, March 1989–March 1993; group 2, March 1993–June 1996.

Table 5. Type of assistance provided by ventricular assist device

	BioMedicus (n = 8)	Abiomed (n = 13)	Thoratec (n = 55)	Novacor (n = 17)	HeartMate (n = 9)	Medos (n = 1)
LVAD	6	7	30	17	9	0
BVAD	2	6	24	0	0	0
RVAD	0	0	1	0	0	1

The number of patients was 101. Two patients received two devices each.
LVAD, left ventricular assist device; BVAD, biventricular assist device; RVAD, right ventricular assist device.

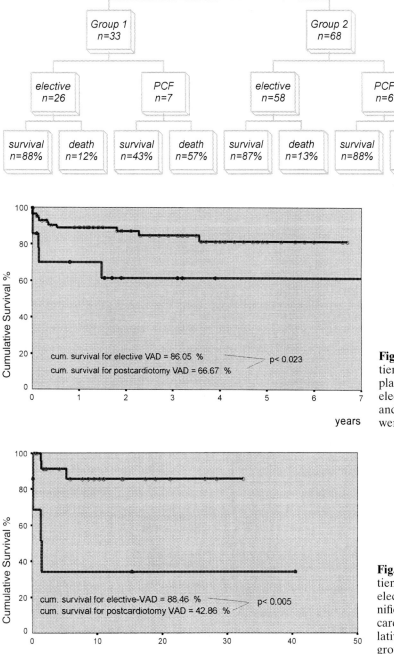

Fig. 10. Outcome for the recipients who received VAD support. The survival rate of the transplant recipients who were bridged electively was quite high in both groups (88% in group 1 and 87% in group 2). *PCF*, postcardiotomy cardiac failure

Fig. 11. The actuarial survival rates of the patients who were bridged prior to heart transplantation. The cumulative survival rates for the electively bridged patient group (*upper trace*) and the postcardiotomy group (*lower trace*) were 86% and 67%, respectively; $P < 0.023$

Fig. 12. The actuarial survival curve in 33 patients of group 1. The survival rate of the electively bridged patients (*upper trace*) is significantly higher than that of the postcardiotomy cardiac failure patients (*lower trace*). The cumulative survival rates were 88.5% for the elective group and 42.9% for postcardiotomy group: $P < 0.005$

difference was statistically not significant because of the small number of patients in both groups (group 1, $n = 7$, and group 2, $n = 6$).

The actuarial survival rates of the patients who were bridged prior to heart transplantation are shown in Fig. 11. The survival rates in the electively bridged patients and the postcardiotomy group were 86% and 67%, respectively. The difference is statistically significant ($P < 0.023$).

The actuarial survival curve in 33 patients (group 1) is depicted in Fig. 12. The survival rate of the electively bridged patients was significantly higher than that of the postcardiotomy patients. In contrast, for the respective actuarial survival curves for group 2, there was no statistically significant difference between these groups (Fig. 13).

Discussion

A few weeks after implantation of a device providing mechanical ventricular support, the general condition of the patient recovers rapidly, so that they are able to

Table 6. Characteristics of ventricular assist devices

	Disadvantages	Advantages
BioMedicus	Nonpulsatile Anticoagulation	Easy installation
Abiomed/Medos	Thromboembolism Anticoagulation	BVAD
Thoratec	Preclotting Evacuation Mobilization	BVAD
Novacor	Thromboembolism LVAD	Easy mobilization
HeartMate	Hazard connections LVAD	Easy mobilization Low thromboembolism

walk around in the hospital. Almost all of the patients underwent at least one cardiopulmonary resuscitation [8–11].

In Table 6, advantages and disadvantages of the different types of device are described. BioMedicus has the advantage of easy installation, but the disadvantages of non-pulsatile flow and the need for anticoagulation. The paracorporeal devices such as the Abiomed, Medos, and Thoratec systems can be used for biventricular support, but also have the disadvantages that they need anticoagulation and they have a higher rate of thromboembolism. The implantable and wearable devices such as the Novacor and HeartMate have the advantages of early mobilization of the patients and long-term support; however, device-related complications have been reported in several cases: degeneration of inflow and outflow valves and thrombus formation in a Novacor pump (Fig. 14); air embolism due to leakage of the HeartMate connectors; and spontaneous rupture of the outflow Dacron prosthesis of a HeartMate.

The use of the Thoratec pump is indicated for bridging to transplantation, especially in patients with

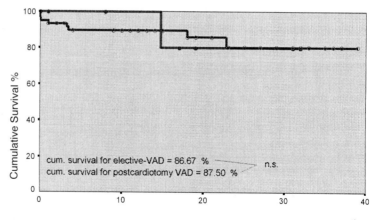

Fig. 13. The actuarial survival curve in 68 patients of group 2. There is no statistically significant difference between the patient groups: electively bridged (*open circles*) and postcardiotomy cardiac failure (*closed circles*)

cum. survival for elective-VAD = 86.67 %
cum. survival for postcardiotomy VAD = 87.50 %   n.s.

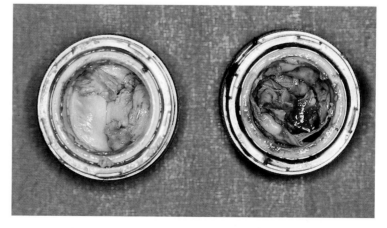

Fig. 14. Inflow and outflow valve degeneration and thrombosis in a Novacor pump

biventricular cardiac failure. Also, the Thoratec is useful for recovery from postcardiotomy cardiac failure in patients who are potential candidates for heart transplantation. However, due to the increasing waiting time of recipients and the low complication rate, we recommend use of the Novacor or HeartMate pump systems for bridging to transplantation. The BioMedicus, Abiomed, and Medos pump systems should be applied for temporary use in transplant recipients.

Totally implantable artificial hearts have been developed by several groups, and successful vivo studies have been performed during the last 10 years [12]. Due to the shortage of donor organs, further development of totally implantable devices for clinical use is imperative and urgent.

Conclusion

We can conclude that the ventricular assist device is an important tool for treating patients suffering from severe cardiac failure and waiting for transplantation. Due to the long waiting time, the need for VAD application has increased markedly in recent years (7.3% in group 1 vs 21.7% in group 2).

The early mortality rate of the recipients in group 2 was significantly lower than that in group 1 (5.2% vs 8.7%). One of the explanations for the marked decrease in the mortality rate could be the better general condition of the patients who are supported by a VAD. Because of potential device-related complications such as thromboembolism, rupture and acute bleeding from the device, and mechanical failure, the clinical application of VAD should be allowed when heart transplantation is established as a routine treatment in patients with end-stage cardiac failure.

References

1. Norman JC, Cooley DA, Kahan BD, Keats AS, Massin EK, Solis RT, Luper WE, Brook MI, Klima T, Frazier OH, Hacker J, Duncan JM, Dasco CC, Winston DS, Reul GJ (1978) Total support of the circulation of a patient with postcardiotomy stone-heart syndrome by a partial artificial heart (ALVAD) for five days followed by heart and kidney transplantation. Lancet I:1125–1127

2. DeBakey ME (1971) Left ventricular bypass pump for cardiac assistance. Clinical experiences. Am J Cardiol 27:3–11

3. Cooley DA, Liotta D, Hall GL, Bloodwell RD, Leachman RD, Milam JD (1969) Orthotopic cardiac prosthesis for two-staged cardiac replacement. Am J Cardiol 24:723–730

4. Kolff WJ, DeVries WC, Joyce LD, Olsen DB, Jarvik RK, Nielsen S, Hastings L, Anderson J, Anderson F, Menlove R (1984) Lessons learned from Dr. Barney Clark, the first patient with an artificial heart. In: Atsumi K et al. (eds) Progress in artificial organs — 1983, Cleveland, ISAO Press, pp 165–174

5. Portner PM, Oyer PE, Pennington DG, Baumgartner WA, Griffith BP, Frist WR, Magilligan DJ, Noon GP, Ramasamy N, Miller PJ, Jassawalla JS (1989) Implantable electrical left ventricular assist system: Bridge to transplantation and the future. Ann Thorac Surg 41:142–150

6. Kormos RL, Borovetz HS, Gasior T, Antaki JF, Armitage JM, Pristas JM, Hardesty RL, Griffith BP (1990) Experience with univentricular support in mortally ill cardiac transplant candidates. Ann Thorac Surg 49:261–272

7. McCarthy PM, Portner PM, Tobler HG, Starnes VA, Ramasamy N, Oyer PE (1991) Clinical experience with the Novacor ventricular assist system. J Thorac Cardiovasc Surg 102:578–587

8. Minami K, Posival H, El-Banayosy A, Körner MM, Schröfel H, Körfer R (1995) Mechanical ventricular support in postcardiotomy cardiac failure. In: Akutsu T, Koyanagi H (eds) Heart replacement. Artificial heart 5 Springer, Tokyo, pp 167–171

9. Minami K, El-Banayosy A, Posival H, Seggewiß H, Murray E, Körner MM, Körfer R (1992) Improvement of survival rate in patients with cardiogenic shock by using nonpulsatile and pulsatile ventricular assist device. Int J Artif Organs 15:715–721

10. Körfer R, El-Banayosy A, Posival H, Minami K, Kizner L, Arusoglu L, Körner MM (1996) Mechanical circulatory support with the thoratec assist device in patients with postcardiotomy cardiogenic shock. Soc Thorac Surg 61:314–316

11. El-Banayosy A, Posival H, Minami K, Arusoglu L, Kizner L, Breymann T, Seifert D, Körner MM, Körtke H, Fey O, Körfer R (1996) Mechanical circulatory support: lessons from a single centre. Perfusion 11:93–102

12. Nosé Y (1991) Toward a totally implantable artificial heart: development status at Cleveland Clinc. Artif Heart 3:147–165

Discussion

Dr. Reul:

Dr. Minami, I have a very simple question: What was the criterion for dividing your patients into two groups? Was it new technology since 1993, or what was the actual reason?

Dr. Minami:

Yes, I can say that. As you have seen in our data, we implanted in the second group more sophisticated ones, especially for bridging for transplantation. They are Novacor and TCI. That's why I have tried to analyze the data, how is the early mortality of the total patient?

Dr. Matsuda:

What is the most important factor to improve the results in the bridge group?

Dr. Minami:

Early mobilization of the patient; the cardiac support is much more efficient. If they could be mobilized after 1 week, the condition of the patient becomes much better.

Dr. Nonoyama:

Dr. Nonoyama from the Heart Institute of Japan. I'd like to ask about your strategies for selecting assist devices. Your group reported that patients with the Abiomed assist device had lower survival rates compared to the HeartMate- or Novacor-implanted patients. Today you mentioned only the difference in the supporting period, not the difference in type. So, could you tell me your latest opinion and impression about Abiomed as a device, or your strategies?

Dr. Minami:

Yes, especially in the first group, which is our first experience. But we can say retrospectively the patient who be on an Abiomed assist device could be supported up to 3 weeks maximum, whereas, with other devices, you can wait up to 3 months, 4 months, so that the patient's general condition would be better. We have transplanted the patient in early times with dysfunction of the liver or kidney because recovery of their hemodynamics was not sufficient.

Dr. Nonoyama:

But I think your group reported that the reason why the Abiomed patient had a lower survival rate is because of their limited capacity, flow capacity, with the Abiomed device, less than 5 liters per minute.

Dr. Minami:

Which manner of capacity? Capacity of what?

Dr. Nonoyama:

Abiomed has a limited capacity, less than 5.0 or 4.8 liters per minute, I think. Your group reported that reason, so I'd like to ask your new strategy for selection for these types of patients.

Dr. Minami:

Just a short comment. Today, we don't implant Abiomed for the bridging, because you have no chance to get a heart between the 2 weeks or 2 months. You have to wait up to 300 days, and then you have to choose the more sufficient one, like the Novacor or TCI. Today we use Abiomed for postcardiotomy cardiac failure.

Speaker:

I am always surprised when I see your or *Dr. Hertz's data* from Berlin about the high number of bridged patients. Our program is also not so small. We have about 650 transplants, but the number of bridged patients in our program is much lower than 5%. I think that one of the differences between your program and our program is that we have a very aggressive policy in pharmacologic bridging. A lot of our patients, they have implantable prostaglandin pumps, implanted pumps with dopamine, and so on, long-term implantable pump. We have also a very intensive and very extensive electrical bridging. All these methods — they are also not cheap, but they are not as expensive as all these bridged patients, in my opinion. My question is, do you have in this group of patients — have you any comparison with such methods as implantable prostaglanding pumps, implantable dopamine pumps with adrenergic substances? And my second question is, in one of your slides, you stated that the difference between the Novacor and the TCI is the lower thromboembolic rate with the TCI. Have you any data from your own patient material in this regard?

Dr. Minami:
For the second question, we have no thromboembolism with TCI. Actually we have done this in 12 cases. Up to now, we have no case with thromboembolism. And in the Novacor case we have up to now one definitive embolism complication and a second one is maybe related to the device. I would like to comment on your second question about the higher implantation rate of VAD in our hospital compared to other groups. We have lots of patients, more than 400 patients, who are waiting for transplantation today, with an average waiting time of 273 days. All of the patients have maximal medical support, sometimes including intra-aortic balloon pump and PDA III inhibitors and so on. As you have seen in our cases, the need of the assist device is indeed increased year by year. That is my comment, but we have no scientific complied studies with/without transplant or device, but maybe we can do that later on.

Dr. Olsen:
Olsen, University of Utah. You listed a large number of patients waiting on your transplant list and you listed also those that were bridged and those that were transplanted and those that died, and they didn't add up to the ones on the transplant list. What happens to the balance? Are they carried forward all the time?

Dr. Minami:
No, the patients who died on the device were not listed. In the first group (March 1989–March 1993) we have only 33 patients who were supported by the device and transplanted, whereas in the second group (March 1993–June 1996), 68 patients.

Dr. Olsen:
So the number of patients who were on the waiting list who actually died was not included in your data.

Mechanisms of Exercise Response in Denervated Heart After Transplant

Mitsuhiro Hachida, Satoshi Saitou, Masaki Nonoyama, Hironobu Hoshi, Naoji Hanayama, Akihiko Ohkado, Yukihiro Bonkohara, Tomohiro Maeda, and Hitoshi Koyanagi

Summary. Mechanisms through which the denervated heart responds to supine exercise were assessed in various ways in seven cardiac transplant recipients, 1–37 months after surgery. The results were compared with those in 15 normal subjects. The heart rate at rest and after exercise in transplant patients was 30% higher than normal ($P < 0.01$). Although cardiac output at rest was similar in both groups, early in exercise the means by which cardiac output increased in the transplant patients differed from normal. In the transplant recipients during the early stage of exercise, the blood norepinephrine level was significantly elevated, and the percent fraction shortening and velocity of circumferential fiber shortening (Vcf) was also higher than in normal subjects with an approximately similar heart rate. The level of atrial natrium diuretic peptide was also significantly increased during exercise by augmented preload ($P < 0.01$). These results support the concept that in the transplanted heart, there are increases in cardiac output via mechanisms different from those in normal hearts.

Key words: Heart transplantation — Posttransplant exercise — Denervated heart

Introduction

With the continued improvement in the long-term survival of orthotopic cardiac recipients, heart transplantation has become widely employed for the treatment of intractable heart failure. However, patients with a heart transplant remain subject to problems that may ultimately affect denervated graft function [1]. In denervated heart, the cardioacceleratory response to exercise is reported to be delayed [2]. In the present study of cardiac transplant recipients, we assessed their cardiac function during exercise, and mechanisms of functional capacity after the cardiac transplantation were studied.

Methods

Patient Selection

Seven cardiac transplant recipients ranging in age from 17 to 52 years were studied (Table 1). All patients underwent heart transplantation at the University of California, Los Angeles (UCLA) Medical Center and were followed postoperatively in our institute. Patients were studied from 12 to 61 months postoperatively at the time of evaluation. They had been rejection-free for at least 6 months. The hemodynamic parameters and left ventricular dimensions in these patients may be considered representative of the functional capacity of the transplanted human heart in the late postoperative period.

In the control group, the subjects (all male) ranged from 23 to 39 years old, and were healthy volunteers.

Evaluation Protocol

The exercise test was performed at the time of biopsy. Pulmonary arterial pressure, cardiac output, and pulmonary wedge pressure were continuously measured during exercise using a Swan-Gantz catheter. Exercise were initiated with a workload of 25 W and was increased by 25 W every 5 minutes. The heart rate and cardiac output were recorded in the final minute of each stage. The data after exercise were also obtained at 5 and 10 minutes after exercise. Blood samples were taken at each stage of exercise, and the concentrations of norepinephrine and atrial natrium diuretic peptide (ANP) were measured. Echocardiography, the left ventricular dimensions during diastolic and systolic phases, the percent fraction shortening, and the velocity of circumferential fiber shortening (Vcf) were measured by computer analysis, before and after exercise using the Master Two-step exercise test.

Statistical Analysis

Results are given as the mean ± SEM. Changes between rest and exercise were analyzed using a paired t-test. Differences between normal and transplant subjects were assessed by a two-tailed unpaired t-analysis. A probability value of less than 0.05 was considered significant.

Department of Cardiovascular Surgery, The Heart Institute of Japan, Tokyo Women's Medical College, 8-1 Kawada-cho, Shinjuku-ku, Tokyo 162, Japan

Table 1. Patients' characteristics

Patient	Age (years)	Sex	Transplant date	Immunosuppressants
1	51	Male	2 March 1993	Cyclosporin-A, azathioprine, prednisolone
2	26	Male	26 July 1993	Tacrolimus, azathioprine, prednisolone
3	17	Female	24 February 1995	Cyclosporin-A, prednisolone
4	24	Male	5 May 1995	Cyclosporin-A, azathioprine, prednisolone
5	40	Male	1 June 1995	Cyclosporin-A, azathioprine, prednisolone
6	21	Male	7 September 1995	Tacrolimus azathioprine, prednisolone
7	35	Male	15 March 1996	Cyclosporin-A, azathioprine, prednisolone

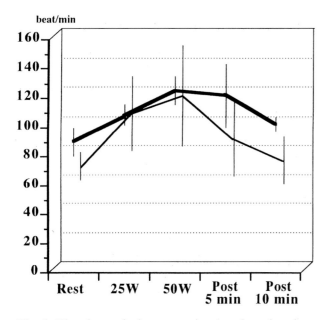

Fig. 1. The change in heart rate in transplanted patients (*thick line*) and normal subjects (*thin line*) during exercise. *25 W*, *50 W*, workload; *Post*, after finish of exercise; *error bars*, ± one SEM

Results

Hemodynamic Changes

At rest, the heart rate in transplanted recipients was 90.4 ± 9.8 beats/min compared with 74 ± 8.7 in normal patients. During the first stage of exercise (25 W), the heart rate among transplant recipients increased only 20.4% compared with a 34.9% increase in the normal subjects. The heart rate among the transplant patients increased slowly, and at the peak of exercise reached a level of 22.5% higher than at baseline. In normal subjects, exercise caused a more marked increase in heart rate, up to double the resting rate (Fig. 1). Similarly, on termination of exercise, the heart rate quickly returned to near baseline level in normal subjects, whereas among the transplant recipients, the heart rate 10 minutes after exercise was still 113.7% of the baseline level.

The cardiac output during the exercise was increased in transplant recipients in both groups (Fig. 2). There was a statistically significant difference between the two groups at 5 minutes after exercise ($P < 0.01$). Norepinephrine concentrations at rest averaged 120 ± 32.8 pg/ml in the normal group and 251 ± 63.8% pg/ml in the transplant group ($P < 0.05$). Norepinephrine significantly increased with exercise to 1211 ± 735.9 pg/ml in the transplant group at the 50 W level, but a less marked increase, to 215 ± 112 pg/ml, occurred in the normal group. Thus, the higher level of blood catecholamine may be the main source of increased contractile function during exercise in the transplant group.

Also, the plasma level of ANP was increased by exercise to a much greater extent in transplant patients than in normal subjects (Fig. 3).

On echocardiography, the left ventricular dimensions during diastolic and systolic phases were not significantly changed before and after exercise in either group. There were no statistical differences between the groups at rest or exercise.

Discussion

The first hemodynamic evaluations during exercise in human cardiac transplant recipients were reported by Carleton et al. [3]. Their data suggested that cardiac performance at rest and with mild exercise could vary appropriately with oxygen demand in the absence of innervation, and was regulated almost exclusively by variations in left ventricular filling. Leachman et al. likewise noted near-normal resting hemodynamic parameters in human cardiac recipients and described delayed but normal increases in heart rate [4]. However, Campeau et al. reported abnormalities of left ventricular function both at rest and during exercise in cardiac transplant patients [5]. Specifically, they noted an abnormally high left ventricular end-diastolic pressure and subnormal changes in left ventricular stroke work and tension-time indexes in response to moderate exercise. More recently, Hosenpud et al. demonstrated that a high heart rate,

Fig. 2. Plasma norepinephrine level (**a**) and cardiac index (**b**) during exercise. *Thick lines*, transplant; *thin lines*, normal

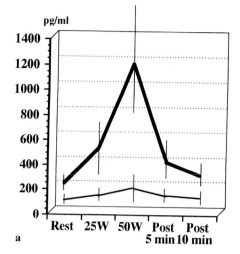

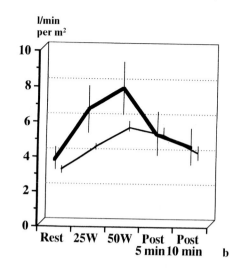

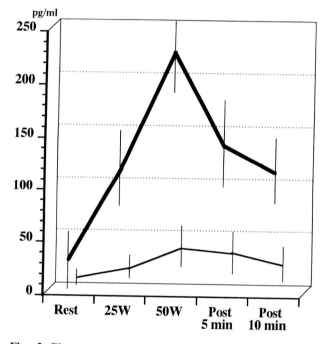

Fig. 3. Plasma concentration of atrial natrium diuretic peptide (ANP) during exercise. *Thick lines*, transplant; *thin lines*, normal. The level of ANP in plasma of transplant patients after 50 W exercise was significantly higher than that after 25 W exercise ($P = 0.076$)

relatively low stroke volume, and elevated filling pressures could be expected, especially when a small donor heart fails to adapt to a large recipient [6]. Pump failure and sympathetic denervation in themselves were considered possible causes of depressed performance. However, all of these studies consequently remain controversial.

Our data indicated the ability of the transplanted heart to increase its heart rate and cardiac output in response to moderate exercise. The response of both heart rate and Vcf was correlated with circulating plasma norepinephrine levels. This is the first direct demonstration of a humoral adrenergic mechanism underlying the adaptation of the transplanted human heart to vigorous exercise. This response may be enhanced by the increased sensitivity of the denervated heart to catecholamine [7].

This study has demonstrated that the initial increase in cardiac output with exercise in cardiac transplant recipients is achieved by augmentation of preload. Clark et al. demonstrated that the participation of peripheral regulatory factors is important in the cardiac output response to exercise [8]. The increase of venous return may influence the right atrial volume during exercise. In our studies, the elevation in ANP level during early stages of exercise in transplant patients is significant. This may be evidence for a unique dependence of the transplanted heart on preload, and is distinctly different from the behavior of the normally innervated, intact heart, in which heart rate and contractility changes are paramount during early exercise. Therefore, we suggest that the augmentation of preload volume during exercise in transplant hearts may be very important for adaptig the circulatory volume; therefore, an excessively small transplanted heart may have insufficient functional capacity during exercise. This hypothesis needs further investigation.

In conclusion, the humoral adrenergic mechanisms dominated during exercise in the transplanted heart, as manifested by striking increases in the heart rate, cardiac output, and velocity of circumferential fiber shortening, linked to a rising plasma norepinephrine level.

References

1. Pope SE, Stinson EB, Daughters GT, Schroeder JS, Ingels NB, Alderman EL (1980) Exercise response of the denervated heart in long-term cardiac transplant recipients. Am J Cardiol 46:213–218
2. Donald DE, Shepherd JT (1963) Response to exercise in dogs with cardiac denervation. Am J Physiol 25:393–400
3. Carleton RA, Heller SJ, Najafa H, Clerk JG (1969) Hemodynamic performance of a transplanted human heart. Circulation 40:447–452
4. Leachman RD, Leatherman LL, Rochelle DG (1969) Physiologic behavior of the transplanted heart in human size recipients (abstract). Am J Cardiol 23:123–124
5. Campeau L, Posipisil L, Grondin P, Dyrda I, Lepage G (1970) Cardiac catheterization findings at rest and after exercise in patients following cardiac transplantation. Am J Cardiol 25:523–528
6. Hosenpud JD, Pantely GA, Morton MJ, Norman DJ, Cobanoglu AM, Starr A (1989) Relation between recipient: donor body size match and hemodynamics three months after heart transplantation. J Heart Lung Transplant 8:241–243
7. Lurie KG, Bristow MR, Reitz BA (1983) Increased β-adrenergic receptor density in an experimental model of cardiac transplantation. J Thorac Cardiovasc Surg 86:195–201
8. Clark DA, Schroeder JS, Griepp RB (1969) Cardiac transplantation in man: review of first three years' experience. Am J Cardiol 40:447–452

What Will Happen to Permanent Left Ventricular Assist Device Recipients? Clues from Long-Term Outcomes of Heterotopic Heart Transplants

Osamu Tagusari[1], Akihiko Kawai[1], Kenji Yamazaki[1], Masayuki Miyagishima[1], Si M. Pham[1], Brack G. Hattler[1], Srinivas Murali[2], Bartley P. Griffith[1], and Robert L. Kormos[1]

Summary. Donor organ shortage and successful experience with left ventricular assist devices as a bridge to transplantation have prompted us to consider a permanent alternative to transplantation. However, we have little information on the long-term follow-up, because the left ventricular assist device has been used as a bridge to transplantation for a period of just over one year. In recipients of a left ventricular assist device, the potential heart-related complications expected include arrhythmia, thromboembolism, valvular heart disease, and progression of ischemic heart disease. Heterotopic heart transplantation (in which the native heart is retained) may be a good model to study long-term pathophysiological processes in the native heart. We analyzed the prevalence of native-heart-related complications in heterotopic heart transplantation to help in predicting the performance of the native heart in patients with a permanent left ventricular assist device. Between December 1984 and December 1994, 16 patients (13 men, 3 women, 37–60 years old) underwent heterotopic heart transplantation at the University of Pittsburgh. The indication for heterotopic heart transplantation in all recipients was pulmonary hypertension unresponsive to vasodilators. The one- and five-year survival rates after transplantation were 81% and 44%. Pulmonary hemodynamics improved significantly after the operation. The actuarial percentages of patients free of complications related to the native heart after one and four years were, respectively: ventricular arrhythmia: 85%, 75%; ischemic heart disease: 85%, 64%; and valvular heart disease: 100%, 88%. The actuarial freedom from all these complications was 70% after one year and 50% after four years. These results will give us an indication of the native heart performance to expect in the patient with a permanent left ventricular assist device.

Key words: Heterotopic heart transplantation — Left ventricular assist device — Arrhythmia — Valvular heart disease — Ischemic heart disease

Introduction

Donor organ shortage and successful experience with left ventricular assist devices (LVAD) as a bridge to transplantation have prompted us to consider a permanent alternative to transplantation [1–4]. However, we have little information on the long-term follow-up, because the LVAD has been used as a bridge to transplantation for a period of just over one year. Potential heart-related complications in permanent LVAD include arrhythmia, thromboembolism, valvular heart disease (VHD), and progression of ischemic heart disease (IHD).

The first heterotopic heart transplant (HHT) in human was performed by Barnard and Losman in 1974 [5]. In this technique, the donor heart is connected in parallel with the recipient heart. As a result, recipients continue to have risks originating from the native diseased heart, such as arrhythmia, angina, thromboembolism, and valvular regurgitation [6–13]. This situation is similar in the LVAD recipient. We analyzed the prevalence of native-heart-related complications in HHT to obtain information on the native heart performance to expect in permanent LVAD recipients in the future.

Patients and Methods

Patient Demographics

Between December 1984 and December 1994, we performed 528 heart transplantations. Of these patients, 16 (3%) underwent HHT. Their ages ranged from 37 to 60 years old (51 ± 7). There were 13 men and 3 women. The indications for transplantation included ischemic heart disease in twelve patients (75%), idiopathic cardiomyopathy in three patients (18.8%), and valvular heart disease in one patient (6.2%). The indication for HHT in all recipients was pulmonary hypertension unresponsive to vasodilators [14]. Preoperative catheterization findings are listed in Table 1. The mean follow-up was 4.1 years (range, 1 day–11.5 years).

Operation and Postoperative Management

HHT was performed according to a technique previously described [15]. We prefer to use the donor's descending thoracic aorta to interpose between the donor and recipient pulmonary arteries due to the experience of synthetic pulmonary artery graft infec-

Departments of [1]Surgery and [2]Cardiology, University of Pittsburgh School of Medicine Pittsburgh, PA 15213, USA

tion [16] (Fig. 1). We used a woven Dacron graft for eleven patients, and the donor's descending thoracic aorta for five patients. One patient underwent mitral valve replacement on the native heart combined with HHT. The baseline immunosuppression was achieved using azathioprine, corticosteroids, and cyclosporine (CsA) or tacrolimus (FK 506), as described [17]. Thirteen patients were given CsA and two, FK 506. One patient switched from CsA to FK 506 due to persistent acute rejection. Anticoagulation was used routinely with warfarin sodium (Coumadin) in all patients.

Statistics

Results are expressed as mean ± standard deviation. Hemodynamic results were compared using the paired t-test. Values of P less than 0.05 were considered to be statistically significant. Actuarial survival and actuarial freedom from complications were both calculated using the Kaplan-Meier product-limit method.

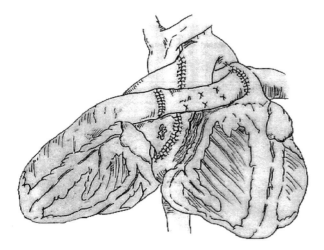

Fig. 1. Heterotopic heart transplantation using donor descending thoracic aorta to interpose between the donor and recipient pulmonary arteries

Results

Survival

Hospital death (death within 30 postoperative days or before hospital discharge) occurred in 3 of 16 patients (18.8%). The cause of death varied — primary graft failure, infection, or acute renal failure. Late death occurred in 7 patients, the major cause being infection (4). Other deaths were due to chronic rejection (1), malignancy (1), and unknown causes (1). The actuarial one-year survival after HHT was 81.2%, and the actuarial five-year survival after HHT was 43.8% (Fig. 2).

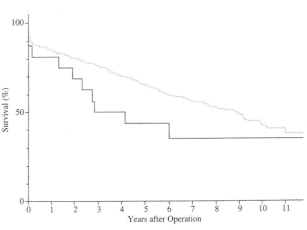

Fig. 2. Actuarial survival of patients after heterotopic heart transplantation (HHT; *solid line*) or orthotopic heart transplantation (*dotted line*). Between December 1984 and December 1994, we performed 528 heart transplantations. Of these patients, 16 (3%) underwent HHT. The one and five-year rates of survival were 81.2% and 50.0%, which can be compared to survivals of 85.4% and 70.2% obtained in patients treated by orthotopic transplantation during a similar period of time

Table 1. Cardiac hemodynamic profile before and after heterotopic heart transplantation

	Before HHT	After HHT	P value
PAP (systolic) (mmHg)	71 ± 10	33 ± 7	<0.0001
PAP (diastolic) (mmHg)	37 ± 7	16 ± 3	<0.0001
PAP (mean) (mmHg)	49 ± 5	23 ± 4	<0.0001
PVR (Wood units)	5.3 ± 2.0	2.5 ± 0.6	<0.0001
PCW (mmHg)	29 ± 5	10 ± 5	<0.0001
TPG (mmHG)	19 ± 6	13 ± 3	=0.002
Cardiac output ($l \cdot min^{-1}$)	4.0 ± 1.5	5.3 ± 1.1	=0.0041
Cardiac index ($l \cdot min^{-1} \cdot m^{-2}$)	2.1 ± 0.7	2.8 ± 0.6	=0.0027

HHT, heterotopic heart transplantation; PAP, pulmonary arterial pressure; PVR, pulmonary vascular resistance; PCW, pulmonary capillary wedge pressure; TPG, transpulmonary pressure gradient.

Hemodynamic Results

Preoperative and postoperative catheterization findings are listed in Table 1. There were significant decreases in pulmonary artery pressures, the transpulmonary pressure gradient, and the pulmonary vascular resistance. Cardiac output and the cardiac index improved after 3–6 months.

Native-Heart-Related Complications

The actuarial freedom from arrhythmia (sustained ventricular tachycardia or ventricular fibrillation) related to the native heart was 85.1% after one year and 74.5% after four years (Fig. 3). One patient underwent catheter ablation 82 months after the transplantation. Only one patient experienced episodes of ventricular tachycardia before the operation.

The actuarial freedom from IHD (unstable angina or myocardial infarction) related to the native heart was 85.1% after one year and 63.8% after four years (Fig. 3). One patient underwent percutaneous transluminary coronary angioplasty for the native heart at 79, 81, and 103 months after the transplantation.

As for VHD, one patient, whose underlying disease was end-stage ischemic heart disease, needed native cardiectomy after 46 months to resolve refractory congestive heart failure due to the progression of native aortic and mitral regurgitation. The actuarial freedom from VHD related to the native heart was 100% after one year and 87.5% after four years (Fig. 3).

The actuarial freedom from all complications related to the native hear was 70.1% after one year and 50.1% after four years (Fig. 4).

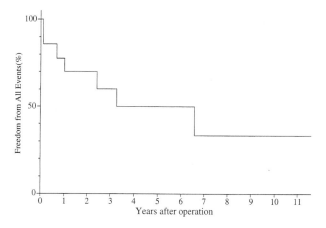

Fig. 4. Actuarial freedom from all complications related to the native heart. The actuarial freedom from all complications related to the native heart excluding thromboembolism was 70.1% after one year and 50.1% after four years.

Conclusions

Arrhythmia, thromboembolism, VHD, and IHD of the native heart are potential complications for future recipients of a permanent LVAD. The cause of thromboembolism in an LVAD recipient is usually related to the device, whereas in the recipient of a HHT the cause is a poorly contracting and dilated recipient left ventricle. However, each of these complications of the native heart, except thromboembolism, is due to the deterioration of the diseased native heart, in the recipients of either LVAD or HHT. Thus, HHT may be a useful model to predict native-heart-related complications in recipients of a permanent LVAD.

This study showed that the long-term frequency of complications related to the native heart in HHT is higher than we expected. There are several limitations of this study. First, our study consisted of only 16 HHT patients and all of them were complicated with pulmonary hypertension. Second, in HHT, the donor heart, where access is via the left atrium, is only a partial support for the recipient heart, in contrast to the LVAD, where access is via the left ventricle. Third, HHT patients require immunosuppression, whereas permanent LVAD recipients are expected to have normal immune function. However, we believe that the long-term performance of the diseased native heart will be a key indicator to predict morbidity and mortality in recipients of a permanent LVAD.

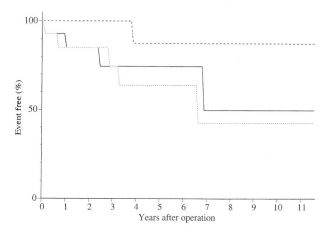

Fig. 3. Actuarial freedom from arrhythmia (*solid line*), ischemic heart disease (*dotted line*), or valvular heart disease (*dashed line*), related to the native heart

References

1. Griffith BP, Kormos RL, Nastala C, Winowich S, Pristas JM (1996) Results of extended bridge to transplantation: window into the future of permanent ventricular assist devices. Ann Thorac Surg 61:396–398

2. Pennington DG (1996) Extended support with permanent system: percutaneous versus totally implantable. Ann Thorac Surg 61:403–406
3. Kormos RL, Murali S, Amanda M, Armitage JM, Hardesty RL, Borovetz HS, Griffith BP (1994) Chronic mechanical circulatory support: rehabilitation, low morbidity, and superior survival. Ann Thorac Surg 57:51–58
4. Frazier OH, Macris MP, Myers TJ, Duncan JM, Radovancevic B, Parnis SM, Cooley DA (1994) Improved survival after extended bridge to cardiac transplantation. Ann Thorac Surg 57:1416–1422
5. Barnard CN, Losman JG (1975) Left ventricular bypass. S Afr Med J 48:303–312
6. Losman JG, Curcio A, Barnard C (1978) Normal cardiac function with a hybrid heart. Ann Thorac Surg 26:177–184
7. Cooper DKC, Novitzky D, Reichart B, Becerra E (1986) Are there indications for heterotopic heart transplantation in 1986? A 2- to 11-year follow-up of 49 consecutive patients undergoing heterotopic heart transplantation. Thorac Cardiovasc Surgeon 34:300–304
8. Alexopoulos D, Yusuf S, Bostock J, Johnston JA, Sleight P, Yacoub MH (1988) Ventricular arrhythmias in long term survivors of orthotopic and heterotopic cardiac transplantation. Br Heart J 59:648–652
9. Desruennes M, Muneretto C, Gandjbakhch I, Kawaguchi A, Pavie A, Bors V, Piazzs C, Rabago G, Leger P, Vaissier E, Cabrol C (1989) Heterotopic heart transplantation: current status in 1988. J Heart Transplant 8:479–485
10. Neerukonda SK, Schoonmaker FW, Nampalli VK, Narrod JA (1992) Ventricular dysrhythmia and heterotopic heart transplantation. J Heart Lung Transplant 11:793–796
11. Allen MD, Naasz CA, Popp RL, Hunt SA, Goris ML, Oyer P, Stinson EB (1988) Noninvasive assessment of donor and native heart function after heterotopic heart transplantation. J Thorac Cardiovasc Surg 95:75–81
12. Akasaka T, Lythall D, Cheng A, Yoshida K, Yoshikawa J, Mitchell A, Yacoub MH (1989) Continuous aortic regurgitation in severely dysfunctional native hearts after heterotopic cardiac transplantation. Am J Cardiol 63:1483–1488
13. Hildebrandt A, Reichenspurner H, Gordon GD, Horak AR, Odell JA, Reichart B (1990) Heterotopic heart transplantation: mid-term hemodynamic and echocardiographic analysis — the concern of arteriovenous-valve incompetence. J Heart Transplant 9:675–681
14. Villanueva FS, Murali S, Uretsky BF, Reddy PS, Griffith BP, Hardesty RL, Kormos RL (1989) Resolution of severe pulmonary hypertension after heterotopic cardiac transplantation. J Am Coll Cardiol 14:1239–1243
15. Griffith BP, Kormos RL, Hardesty RL (1987) Heterotopic cardiac transplantation: current status. J Cardiac Surg 2:283–289
16. Reddy SCB, Katz WE, Medich GE, Gasior TA, Quinlan JJ, Pham SM, Ziady GM, Kormos RL (1994) Infective endocarditis of the pulmonary artery conduit in a recipient with a heterotopic heart transplantation: diagnosis by transesophageal echocardiography. J Heart Lung Transplant 13:139–141
17. Pham SM, Kormos RL, Hattler BG, Kawai A, Tsamandas AC, Demetris AJ, Murali S, Fricker FJ, Chang HC, Jain AB, Starzl TE, Hardesty RL, Griffith BP (1996) A prospective trial of tacrolimus (FK-506) in clinical heart transplantation: intermediate-term results. J Thorac Cardiovasc Surg 111:764–772

Discussion

Speaker:
I would like firstly to congratulate the two excellent presentations. I have two questions, one for each presentations. I agree with you that, due to lack of donors, it's necessary for us to use a not-optimal donor. But we have to choose the recipients carefully when we use a not-optimal donor. You said that you used bad donors but you never said to which recipient you give the bad donors. Because if you give bad donors to bad recipients, generally the result is certain.

Dr. Furukawa:
I agree that if you put a perfectly good 20-year-old heart in someone who is 65 years old and deconditioned and is not doing very well, that heart has no chance to do well. What we try to do is, in those patients, say a 65-year-old gentleman who has ischemic heart disease, has had a CABG, now has ischemic cardiomyopathy, we would try to, rather than "waste a 20-year-old" heart, we'd try to use a 50-year-old heart or above, knowing that there is a higher risk of coronary artery disease. We're not in the business of giving immortality. We are just trying to give them time, just like everybody else. One year, two years, three years of better-quality life outside the hospital. These people are otherwise sitting in a hospital on inotropic support or perhaps on a balloon pump or perhaps on a ventricular assist device. So, it's hard to say who do we put these hearts into. I can tell you who I don't put them into: the undersized hearts, the less than, say, 0.5 weight ratio. I would not put them into someone who has pulmonary vascular hypertension, obviously. But, in someone who has normal pulmonary vascular resistance, I put them in and, yes, you have to keep them sedated for a longer period of time; yes, there are more management issues, but they do just fine postoperatively long-term. And, again, what we're trying to accomplish is to buy them time.

Speaker:
I totally agree with you. My second question is on your second presentation. You have insisted on the interests of new techniques with total excision of the heart and you have said you prefer bicaval technique rather than total excision due to lung procurement. In prac-

tice, it's only unfortunately for lung transplantation, it's only in a few circumstances, and with your technique, you really reduce the left atrium. What is the advantage of using bicaval and not using total excision when you can?

Dr. Furukawa:
I don't think I said that I would prefer to do a bicaval versus a total. I would prefer to do a bicaval versus the standard technique. But I also do lung transplants, and if we're procuring both lungs and heart, yes, we have no problem doing the total orthotopic heart transplant technique. But, because of where I work and how many transplant centers are around, we, up to now, have preferred or used the bicaval technique, just out of ease and have now recently gone on to do it more preferentially to do a total orthotopic heart transplant.

Speaker:
May I ask one question, Dr. Furukawa? In the bicaval anastomosis, one of this disadvantages of the technique is stenosis of, especially, the superior vena cava. Have you seen it in some cases?

Dr. Furukawa:
We have, as I said, done over a hundred of these, and have not yet, knock on wood found a problem with stenosis. We line up, we put a stay suture on one side, and we have been able to avoid superior vena caval stenosis. Yes, it has been described but we have not yet experienced that.

Dr. Kormos:
Kormos, University of Pittsburgh. This is for Dr. Furukawa. You know, the cardiac transplant research data, the cardiology transplant research data base, as well as, you know, ISHLT database, both show that older recipient actuarial survival is reduced. It also shows that using older donors reduces actuarial survival. What you are suggesting is to combine those two independent risk factors with the possibility of reducing actuarial survival even more. And, you know, what you've shown is 1-year and 30-day survival. I think we have to be very careful when you're talking about any procedure which ultimately is meant to increase sur-

vival as much as possible. And I think I disagree with you that, you know, it's fine to say we're not in the business of immortality, but you're got to be very careful. There's a lot of 65-year-olds out there who may disagree with you, that they will accept a suboptimal donor and why can't they be on the good donor list?

Dr. Furukawa:

I agree. I should preface it in saying that with all these "older," it's not just the "age of the recipient" that we're talking about. We're talking about some of these patients who otherwise cannot get a ventricular assist device, for insurance reasons or just that the patient is not, or their families are not, capable of using those devices. And if they are in extremis we will use whatever is available to them, whether it be greater than 50 years of age. We have no other mode of therapy for those patients. And that's how we came up with about 10 or 12 patients that are listed there. I totally agree. If I had a 65-year-old well-maintained man or woman, I would not deliberately go and try to place — O.K., he or she is over 65; I'm only going to put a 50. . . . No. If that's what I made it sound like, that's not what I was trying to say. These are patients that are in actuality in extremis and, for whatever reasons, we don't like to put in ventricular assist devices if they've already had two or three CABGs. Just the mortality from that operation for us is extremely high, so it's more of a last-ditch effort and then we put it up there because, yes, in some ways, these patients can be helped. It's not ideal, but it's the best we have for those patients at the present time.

Dr. Wolner:

Wolner, Vienna. Perhaps I can contribute a little bit to your discussion. We just finished a multivariate analysis of 600 transplant heart patients as a single-center experience. Which factors have an influence on the late outcome? And in this study we found that donor-related factors don't have any influence. They are only recipient-related influences. The most important factor we if such a patient has a resuscitation at any time before the transplantation. Second is where he is coming from: ICU, regular ward, from home. And third, some metabolic factors. It will be published soon. The long-term outcome has nothing to do with donor age, ischemic time, or other factors. And the second thing I want to tell you, in our experience, we have also done a lot of bicaval anastomosis. You have less trouble with the sinus rhythm and you have less tricuspid insufficiency. But we had one case with superior vena cava stenosis which was treated by interventional radiology.

Part III
Biomaterials

Blood Compatibility
Device-Related Problems

Biomaterials: Facts and Fiction

Pierre M. Galletti

Summary. Worldwide, 30–50 million men and women benefit from implanted devices. Therefore, the clinical experiences with synthetic materials in intimate contact with human cells and tissues exceeds by three orders of magnitude the number of laboratory animals sacrificed in the elusive quest for "biocompatibility." Furthermore, the much longer duration of observation characteristic of human implants, compared to animal studies, adds two orders of magnitude to the superiority of clinical and anatomopathological experience over laboratory animal studies. This glaring disparity must be kept in mind in the assessment of materials through in vitro and small animal studies, and the regulatory agencies' pronouncements based on such evidence. Another sobering fact is that over 95% of the materials utilized for implants are standard commercial substances originally developed for industrial purposes. Those products which have been found to be appropriate for a specific medical device are labeled "biomaterials" (or more modestly, materials for medical use) on the grounds of established specifications and quality control, supported by continuing feedback from the clinical experience. The major obstacle to the advent of custom-designed biomaterials is that the medical device market is so small (not in numbers of implants and impact on health care budgets, but in the quantity of material used per implant) that large-scale production and amortization of industrial production expenditures is well nigh impossible for truly novel substances. In litigious countries such as the USA, suppliers are pulling out of the market because of the excessive cost of defending against legal action when materials allegedly fail in the body environment. Against this background, biomaterials science is bravely searching for new solutions to old problems. The ill-defined property of biocompatibility is slowly making way for the notion of *bioacceptance* as we expand our knowledge of the cellular aspects of tissue–material interactions. Bioacceptance can seek two diametrically opposed end points: *biointegration*, meaning that the material and the surrounding living structures form a continuum with stable, low-grade interactions; and *biopassivation*, meaning that the material is hardly recognized by surrounding body fluids or tissues and that its stealth characteristics can persist for clinically meaningful periods of use.

Key words: Biomaterials — Clinical evaluation — Bioacceptance — Biointegration — Biopassivation

Artificial Organ Laboratory, Box G-B393, Brown University, Providence, RI 09212, USA

Introduction

Concern for materials has been a constant in the design and evaluation of artificial hearts and cardiac assist devices. The relative inadequacy of currently available materials constitutes a limitation on the scope of application of these devices, much as it has been, and remains, a limitation on the utilization of other artificial organs.

The purpose of this chapter is to present a global view of the "biomaterial" challenge, how it has evolved, what we have learned, and what we can expect in the next phase of progress.

Materials and Devices

Interest in materials to serve a medical purpose started empirically. Witness the ancient art of malleable gold plates to repair skull defects, the crafting of molded and painted glass spheres to substitute for a lost eye in the orbital socket, and the shaping and dying of boiled leather (collagen!) to fashion external prostheses and hide missing noses and ears. High hopes were born, and important promises made, 50 years ago when the productive interplay between chemistry and materials science gave us new polymers, metal alloys, and ceramics, which seemed initially to resolve all challenges of artificial organs and prosthetic implants.

However, in developing replacement parts for organs and tissues since the 1950s, engineers and doctors soon found out that obstacles would arise not so much from the inadequacy of chemical and mechanical properties of the materials used, as from unexpected, untoward biological reactions when these materials were exposed to living tissues. Problems arose with the structural integrity, performance, and endurance of materials in the warm, moist, salty, and highly corrosive environment of the human body over clinically meaningful periods of time. Cellular changes appeared in proximity to material alterations, and therefore the two observations were thought to be related. The unifying concept of biocompatibility was introduced to address this challenge.

103

Biocompatibility

Biocompatibility defines a new type of design constraint which has become a dominant consideration in the development of artificial organs. As observed by Tirrell et al. [1], "materials science has made important contributions to medicine, but the discipline has yet to draw on biology in the same way that it has absorbed people, ideas and skills from chemistry and physics."

Indeed, the efficacy of a man-made replacement part involves much more than the hemobiologic compatibility of the materials of which it is made. Artificial organs must be compatible with the available space and the contiguous structures in the location for which they are intended (*anatomic compatibility*). They must match the mechanical properties and dynamic behavior of the tissues to which they are attached (*mechanical* and *hemodynamic compatibility*). These requirements typically dictate the choice of construction materials for individual replacement parts. As a result, there are real limits to the concept of biocompatibility as a general property of a given composition of matter, whatever the use to which it may be put. The chemical composition and the finish of a particular substance to be placed in a living environment are but two determinants of its compatibility.

Historically, the value judgments addressing tissue–material interactions and in vivo material degradation were first cast in negative terms (Didisheim [2]). For instance, an early pioneer, Bruck [3], stated that materials can be called biocompatible if they "do not cause deleterious changes in body fluids or tissues with which they come in contact, and do not deteriorate in the biological environment." Later, the Clemson Advisory group [4] defined biomaterial as "a systematically pharmacologically inert substance designed for implantation or incorporation with living tissue," stressing through the word "inert" the absence of interactions as the principal design goal. In 1982, a NIH Consensus Development Conference on Clinical Applications of Biomaterials (Galletti and Boretos [5]) initially defined biomaterials as "substances which can be placed in intimate contact with living structures without harmful effects," stressing again negative evidence as the hallmark of biocompatibility. The same multidisciplinary group then moved to a simpler and more pragmatic formulation: "substances which can be successfully incorporated in devices of medical interest." This view was later echoed and amplified by a European group (Williams [6]), which characterized biocompatibility as "the ability of a material to perform with an appropriate host response in a specific application."

The positive definition of biocompatibility introduced two new elements into the conceptualization of biomaterials: (1) the recognition of positive interactions with the surrounding tissues, rather than negative outcomes, as the litmus test of biocompatibility; and (2) the unavoidable reference to devices in which biomaterials are processed or shaped to serve a specific function. In other terms, biocompatibility is no longer seen as a general property of a chemically defined material for medical applications, but a specific quality of that material which gives it desirable characteristics with the shape and surface treatment used for a specific device application. While material choice can be the key to success or failure of a device, proper functioning of the device is a necessary condition for evaluating the adequacy of its component materials. Successful long-term evaluation of the biomaterial depends upon the long-term integrity of the device in which it is used.

Facts and Fiction

The concept of biocompatibility often appears fuzzy and ill-defined because it is difficult to separate in the literature experimental facts from wishful thinking; documented observations from generalizations which have yet to stand the test of time; highly controlled, often short-term studies from life-long projections and hypotheses which have yet to be falsified. Taken together, benchtop, animal, and clinical observations point to the following empirical conclusions (Table 1).

A number of factors contribute to the limitations of materials as building blocks of devices:

— Thrombus formation in contact with blood
— Protein gel accumulation from biological fluids
— Chronic inflammatory reaction around implants
— Excessive scar formation in the healing period
— Material or tissue capsule calcification or ossification
— Biofilm formation and susceptibility to infection

Table 1. Materials: facts and fiction

1. The overwhelming majority of materials used in medical devices and implants are standard commodity substances developed for industrial purposes.
2. Biocompatibility is not an inherent property of a particular composition of matter, but depends upon the shape, finish, fabrication techniques, and choice of application of a particular material.
3. Material characteristics and device design features are interactive and therefore must be evaluated simultaneously over a clinically relevent period of time.
4. Biologic reactivity to specific materials is species-, site-, and time-dependent. In humans, a notoriously "mongrel" species, it can vary substantially from one individual to another.

— Material degradation with particulate release
— Progressive loss of mechanical properties

It is instructive to reflect on the information that can be gathered through systematic labors by investigators versus the wealth of often unorganized data derived from clinical observations (Table 2).

Clinical experience covering several decades is needed to evaluate materials for permanent implants, and some of the decay only manifests itself after several years of interactions with body fluids or tissues. The difference between biomaterials studies and device studies is summarized in Table 3.

In a case of failure of an implantable device, the fault is usually attributed to the materials of which the device is made, rather than to the host, on the assumption that all human subjects present the same reaction to a given clinical substance. There is no factual evidence that such a generalization applies to the relatively inert polymers, metals, or ceramics used in medical devices. Neglect of the host role rather reflects our inability to predict how individual biological characteristics may translate in terms of tissue–material interactions. Finding out whether personalized predictive tests could improve bioacceptance in the clinical setting is a challenge for the next generation of investigators.

Table 2. Evaluation of biomaterials: animal vs clinical

Animal	Clinical
10^4–10^5 Small animal experiments	3×10^6 Patients per year
10^3–10^4 Large animals in the USA	
10^4 Implanted animals observed at any one time	20×10^6 Living implant patients
Median duration of implantation expressed in weeks or months	Median duration of implantation measured in years
Planned retrieval allows systematic evaluation	Random retrieval complicates interpretation
Focus is on the early phase of tissue–material interactions	Focus is on the late stages of tissue–material interactions
Relevant for toxicology, mutagenicity, and carcinogenicity (chemical properties)	Relevant for material durability, decay, and release of particulate matter (physical properties)

Table 3. Biomaterials versus devices

Biomaterials	Devices
Defined primarily by chemical composition	Defined primarily in operational terms
Single composition of matter (occasionally composites)	Generally an assembly of several processed materials
Focus on material–tissue interface	Focus on overall device function

The clinical success of biomaterials is altogether remarkable, considering how limited is our understanding of the physical and biological mechanisms underlying tissue–material interactions. Indeed, the most substantial conclusion one can draw from a review of the record of literally millions of clinical implants is how few major accidents have been reported, and how uncommon and benign, in general, have been the side effects of implanting substantial amounts of synthetic materials into the human body. In a medical culture uncritically dominated by the fear of toxicity of foreign agents, the implant experience in man over more than 30 years casts some doubts about the clinical meaning of toxicity data obtained in animals with a much shorter life expectancy.

Bioacceptance

One way to conceptualize the human body's acceptance of devices, as distinct from materials, is to observe that there are two final pathways through which an implant can remain functional in a living environment (Fig. 1): once the initial sequence of events mediated first passively by molecular diffusion and adsorption, then through the inflammatory and immune responses to the implant, have run their course (typically over a period of weeks to months — right side of Fig. 1), the global adaptive response of the body can stabilize either through passivation or integration of the foreign object (left side of Fig. 1). The ultimate goal, permanent bioacceptance and continuing functional performance of the device, can be achieved with either strategy.

The initial interactions with the body environment are qualitively the same for all materials, but vary enormously in intensity according to material bulk properties, surface finish, macro- and microgeometry, animal species, and site of implantation. The later interactions are most favorable when they take the characteristic paths of either biopassivation or biointegration of the foreign body. Clinical experience has pinpointed the success of two alternative strategies for biomaterials in a living environment. Nonetheless, complications associated with infection, calcification, and carcinogenesis must be taken into account. However, it may well be that biological characteristics of the recipient, and not just those of the material alone, are the primary determinants of such outcomes.

Altogether, the blurred concept of biocompatibility of materials is progressively making way for the notion of bioacceptance of devices, meaning the ability of a man-made construct to perform indefinitely with an appropriate host response in a specific application (Fig. 2).

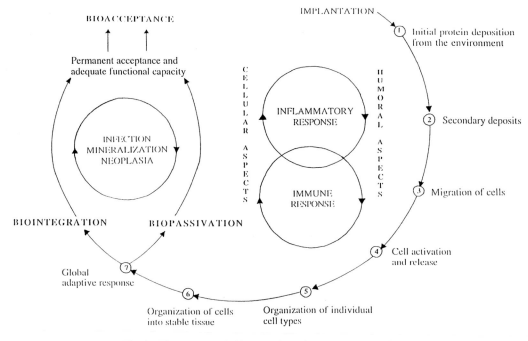

Fig. 1. Tissue–material interactions in long-term implants

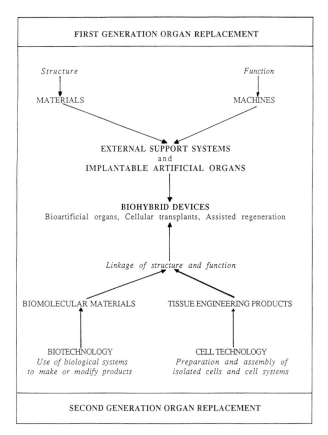

Fig. 2. Biomaterials in organ replacement

The Case of Hemocompatibility

Hemocompatibility means compatibility with blood, the primary fluid in the cardiovascular system. Operationally, blood can be considered as a heavily packed suspension of more or less differentiated cells in an electrolyte solution, containing a high concentration of complex proteins, lipids, and peptides, as well as numerous other bioactive substances. Blood is characterized by a remarkably stable composition despite rapid circulation through a variety of chemical reactors through which water and solutes are continuously added or removed. Hemocompatibility is critical for cardiovascular devices, which almost always contact blood. The elusive pursuit of hemocompatibility has taught us much of what we know in terms of tissue–material interactions. In brief:

a) All materials in contact with body fluids undergo almost instantaneous surface modifications which alter the original properties of their superficial layer, and in some cases, the bulk of the substance.
b) All body fluids and tissues in contact with foreign materials undergo a dynamic sequence of alterations which evolve over weeks or months, and may never cease.

The material–tissue interactions change with age and are subject to complicating effects of disease or trauma. Therefore, the notion of hemocompatibility is relative, statistical, and evolving. The most recent review of the field [7] admits that "in general, current tests for preclinical evaluation of biomaterials, devices, and their interactions with blood and tissues do not adequately predict the clinical behavior of devices."

This does not mean that bench tests and evaluation in laboratory animals are useless. They serve as screens, and eliminate most substances from further consideration. Witness the fact that out of over a million chemical compounds synthesized by chemists, only a few dozen have found their way into cardio-vascular devices. The International Organization for Standardization [8] has recommended that tests for hemocompatibility be conducted in each of five categories: thrombosis, blood coagulation, platelet and platelet functions, hematology, and immunology. However, in view of the limitations of these tests in predicting the clinical effectiveness of devices, "pass–fail" criteria for each test were specifically omitted from the standard. This prudent decision illustrates the current lack of consensus about what constitutes hemocompatibility.

Outlook for Biomaterials

The history of science shows that when medical progress is based on the accumulation of negative evidence, operational difficulties have to be resolved pragmatically rather than on the basis of theory, at least until broad generalizations or "laws" allow reliable predictions through the convergence of physical, chemical, or biological findings.

Biomaterials science has not yet reached that stage. However, things are beginning to change. Spurred in part by advances in protein chemistry and molecular biology, in part by the uniquely American phenomenon dubbed the "biomaterials availability crisis" [9,10], scientists and managers have started reflecting on the ambiguity of the concept of biomaterials, and the nature of materials for implantable devices. As expectations are redefined, new principles are promulgated to address material–tissue interactions, and new materials or processing strategies are emerging (Table 4).

The technology of artificial organs has now accumulated 40 years of clinical experience and sorted out the

Table 4. New classes of biomaterials

Bioinert materials
⟶ Bioreactive materials
⟶ Bioactive materials
⟶ Biomimetic materials
⟶ Biomolecular materials

problems with many of its constituent materials. Since acceptable solutions have been found to meet the most pressing needs of device manufacturers, the emphasis has progressively shifted toward fundamental studies in four major directions:

1. Characterization of the physical and chemical properties of implants which seem relevant for long-term performance in the biological environment, and comparison of control data from virgin materials with values obtained after actual exposure to body fluids and tissues

2. Characterization of the biological mechanisms involved in tissue–material interactions, both in the initial contact and in the chronic, or stabilized, phase of the interaction

3. Attention to distant as well as local host responses, meaning consideration of the potential for systemic effects of the implant, such as thromboembolism, toxicity, hypersensitivity, or immunological activation or inhibition

4. Synthesis of new materials which respond to the specifications derived from biological studies, and to a conjoint definition of material goals and tissue-response goals in terms of biostability, bioresorption, and biointegration

Biopassivation and biointegration are sought through the application of a variety of technologies:

— Material surface coatings to impart biological properties
— Material surface modifications to limit or promote material–tissue interactions
— Synthetic scaffolds as templates for cell proliferation or differentiation
— Grafting or inclusion of bioactive molecules in the bulk of biomaterials
— Grafting or inclusion of living cells on synthetic polymers (tissue-engineered devices)

Biomaterials for Bioartificial Organs

The first generation of artificial organs, which emerged around the middle of the 20th century, exemplified the combination of *machines*, designed to fulfill a specific function, with specially chosen *materials* to fabricate the desired structure and interact as desired with body fluids or tissues (Fig. 2). This approach still dominates the technology of clinical organ replacement. However, a second generation of artificial organs is currently going through a long gestation period. Biotechnology allows the precise control of molecular and supramolecular structures and promises new classes of materials with properties engineered for specific purposes. One of the purposes is matching

Table 5. Classical devices versus bioartificial organs

Classical devices	Bioartificial organs
Primary effect results from man-made design	Primary effect results from the potential of living tissue
Materials and design are key determinants of function	Materials and design are supportive elements of function
Performance is limited by design and availability of man-made components	Performance is further limited by survival or proliferation of living elements
Host tissue–material interaction is a major determinant of long-term performance	Host cell vs transplanted cell as well as tissue–material interactions are the key elements of functional effectiveness

bioactive substances on the surface of materials with corresponding receptors on the surfaces of living cells cultured and sometimes genetically modified to enhance their affinity for the *biomolecular materials*. Such substances, made possible by advances in cell technology, are known as *tissue-engineered products*. They are the building blocks of hybrid artificial organs, or *bioartifical* organs, a new form of organ replacement therapy which features elements of:

— *Standard transplantation*: Involves the surgical introduction of autologous, allogeneic, xenogeneic, or genetically engineered cells into the patient's body.
— *Implantable devices*: Design and structures are man-made and do not necessarily resemble the natural organ.
— *Biomaterials*: Man-made, custom-designed substances which are needed to provide a scaffold, template, or envelope for the transplanted cells.
— *Drug delivery systems*: Some bioartifical organs exert their effects through the release of bioactive molecules and obey a cell mass plus physiologic effect paradigm.

The distinguishing features of bioartifical organs, as compared with classical medical devices, are summarized in Table 5.

Conclusion

Because of the difficulty of developing entirely new materials for medical use, the current trend is to apply biotechnology to achieve better matching with the host. Strategies include: surface modifications to promote or limit interactions with cells and their secretion products; the grafting of biologically active molecules on synthetic materials to guide and control those interactions; the design of tissue-engineering products incorporating living cells in synthetic compounds; and the preparation of synthetic scaffolds or templates for inducing tissue regeneration, using either durable or bioresorbable materials. These avenues all involve a lengthy and expensive iterative process, and are unlikely to enter clinical practice in the next few years [11,12].

Two major obstacles will delay the availability of truly novel materials: the difficulty of identifying specific technological advances which correspond to a broad commercial opportunity; and the disincentive for major chemical companies to fabricate substances with a limited market, not much value-added leeway, and a high liability potential (at least in the USA). Whether "boutique" chemical manufacturers will muster the resources and the will to step into the breach remains to be seen.

References

1. Tirrell JG, Fournier MJ, Mason TL, Tirrell DA (1994) Biomolecular materials. Chem Eng News, 19 December:40–51
2. Didisheim P (1993) An approach to biocompatibility. Cardiovasc Pathol 2:1S–2S
3. Bruck SD (1972) Biomaterials in medical devices. ASAIO Trans 18:1–7
4. Black J (1982) The education of the biomaterialist. J Biomed Mater Res 16:159–167
5. Galletti PM, Boretos JW (1983) Report on the Consensus Development Conference on clinical applications of biomaterials. J Biomed Mater Res 17:539–555
6. Williams DF (1988) Consensus and definitions in biomaterials. In: Progress in biomedical engineering, vol 8. Elsevier, Amsterdam, pp 11–71
7. Harker LA, Ratner BD, Didisheim P (eds) (1993) Cardiovascular biomaterials and biocompatibility. Cardiovasc Pathol 2(Suppl):1S–224S
8. International Organization for Standardization (1992) ISO 10993-4: Biologic evaluation of medical devices, Part 4. Selection of tests for interactions with blood. Geneva
9. Hill JD (1994) An impending crisis involving biomaterials. Ann Thorac Surg 58:1571
10. Galletti PM (1996) Biomaterials availability in the U.S. J Biomed Mater Res 32(3):289–291
11. Galletti PM (1996) Medical device innovation and the public interest. ASAIO Journal May–Jun 1997 43(3):127–131
12. Greco RS (1994) Implantation biology. CRC, Boca Raton, pp 1–418

Discussion

Dr. Teoh:

My name is Teoh, from the Biomat Center at the National University of Singapore. I agree with you and I think you did mention very well that over the two decades we have realized that there are many materials that are not really biocompatible in that sense. And you have made a very important point that the word "biocompatible materials" needs perhaps to be redefined, and you have used the word "bioacceptable material," which I thought was an interesting adjective. There is a group of people in the biomaterials community, especially in our center, who used to avoid the word "biocompatible material" but introduced the word "biotolerant material" as we realize that our body is highly tolerant to a number of tortures in the use of raw materials. I just would like to ask for your comments on this word "biotolerant material."

Dr. Galletti:

Is it for polymer, the word you are saying?

Dr. Teoh:

It can be polymer, it can be metals, it can be ceramics.

Dr. Galletti:

Well, my first observatoin would be that, if you read the history of biomaterials, up to about 1980 almost every defintion of biocompatibility was expressed in negative terms. A biomaterial was a material which did not do something — did not elicit a reaction. It's only since about 1982 or '83 that the perspective has changed, leading to the one you are proposing, that we should try to define compatibility in positive terms, the ability of the material to act and interact within the body, or in some situation to develop "stealth" characteristics, that is to say, develop such characteristics that it will be ignored. My general philosophy is that when we are developing materials we have to make a choice from the beginning, which one is going to be best in a particular application. Are we trying to be better off by essentially making the material as invisible to the body as possible? Of course it's never going to be totally invisible. Are we going to be better off eventually by making the material interact, integrate, and essentially relate directly to the environment? I think the two strategies are actually possible. Some of the slides I used showed the extreme of that range, biopassivation and biointegration. It's never possible to go to the absolute extreme. I don't think there is ever going to be a material which the body will ignore forever, nor do I think that there will be a material which the body will fully accept without any negative reaction. In that sense, your proposal is a construtive one because it stresses the positive in the definition of biomaterials.

Dr. Sakurai:

Concerning the evolution of biomaterials, I'd like to introduce you to a movement in Japan. About 10 years ago, we created a new concept of intelligent biomaterials. So, intelligent means that inside of the molecular architecture of materials, some new function is incorporated. Usually the most important characterstic of the biomolecule is adaptability, I think, so they can detect some change of environment and change the conformation or change the function and then adapt to change of environment. So, regrettably, the synthetic materials do not have adaptability. But our concept of intelligent biomaterials is that they have some kind of adaptability so they can detect some change of environment; and according to that signal they change conformation or structure and function and they can release some effective action.

Dr. Galletti:

I think that what you're pointing to is a very important movement in the philosophy of materials, what you call intelligent biomaterials, some people call them smart biomaterials. And I think what this points to is that all artifical organs which we have created so far do not adapt to the process of growth and aging of the human body. And will we ever be able to develop such organs which really can live and age gracefully with us? Fundamentally one would have to start with the materials themselves by introducing in the materials the molecular recognition mechanism and the molecular adaptation mechanism, so I think starting with intelligent biometerials is the right way to do it.

Calcification and Thrombus Formation on Polymer Surfaces of an Artificial Heart

Kou Imachi[1], Yusuke Abe[1], Tsuneo Chinzei[1], Kunihiko Mabuchi[2], Kazunori Baba[1], Hiroyuki Matsuura[3], Akimasa Kouno[1], Toshiya Ono[1], Shuichi Mochizuki[1], Yan-Pin Son[1], Kaoru Imanishi[4], and Iwao Fujimasa[5]

Summary. Calcification and thrombus formation are still important problems in artificial heart research. The calcification and thrombus formation generated in artificial heart blood pumps, driven without anticoagulant for 312 days as the left side and 414 days as the right side, were analyzed in this study. A thrombus was observed at the circumference of the sac in the 312-day pump, but it was not associated with calcification. Several phenomena were observed on the polymer membrane valves (jellyfish valves) incorporated into the blood pump: plastic deformation of the valve membrane by creep fatigue; no calcification of stationary parts such as spokes and the center of the membrane; calcification of the particular portion which received repeated stretching stress; and no association of calcification with thrombus. The calcification of the valve area which received repeated stretching force might be explained as follows. Repeated stretching forces extend the polymer membrane, causing some loosening between polymer molecules and generating microgaps. Blood proteins and phospholipids invade these microgaps, which then attract Ca^{2+} ions followed by phosphate ions(PO_4^{2-}) leading to the formation of calcium phosphate complexes.

Key words: Artificial heart — Cardiac valve prosthesis — Calcification — Thrombus formation — Polyurethane

Introduction

Although the blood compatibility of the artificial heart has greatly improved since segmented polyurethanes and their copolymers such as Biomer and Avcothane have been developed, thrombus formation and calcification in the blood pump are still important problems [1,2]. However, the mechanism leading to these complications has not been elucidated.

Recently, we have succeeded in maintaining a goat for 532 days with a total artificial heart. In this experiment, the left and the right side blood pumps were each exchanged for a new one on the 312th day and 414th day, respectively. The objective of this study was to analyze the thrombus formation and calcification in these blood pumps to clarify the long-term mechanism of calcification and thrombus formation on the artificial heart polymer surface.

Materials and Methods

The blood pump used in this experiment was a sac type with a 60-ml sac volume [3]. The blood pump was made of polyvinyl chloride paste resin (PVC) and its blood contacting surface was coated with KIII (developed by Nippon Zeon, Tokyo, Japan). Jellyfish valves were installed in each blood pump. In this animal, the sac used as the right side pump had previously been used for one week and fixed with phosphate-buffered glutaraldehyde. The four cannulae for the right and left atrium, pulmonary artery, and descending aorta, were also made of PVC and coated with KIII. Each inflow cannula had a cuff made of expanded polytetrafluoroethylene (EPTFE) to anastomose with the atrium. The aortic cannula was molded in one piece with an EPTFE vascular graft at its end to allow an end-to-side anastomosis to the descending aorta.

KIII is a copolymer of polyether-polyurethane with polydimethylsiloxane, made using a silane coupling agent. Although it has the same composition as Cardiothane, its polydimethylsiloxane particles are finer than in Cardiothane and well dispersed into the polyurethane, making a so-called interpenetrating polymer network (IPN) structure. It shows fairly good antithrombogenicity.

The jellyfish valves were home-made polymer membrane valves developed for an artificial heart [4–8]. Their structure is simple: a thin flexible polymer membrane adhered at the center of the valve seat, with 12 spokes to prevent prolapse when it closes. The valve seat (outer and inner diameter, 20mm and 18mm, re-

[1]Department of Biomedical Engineering, Graduate School of Medicine, The University of Tokyo, 7-3-1 Hongo, Bunkyo-ku, Tokyo 113, Japan
[2]Center for Collaborative Research and [3]Research Center for Advanced Science and Technology, The University of Tokyo, 4-6-1 Komaba, Meguro-ku, Tokyo 153, Japan
[4]Second Hospital, Tokyo Women's Medical College, 2-1-10 Nishi-Ogu, Arakawa-ku, Tokyo 116, Japan
[5]Graduate School of Policy Science, Saitama University, 255 Shimo-Okubo, Urawa, Saitama 338, Japan

spectively) was made of two liquid reacted urethane by a casting method, and coated with KIII. The valve membrane (50–70μm thick) was made of KIII by a casting method. The performance of the jellyfish valve is superior to that of the Björk-Shiley valve with the same orifice diameter, when assessed by maximum pump flowrate, regurgitant flow, and leakage flow. The antithrombogenicity of this valve was sufficient without use of anticoagulant for about 4 months.

A female goat of 47.6kg body weight was used in this experiment [9]. The natural heart was resected under extracorporeal circulation and the right and left blood pumps were connected to the right atrium, pulmonary artery, left atrium, and descending aorta through four cannulae. The blood pumps were placed paracorporeally on the chest wall to allow observation of pump movement, blood oxygenation, and thrombus formation, and to exchange the blood pump if needed. Neither anticoagulant nor any antiplatelet agent were administered systemically in this experiment after the surgical operation. Only the pressure measurement lines needed for artificial heart control were maintained by small amounts of pressurized, heparinized saline drip.

When the blood pump needed to be changed, heparin was infused intravenously and the pumping was only stopped for 30–40s. The retrieved blood pump was rinsed gently with saline several times and fixed with phosphate-buffered 2.5% glutaraldehyde for several hours. It was dried in a clean room after rinsing with distilled water. The calcification in the

blood pump was analyzed using a microscope and an X-ray microanalyzer loaded on a low-vacuum scanning electron microscope (SEM).

Results

The goat survived normally for 532 days until it died because of mismanagement of a pressure measurement line. During that period, the left blood pump was exchanged for a new one on the 312th pumping day, because thrombus had formed in the sac by the 306th day. Thrombus formation was also observed in the right side blood pump on the 380th pumping day and the pump was changed on the 414th day.

Figure 1 shows the left side blood pump, removed on the 312th day. Thin-layered thrombus was observed at the circumference of the sac. No thrombus was found around the jellyfish valve. However, by analyzing the jellyfish valves, the following phenomena were elucidated. The valve membrane deformed plastically. It expanded to the upper stream side between the spokes, which was interpreted as due to a creep fatigue phenomenon. A perforation of the membrane between the spokes was observed on the outlet valve. Innumerable white scratches were seen on the membrane located on the spokes. These white scratches were greater in number on the inlet valve membrane, resulting in crystallization. Figure 2 shows the macroscopic view of the jellyfish valve taken out on the 312th day. By SEM and X-ray microanalyzer

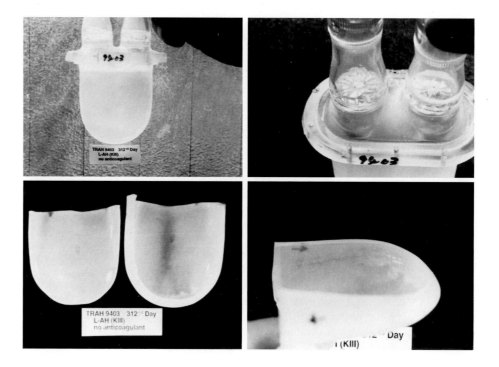

Fig. 1. Blood pump driven for 312 days. *Upper* two figures, exterior view; *lower* two figures, interior view

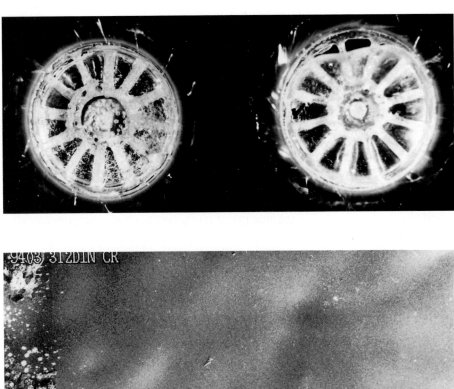

Fig. 2. Macroscopic view of the jellyfish valve after 312 days' pumping: *left*, inlet valve; *right*, outlet valve

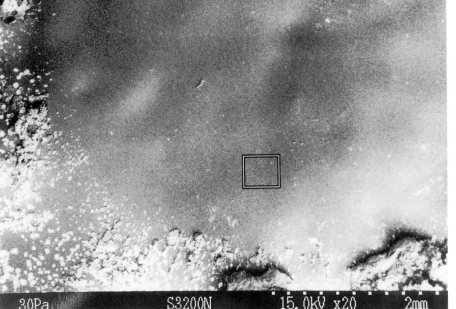

Fig. 3. Scanning electron micrograph [×20] of the center of the jellyfish valve membrane driven for 312 days

analysis, the white scratches were identified as crystals of calcium phosphate. No thrombus or calcification was found at the center of the membrane which did not move (Fig. 3). Calcification mainly occurred on the spokes on the downstream side of the valve membrane (the other side of the valve seat). Calcification also appeared between the spokes on the upper stream side of the membrane (valve seat side). No calcification could be detected in the thrombus formed in the sac.

Figure 4 shows the blood pump taken out on the 414th day. Heavy thrombus had formed at the circumference of the sac; part of it reached up to the outlet, passing through the outlet jellyfish valve. No calcification was detected on the thrombus. However, a small calcification was found beneath the thrombus when it

was taken off, as shown in Fig. 5. Figure 6 shows the inlet jellyfish valve taken out on the 414th day. Its condition was almost the same as that of the 312-day valve.

Discussion

In short, we made the following observations:

1) Thrombus suddenly formed in the left and right sacs after 10–12 months.
2) No calcification was observed in the left sac; however, small areas of calcification were detected beneath the thrombus in the right sac.

Fig. 4. Blood pump driven for 414 days. **a–c** thrombus formed in pump; **d** thrombus attached to jellyfish valve

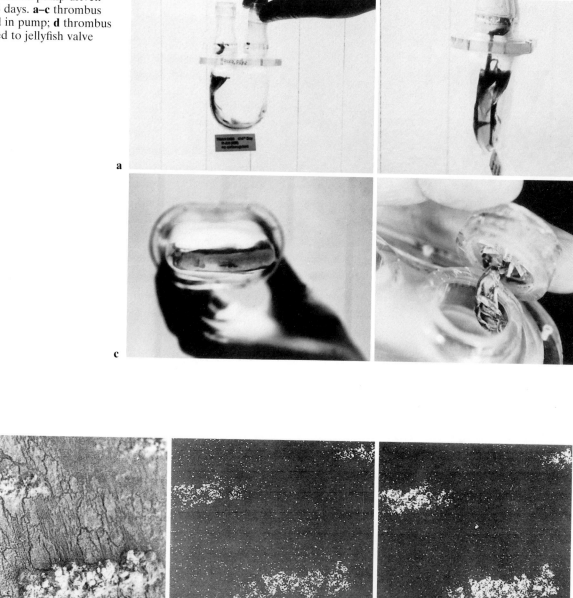

Fig. 5. Calcification found beneath the thrombus in the sac. **a** Scanning electron micrograph [×120]; **b** phosphate and **c** calcium analysis by X-ray microanalyzer [×120]

3) The jellyfish valves deformed plastically, expanding to the upstream side between the spokes.

4) Calcification was observed on all of the jellyfish valves, but it was not associated with thrombus formation.

5) No calcification was observed on the stationary parts of the jellyfish valves, such as the central portion of the valve membrane, the valve seat, and the spokes.

6) Calcification on the downstream side of the valve membrane was concentrated to the portions located on the spokes. On the upstream side of the valve membrane, calcification was observed between the spokes.

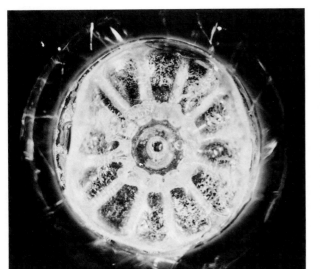

Fig. 6. Macroscopic view of the inlet jellyfish valve after 414 days' pumping

Since segmented polyurethane and its copolymers have been applied to the artificial heart blood pump, the antithrombogenicity of the blood pump has been greatly improved, resulting in longer survival of animals with the artificial heart. However, as survival extends, new problems have occurred: namely, thrombus formation and calcification after several months. Thrombus formation in the blood pump has often been observed at particular points such as junction lines of valves and connectors, the diaphragm–housing junction (D-H junction), and the circumference of the sac. The cause of thrombus formation is thought to be macro-scopic or microscopic stagnation of blood flow [3]. Efforts have been made to minimize these gaps and to change the configuration of the sac. The jelly-fish valve was developed to allow seamless incorporation into a blood pump. Although these efforts have proven effective in preventing thrombus formation in the blood pump, the problem has not been completely solved. In this experiment, a thrombus suddenly appeared in the sac after 308 pumping days in the left side and 380 pumping days in the right side. Several factors may explain this phenomenon: a change in the surface properties of the polymer surface due to long-term mechanical stress, environmental effects of blood contact, or alterations of blood properties such as changes in hematocrit, platelet activity, etc. From our experience, the hematocrit appears to be one of the most significant factors in thrombus formation. Most animals with a total artificial heart, in every laboratory, have shown a mild degree of anemia. Recently, we succeeded in improving their condition by changing the control method for the artificial heart (see the

chapter by Y. Abe et al., in this volume). The hematocrit in our goats with a total artificial heart, including the one in the present report, returned to preoperative values 1–2 months after the surgical operation. The problem of thrombus formation in the blood pump became more severe with the recovery of the hematocrit. However, this does not fully explain why thrombus formed after such a long delay.

Concerning calcification on the blood pump surface, it is well known that calcification often occurs at the stress concentration sites [10,11]. Although microcrack generation by stress concentration is one of the most probable causes of calcification, the mechanism has not yet been clarified. This study shows that calcification did not occur in stationary parts such as the center of the valve membrane and the spokes. Calcification occurred mainly where the valve membrane received repeated stretching stress. This leads us to propose the following hypothesis: when segmented polyurethane is subjected to repeated stretching stresses, it is extended and some loosening between the molecules occurs in the soft segment domains. Blood proteins and/or phospholipids invade these microgaps between loosened polymer molecules, and these attract Ca^{2+}ions followed by phosphate ions (PO_4^{2-}) to allow the formation of a complex. Several observations support this hypothesis. In general, when we studied the cross-section of a calcified polymer, we found that the calcified deposits had penetrated into the polymer. Vašků also found by SEM analysis that some calcified particles were trapped inside the driving diaphragm [12].

The hypothesis suggests how to protect against calcification on the jellyfish valve. One approach is to thicken the valve membrane and another is implantation of an ion such as carbon or gold on the membrane surface. The former can delay the creep fatigue of the membrane and the latter can prevent the invasion of blood protein and phospholipid into the membrane.

References

1. Boretos JW (1968) Segmented polyurethane: a polyether polymer. J Biomed Mater Res 2:121–130
2. Nyilas E (1972) Development of blood compatible elastomer. J Biomed Mater Res Symp 3:97–127
3. Imachi K, Fujimasa I, Miyake H, Takido N, Nakajima M, Motomura K, Kouno A, Ono T, Atsumi K (1981) Evaluation of antithrombo-genicity, durability, and blood compatibility of an artificial heart system for more than 100 days. Artif Organs 5(Suppl):423–429
4. Imachi K, Fujimasa I, Mabuchi K, Chinnzei T, Abe Y, Maeda K, Imanishi K, Kouno A, Ono T, Atsumi K (1988) A newly designed jellyfish valve for an artificial heart blood pump. ASAIO Trans 34:726–728
5. Imachi K, Mabuchi K, Chinnzei T, Abe Y, Imanishi K, Yonezawa T, Maeda K, Suzukawa M, Kouno A, Ono T,

Fujimasa I, Atsumi K (1989) In vitro and in vivo evaluation of a jellyfish valve for practical use. ASAIO Trans 35:298–301

6. Imachi K, Mabuchi K, Chinzei T, Abe Y, Imanishi K, Suzukawa M, Yonezawa T, Kouno A, Ono T, Nozawa H, Atsumi K, Fujimasa J (1991) Blood compatibility of the jellyfish valve without anticoagulant. ASAIO Trans 37:220–222

7. Imachi K, Mabuchi K, Chinzei T, Abe Y, Imanishi K, Yonezawa T, Kouno A, Ono T, Nozawa H, Isoyama T, Atsumi K, Fujimasa I (1992) Fabrication of a jellyfish valve for use in an artificial heart. ASAIO J 38:237–242

8. Imachi K, Mabuchi K, Chinzei T, Abe Y, Imanishi K, Yonezawa T, Nozawa H, Isoyama T, Kouno A, Ono T, Atsumi K, Fujimasa I (1993) The jellyfish valve: a polymer membrane valve for the artificial heart. In: Akutsu T, Koyanagi H (eds) Heart replacement: Artificial heart 4. Springer, Tokyo, pp 41–44

9. Atsumi K, Fujimasa I, Imachi K, Nakajima M, Tsukagoshi S, Mabuchi K, Motomura K, Kouno A, Ono T, Miyamoto A, Takido N, Inou N (1985) Long-term heart substitution with an artificial heart in goats. ASAIO J 8:155–165

10. Levy RJ, Schoen FJ, Anderson HC, Harasaki H, Koch TH, Brown W, Lian JB, Cumming R, Gavin JB (1991) Cardiovascular implant calcification: a survey and update. Biomaterials 12:707–714

11. Imachi K (1986) Long-term use of artificial heat without anticoagulant. In: Nosé Y, Kjellstrand C, Ivanovich P (eds) Progress in artificial organs—1985. ISAO Press, Cleveland, pp 319–326

12. Vašků J (1986) Total artificial heart research in Czechoslovakia: patho-physiological evaluation of long-term experiments performed from 1979 to 1985. In: Akutsu T (ed) Artificial heart 1. Springer, Tokyo, pp 161–179

Discussion

Dr. Galletti:
Did you detect any cellular components in this calcium deposit?

Dr. Imachi:
No, I did not find any.

Dr. Vasku:
My question is to Professor Imachi. Do you think that there is a great difference between calcification of collagen, of cartilage, of bone, and of biomaterials? Is it, according to your opinion, a big difference?

Dr. Imachi:
I don't know if there is calcification in the collagen, but I expect that some mechanism will be the same.

Dr. Vasku:
Yes, I think I agree with you, because there may be, in some details, some differences in these kinds of calcifications but they have some common denominators that's great feedback. These are inhibitors of calcifications, and they work. Because, for example, if we have patients with scleroderma it means that all pyrophosphates are removed from the skin due to extreme activity of phosphatases. So, this is a problem which we must think about even in the artificial biomaterials.

Dr. Imachi:
Yes, I think so.

Dr. Vasku:
It is, for example, different from dystrophic calcification. Due to dead and decomposed cells and mitochondria calcium, it goes very quickly, without any plan. But calcification due to matrix vesicles is very complicated and goes in two phases: they are the start of calcifying nucleation and its regulation by phosphatases, which are produced in the intravesicular matrix.

Dr. Kataoka:
Related to your work, I would like to emphasize the work done by Professor Takahara in Kyushu University. They studied the relationship between the calcification and phospholipid uptake in some polyurethane compounds. Their conclusion is that a relationship exists, and this is related to the microarchitecture of the polyurethane compounds. So, I would like to know, have you observed a difference in phospholipid uptake in different materials which you used for this jellyfish valve?

Dr. Imachi:
No, our experience is only for one material.

Dr. Kataoka:
Is that pure polyurethane or copolymers?

Dr. Imachi:
It's a copolymer of the polyurethane with poly-dimethyl siloxane. It's similar to Avcothane, made by the Nippon Zeon Company.

Dr. Kataoka:
I think it must be interesting to see the relationship between the microarchitecture and possible uptake of phospholipids in your system.

Dr. Imachi:
Yes, I want to do that, but it needs a very long time, so it's a very difficult experiment.

Dr. Vasku:
I agree, it's very important, because acidic phospholipids in vesicular matrix initiate the whole process of calcification by attacking the calcium.

Dr. Watson:
What's the amount of mechanical strain at the sites of calcification?

Dr. Imachi:
You mean the creep expansion?

Dr. Watson:
The strain during opening-closing.

Dr. Imachi:
Originally the membranes were flat. And the height of the spokes is 2mm, so it stretched maximally more than 1.5mm, as shown in the slide.

Dr. Watson:
So, what is the percent strain then?

Dr. Imachi:
What should I say about percent?

Dr. Watson:
We can discuss my question later.

Dr. Reul:
Dr. Reul from Aachen, Germany. When you use these valves in the animals you apparently had progressive stiffening. Is it due to calcification? And you also mentioned that you had no thrombus formation. How do you explain that, and you should have lots of flow separation and stagnation areas when the valve gets stiff, and still you got no thrombosis. What is your explanation for that?

Dr. Imachi:
You mean on the calcification?

Dr. Reul:
I mean, due to the calcification you got stiffening of the valves where it didn't open fully, and you must have some areas of stagnation and so on.

Dr. Imachi:
I do not believe the membrane is so stiff. The membranes are very thin. So if it is calcified it can be fully opened and closed, because in the animal experiments we did not need to increase the driving pressure.

Dr. Reul:
So the function was not impaired by a calcification?

Dr. Imachi:
Yes, that's correct.

Surface Modification Techniques for the Artificial Heart

Masahiro Waki[1], Chisato Nojiri[2], Hidekazu Hayashi[1], Takayuki Kido[2], Noboru Saito[2], Tomoko Sugiyama[2], Kazuhiko Ishihara[3], Nobuo Nakabayashi[3], Akio Kishida[4], Mitsuru Akashi[4], Kiyotaka Sakai[1], and Tetsuzo Akutsu[2]

Summary. We evaluated different surface modification techniques for polymeric materials used in the artificial heart. Proposed approaches to design nonthrombogenic polymer surfaces include (1) phase-separated micro-domain surfaces, (2) hydrophilic surfaces. (3) surfaces incorporating a bioactive molecule and (4) biomembrane-like surfaces. We have developed several in situ surface modification techniques to improve the blood compatibility of the blood-contacting surfaces of medical devices, including HEMA-styrene block copolymer (HEMA-st) coating, polyethylene glycol (PEG) grafting, human thrombomodulin (h-TM) and heparin (HEP) immobilization, and 2-methacryloyl oxyethyl phosphorylcholine (MPC) copolymer coating, each onto a segmented polyurethane (PU) surface. These surface-modified PUs were evaluated using an epifluorescent video microscope (EVM system) combined with a parallel plate flow cell for assessing in vitro platelet adhesion and activation and complement activation. All surfaces showed significantly lower platelet adhesion than nontreated PU, with the following ranking: HEMA-st $\geqq$ MPC > h-TM $\fallingdotseq$ HEP $\geqq$ PEG > PU. As for complement activation, h-TM and HEP showed the least C3a production, which we attributed to their inherent inhibitory effects on complement activation. HEP, PEG, or MPC copolymer treatments were applied in situ to the blood-contacting surfaces of artificial hearts made of PU, and evaluated ex vivo using 1-month implantation of the left ventricular assist devices in sheep. The preliminary results of ex vivo evaluations tend to confirm the in vitro results.

Key words: Surface modification — Epifluorescent video microscopy — Polyurethanes — Platelet adhesion — Blood compatibility

Introduction

Segmented polyurethanes (PU) are currently being used to fabricate various medical devices, such as artificial hearts and pacemaker leads, because of their good mechanical properties. However, the limited blood compatibility of PU remains a problem, especially for long-term in vivo application.

Hypotheses proposed to design nonthrombogenic polymer surfaces include: (1) phase-separated microdomain surfaces, (2) hydrophilic surfaces, (3) surfaces incorporating bioactive molecules and (4) biomembrane-like surfaces. We have developed surface modification techniques to improve the blood compatibility of PU according to these hypotheses. These include: (1) 2-hydroxyethyl methacrylate (HEMA)–styrene block copolymer (HEMA-st) coating; (2) polyethylene glycol (PEG)grafting; (3) human thrombomodulin (h-TM) and heparin (HEP) immobilization; and (4) 2-methacryloyl oxyethyl phosphorylcholine (MPC) copolymer coating.

In this study, we evaluated these surface-modified PUs using an epifluorescent video microscope combined with a parallel plate flow cell (EVM system) for in vitro platelet adhesion/activation and complement activation. HEP, PEG, or MPC were applied to blood-contacting surfaces of an artificial heart pump made of PU, and evaluated ex vivo for 1 month using sheep with modified left ventricular assist devices (LVAD). Nontreated PU was used as a control in both in vitro and ex vivo experiments.

Materials and Methods

Surface Modification

HEMA-Styrene Coating
An amphiphilic ABA-type block copolymer composed of 2-hydroxyethyl methacrylate (HEMA) and styrene (HEMA-st) was synthesized by a coupling reaction of oligo-HEMA with oligostyrene. HEMA-st is known to have hydrophilic/hydrophobic microdomain structures tens of nanometers in size. The excellent nonthrombogenicity of HEMA-st, and details of its synthesis and characterization, have been reported previously [1–3]. The PU surfaces were coated three times by applying a 1% w/v HEMA-st solution in N,N'-dimethylformamide (DMF), followed by air drying at 40°C for 24h.

[1] Waseda University, Tokyo 169, Japan
[2] Terumo Corporation R&D Center, 1500 Inokuchi, Nakai-machi, Ashigarakami-gun, Kanagawa 259-01, Japan
[3] Tokyo Medical and Dental University, Tokyo 113, Japan
[4] Kagoshima University, Kagoshima 890, Japan

PEG Grafting

Photoreactive PEG (MW = 1360; Union Carbide Chemicals and Plastics, Tokyo, Japan) was prepared by reaction of PEG with p-azidobenzoyl chloride (Tokyo Kasei, Tokyo, Japan). A photoreactive *p*-azidophenyl-derivatized PEG solution (0.1% w/v in ethanol) was coated on PU surfaces and washed with a 10% v/v ethanol solution, followed by air drying. The samples were then irradiated by ultraviolet (UV) light using a UV generator (HLS 100U; Hoya-Schott, Tokyo, Japan). Upon UV light irradiation, the azidophenyl group is converted to a highly reactive nitrene which immediately reacts with the neighboring hydrocarbons of PU covalently Details of the photoreaction has been described elsewhere [4].

h-TM Immobilization

Thrombomodulin (TM) is a newly described endothelial-cell-associated protein that functions as a potent natural anticoagulant by converting thrombin from a procoagulant protease to an anticoagulant [5]. In this study, we prepared PU grafted with poly (acrylic acid) (PAAc, Wako Pure Chemicals, Osaka, Japan) using corona discharge. Then, PAAc-grafted PU was immersed in mixture of h-TM (Asahi Chemical Industry, Tokyo, Japan) and water-soluble carbodiimide (Nakalai Tesque, Kyoto, Japan) solution. The immobilization reaction was performed at 4°C for 24h. After a predetermined time, the modified surface was repeatedly washed with phosphate-buffered saline (PBS, pH = 7.4) and freeze dried [6].

HEP Immobilization

PU was first treated with ozone gas, and poly (ethyleneimine) (PEI) was grafted onto the surfaces through a coupling reaction between the peroxide on the PU surface and the NH_2 group of the PEI. HEP was then covalently attached to the spacer by glutaraldehyde, followed by the reduction of the Schiff's base. The PU with immobilized HEP was washed with distilled water to remove unreacted reagents, then air-dried at room temperature [7–9].

MPC Copolymer Coating

Recent studies have demonstrated that MPC copolymers have excellent nonthrombogenic properties by virtue of reducing protein adsorption and cell adhesion. Since the MPC copolymers have a typical phospholipid polar group, they have a strong affinity for phospholipid molecules in plasma; phospholipids are therefore adsorbed on the MPC copolymer surfaces to form a "self-assembled biomimetic membrane", thereby inhibiting protein adsorption and cell adhesion/activation on the surface of the material [10].

In this study, we synthesized three methacrylates, having butylurethane, benzylurethene, or phenylure-thane in the side chain. One of these methacrylates, butylmethacrylate (BMA), was copolymerized with MPC to form the the MPC copolymer. The PU surfaces were modified by coating with a 0.5% w/v MPC copolymer solution in ethanol. The urethane moieties of this copolymer had been proven to have strong affinity for PU, and the coating layer formed by this copolymer was highly stable in water [11].

In Vitro Blood Compatibility

Figure 1 shows a schematic diagram of the epifluorescent video microscope (EVM) system. The surface-modified PUs were evaluated using EVM combined with a parallel plate flow cell. A surface-modified PU film was mounted on the flow cell Initially, PBS (pH 7.4) was passed through the flow cell via poly (vinyl) chloride (PVC) tubing connected to the flow cell for 1h at a wall shear rate of $100s^{-1}$. The luminal surfaces of the PVC tubing (1.8mm inner diameter 90cm total length) were coated with a PU solution and modified using the same methods as for PU films. Whole human blood was drawn from healthy donors, anticoagulated with heparin (2U/ml), then immediately incubated with the fluorescent dye Mepacrine (5mM) for 30min at 37°C for platelet labeling. The blood was substituted for the PBS in the flow cell, and then passed through for 20min. The flow cell was set to be irradiated by the excited light at the center of the flow cell intermittently for 2s every minute to prevent photo enhancement. A camera coupled with the device and mounted on an epifluorescent microscope transmitted the image of platelets to a hard disk which allowed subsequent analysis by an image processor. From this, the ratio of the surface area of the test materials to the adherent platelet area was calculated. Nontreated PU was used as a control. The blood that had passed through the flow cell was collected and centrifuged at $2000 \times g$ for 30min, then the supernatant platelet activation β-thromboglobulin (β-TG) and complement activation (C3a) levels were measured by enzyme immunoassay and radio immunoassay, respectively, and compared with the samples prior to the EVM experiment [7,12].

Ex Vivo Evaluation

HEP, PEG, and MPC were applied in situ onto blood-contacting surfaces of artificial hearts made of PU and evaluated for 1 month in a sheep ex vivo model using a 20-cm^3 diaphragm-type artificial heart pump (LVAD). Eleven sheep weighing between 29 and 86kg were anesthetized with ketamine, intubated, and mechanically ventilated. Anesthesia was maintained with enflurane (Ethrene; Abbott Laboratories, North Chicago, IL, USA). The Dacron outflow graft (C.R. Bard, Tewksburg, MA, USA) was sutured to the descending

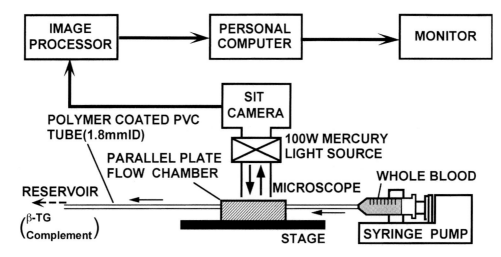

Fig. 1. Epifluorescent video microscopy (EVM) experimental apparatus. The flow chamber was mounted on the stage of the microscope. The syringe pump controlled the flow rate. The mercury are light source of the microscope was modulated by the insertion of a $\frac{1}{16}$% neutral density filter. SIT, silicon intensified targee; β-*TG*, β-thromboglobulin

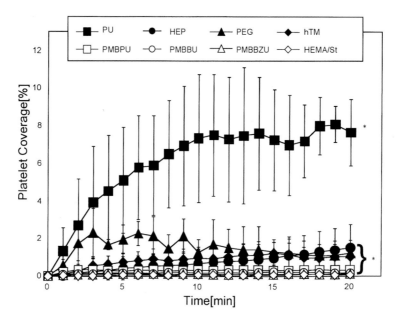

Fig. 2. Time course of platelet coverage on materials during a 20-min EVM experiment. Platelet adhesion was expressed as the percentage area of platelet coverage on the basis of 0.03 mm^2 of the substrate area. *PU*, segmented polyurethane. Coated PU: *HEP*, heparin; *PEG*, polytehylene glycol; *hTM*, human thrombomodulin; PMBPU, MPC copolymer having phenylurethane in the side chain; PMBBU, MPC copolymer having buthylurethane in the side chain; PMBBZU, MPC copolymer having benzylurethane in the side chain

aorta and the inflow cannula was inserted into the left atrium through a cuff sutured to the left atrial appendage. The bypass flow was maintained between 1.5 and 2 l/min throughout the experiment. The pumps were removed after 1 month or when interdevice thrombus was detected. The pumps were then perfusion-washed with saline, soaked in Kornovsky's fixative, and analyzed by a scanning electron microscope (SEM, Model JSM-840, JEOL, Tokyo, Japan).

Results

In Vitro Evaluation

Figure 2 shows the platelet adhesion behavior over time for the modified PU. All surfaces showed signifi-

Fig. 3. The effect of materials on **a** β-thromboglobulin (β-TG) release from platelets and **b** C3a producton after a 20-min EVM experiment. Coatings were as for Fig. 2

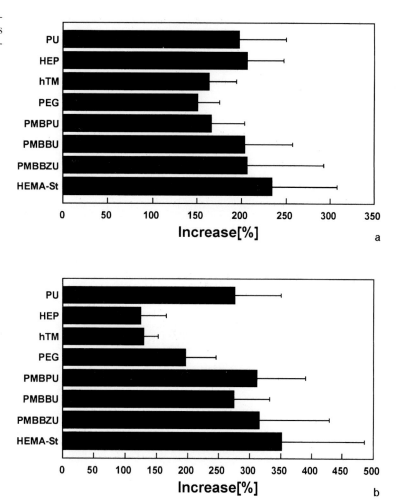

cantly lower platelet adhesion than to PU with the following ranking: HEMA-st showed the least platelet adhesion; MPC copolymers were comparable to HEMA-st; at slightly higher platelet adhesion levels, h-TM and heparin showed nearly the same behavior; and PEG showed significantly more platelet adhesion during the initial 5 min than the others. Figure 3 shows the effect of the materials on β-TG released from platelets and C3a production after a 20-min perfusion. Surface modification with h-TM or heparin resulted in the least C3a production, perhaps because of the inherent inhibitory effects of these molecules on complement activation [13].

Ex Vivo Evaluation

Figure 4 shows the photographs and SEM pictures of the control and the surface-modified LVAD pumps after 1 month. The control pump (Fig. 4a) demon-strated considerable amounts of microthrombi along the diaphrgm-housing (D–H) junction. For the control pump, thrombus formation in these areas usually developed within one month, and occasionally within a few days. SEM pictures of a control pump showed occasional platelet depositions with distorted morphologies and aggregates on the diaphragm and housing. On the other hand, heparinized (Fig. 4b) and MPC copolymer-coated (Fig. 4c) pumps showed very clean surfaces without detectable thrombi, and SEM pictures of these surfaces demonstrated significantly less platelet adhesion and activation compared with the control pump. The PEG-grafted pump (Fig. 4d) developed thrombi along the D–H junction and at the outflow valve after 1 month's implantation, and SEM pictures showed a significantly larger quantity of adhered platelets and microthrombi when compared to the heparinized and MPC-coated pumps, although the amount of platelet adhesion was much less than that of the control pump.

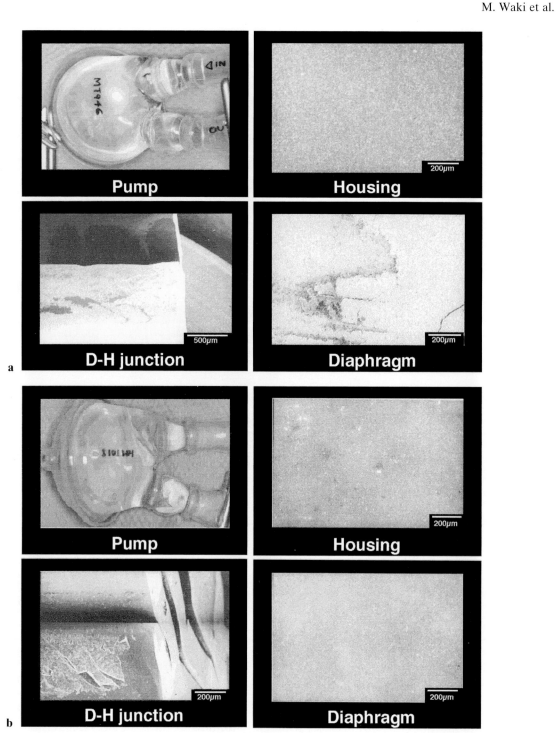

Fig. 4a–d. The photographs and scanning electron micrographs (SEM) of surface-modified left ventricular assist device (LVAD) pumps after a 1-month implantation. **a** The photograph and SEM of the nontreated pump. There were many microthrombi along the diaphrgm-housing (D–H) junction, and platelet depositions with distorted morphologies and aggregates were observed on the diaphragm and housing. **b** The photograph and SEM of the heparinized pump. HEP-immobilized surfaces were very clean, without detectable thrombi, and there was significantly less platelet adhesion and activation compared with the control pump. **c** The photograph and SEM of the MPC-

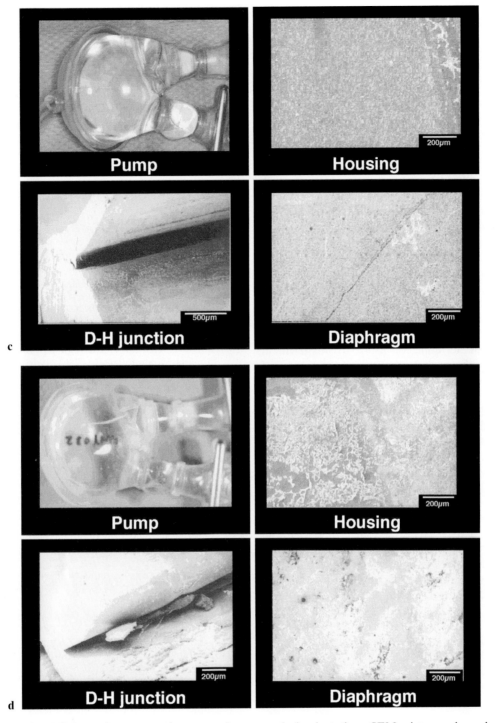

coated pump. The MPC-copolymer-coated pump also showed very clean surfaces comparable to heparin-immobilized surfaces. **d** The photograph and SEM of the PEG-grafted pump. The PEG-grafted pump developed thrombi along the D–H junction and at the outflow valve after a 1-month implantation. SEM pictures showed significantly more adhered platelets and microthrombi when compared with the heparinized and MPC-coated pumps, although the amount of platelet adhesion was much less than that on the control pump

Discussion

In this study, we selected four surface modification techniques to improve the blood compatibility of PU, and evaluated these in both in vitro and ex vivo experiments. The HEMA-st coating showed the highest resistance to platelet adhesion in in vitro EVM experiments. However, this type of coating was not suitable for the moving diaphragm of a diaphragm-type artificial heart pump because of its poor mechanical properties and the need for an organic solvent which deforms the shape of the pump components. h-TM immobilization using corona discharge was also difficult to apply in situ in medical devices with a complex design such as artificial hearts, since the corona discharge might not activate all the inner surfaces of the fabricated devices. On the other hand, PEG grafting using photoreaction, heparin immobilization using ozone oxidation, and coating with MPC copolymers from an ethanol solution, can provide uniform in situ surface modification on medical devices with a complex design. Of these coatings, PEG showed the highest level of platelet adhesion in in vitro experiments and generated the greatest amounts of thrombi in a 1-month ex vivo LVAD experiment in sheep. HEP immobilization using ozone oxidation and MPC coating both resulted in low platelet adhesion as well as improved blood compatibilities in ex vivo experiments, compared with PEG grafting and the control surface. Furthermore, these techniques appeared suitable for in situ surface modification onto medical devices, even those of a complex design.

In vitro methods to evaluate the blood compatibility of various biomaterials are useful to predict the in vivo performance of these materials, since in vivo studies are time-consuming and costly. In this study, we observed a good correlation between the results of in vitro EVM experiments and ex vivo evaluations using sheep connected for 1 month to a surface-modified LVADs. The EVM system proved to be an excellent and sensitive in vitro evaluation method for predicting the ex vivo blood compatibility of biomaterials.

Conclusion

Surface-modified PUs were evaluated in vitro using an EVM system and ex vivo in a sheep model with long-term LVAD connection. The results showed that:

1. All modified surfaces showed significantly lower platelet adhesion compared with control PU, and the ranking was as follows: HEMA-st ≧ MPCs > h-TM ≒ HEP ≧ PEG > PU.

2. HEMA-st showed the least platelet adhesion.
3. The MPC copolymer coating also showed a low level of platelet adhesion, comparable to HEMA-st.
4. Both h-TM and HEP surfaces gave the least C3a production, because of their inherent inhibitory effects on complement activation.
5. The preliminary results of ex vivo experiments confirmed those of in vitro evaluations.

References

1. Okano T, Nishiyama S, Shinohara I, Akaike T, Sakurai Y, Kataoka K, Tsuruta T (1981) Effect of hydrophilic and hydrophobic microdomains on mode of interaction between block copolymers and blood platelets. J Biomed Mater Res 15:393–402
2. Nojiri C, Okano T, Grainger D, Park GK, Nakahama S, Suzuki K, Kim SW (1987) Evaluation of nonthrombogenic polymers in a new rabbit A-A shunt model. ASAIO Trans 33:596–601
3. Okano T, Aoyagi T, Kataoka K, Abe K, Sakurai Y, Shimada M, Shinohara I (1986) Hydrophilic-hydrophobic microdomain surfaces having an ability to suppress platelet aggregation and their in vivtro antithrombogenicity. J Biomed Mater Res 20:919–927
4. Matsuda T, Inoue K, Ozeki E, Akutsu T (1990) Novel surface modification technology based on photoreactive chemistry. Artif Organs 14:193–195
5. Kishida A, Ueno Y, Maruyama I, Akashi M (1994) Immobilization of human thrombomodulin onto biomaterials — comparison of immobilization methods and evaluation of antithrombogenicity ASAIO J 40:840–845
6. Akashi M, Maruyama I, Fukudome N, Yashima E (1992) Immobilization of human thrombomodulin on glass beads and its anticoagulant activity. Bioconjug Chem 3:363–365
7. Nojiri C, Kuroda S, Saito N, Park KD, Hagiwara K, Sensyu K, Kido T, Sugiyama T, Kijima T, Kim YH, Sakai K, Akutsu T (1995) In vitro studies of immobilized heparin and sulfonated polyurethane using epifluorescent video microscopy. ASAIO J 41:389–394
8. Park KD, Okano T, Nojiri C, Kim SW (1988) Heparin immobilization onto segmented polyurethaneurea surfaces — effect of hydrophilic spacers. J Biomed Mater Res 22:977–992
9. Fujimoto K, Takebayashi Y, Inoue H, Ikada Y (1993) Ozone-induced graft polymerization onto polymer surface. J Polymer Sci 31:1035–1043
10. Ishihara K, Ueda T, Nakabayashi N (1990) Preparation of phospholipid polymers and their properties as polymer hydrogel membranes. Polymer J 22:355–360
11. Ishihara K, Hanyuda H, Nakabayashi N (1995) Synthesis of phospholipid polymers having a urethane bond in the side chain as coating material on segmented polyurethane and their platelet adhesion-resistant properties. Biomaterials 16:873–879

12. Kawagoishi N, Nojiri C, Sensyu K, Kido T, Nagai H, Kanamori T, Sakai K, Koyanagi H, Akutsu T (1994) In vitro evaluation of platelet/biomaterial interactions in an epifluorescent video microscope combined with a parallel plate flow cell. Artif Organs 18:588–595

13. Weiler JM, Yurt RW, Fearon DT, Austen KF (1978) Modulation of the formation of the amplification convertase of complement, C3b, Bb, by native and commercial heparin. J Exp Med 147:409–421

Discussion

Dr. Imachi:
I have one question. What kind of polyurethane did you use in this experiment? In my impression, the antithrombogenicity of this polyurethane is worse than that of conventionally used polyurethane.

Dr. Waki:
We used polyurethane Tecoflex EG 80-A.

Dr. Imachi:
And did you use other polyurethanes? Only one kind of polyurethane as a control?

Dr. Waki:
Tecoflex was used in the EVM system. For ex vivo evaluation, we used Pellethane.

Dr. Nojiri:
I'd like to add my comment. We already evaluated several kinds of polyurethanes, including Tecoflex, Biomer TM3, and Pellethane. We evaluated all these polyurethanes in the EVM system, and the result was that the Tecoflex was the best. That's why we used the Tecoflex as a control.

Dr. Harasaki:
Dr. Waki, I would like to ask about your platelet adhesion test on the various surfaces. What kind of test method did you use when you expressed the platelet coverage in percent?

Dr. Waki:
Using an image processor and a personal computer.

Dr. Harasaki:
And SEM?

Dr. Waki:
No. Video imaging.

Dr. Harasaki:
I think the platelet is labeled by fluorescence. Is that so?

Dr. Waki:
Platelets were labeled with fluorescent dye and incubated for 30 minutes. Platelet adhesion was observed every 1 minute for 20 minutes, in real time.

Dr. Harasaki:
Oh, every 1 minute for 20 minutes.

Dr. Waki:
Yes.

Durability of Endothelial Cell Monolayers Inside a Beating Cardiac Prosthesis

Victor V. Nikolaychik, Matthew D. Silverman, Mark M. Samet, Dawn M. Wankowski, and Peter I. Lelkes

Summary. Thromboembolic complications associated with the use of cardiac prostheses might be alleviated by lining the blood-contacting surfaces of these devices with a functional monolayer of endothelial cells. In the current study, we tested our hypothesis that precoating textured surfaces of artificial ventricles with various plasma proteins could enhance the resistance of endothelial cell monolayers to hemodynamic forces generated within an in vitro mock circulatory loop system. Bovine jugular vein endothelial cells were grown to confluence on the luminal surface of artificial ventricles constructed of textured, medical grade polyurethane (Biospan), which had been precoated with either fibronectin or plasma cryoprecipitate. Following 7 days of culturing under static conditions, the endothelialized ventricles were connected to a mock loop system, and exposed to pulsatile flow for 6 and 24h (60bpm, 3.2l/min mean flow rate, 150mmHg ejection pressure). Retention of endothelial cells was evaluated by Alamar Blue assay before and after each run. Monolayer integrity and additional morphometric parameters were also assessed by direct visualization, employing various light and electron microscopic techniques. In ventricles which had been precoated with fibronectin, Alamar Blue assay indicated cellular retention to be 77% ± 4% and 72% ± 5% of static controls, after 6 and 24h, respectively. In marked contrast, cryoprecipitate-coated ventricles retained over 90% of their endothelial cell lining through 24h of exposure to physiological hemodynamic conditions. These findings were confirmed by visual inspection. Our study demonstrates the feasibility of maintaining an intact endothelial surface in a beating ventricular prosthesis, and that the durability of the cell layer is highly dependent upon the selection of biomaterial surface topography and protein coating.

Key words: Artificial heart — Ventricular assist device — Cell–biomaterial interactions — Endothelialization

Introduction

The successful clinical use of permanently implanted cardiac prosthetic devices, such as total artificial hearts or ventricular assist devices (VADs), continues to be thwarted by problems of hemocompatibility mani-

Laboratory of Cell Biology, Department of Medicine, University of Wisconsin Medical School, Milwaukee Clinical Campus, Sinai Samaritan Medical Center, P.O. Box 342, Milwaukee, WI 53201-0342, USA

fested primarily in their tendency to initiate unwanted coagulation [1]. Previous studies suggest that the hemocompatibility of cardiovascular prostheses can be significantly improved by lining their blood-contacting surfaces with a functional monolayer of autologous endothelial cells (EC) [2–4]. In recent years, we have cultured EC monolayers in cell culture chambers modeled after human ventricles, and have subjected them to complex flow fields, cyclic strain, and elevated hydrostatic pressure to test the effects of these hemodynamic parameters on various cellular functions [5–7]. We also described the advantages of using rough, textured polyurethane (PU) surfaces rather than smooth ones for the purpose of endothelialization [4], and of precoating biomaterials with a plasma cryoprecipitate-based provisional matrix [8]. Additionally, new approaches have been characterized for rotational seeding of PU ventricles [9], and for continual, nondestructive evaluation of EC coverage in such devices [10]. In this communication, we compare the effect of various biomaterial precoatings on the durability of bovine jugular vein endothelial cell (BJVEC) monolayers tested under simulated physiological hemodynamic conditions, inside a beating ventricular prosthesis.

Materials and Methods

Endothelial Cell Isolation, Culture and Seeding

Bovine jugular vein EC were isolated, cultured, and subsequently seeded according to established procedures [9,11], and were used between passages 5 and 9. Cells grown in PU ventricles had their medium replaced after seeding, and every third day thereafter.

Polyurethane Ventricles

Based on the design and function of the Milwaukee Heart [12] polyurethane ventricles were fabricated from a textured medical-grade PU (Biospan, Polymer Technology Group, Emeryville, CA, USA) by the lost-wax technique. Following insertion into the VAD casing, ventricles were coated with either bovine plasma cryoprecipitate (2 mg/ml) or bovine plasma fibronectin (20 μg/ml), and were then seeded with BJVEC (4–6×10^7 cells/125 ml medium, 3 h) on a pitch-yaw rotation apparatus at 10 rotations/h [11].

Mock Loop System

Design and operation details of the mock loop system have been previously described in detail [11]. Pulsatile flow parameters used in this study were 60 bpm, 3.2 l/min mean flow rate, and 150 mmHg maximum ejection pressure.

Cell Quantification

Cell retention on the luminal surface of ventricles was assessed every third day during up to 12 days of static culturing conditions, and immediately prior to and after mock loop testing, by the Alamar Blue (AB) assay [10]. Additional morphometric data were obtained by 3-(4,5-dimethylthiazol-2-yl)-2,5-diphenyl tetrazolium bromide (MTT) staining of cellular/PU interaction [13], and by visual evaluation using light and scanning electron microscopy (SEM) [11].

Experimental Design

After 7 days of static culture, fully assembled endothelialized VADs were connected to the mock loop system, and were run for either 6 or 24 h under the aforementioned dynamic conditions. In all experiments, identical VADs maintained under static conditions served as controls.

Statistical Analysis

All experiments were repeated at least four times. Numerical data are presented as mean ± SD. The significance of variability between the various experimental groups was determined by ANOVA testing, with $P < 0.05$ considered statistically different.

Results

Low-power stereomicroscopic examination of the surface of untreated, textured PU ventricles revealed abundant, randomly dispersed cavities of varying dimensions, ranging from 50 to 200 μm in diameter (Fig. 1a). They differed from each other in width, length, and angle of inclination, and had no particular orientation relative to the main axis of the ventricle (Fig. 1b).

After 3 h of rotational EC seeding, in line with previous observations using other cell types [11], the efficacy of seeding was ≈50% on fibronectin coating and

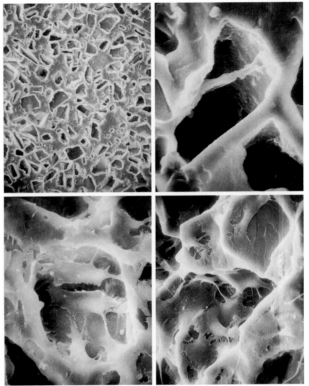

a,b

c,d

Fig. 1. Scanning electron microscopic view of the luminal surface of a ventricle. Untreated porous surface at **a** low, and **b** high magnification (×80, ×640, repectively); **c** high magnification (×640) of a confluent monolayer of bovine jugular vein endothelial cells (BJVEC) grown on a plasma cryoprecipitate-coated surface prior to pumping; **d** BJVEC on a plasma cryoprecipitate-coated sample obtained from a ventricle after 24 h of pumping

≈60% on plasma cryoprecipitate coating, based on evaluation of unattached BJVEC in aliquots of cell-seeding media. At this time, attached cells were primarily localized within the pores, and surface coverage was estimated to be ≈40%–50%. By three days after seeding, the monolayers in the ventricles had reached confluence on both the fibronectin- and cryoprecipitate-coated surfaces (Fig. 2a). After attaining confluence, EC monolayer densities remained constant for 12 days under static conditions, and cell coverage on PU ventricles was uniform and complete in both groups. The EC monolayer appeared densely packed, with randomly oriented cells covering both the hills and valleys of the textured scaffold. There was no evidence of cell sprouting, aggregation, or bilayer formation atop either PU coating, as evaluated by both light and electron microscopy. Figure 1c shows a typical SEM view of an EC monolayer grown on cryoprecipitate-coated PU, at the initiation of a 24-h mock loop experiment.

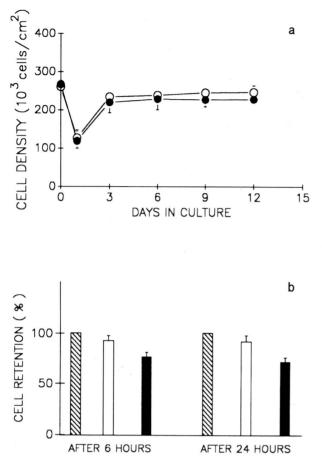

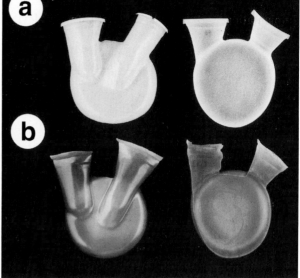

Fig. 2. Alamar Blue determination of **a** cell densities of BJVEC monolayers grown under static conditions on select surface coatings, and **b** cell retention after 6 and 24h of pumping, as compared to static controls (*hatched bars*). *Open circles/white bars*, cryoprecipitate-coated surface; *closed circles/black bars*, fibronectin-coated surface

Fig. 3. 3-(4,5-dimethylthiazol-2-yl)-2,5-diphenyl tetrazolium bromide (MTT)-formazan stained ventricles. **a** Nonendothelialized polyurethane (PU) ventricle does not display any staining. **b** Typical staining of PU surface with firmly attached cells after 24h of pumping. Minimal cell loss can be noticed (*light spots*), especially in the vicinity of mitral and aortic valve sites. This image is in accordance with cell-density readings obtained by the Alamar Blue (AB) assay

After 7 days of culturing under static conditions, endothelialized VADs were connected to the mock loop system for 6 or 24h. Following 6h of continuous pumping, the AB assay indicated that the number of EC retained on fibronectin-coated PU was 77% ± 4% of that observed in static controls (Fig. 2b, $P < 0.005$, $n = 5$). After 24h of hemodynamic simulation, the percentage of EC attached to PU/fibronectin was further reduced, with only 72% ± 5% of the initially intact EC monolayer remaining attached to the luminal surface ($P < 0.005$ vs static controls, $n = 4$). In strong contrast to the data obtained on fibronectin coatings, EC monolayers generated on plasma cryoprecipitate-coated PU were highly resistant to damage and denudation caused by the flow, pressure, and straining forces experienced inside the beating ventricle. Remarkably, after 6 and 24h of hemodynamic simulation, there was no significant loss of cells, with 92% ±

3% and 92% ± 4%, respectively, of the initial EC monolayer remaining intact and attached to the ventricle luminal surface (Fig. 2b, $P > 0.5$ vs static controls, and $n = 5$ in both cases). The marked enhancement of cryoprecipitate vs fibronectin coating to withstand the various dynamic forces associated with the mock loop circuitry was highly significant ($P < 0.01$ and $n = 4$–6 at both time points).

Visual examination of MTT staining of cellular/PU interactions within ventricles supported the results obtained by AB measurements (Fig. 3). This assay allows evaluation of both the extent of surface coverage by cells, and of their firmness of attachment to the substratum [13], with colorless sites indicative of complete denudation, and variable-intensity staining providing a measure of the strength of EC attachment. Additionally, routine light microscopic inspection of $KMnO_4$/toluidine blue-stained samples which were excised from various regions of the ventricle confirmed negligible EC denudation on cryoprecipitate-coated PU. High-resolution SEM visualization of the endothelialized cryoprecipitate-coated surfaces (Fig. 1d) revealed close apposition of densely packed and tightly attached cells, suggesting the in vitro establishment of a durable endothelial monolayer.

Discussion

Implantation of cardiovascular prosthetic devices, from small caliber grafts to total artificial hearts, often results in aberrant hemostasis and thrombotic complications due to the biological incompatibility between their luminal surfaces and the blood which circulates within them. Although great improvements in biomaterial design and composition have been accomplished, none developed to date posses all of the necessary functional traits (e.g., nonthrombogenicity and nonimmunogenicity), of the native quiescent vascular endothelium which they, ideally, would closely mimic. Endothelialization of vascular prostheses, as a potential means of alleviating postimplantation thrombotic complications, was introduced nearly 20 years ago [2,3]. In subsequent years, advances in our ability to culture and study EC in vitro, to create improved biomaterials and vascular prosthetic designs, and to develop advanced laboratory models of the in vivo hemodynamic environment have been merged to make possible rapid progress in evaluating the practicality of this concept [14–18].

Requisite for successful endothelialization of permanent vascular prostheses is the construction of their blood-contacting surfaces with materials upon which EC can form continuous monolayers that are highly resistant to the physical forces present in the circulation. Currently, polyurethanes offer the greatest potential for success in this capacity, as they are inexpensive, nontoxic, nonimmunogenic, resistant to degradation, and can support EC proliferation [19–22].

In a previous report, we detailed the importance of the surface texture of the PU scaffolding in optimizing EC growth and monolayer maintenance [4,9,11]. In the current study, we found that precoating the lumen of textured PU ventricles with autologous plasma proteins significantly enhanced cellular retention in a simulated hemodynamic environment, and that the degree of augmentation was highly dependent upon which proteins were employed. After 24h testing in the mock circulatory loop system, EC monolayers grown inside cryoprecipitate-treated VADs remained essentially intact, while substantial denudation occurred inside VADs which were precoated with purified fibronectin alone. Thus, it is apparent that the selection of substratum composition is pivotal in maximizing cellular retention in VADs experiencing typical cardiac flow conditions. In both cases, however, the majority of total cell loss sustained occurred within 6h after the onset of physiological pulsatile flow, and did not increase significantly in the subsequent 18h. This is in agreement with earlier findings, both in mock loop systems [14,15] and following in vivo implantation [16–18] of such devices. The combination of a porous PU

surface with a tightly juxtaposed multiprotein layer holds promise for further improving the durability of the EC monolayer. Considerable amounts of cryoprecipitate can be adsorbed to the textured PU surface. This could be spiked with various defined attachment and/or growth factors, should they prove advantageous in maintaining monolayer integrity, and serve as a reservoir for their long-term availability or gradual release.

To date, most studies which have sought to assess the efficiency of endothelialization have relied upon end-point techniques which mandate experimental termination. In the current study, besides using classical histological and SEM techniques for evaluating cell numbers, we also employed the AB assay, which provides a nondestructive method for the continual monitoring of the EC monolayer status in long-term experiments. It has proven to be highly reproducible, as verified by different archetypal techniques, and has the unique advantage of not precluding or interfering with subsequent functional investigations. Additionally, we have also employed MTT staining to provide information on both the extent of EC coverage and the firmness of cellular attachment to the PU substratum. By using a diverse variety of visualization/quantification methods, we are better able to discern critical morphometric parameters which exist within endothelialized prostheses.

From our experience, allowing time for an EC monolayer to "mature" beyond its initial attainment of confluence results in a lining which is much more resistant to denudation. Quiescence in a confluent EC monolayer is not tantamount to biological inactivity, but rather indicates a shifting in the functional priorities of the cells. After reaching confluence, EC continue to reevaluate and reorganize their associations with both one another and with their substratum. They express adhesion molecules on their surfaces, and deposit a complex extracellular matrix which is neither inert nor static, but instead is biologically multipotent and is continually remodeled. Their cytoskeletal network is reorganized, and intercellular communication is facilitated by the development of both extensive cell–cell contacts and autocrine/paracrine networks. Although the exact mechanism(s) by which time in culture increases resistance to monolayer damage by hemodynamic challenge is unclear, it appears that at least 6 days is necessary to provide maximum protection.

Selection of an appropriate source of EC for endothelialization is of obvious importance. We have previously compared performance of bovine EC derived from both the arterial and venous circuitry [11] and were unable to distinguish differences in their suitability, with respect to cell retention in a simulated hemodynamic environment. In this study, the accessibility of jugular vein for the isolation and propagation of autologous EC, without undue compromise to the overall patency of the animal's circulation, affords us with a practical source of cells for furthering these studies. Another potential source of large numbers of EC is the microcirculation, particularly the abundant capillary networks within adipose tissue. Albeit an attractive candidate, several barriers must be overcome prior to testing this approach. The availability of sufficient quantities of adipose tissue in young, lean animals presents the first obstacle. Efficient techniques for large-scale culturing of highly enriched adipose microvascular EC are still in development. Additionally, the functional profile of microvascular EC is not as well characterized as that of EC derived from the macrovasculature, and requires further investigation.

Although certainly encouraging, it must be recognized that the ability to establish a viable EC monolayer, which can endure the physical impositions inherent to the cardiac/arterial circulatory system, is not the endpoint to achieving successful endothelialization of cardiovascular prostheses. The next logical step is the thorough characterization of the biological functioning of these autologously transplanted EC. It remains to be demonstrated that, in the long-term in vivo scenario, these cells will continue to exhibit the antithrombotic and fibrinolytic traits which we desire (and optimistically expect) of them.

Acknowledgments. Special thanks to Mrs. I. Hernandez for her technical expertise in conducting the SEM studies. This work was supported in part by grants in aid from the Milwaukee Heart Research Foundation and from the American Heart Association, Wisconsin Affiliate.

References

1. Menconi MJ, Pockwinse S, Owen TA, Dasse KA, Stein GS, Lian JB (1995) Properties of blood-contacting surfaces of clinically implanted cardiac assist devices: gene expression, matrix composition, and ultrastructural characterization of cellular linings. J Cell Biochem 57:557–573
2. Wechezak AR, Mansfield PB (1979) Environmental influence of endothelial surface characteristics. Scanning Electron Microsc 3:857–864
3. Herring M, Gardner A, Glover J (1978) A single-staged technique for seeding vascular grafts with autogenous endothelium. Surgery 84:498–504
4. Lelkes PI, Samet MM (1991) Endothelialization of the luminal sac in artificial cardiac prostheses: a challenge for both biologists and engineers. J Biomech Eng 113:132–142
5. Lelkes PI, Samet MM (1991) Pulsatile flow and EC morphology in a VAD-like chamber. ASAIO J 37:M315–M316
6. Manolopoulos VG, Lelkes PI (1993) Cyclic strain and forskolin differentially induce cAMP production in phenotypically diverse endothelial cells. Biochem Biophys Res Commun 191:1379–1385
7. Silverman MD, Manolopoulos VG, Unsworth BR, Lelkes PI (1996) Tissue factor expression is differentially modulated by cyclic mechanical strain in various human endothelial cells. Blood Coagul Fibrinolysis 7:281–288
8. Nikolaychik VV, Samet MM, Lelkes PI (1994) A new, cryoprecipitate-based coating for improved endothelial cell attachment and growth on medical grade artificial surfaces. ASAIO J 40:M846–M852
9. Samet MM, Wankowski DM, Nikolaychik VV, Lelkes PI (1994) Endothelial cell seeding with rotation of a ventricular blood sac. ASAIO J 40:M319–M324
10. Nikolaychik VV, Samet MM, Lelkes PI (1996) A new method for continual quantitation of viable cells on endothelialized polyurethanes. J Biomater Sci Polym Ed 7(10):881–891
11. Nikolaychik VV, Wankowski DM, Samet MM, Lelkes PI (1996) In vitro testing of endothelial cell monolayers under dynamic conditions inside a beating ventricular prosthesis. ASAIO J 42:M487-M494
12. Gao H, Smith LM, Krymkowski MG, Kohl RJ, Schmidt DH, Christensen CW (1992) In vitro assessment of the Milwaukee Heart and right to left balance. ASAIO J 38:M722–M725
13. Nikolaychik VV, Samet MM, Wankowski DM, Lelkes PI (1996) A method for evaluation of surface coverage and firmness of cell attachment in endothelialized cardiac prostheses (abstract). ASAIO J 42(2):20
14. Eskin SG, Sybers HD, O'Bannon W, Navarro LT (1982) Performance of tissue cultured endothelial cells in a mock circulatory loop. Artery 10:159–171
15. Schneider PA, Hanson SR, Price TM, Harker LA (1988) Durability of confluent endothelial cell monolayers on small-caliber vascular prostheses in vitro. Surgery 103:456–462
16. Zilla PP, Fasol RD, Deutsch M (1987) Endothelialization of vascular grafts. Karger, Basel, pp 1–258
17. Greisler HP, Johnson S, Joyce K, Henderson S, Patel NM, Alkhamis T, Beissinger R, Kim DU (1990) The effects of shear stress on endothelial cell retention and function on expanded polytetrafluoroethylene. Arch Surg 125:1622–1625
18. Gosselin C, Vorp DA, Warty V, Severyn DA, Dick EK, Borovetz HS, Greisler HP (1996) ePTFE coating with fibrin glue, FGF-1, and heparin: effect on retention of seeded endothelial cells. J Surg Res 60:327–332
19. Ward RS, White KA, Wolcott CA (1993) Thermoplastic siloxane–urethane copolymer development (abstract). Proceedings AAMI Cardiovascular Science and Technology Conference, AAMI, Arlington, VA, USA, p 129
20. Okoshi T, Soldani G, Goddard M, Galletti PM (1996) Microporous polyurethane inhibits critical mural thrombosis and enhances endothelialization at blood-contacting surface. In: Akutsu T, Koyanagi H (eds) Heart replacement: artificial heart 5. Springer, Tokyo, pp 47–51
21. Bruck SD (1991) Biostability of materials and implants. J Long-Term Effects Med Implants 1:89–106
22. Lin H, Sun W, Mosher DF, García-Echeverría C, Schaufelberger K, Lelkes PI, Cooper SL (1994) Synthesis, surface, and cell-adhesion properties of polyurethanes containing covalently grafted RGD-peptides. J Biomed Mater Res 28:329–342

Evaluation of a Newly Developed, Heparin-Bonded Artificial Lung in Chronic Animal Experiments

Yoshiaki Takewa[1], Eisuke Tatsumi[1], Kazuhiro Eya[1], Yoshiyuki Taenaka[1], Takeshi Nakatani[1], Toru Masuzawa[1], Takashi Nishimura[1], Takashi Ohno[1], Yoshinari Wakisaka[1], Koki Takiura[1], Makoto Nakamura[1], Seiko Endo[1], Y.-S. Sohn[1], Hisateru Takano[1], Takehiko Okamoto[2], Takumi Yoda[2], Yasujirou Ohara[2], and Soichi Tanaka[2]

Summary. Our artificial lung (AL) for long-term extracorporeal membrane oxygenation (ECMO) consists of a special membrane in which micropores on the outer surface of the hollow fibers are blind-ended to eliminate direct blood–gas contact, and the entire blood-contacting surface is treated with covalent heparin binding to promote antithrombogenicity. Chronic performance of the AL was evaluated for gas-exchange function and thromboresistant properties in four goats weighing 28–36kg, using a venoarterial bypass circuit perfused by means of a pneumatic ventricular assist device for up to 14 days. Serum leakage was completely prevented in all the devices throughout the experimental period. With 3.3–4.2 l/min of blood flow and 10–15 l/min of oxygen flow, the AL transferred 166 ± 25 ml/min of oxygen and 116 ± 41 ml/min of carbon dioxide. Platelet counts and antithrombin III levels significantly decreased during the initial 3 days but rebounded thereafter. Only in one AL was macroscopic thrombus formation observed, presumably related to severe infection. Scanning electron microscopy showed the surface of hollow fibers to be free of thrombus, while fibrin deposits were observed in all devices, mainly on the polyester threads used for weaving the hollow fibers. These results indicate that our new AL can be used for prolonged ECMO, although further improvement in thromboresistant properties should be achieved.

Key words: Artificial lung — Heparin bonding — Antithrombogenicity — Prolonged extracorporeal membrane oxygenation

Introduction

The artificial lung is widely used for extracorporeal membrane oxygenation (ECMO) and percutaneous cardiopulmonary support (PCPS) [1]. It may also in the future serve as a bridge to lung or heart-lung transplantation [2,3]. Thus, the demand for extended use in the order of days to weeks is increasing. However, current devices present several major problems for prolonged use, such as serum leakage, destruction or consumption of blood components, and thromboembolism. To solve these problems, we have developed an artificial lung which prevents serum leakage and possesses good hemocompatibility. The purpose of this study is to evaluate this newly developed artificial lung in a series of long-term animal experiments.

Materials and Methods

The newly developed artificial lung is made of special polyolefin hollow fibers modified to prevent serum leakage [4]. In the membrane, micropores are blind-ended to create a thin, dense layer of less than 1 μm thickness and thereby eliminate direct blood–gas contact (Fig. 1). Structural specifications for this artificial lung are basically the same as for the Menox EL 6000 (Kuraray, Kurashiki, Japan) — i.e., a 1.2 m^2 membrane surface area, a 140 ml priming volume, and an extraluminal blood flow arrangement. For our experiments, the entire blood-contacting surface was treated with a new covalent heparin-bonding method to provide long-term antithrombogenicity (Fig. 2). Polyethyleneimine and silane were used as spacers so that heparin was immobilized onto the blood-contacting surface by covalent bonding only, which keeps heparin on the surface for longer than ionic bonding.

In four adult goats weighing from 28 to 36 kg, a biventricular bypass system with two ventricular assist devices [5] was surgically implanted in a paracorporeal fashion. Two weeks later, the extracorporeal circuitry was changed to venoarterial bypass without anesthesia. The right drainage cannula and the left return cannula were connected to the same ventricular assist device for venoarterial bypass and the artificial lung was inserted in the blood return line (Fig. 3). No systemic anticoagulation was used except for minute amounts of heparin in the infusion lines.

Gas-exchange performance was evaluated for oxygen transfer rate ($\dot{V}O_2$) and carbon dioxide removal rate ($\dot{V}CO_2$), using a blood gas analyzer (ABL 500, Radiometer, Copenhagen, Denmark) and measuring bypass flow with an electromagnetic flowmeter (MF-200, Nihon Kohden, Tokyo, Japan). Changes in blood components (including platelet counts and plasma free

[1] Department of Artificial Organs, National Cardiovascular Center Research Institute, 5-7-1 Fujishiro-dai, Suita, Osaka 565, Japan

[2] Medical Research and Development, Kuraray Co., Ltd., 1621 Sakazu, Kurashiki, Okayama 710, Japan

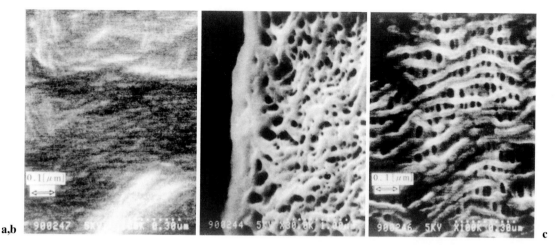

Fig. 1. Electron microscopic views of the special polyolefin hollow fiber membrane: outer surface (**a**), cross section (**b**), and inner surface (**c**). Micropores are blind-ended at blood-contacting surface to prevent serum leakage

Table 1. Summary of chronic animal experiments

Experiment no.	Body weight (kg)	Duration of ECMO (days)	Bypass flow rate (l/min)	O$_2$ flow rate (l/min)
1	28	14	3.3–3.9	15
2	36	9	3.8–4.2	15
3	36	8	3.3–3.8	15
4	30	7	3.4–3.9	10–15

ECMO, extracorporeal membrane oxygenation.

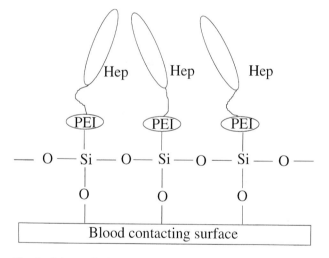

Fig. 2. Schematic drawing of surface treatment of the artificial lung. The entire blood-contacting surface was treated with covalent heparin bonding to provide good and long-term antithrombogenicity. *Hep*, heparin; *PEI*, polyethyleneimine; *Si*, silane; *O*, oxygen

hemoglobin) and coagulation factors [prothrombin time (PT), activated partial thromboplastin time (APTT), fibrinogen, fibrinogen degradation products (FDP), antithrombin III, and antiplasmin] were evaluated. At the end of experiment, the blood-contacting surface of each artificial lung was inspected macroscopically and scanning electron microscopic observations were made.

Results

The duration of venoarterial ECMO ranged from 7 to 14 days (Table 1). The bypass flow rate ranged from 3.3 to 4.2 l/min. Serum leakage was completely prevented in all the artificial lungs throughout the experiments. Under 10–15 l/min of oxygen flow rate, the artificial lung showed rates of 166 ± 25 ml/min of oxygen transfer, and 116 ± 41 ml/min of carbon dioxide removal (Fig. 4). These levels were maintained throughout the experiment.

No significant elevation was observed in plasma free hemoglobin levels. Platelet counts decreased during the initial 3 days from a prebypass level of 44.7 ± 8.2 to $23.4 \pm 6.8 \times 10^4/\mu l$. However, they rebounded thereafter, and reached $33.3 \pm 13.7 \times 10^4/\mu l$ on the 7th day (Fig. 5). With respect to coagulation factors, PT and APTT were maintained at rather constant levels (Fig. 6). Levels of fibrinogen and FDP remained within the normal range throughout the experiments, although a slight decrease in fibrinogen and a slight increase in FDP were seen on the first and second day (Fig. 7).

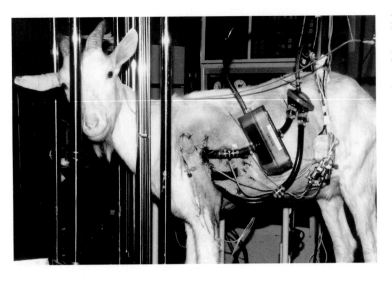

Fig. 3. View of chronic animal experiment. Venoarterial extracorporeal membrane oxygenation (ECMO); right uptake and left return cannulae, single ventricular assist device, and an artificial lung interposed in the return cannula

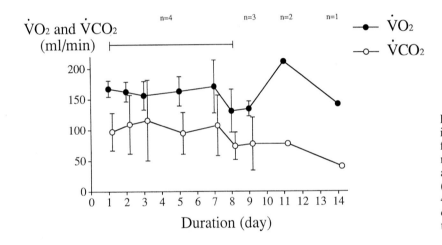

Fig. 4. Gas-exchange performance during the experiment. $\dot{V}O_2$, oxygen transfer rate; $\dot{V}CO_2$, carbon dioxide removal rate; *Duration*, duration of ECMO. This artificial lung maintained sufficient $\dot{V}O_2$ (166 ± 25 ml/min) and $\dot{V}CO_2$ (116 ± 41 ml/min). Values are mean $\pm$ SD. The oxygen flow rate was 10–15 l/min, and the blood flow rate was 3.3–4.2 l/min

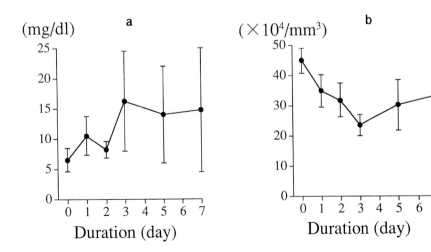

Fig. 5. Changes in blood components: **a** plasma free hemoglobin; **b** platelet count. No significant change was observed in plasma free hemoglobin level. Platelet counts slightly decreased during the initial 3 days, but increased thereafter. Values are means $\pm$ SE

Fig. 6. Changes in coagulation factors (1).
a Prothrombin time; **b** activated partial
thromboplastin time. Both were
maintained at rather constant levels.
Values are means ± SE

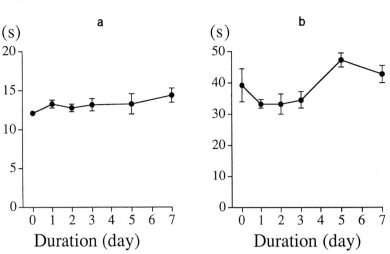

Fig. 7. Changes in coagulation
factors (2). **a** Fibrinogen;
b Fibrinogen degradation products
(FDP). A slight decrease of
fibrinogen and slight increase of
FDP were seen on the first and
second day, but these levels were
kept within normal range
throughout the experiments.
Values are means ± SE

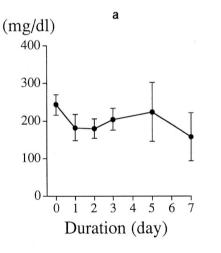
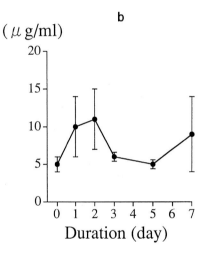

Fig. 8. Changes in coagulation factors (3).
a Antithrombin III; **b** antiplasmin. The
antithrombin III level decreased during
the initial 3 days. No significant change
was seen in the antiplasmin level. Values
are means ± SE

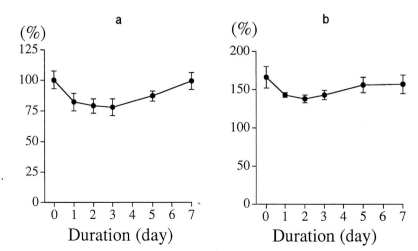

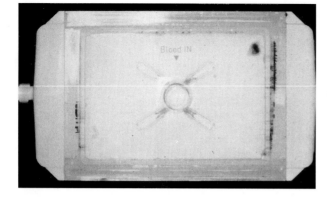

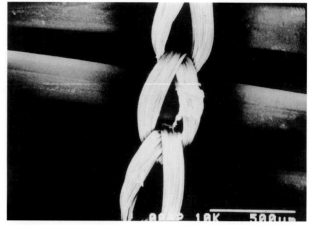

Fig. 9. The artificial lung after 14 days of use without systemic anticoagulation. Almost all the blood-contacting surface was found to be free of macroscopic thrombi except margins and a corner

Fig. 10. Scanning electron microscopic view of the hollow fibers after the experiment. The surface of the hollow fibers was found to be free of thrombus, while fibrin deposition was observed on the polyester weaving threads

Antithrombin III decreased from 100% ± 13% of the prebypass level to 79% ± 12% the 3rd day of the bypass. No significant change was seen in the antiplasmin level (Fig. 8).

Moderate thrombus was observed macroscopically at the end of the experiment in one case where the animal suffered from severe infection. However, three out of four artificial lungs were almost free of thrombus formation (Fig. 9). The blood-exposed surface of the hollow fibers in these three cases was also found to be free of thrombus by scanning electron microscopy (Fig. 10), while fibrin deposits were consistently observed on the polyester weaving threads which transversely anchored the hollow fibers.

Discussion

One of the major requirements for long-term use of artificial lungs is to maintain sufficient gas-exchange performance. In the current artificial lungs using microporous membranes, gas-exchange function deteriorates over several days because of: (1) serum leakage through the microporous membrane, (2) progressive flow channeling among hollow fibers [6], (3) condensation of water vapor in the hollow fiber lumen, and (4) covering of the membrane surface with a protein layer or blood cells. In our newly developed artificial lung, serum leakage was completely prevented throughout the experiments by employing a novel composite gas-exchange membrane. Flow channeling inside the artificial lung was circumvented by the vertical weaving threads which anchored the hollow fibers at uniform intervals. The dew in the hollow fibers was blown off periodically with compressed gas. Macroscopic and electron microscopic observations showed that adhesion of blood cells to the membrane surface could be successfully avoided by covalent heparin-

bonding treatment. Consequently, the artificial lung maintained a stable gas-exchange function for up to 14 days, thus exhibiting the potential for long-term use in terms of gas exchange performance.

Another requirement for long-term use of the artificial lung is good blood compatibility. In the present study, the levels of most blood components and clotting factors were maintained within the normal range. Decreases in platelet counts and antithrombin III were temporary and acceptable. Consumption of blood coagulation factors in prolonged ECMO is generally caused by contact of the blood with a large material surface, as well as mechanical destruction by the blood pump. In our ECMO system, the blood-contacting surface area was minimized by employing a compact design and a short circuit without accessory parts such as a heat exchanger. The ventricular assist device used as blood pump system may also have contributed to limiting blood cell destruction, as compared with roller pumps or centrifugal pumps [7,8].

Nonthrombogenicity of artificial lungs is another important requirement for long-term use. In the present series of experiments, three out of four devices were found to be free of thrombus by macroscopic observation. Clotting formation observed in one case was presumably related to as severe infection. Overall, the newly developed artificial lung demonstrated satisfactory antithrombogenic properties in chronic animal use under standard perfusion conditions. However, fibrin deposits were consistently found by microscopic observation, primarily on the polyester weaving threads, but rarely on the hollow fiber surface. It is likely that local flow stagnation was the responsible factor. It may also be that heparin bonding to the weaving threads was insufficient, compared with the hollow fibers. Elimination of the weaving threads may help to improve the antithrombogenic properties of the gas-exchange device.

Conclusions

1. The newly developed artificial lung demonstrated satisfactory long-term gas-exchange performance for up to 14 days.
2. Levels of blood components and coagulation factors were maintained within acceptable limits.
3. The newly developed artificial lung shows a potential for long-term use, although thromboresistant properties should be further improved for use in the absence of systemic anticoagulation.

Acknowledgment. This work was supported in part by a grant from the Human Science Promoting Foundation.

References

1. Ichiba S, Bartlett RH (1996) Current status of extracorporeal membrane oxygenation for severe respiratory failure. Artif Organs 20:120–123
2. Nido PJ, Armitage JM, Fricker FJ, Shaver M, Cipriani L, Dayal G, Park SC, Siewers RD (1994) Extracorporeal membrane oxygenation support as a bridge to pediatric heart transplantation. Circulation 90:II-66–II-69
3. Jurmann IJ, Schaefers H-J, Demertzis S, Haverich A, Wahlers T, Borst HG (1993) Emergency lung transplantation after extracorporeal membrane oxygenation. ASAIO J 39:M448–M452
4. Akasu H, Anazawa T (1990) Development of a membrane oxygenator using novel polyolefin hollow fibers with blind-ended micropores. Jpn J Biomater 8:141–147
5. Takano H, Nakatani T, Taenaka Y (1993) Clinical experience with ventricular assist systems in Japan. Ann Thorac Surg 5:250–256
6. Tatsumi E, Takewa Y, Akagi H, Taenaka Y, Eya K, Nakatani T, Baba Y, Masuzawa T, Wakisaka Y, Toda K, Miyazaki K, Nishimura T, Ohno T, Takano H, Mimura R, Tanaka S (1996) Development of an integrated artificial heart-lung device for long-term cardiopulmonary support. ASAIO J 42:M827–M832
7. Tatsumi E, Eya K, Taenaka Y, Nakatani T, Baba Y, Masuzawa T, Wakisaka Y, Toda K, Miyazaki K, Takano H (1995) Long-term cardiopulmonary support with a composite artificial heart-lung system. ASAIO J 41:M557–M560
8. Tatsumi E, Taenaka Y, Nakatani T, Akagi H, Sekii H, Yagura A, Sasaki E, Goto M, Nakamura H, Takano H (1990) A VAD and novel high performance compact oxygenator for long-term ECMO with local anticoagulation. ASAIO Trans 36:M480–M483

Discussion

Dr. Teoh:
My name is Teoh from Biomat Center, National University of Singapore. The question is for Dr. Nikolaychilk. You mentioned that you use a rotation method for seeding of the endothelial cells. Is this a typical two-axia rotation machine, or is it a single-axis rotation machine?

Dr. Nikolaychik:
We have been using a two-axis rotation apparatus which covers all three angular degrees of freedom, i.e., yawing, pitching, and rolling motions.

Dr. Teoh:
We have been doing a lot of rotation molding of medical devices, ranging from the left ventricular assist device to artificial limbs in Singapore. And we realize that the speed ratio is very imporant in order for complete coverage of the solution. May I know the speed ratio you are using for your rotation molding?

Dr. Nikolaychik:
The two-axis rotation apparatus was designed to operate at a fixed speed ratio of 1:0.9, main vs. secondary,

respectively. For seeding purposes we have been operating the main axis of the apparatus at 10 rotations per hour. Now, I agree with you that the speed of rotation is a very important parameter, and you have to play between the devil and the deep blue sea. At low speeds one obtains cell aggregation on and nonuniform coverage of the surface. On the other hand, at high speeds one gets into problems of low efficiencies of attachment and, most likely, cell damage. Hence, 10 rotations per hour is a good compromise.

Dr. Nosé:
Nosé, Baylor. Dr. Takewa, excellent presentation, and I would like to ask one question. Did you have any control study without a heparin-coated oxygenator?

Dr. Takewa:
No, I have no control studies. If we use a nonheparin-coated oxygenator without anticoagulant therapy, we cannot follow longer-term experiments more than one day.

Alumina Ceramic and Polyethylene: Materials for the Double Pivot Bearing System of an Implantable Centrifugal Ventricular Assist Device

Yoshiyuki Takami, Tadashi Nakazawa, Kenzo Makinouchi, Julie Glueck, Robert Benkowski, and Yukihiko Nosé

Summary. To achieve the development of a centrifugal blood pump for long-term implantation, the Gyro C1E3 pump was designed with a double pivot bearing system to remove the need for seals. Based upon this pump design, an implantable centrifugal ventricular assist device (VAD; Gyro PI) is currently being developed. Alumina ceramic (Al_2O_3) and ultrahigh molecular weight polyethylene (UHMWPE) are used for the male and female pivots for this pump respectively. Since the double pivot bearing system is the most critical component in this pump design, these components were studied in terms of durability, spinning stability, and biocompatibility.

Durability was examined by measuring the wear rate of the pivots in in vitro studies of the C1E3 pump. Spinning stability was examined by evaluating the degree of vibration of the working pump with a piezoelectric accelerometer. Basic biocompatibility was examined in tests for systemic toxicity, irritation, sensitization (guinea pig maximization test), mutagenicity (Ames test), hemolysis, and thrombogenicity.

In the wear measurements, the amount of the initial wear was $60\,\mu m$, followed by a sustained wear rate of $0.18\,\mu m/10^6$ rotations, indicating a 6-year life expectancy of the bearings of the Gyro PI as a left VAD. In the vibration study, the pump with Al_2O_3 and UHMWPE pivots exhibited less vibration than pumps with SiC pivots. In biocompatibility tests, samples of the Al_2O_3 and UHMWPE demonstrated no significant differences from the negative controls.

We conclude that Al_2O_3 and UHMWPE are a good combination of materials for the biocompatible, durable, and stable bearing system of an implantable centrifugal pump.

Key words: Alumina ceramic — Polyethylene — Centrifugal blood pump — Ventricular assist device

Introduction

The mean waiting time for heart transplantation was reported to be 245 days in 1993 [1]. Insufficient supply of donor organs makes the role of the chronic mechanical circulatory support, especially the ventricular assist device (VAD), very important. Now, several VADs are available for long-term clinical use, including extracorporeal [2,3] and implantable VADs [4,5]. All of them are, however, pulsatile VADs whose potential disadvantages may include high cost, large size, and relative complexity. The cost per patient transplanted after mechanical support was reported to be over $80000, which was higher than that after pharmacological treatment [6]. To replace the pulsatile VAD, development of a continuous flow VAD has been expected, based upon its predicted cost-effectiveness, small size, and easy controllability. Centrifugal pumps have been used as a VAD both for postcardiotomy ventricular failure and as a bridge to cardiac transplantation [7,8]. Although the clinical outcomes with the centrifugal mechanical support were comparable to that with the pulsatile support, the lifetime of the pump is limited to 3 days due to blood seepage into the pump housing and thrombus formation around the shaft.

Since 1991, we have been developing a completely seal-less design for a long-term centrifugal pump [9–14]. To obtain a completely seal-less pump casing, a double pivot bearing system was adopted together with a magnetic coupling system. In addition, special "eccentric inlet port" was designed for the double pivot bearing system so there would be no obstacles in the blood path [11,14]. It has been demonstrated that this pivot-bearing-supported Gyro C1E3 centrifugal pump (Fig. 1) can be used not only for cardiopulmonary bypass but also for a 1-month extracorporeal VAD [12,13]. To be incorporated into an implantable centrifugal ventricular assist system, the C1E3 is being miniaturized and modified to a permanently implantable model of Gyro pump (Gyro PI) based on the same design concept as the C1E3 [15] (Fig. 1). Even if modified, however, the double pivot bearing system is still the most critical point of the Gyro PI. We have adopted alumina ceramic (Al_2O_3) for the male pivot and ultra high molecular weight polyethylene (UHMWPE) for the female pivot in the double pivot bearing system (Fig. 2). Although the Al_2O_3 ceramic — UHMWPE combination has proven to be clinically reliable over 10 years in artificial joints [16], there has been little experience in using these materials in a blood-contacting device. The present study investigated Al_2O_3 ceramic and UHMWPE as materials for

Department of Surgery, Baylor College of Medicine, One Baylor Plaza, Houston, TX, 77030, USA

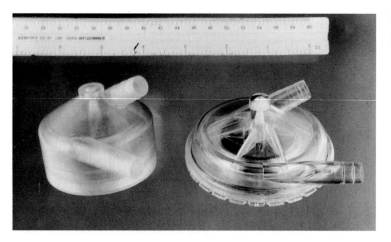

Fig. 1. Pivot-bearing-supported Gyro centrifugal blood pumps (*right*, Gyro PI; *left*, Gyro C1E3). *Scale*: cm (*upper*), inches (*lower*)

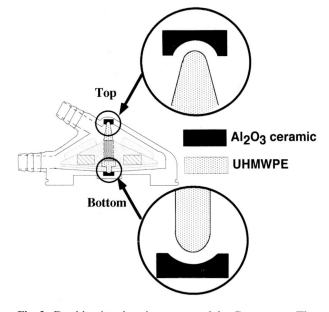

Fig. 2. Double pivot bearing system of the Gyro pump. The male pivots are alumina (Al_2O_3) ceramic and the female pivots are ultra high molecular weight polyethylene (*UHMWPE*)

the pivot bearings, in terms of durability, spinning stability, and basic biocompatibility, using the C1E3 pump.

Materials and Methods

Wear Measurement

According to the previously reported method [17], three C1E3 pumps with different pivot materials were compared: (1) a pump with the male and female pivots

made of silicon carbide ceramic (SiC); (2) a pump with SiC male and UHMWPE female pivots; and (3) a pump with Al_2O_3 male and UHMWPE female pivots. After pump operation with bovine blood at a rotational speed of 3000 rpm (6 l/min against a pressure of 500 mmHg), the total wear of the four pivots, including male and female pivots, was measured using a dial gauge (Mitsutoyo MFG., Tokyo, Japan) at room temperature. The wear of the male pivot was defined as a decrease in height, while the wear of the female pivot was defined as an increase in depth. Cumulative rotation was defined as the product of the rotational speed times the running time of the pump.

Vibration Measurement

After the wear measurement, three C1E3 pumps with different pivot materials were compared. A piezoelectric accelerometer (Isotron Conditioner 4416B, Endevco, San Juan Capistrano, CA, USA) was mounted on the top of the pump housing to detect axial acceleration caused by the pump running. When the pumps were operated with 37% (v/v) glycerol at 2700 rpm (10 l/min against 250 mmHg), the ongoing vibration detected by the accelerometer was electrically transformed to a digitizing oscilloscope (TDS 420, Tektronix, Beaverton, OR, USA) to analyze the waveform of the fast Fourier transform.

Biocompatibility Tests

Systemic Toxicity

To test for systemic toxicity [18], eight pieces of the sterile test material were extracted with 22.4 ml of the extracting medium (normal saline solution for intravenous (IV) and sesame oil for intraperitoneal (IP) injection). An additional sterile tube was filled with 22.4 ml of the same medium to serve as a blank. Five mice were each injected IV and IP with 50 ml/kg of one extracted sample or blank and were observed.

Irritation

To test for irritation [18], a 0.2-ml portion of one of the sample extracts was injected intracutaneously at each of five sites in rabbits. A 0.2-ml portion of the corresponding blank was also injected. The injection sites were examined and scored from 0 to 4 for erythema, eschar formation, edema, and necrosis.

Sensitization (Guinea Pig Maximization Test)

The guinea pig maximization test [19] involved twenty-seven Hartley albino guinea pigs divided into four groups: twelve test animals, five positive controls, and five negative controls. As a negative control, a vehicle blank was incubated under the same conditions as the test material. As a positive control, a 0.1% solution of dinitrochlorobenzene (DNCB) in 9.5% ethanol was employed.

Induction Phase. The test material extracts and the controls were injected into the animals intradermally (ID). Seven days after the ID injections, the dosing patches were administered topically over the same area as the ID injections. The topical exposure lasted 48 h.

Challenge Phase. Fourteen days after the topical administration, the animals were exposed to the test extracts and control solution on hill top chambers, which were applied to untreated sites and allowed to remain there for 24 h. Skin responses at the challenge sites were scored from 0 to 3, 24 and 48 h after removal of the patches.

Mutagenicity (Ames Test)

The Ames test [20] was carried out with five strains of *Salmonella typhimurium* (TA97A, 98, 100, 102, and 1535) with the desired properties. Six grams of the sample was extracted in 30 ml of saline at 50°C for 72 h. The overnight broth culture (10 ml) of the bacterial tester strains was added to the top agar, and 2 ml of this mixture was transferred to sterile tubes. The sample extract (0.1 ml) was added to each tube and tested with and without 0.5 ml of the S-9 activation system (Organon Teknika, Durham, NC, USA) which was used to detect the mutagens from byproducts of the test samples. Positive controls were performed using sodium azide, 4-nitro-*o*-phenylene-diamine, and 2-aminofluorene. The criterion for a mutagen was a more than twofold increase over the spontaneous reversion rate.

Hemolysis (Direct Contact)

The test material (2.0 g) was transferred into the test tubes with 10 ml of 0.9% NaCl. The 0.9% NaCl was used for negative controls and 10% of sterile water for irrigation was used for positive controls. After 0.2 ml of rabbit blood was added and incubation carried out at 37°C for 60 min, each tube was centrifuged at 2000 rpm for 10 min. The absorbance (A) of the supernatant was measured at 545 nm on a spectrophotometer. The % hemolysis was calculated using the following formula, where A is absorbance:

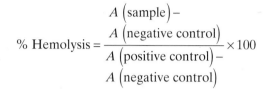

$$\% \text{ Hemolysis} = \frac{A\left(\text{sample}\right) - A\left(\text{negative control}\right)}{A\left(\text{positive control}\right) - A\left(\text{negative control}\right)} \times 100$$

Thrombogenicity (Recalcification Method)

A total of 19.5 g of the sample was extracted in 32.5 ml of saline at 70°C for 24 h. An extract of polypropylene beads was tested as a negative control, and glass beads were included as a positive control. Plasma (0.2 ml) and sterile saline (0.2 ml) were added to each sample and control tube. Calcium chloride (0.2 ml) was then added to each tube. Results were reported as clotting time in seconds for each tube at 37°C.

Results

Wear

Figure 3 shows the wear measurements for three pumps with pivots of different materials. The pump with SiC–SiC pivots demonstrated initial wear of about 230 μm and a sustained wear rate of about 4.0 μm per one million rotations. The pump with SiC–UHMWPE pivots demonstrated initial wear of about 80 μm and a wear rate of about 0.16 μm per one million rotations. The pump with Al_2O_3–UHMWPE pivots demonstrated initial wear of about 60 μm and a wear rate of about 0.18 μm per one million rotations.

Vibration

Figure 4 shows the fast Fourier transform waveforms of the vibration signals caused by three pumps with pivots of different materials. In this figure the horizontal axis is the frequency in Hertz, and the vertical axis is the amplitude in millivolts of the detected vibration signals (the voltage sensitivity of the piezoelectric accelerometer used is 10 mV/g, where g is gravitational acceleration). In the pump with SiC–SiC pivots, the integrated area of the signals (frequency domain) was 1057 g Hz. In the pump with SiC–UHMWPE pivots, the area was 160.6 g Hz. In the pump with Al_2O_3–UHMWPE pivots, the area was 63.9 g Hz. The SiC–

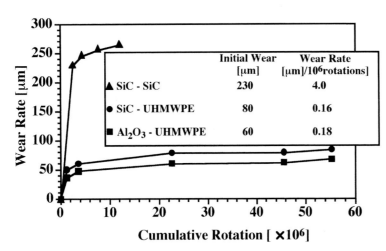

Fig. 3. Results of the wear measurement. Note that the wear on the SiC male–SiC female pivots was much greater than the wear on the pivots with UHMWPE females. There was no significant difference between SiC–UHMWPE and Al$_2$O$_3$–UHMWPE pivots

SiC pump caused significantly more vibration when rotating than the SiC–UHMWPE or Al$_2$O$_3$–UHMWPE pumps. The SiC–UHMWPE pump tended to cause more vibration than the Al$_2$O$_3$–UHMWPE pump, but the difference was not significant.

Biocompatibility Tests

Systemic Toxicity
No toxic signs were observed during a 72-h period in any of the animals treated with the sample extracts of Al$_2$O$_3$ or UHMWPE, or in those treated with the blank. In addition, all of the animals gained weight during the test (mean: Al$_2$O$_3$, 3.8 g; UHMWPE, 4.0 g; blank, 4.6 g).

Irritation
All animals tested remained healthy throughout the test period. The difference between the mean score for each for the sample extracts of the Al$_2$O$_3$ and UHMWPE and corresponding blanks was 1.0 or less (mean scores: Al$_2$O$_3$, 0.5; UHMWPE, 0.7; blank, 0.4).

Sensitization
No toxic signs were observed in any of the test or control animals over the duration of the study. None of the test groups with Al$_2$O$_3$ or UHMWPE or the negative controls exhibited scores higher than 1 (mean scores: Al$_2$O$_3$, 0.33; UHMWPE, 0.5; blank, 0.6). All five positive control animals exhibited sensitization responses to the challenge dose (mean score 2.8).

Mutagenicity
The test results are presented in Table 1. No mutagenic activity was observed with the extracted samples of the Al$_2$O$_3$ or UHMWPE, with or without metabolic activation by S-9. The controls yielded the expected results.

Table 1. *Salmonella* mutagenicity assay tests

Tester	Strains	Revertants per plate (mean ± standard deviation)		
		Negative control	Al$_2$O$_3$	UHMWPE
TA97A	S(−)	158 ± 25	159 ± 17	162 ± 25
	S(+)	161 ± 12	191 ± 11	182 ± 26
TA98	S(−)	30 ± 5	21 ± 3	28 ± 9
	S(+)	36 ± 4	29 ± 4	28 ± 5
TA100	S(−)	131 ± 5	195 ± 9	164 ± 4
	S(+)	224 ± 31	223 ± 19	218 ± 13
TA102	S(−)	353 ± 33	339 ± 26	335 ± 22
	S(+)	351 ± 39	345 ± 22	263 ± 18
TA1535	S(−)	40 ± 1	31 ± 5	35 ± 5
	S(+)	16 ± 1	21 ± 4	16 ± 4

Hemolysis
The test samples of both the Al$_2$O$_3$ and UHMWPE exhibited a % *hemolysis* < 1%.

Thrombogenicity
There was no significant difference between the clotting times for the Al$_2$O$_3$ or UHMWPE samples and the negative control (mean: Al$_2$O$_3$, 216 s; UHMWPE, 193 s; positive control, 115 s; negative control, 214 s).

Discussion

The present study justified Al$_2$O$_3$ and UHMWPE as the materials of choice for the double pivot bearings of the Gyro pump in terms of basic biocompatibility, durability, and spinning stability. The Gyro C1E3 was designed for extracorporeal circulatory assistance including cardiopulmonary bypass and the VAD. Miniaturization of the C1E3 using the same design concepts resulted in the Gyro PI for an implantable

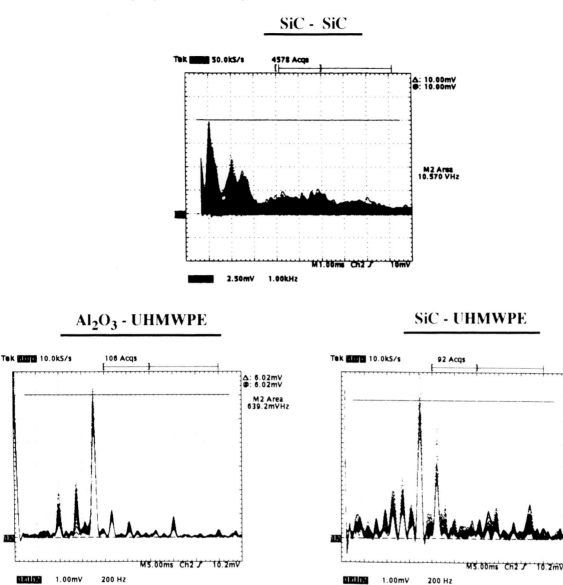

Fig. 4. Results of the vibration measurement. Fast Fourier transform waveforms of the vibration signals caused by pumps containing different combinations of pivot materials under the same conditions (flow rate, 10 l/min; total pressure head, 250 mmHg; rotational speed, 2700 rpm). The horizontal axis is the frequency in Hz, and the vertical axis shows the amplitude in mV of the detected vibration signals. Note that the pump with SiC–SiC pivots caused much more vibration than the pumps with UHMWPE female pivots. There was no significant difference between the SiC–UHMWPE and Al_2O_3–UHMWPE pivots

VAD [15]. The most critical design concept in the Gyro pumps is the double pivot bearing system.

SiC was previously used for both male and female pivots of the Gyro C1E3 [9–11]. As demonstrated in the present study, the combination of SiC male and SiC female was found to be undesirable because of the unstable spinning and higher wear rate, which may be caused by contact and friction between the hard SiC pivots. Consequently, the SiC–SiC pivot system was changed to a combination of SiC male and UHMWPE female. As shown in the present study, SiC–

UHMWPE pivots are superior to SiC–SiC regarding spinning stability and durability. Subsequently, SiC–UHMWPE pivots were changed to Al_2O_3–UHMWPE. This combination has been proven to be clinically reliable in artificial joints for over ten years [16]. In addition, the present study demonstrated that Al_2O_3–UHMWPE is slightly superior to SiC–UHMWPE in terms of spinning stability and durability.

Al_2O_3 ceramic is chemically inert, thermodynamically stable, hydrophilic (highly wettable), and hard (tribologically excellent) [21]. In total hip prostheses,

UHMWPE has proven to be wear resistant with a counterbearing of Al_2O_3 [22]. This finding is in keeping with our data from wear and vibration measurements. The hard and stable Al_2O_3 surface maintains a mirror finish and thus reduces the abrasive wear of UHMWPE. In addition, the highly wettable Al_2O_3 surface has an increased lubricating ability in an aqueous environment and thus reduces the adhesive wear of UHMWPE. Furthermore, Al_2O_3 is more suitable than SiC because Al_2O_3 is more ionic, as demonstrated by the finding that fatty acids produced a friction-reducing adsorbed layer on Al_2O_3 but not on SiC [23].

The wear data from the present study allow us to estimate the lifetime (T) of the double pivot bearing system in the Gyro pump, applying the following equation [17]:

$$T = \frac{W_{max} - W_0}{RPM \cdot WR}$$

where W_{max} is the maximal amount of wear (1240µm), W_0 is the initial wear, RPM is the rotational rate of the pump, and WR is the wear rate. (W_0 and WR are presented in Fig. 3). Since the wear of the double pivot bearing system in the Gyro pump depends only upon the cumulative rotation and the materials of the pivot bearings, we can predict the lifetime of the pivot bearings of the Gyro PI from the wear data on the Gyro C1E3 in this study. In the Gyro PI pump, running at approximately 2000 rpm in left (LVAD) and 1500 rpm in right (RVAD) ventricular assist devices [15], the lifetime of the double pivot bearings is estimated to be over 6 years as a LVAD and 8 years as a RVAD.

In artificial joints, there are concerns that UHMWPE wear causes a foreign body reaction to wear particles and loosening of the prosthetic component [24]. The reaction to UHMWPE wear particles has to be evaluated for the Gyro pump in further studies. However, loosening of the bearings by UHMWPE wear is advantageous for the Gryo pump. This is because more loosening due to wear of the UHMWPE female pivots makes the impeller of the Gyro pump rotate in the top contact position, in which more washout of blood flow beneath the impeller occurs. The rotation of the impeller in the top contact position may enhance the antithrombogenicity of the Gyro pump [17,25].

The present study also demonstrated that Al_2O_3 and UHMWPE have a low potential for systemic toxicity, sensitization, mutagenicity, hemolysis, and thrombogenicity. Although only basic, short-term biocompatibility tests were performed, it is possible to state that Al_2O_3 and UHMWPE are biocompatible as blood-contacting materials. Among these tests, the recalcification method for thrombogenicity may not be enough to confirm the low thrombogenicity of UHMWPE, because the International Standardization Organiza-

tion (ISO) defines UHMWPE itself as the negative control. The previous studies on biocompatibility of Al_2O_3 were performed with bulky implant biomaterial; these studies indicated low carcinogenicity [21], minimal soft-tissue response [24], and no complement C3 activation or chemotaxis [26,27]. As blood-contacting materials, SiC and Al_2O_3 have little hemolytic activity [13,28]. In addition, the Al_2O_3 ceramic heart valves demonstrated excellent antithrombogenicity [29,30]. The thromboresistance of Al_2O_3 may result from a thin, firmly anchored, nonvascular layer of tissue covering the Al_2O_3 surface, and from the electrical charge on the surface that can repel blood cells.

Conclusion

Al_2O_3 ceramic and UHMWPE are the materials of choice for the double pivot bearing system of the Gyro centrifugal blood pump, whether extracorporeal or implantable, from the viewpoint of biocompatibility, durability, and spinning stability.

References

1. Frazier OH (1994) The development of an implantable, portable, electrically powered left ventricular assist device. Semin Thorac Cardiovasc Surg 6(3):181–187
2. Farrar DJ, Hill JD (1993) Univentricular and biventricular Thorate VAD support as a bridge to transplantation. Ann Thorac Surg 55:276–282
3. Champsaur G, Ninet J, Vigneron M, Cochet P, Neidecker J, Boissonnat P (1990) Use of the Abiomed BVS System 5000 as a bridge to cardiac transplantation. J Thorac Cardiovasc Surg 100:122–128
4. McCarthy PM, Portner PM, Tobler HG, Starnes VA, Ramasamy N, Oyer PE (1991) Clinical experience with the Novacor ventricular assist system: bridge to transplantation and the transition to permanent application. J Thorac Cardiovasc Surg 102:578–587
5. Frazier OH (1993) Chronic left ventricular support with a vented electric assist device. Ann Thorac Surg 55:273–275
6. Loisance D, Benvenuti C, Lebrun T, Leclerc A, Tarral A, Sailly JC (1991) Cost and cost–effectiveness of the mechanical and pharmacological bridge to transplantation. ASAIO Trans 37:M125–127
7. Curtis JJ (1994) Centrifugal mechanical assist for postcardiotomy ventricular failure. Semin Thorac Cardiovasc Surg 6(3):140–146
8. McBride LR (1994) Bridging to cardiac transplantation with external ventricular assist devices. Semin Thorac Cardiovasc Surg 6(3):169–173
9. Ohara Y, Sakuma I, Makinouchi K, Damm G, Glueck J, Mizuguchi K, Naito K, Tasai K, Orime Y, Takatani S, Noon GP, Nosé Y (1993) Baylor Gyro pump: A completely seal-less centrifugal pump aiming for long-term circulatory support. *Artif Organs* 17:599–604
10. Ohara Y, Makinouchi K, Orime Y, Damm G, Glueck J, Mizuguchi K, Naito K, Tasai K, Takatani S, Noon GP,

Nosé Y (1994) An ultimate, compact, seal-less centrifugal ventricular assist device: Baylor C-Gyro pump. Artif Organs 18:17–24

11. Ohara Y, Makinouchi K, Glueck J, Sutherland B, Shimono T, Naito K, Tasai K, Orime Y, Takatani S, Nosé Y (1994) Development and evaluation of antithrombogenic centrifugal pump; The Baylor C-Gyro pump eccentric inlet port model. Artif Organs 18:673–679

12. Nakazawa T, Makinouchi K, Ohara Y, Ohtsubo S, Kawahito K, Tasai K, Shimono T, Benkowski R, Damm G, Takami Y, Glueck J, Savage A, Takatani S, Noon GP, Nosé Y (1996) Development of a pivot bearing supported sealless centrifugal pump for ventricular assist device. Artif Organs 20:485–490

13. Takami Y, Makinouchi K, Nakazawa T, Glueck J, Ohara Y, Benkowski RJ, Nosé Y (1996) Hemolytic characteristics of pivot bearing Gyro centrifugal pump (C1E3) in various clinical simulated conditions. Artif Organs 20:1042–1049

14. Takami Y, Andrade A, Nakazawa T, Makinouchi K, Glueck J, Benkowski R, Nosé Y (1997) An eccentric inlet port of the pivot bearing-supported Gyro centrifugal pump. Artif Organs 21:312–317

15. Nakazawa T, Takami Y, Benkowski R, Makinouchi K, Ohtsubo S, Glueck J, Kawahito K, Sueoka A, Schmallegger H, Schima H, Wolner E, Nosé Y (1997) Recent advances in the Gyro centrifugal ventricular assist device. ASAIO J

16. Sugano N, Nishii T, Nakata K, Masuhara K, Takaoka K (1995) Polyethylene sockets and alumina ceramic heads in cemented total hip arthroplasty. A ten-year study. J Bone Joint Surg Br 77:548–556

17. Makinouchi K, Nakazawa T, Takami Y, Takatani S, Nosé Y (1996) Evaluation of the wear of the pivot bearing in the Gyro C1E3 pump. Artif Organs 20:523–528

18. United States pharmacopoeia (1995) 23:1699–1702

19. Wahlberg JE, Boman A (1985) Guinea pig maximization test. Curr Probl Dermatol 14:59–106

20. Maron D, Ames BN (1983) Revised methods for the salmonella mutagenicity test. Mutat Res 113:173–215

21. Christel PS (1992) Biocompatibility of surgical-grade dense polycrystalline alumina. Clin Orthop 282:10–18

22. Davidson JA (1993) Characteristics of metal and ceramic total hip bearing surfaces and their effect on long-term ultra high molecular weight polyethylene wear. Clin Orthop 294:361–378

23. Studt P (1987) Influence of lubricating oil additives on friction of ceramics under conditions of boundary lubrication. Wear 115:185–189

24. Harms J, Mausle E (1979) Tissue reaction to ceramic implant material. J Biomed Mater Res 13:67–87

25. Nakazawa T, Takami Y, Makinouchi K, Benkowski R, Glueck J, Damm G, Nosé Y (1996) Hydraulic assessment of the floating impeller phenomena in a centrifugal pump. Artif Organs 21:78–82

26. Pizzoferrato A, Vespucci A, Ciapetti G, Stea S, Tarabusi C (1987) The effect of the injection of powdered materials on mouse peritoneal cell population. J Biomed Mater Res 21:419–428

27. Remes A, Williams DF (1991) Relationship between chemotaxis and complement activation by ceramic biomaterials. Biomaterials 12:661–667

28. Dion I, Lahaye M, Salmon R, Baquey C, Monties JR, Havlik P (1993) Blood haemolysis by ceramics. Biomaterials 14:107–111

29. Mitamura Y, Mikami T, Yuya T, Matsumoto T, Shimooka T, Okamoto E, Eizuka N, Yamaguchi K (1986) Development of a fine ceramic heart valve for use as a cardiac prosthesis. ASAIO Trans 32:444–448

30. Gentle CR, Tansley GD (1995) Development of a ceramic conduit valve prosthesis for corrective cardiovascular surgery. Biomaterials 16:245–249

Discussion

Dr. Jarvik:
Dr. Jarvik from New York. I have two questions. One, I would assume that the wear was entirely on the ultra high molecular weight polyethylene and not on the alumina. Is that correct? You just said the total amount of wear; you didn't say which of the two materials actually wore. Is that the correct assumption, that it was the polyethylene that wore?

Dr. Takami:
Yes. We evaluated the wear of each pivot, I mean the female pivot and the male pivot, and top and bottom, we measured the full wear. At that time we found that in our combination of alumina and polyethylene the wear occurs mostly in the polyethylene on the top pivots.

Dr. Jarvik:
O.K. That's what one would assume. The other things are: Why did you switch from the silicon carbide? And when you say that you have a calculated life, that assumes that a certain amount of wear will cause some kind of a failure, at that point. What was the kind of failure and what was the amount of wear necessary to determine that you could only go 6 years and after that it would fail? So that's two questions.

Dr. Takami:
The reason to change the silicon carbide to alumina ceramic depends upon the clinical reliability of the artificial joints. In artificial joints, alumina ceramic is used popularly so we changed from the silicon carbide to alumina ceramic. I cannot understand the question.

Dr. Nosé:
Probably I can answer. In order to study endurance characteristics of bearings, we ground a ceramic port, and checked how many microns we ground it before it dislocated. If my memory is correct, it was 80 microns to dislocate, and it took approximately 6 to 8 years to reduce the height of the impeller shaft for 80 microns.

Dr. Jarvik:
To the point where it could dislocate.

Dr. Nosé:
From the female pivot bearing, the male ceramic bearing dislocated.

Dr. Jarvik:
Thank you.

Dr. Teoh:
S.H. Teoh from Singapore. Around 1992 we did an experiment on the seriousness of wear for polyethylene, ultra high molecular polyethylene, Delrin, polyacetyl of various grades, peak and polysulphone. While I agree with you that your conclusion in terms of the wear rate of polyethylene is very low, if you check the publication in ASTM STP 1173 we concluded on the basis of the wear, debris size of ultra high molecular polyethylene is in the range of 100 to 150 microns, compared to, say, Delrin, which is only about 30 microns on the average. Based on the conclusion, we say that in the cardiovascular region such large-size debris, though the wear rate is small, may not be suitable.

Dr. Nosé:
Maybe I should answer. That so-called wear is not totally wear. What happened initially is creep formation. Actually deformation of the female pivot shape occurs, then the gradual wear curve takes place. It is the actual wear. So, essentially, the ceramic particles we produced in 6 years is an extremely small amount, which has proven to be acceptable inside of the body.

Dr. Takami:
We conducted this experiment in very severe conditions, which means more severe than the conditions of the LVAD condition, so it is the accuracy of the wear.

Mr. Siess:
Mr. Siess from the Helmoltz Institute. I just want to comment on your wear test. I mean, you say it's been a severe situation, 500 mmHg and 6 liters, but from what I understand, your pump was usually designed to have a bottom floating state and a top state mode, so once you are here doing your wear tests in a nonpulsatile situation, of course you will have most of

the wear on the top. But does that really relate to any pulsatile location, because once you're talking about a device that should be implanted, of course, you will always have a changing delta pressure, and this will also relate to a changing mode inside of the impeller. So I somehow doubt that 6 years, even though that the test was done under severe conditions, will hold true by the time that you test the pump under pulsatile conditions.

Dr. Takami:
Yes, it is very important, so we have to evaluate the wear in the pulsatile fashion.

Highly Blood-Compatible Surface Consisting of a Silicon-Containing Block Copolymer with Supramolecular Structure

Hotaka Ito[1], Yukio Nagasaki[1], Kazunori Kataoka[1], Masao Kato[1], Teiji Tsuruta[1], Ken Suzuki[2], Teruo Okano[2], and Yasuhisa Sakurai[2]

Summary. With the aim of developing a high-performance membrane-type artificial lung, a novel silicon-containing hydrophilic–hydrophobic block copolymer was prepared using a living anionic polymerization technique. To introduce high oxygen permeability, poly{4-[bis (trimethylsilyl)methyl)styrene]} [poly(BSMS)] was employed for the hydrophobic segment. Poly(2-hydroxyethyl methacrylate) [poly(HEMA)] segment was chosen as a counterpart to maintain high blood compatibility. A poly(BSMS-block-HEMA) [BH(X), where X denotes the mole fraction of BSMS in the copolymer] membrane showed a clear separation of microphase structure when the mole fraction X was more than 30% (cast from toluene solution), while BH(10) showed no marked phase separation, when the respective polymer was cast from a dimethylformamide (DMF) solution. It should be noted that DMF is a poor solvent for the poly(BSMS) segment. From a dynamic light scattering measurement of a DMF solution of BH(10) (0.1% w/v), submicron-sized particles were observed. The BH(10) surface prepared from this DMF solution containing submicron particles showed unique characteristics. The wettability of the BH(10) membrane was much higher than that of the poly(HEMA) surface, despite the introduction of the hydrophobic polymer segment. The equilibrium water content of the BH(10) was also higher than that of poly(HEMA). This may be explained by the supramolecular structure of the BH(10) membrane derived from the particle-casting technique. Also surprising was that the BH(10) surface showed extremely high blood compatibility. Indeed, the rate of adhesion and activation of rabbit platelets on the surface was much lower than on poly(styrene-block-HEMA), which we have shown to have fairly high blood compatibility. From these results, it can be concluded that BH(10) is a promising candidate for a novel blood-compatible material for use in such applications as an artificial lung and as a nonthrombogenic coating material.

Key words: Nonthrombogenic coating material — Poly(BSMS/HEMA) block copolymer — Artificial lung — Microphase separated structure — Contact angle

Introduction

With continually improving technology in medical care, the demand for an efficient artifical lung has been increasing in the fields of prolonged respiratory support and routine cardiopulmonary bypass [1]. The materials used in currently available artificial lungs are microporous polymer membranes such as polypropylene. However, the following problems still remain: (1) severe damage to blood plasma due to the direct contact with oxygen gas; (2) leakage of blood plasma; and (3) lowering of gas-exchange ability due to the occlusion of pores by protein. These problems have impeded its utilization for long-term support. Recently, a membrane-type artificial lung has been developed to solve these problems. Since silicone has fairly high gas permeability, most of the membrane-type devices are fabricated using silicone rubber; however, their blood compatibility is not satisfactory [2,3]. Therefore, there is an urgent need for materials which minimize blood damage while retaining high gas permeability.

With the aim of creating a high-performance artificial lung, we designed a new silicon-containing hydrophilic–hydrophobic block copolymer, which consists of a hydrophobic poly{4-[bis(trimethylsilyl) methyl)styrene]} [poly(BSMS)] segment and a hydrophilic poly(2-hydroxyethyl methacrylate) [poly(HEMA)] segment (Fig. 1) [4]. The block copolymer is denoted BH(X), where X is the mole fraction of BSMS in the copolymer. Our idea was to maintain high oxygen permeability by the introduction of organosilicon moieties within the hydrophobic segment, while retaining the high blood compatibility of the poly(styrene-block-HEMA) surface, previously discovered by our group [5]. If a polymer having both high blood compatibility and high gas permeability can be created, such a polymer can be utilized not only as a nonporous membrane but also as a coating material for porous hollow-fibers. This paper deals with the blood compatibility of the block copolymer, and its surface properties as a membrane.

[1] Department of Materials Science and Technology, Science University of Tokyo, 2641 Yamazaki, Noda, Chiba 278, Japan
[2] Tokyo Women's Medical College, 8-1 Kawada-cho, Shinjuku-ku, Tokyo 162, Japan

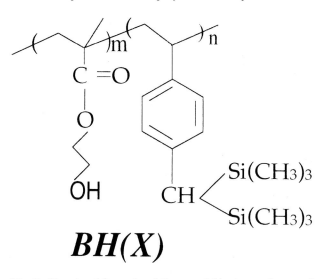

BH(X)

Fig. 1. Structural formula of the novel block copolymer of poly{4-[bis(trimethylsilyl methyl)styrene]} [poly(BSMS)] and poly (2-hydroxyethyl methacrylate) [poly(HEMA)]. The block copolymer is denoted *BH(X)*, where *X* is the mole fraction of BSMS in the copolymer

Materials and Methods

Materials

BSMS was prepared according to our previous paper [6]. The block copolymer samples were prepared by a living anionic polymerization technique [4]. Four samples [BH(10), BH(30), BH(58), and BH(80)] were prepared with molecular weight ranges of 10000–20000.

Properties of BH(X) Membranes

Dynamic contact angle measurements (DCA-20, Orientec, Osaka, Japan) were carried out using the Wilhelmy plate technique [7]. The equilibrium water content was measured by thermal gravimetric analysis (TGA). The samples were measured over a range of temperature from 30°C to 200°C under an argon atmosphere (10°C/min). The water content was defined as $W = (W_s - W_d)/W_s$, where W_s represents the weight of the sample equilibrated with water, and W_d denotes the weight of the sample after the measurement.

Estimation of Blood Compatibility

Preparation of Platelet Suspension. Rabbit platelets were employed for in vitro study (1×10^8 cells/ml). To estimate platelet activation by Ca^{2+} concentration measurement, Fura 2 was incorporated in the cell [8]. Ca ion concentration was adjusted just before the fluorescence measurement by adding $CaCl_2$.

Platelet Adhesion and Intracellular Ca^{2+} Concentration. To known number of polymer coated beads (1.0g, 250–298 µmø) in a plastic microtube, 800µl of the platelet suspension and 500µl of Hank's buffered saline solution (NaCl $8.0 gL^{-1}$, KCl $0.4 gL^{-1}$, KH_2PO_4 $0.06 gL^{-1}$, Na_2HPO_4 $0.12 gL^{-1}$, Glucose $1.0 gL^{-1}$, HEPES $1.19 gL^{-1}$; pH 7.4) were added and the microtube was rotated at ambient temperature for a defined time (ca. 5 rpm). Then, the number of the platelets in the buffer was counted using a Coulter Counter (Model ZBI, Coulter Electronics, Miami, FL, USA). The Ca^{2+} concentration in nonadhered platelets was determined by fluorimetry (CAF100, Japan Spectroscopic, Tokyo, Japan). The cytoplasmic free-Ca^{2+} concentration was calculated as described by Rink et al. [9].

Dynamic light scattering measurements: ADLS was monitored by means of Otsuka DLS-7000 (Otsuka Electronics, Maikata, Japan)

Results and Discussion

We reported previously that a poly(HEMA-block-styrene-block-HEMA) surface (SH(40); styrene 40 mol%) showed fairly high blood compatibility [5]. In this case, the block copolymer surface forms a lamella-type microphase separated structure with submicron dimension which is considered to play an important role in providing blood compatibility. To investigate the surface morphology of BH polymers, a transmission electron microscope (TEM) analysis was carried out. The BH membrane with X > 30% showed clear microphase separation, while BH(10) showed no marked phase separation, when the respective membranes were prepared from dimethylformamide (DMF) solution. It should be noted that DMF is a poor solvent for the poly(BSMS) segment. From a dynamic light scattering (DLS) measurement of a BH(10) solution in DMF, submicron-sized particles were observed. Therefore, a BH(10) membrane prepared from a solution containing submicron sized particles can be expected to have unique characteristics, even though such a surface does not show marked microphase separation. To investigate the characteristics of BH, especially BH(10), in water, the contact angle and water swelling were measured. Figure 2 shows plots of dynamic contact angle vs BSMS content in the copolymer.

The receding contact angle ($\cos(\varphi_R)$) decreased with increasing BSMS content in the block copolymer. The advancing contact angle ($\cos(\vartheta_A)$), however, showed peculiar deviation: $\cos(\vartheta_A)$ for BH(10) was larger than that of poly(HEMA), indicating that the surface hydrophilicity of BH(10) was much greater than that of poly(HEMA), despite the introduction of the hydrophobic polymer segment. The hydrophilicity of

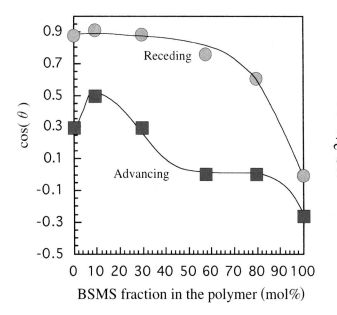

Fig. 2. Change in dynamic contact angles (θ) as a function of BSMS mole fraction in BH(X). *Squares*, advancing dynamic contact angle; *circles*, receding dynamic contact angle

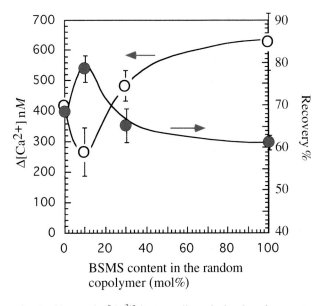

Fig. 3. Change in [Ca^{2+}] in nonadhered platelets (*open circles*) and recovery of platelets *closed circles* as a function of BSMS mole fraction in BH(X). *Bars* represent standard error; $n = 6$; the statistical significance of differences was estimated by the paired *t*-test. $\Delta[Ca^{2+}]$ indicates the increment of Ca^{2+} concentration above the control value (av 200 mM). A control sample of the platelets incubated without beads was used as reference for each measurement. Significant differences were found between BH(10) and poly(HEMA) for platelet recovery ($P < 0.02$) and activation ($P < 0.2$)

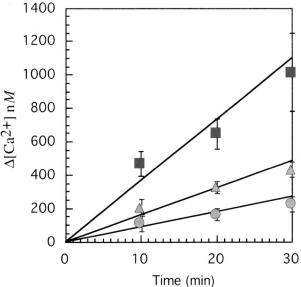

Fig. 4. Time dependence of $\Delta[Ca^{2+}]$ in nonadhered platelets after contact with the block copolymers: BH(10) (*circles*); poly(styrene-block-HEMA) (*triangles*); glass (*squares*). *Bars* represent standard error; $n = 6$; the statistical significance of differences was estimated by the paired *t*-test. The time courses of $\Delta[Ca^{2+}]$ were significantly different between BH(10) and glass ($P < 0.01$) and between BH(10) and poly(styrene-block-HEMA) ($P < 0.2$)

BH(10) was high not only on the surface but also in the bulk. Indeed, the equilibrium water content of BH(10) (ca. 80%) was much higher than that of poly(HEMA) (ca. 30%–40%). This may be explained by the supramolecular structure of the BH(10) membrane being derived from the particle-casting technique.

The extremely hydrophilic surface of BH(10) with polymer tethered chains can be expected to show excellent blood compatibility. Figure 3 shows changes in platelet recovery and Ca^{2+} concentration as a function of BSMS content in the copolymer. BH(10) shows again distinctive behavior in its interaction with platelets. The recovery of platelets after contact with BH(10) was the highest among any of the BH polymers, including poly(HEMA) [10]. Ishihara et al. reported that a high free-water content plays an important role in ensuring a surface highly compatible with blood [11]. The high recovery of platelets indicates a low level of adsorption onto BH(10). The activation of nonadhered platelets, which was estimated by an increase in Ca^{2+} concentration in the platelets, showed a similar relationship to BSMS content: the least activation of platelets was obtained with BH(10) among the members of the BH series including poly(HEMA).

In order to characterize further the blood compatibility of the BH(10) surface, the time course of platelet activation was investigated using BH(10), SH(40), and glass as a positive control (Fig. 4). The Ca^{2+} level increased significantly when platelets contacted with the glass surface, while the increase in Ca^{2+} levels was suppressed in the case of both block copolymers. In particular, the Ca^{2+} level of the platelets after contact with BH(10) was statistically lower than with SH(40) ($P < 0.2$) after 30 min, indicating that BH(10) activates platelets at a slower rate. The difference in the two block copolymers may indicate a new antithrombogenic mechanism on the BH(10) surface. On the basis of these results, it is concluded that the BH(10) membrane obtained from the particle-casting technique showed a new type of supramolecular surface, which possesses high antithrombogenicity. This may be a promising candidate for a novel, blood-compatible material for use in such applications as the artificial lung, and as a nonthrombogenic coating material.

References

1. Terasaki H, Morioka T (1991) Extracoporeal lung and heart assist with the artificial membrane lung in Japan. Artif Organs Today 1:115–127
2. Weathersby PK, Kolobow T, Stool EW (1975) Relative thrombogenicity of polydimethylsiloxane and silicone rubber constituents. J Biomed Mater Res 9:561–568
3. Braley S (1970) The chemistry and properties of the medical-grade silicones. J Macromol Sci Chem A4:529–544
4. Ito H, Taenaka A, Nagasaki Y, Kataoka K, Kato M, Tsuruya T (1996) Silicon-containing block copolymer membranes. Polymer 37:633–637
5. Okano T, Nishiyama S, Shinohara I, Akaike T, Sakurai Y, Kataoka K, Tsuruta T (1981) Effect of hydrophilic and hydrophobic microdomains on mode of interaction between block polymer and blood plateletes. J Biomed Mater Res 15:393–402
6. Nagasaki Y, Tsuruta T (1986) A novel synthesis of styrene derivatives with silylmethyl groups. Makromol Chem Rapid Commun 7:437–439
7. Tingy KG, Ardrade JD, Mcgary CW Jr, Zdrahata RJ (1988) The contact angle and interface energetics. In: Andrade JD (ed) Polymer surface dynamics. Plenum, New York, pp 105–118
8. Grynkiewicz G, Poenie M, Tsien RY (1985) A new generation of Ca^{2+} indicators with greatly improved fluoresence properties. J Biol Chem 260:3440–3448
9. Rink TJ, Smith SW, Tsien RY (1982) Cytoplasmic free Ca^{2+} in human platelets: Ca^{2+} thresholds and Ca-independent activation for shape-change and secretion. FEBS Lett 148:21–26
10. Ito H, Nagasaki Y, Kataoka K, Kato M, Tsuruta T, Suzuki K, Okano T, Sakurai Y (1997) Molecular design of poly(HEMA) brushes and its blood compatibility. Jpn J Anif Organs 16:519–523
11. Iwasaki Y, Fujike A, Kurita K, Ishihara K, Nakabayashi N (1996) Protein adscrption and platelet adhesion on polymer surfaces having phospholipid polar group connected with oxyethylene chain. J Biomater Sci Polym Ed 8:91–102

Development of a Fracture and Wear-Resistant Titanium Graphite Composite

S.H. Teoh[1], R. Thampuran[1], W.K.H. Seah[1], and J.C.H. Goh[2]

Summary. Fracture and wear have been identified as major problems leading to implant loosening, stress shielding, and the ultimate failure of implants. To overcome wear, numerous methods of surface coating have been employed. These have limitations, as the coatings are not able to repair or replenish themselves. The mechanisms of actual in vivo fracture and wear are complex and difficult to study. This is further aggravated by the hostile body environment that makes the biomaterial subject to stress corrosion cracking. Fracture and wear are commonly reported in orthopedic applications, and also cause serious and often lethal failure in mechanical heart valves. This paper reports on the development of a new triphasic titanium composite to overcome these problems. The composite consists of a pure titanium base, a hard titanium carbide phase, and a solid graphite phase. The pure titanium serves as the ductile, fracture-resistant phase while the in situ formation of titanium carbide provides the wear-resistant component. The graphite provides continuous lubrication to both articulating surfaces as the material is worn. A threefold reduction in wear rate has been recorded, as well as a decrease in the coefficient of friction. This composite is therefore a useful material to consider for implant applications.

Key words: Composite biomaterial — Titanium — Graphite — Powder metallurgy

Introduction

Fracture and wear have been identified as major problems associated with implant loosening, stress shielding, and implant failure. To overcome wear, numerous methods of surface coating and hardening have been employed. These methods are not only prohibitively expensive, but a coating is not able to repair or replenish itself. One approach to address the wear problems in heart valves and orthopedic devices is to use materials engineering with ceramics such as alumina and pyrolytic carbon. However, these ceramics have reportedly failed catastrophically despite the best efforts

to minimize defects during manufacture [1]. In this paper, a triphasic composite developed by the controlled heterogeneous sintering of titanium and graphite powders is presented as a candidate biomaterial [2]. The composite comprises a pure titanium matrix and hard titanium carbide and solid graphite phases. The fracture toughness, friction, and wear performance of the composite is compared to sintered pure titanium.

Materials and Methods

Pure titanium (Merck, Germany, mean particle size of 150 μm) and graphite powders (Carbone, USA, mean particle size of 100 μm) were blended, compacted at a pressure of 0.62 GPa and sintered to 1250°C for 2 h in a vacuum at 10^{-5} mbars. The graphite composition in the blend was 8% by weight. The porosity of the 0.62-GPa compacted preparation was about 5% with pore sizes less than 40 μm. Fracture toughness tests were performed in accordance to ASTM E 399.90 for disc-shaped compact tension specimens similar to the one reported previously [3]. The porous compacts were not subjected to a fatigue precrack because pores act as sharp cracks. Friction and wear tests were conducted using the conventional pin-on-disc method on 19-mm diameter disc-shaped specimens [4]. The counterface employed was case-hardened stainless steel (hardner scale of 60 HRc) and the rotational speed of the disc was 30 rpm. All the specimens were subjected to a load of 5 kN.

Results and Discussion

Active diffusion of carbon in titanium leads to the formation of titanium carbide during the sintering of titanium and graphite powders. Pronounced titanium, titanium carbide, and graphite peaks can be observed in the X-ray diffraction (XRD) spectrum of the composite shown in Fig. 1. A schematic diagram of the diffusion of carbon in titanium in the binary powder system is illustrated in Fig. 2. In powder metallurgy, diffusion is controlled by the solubility, curvature, and dislocation gradients between the particles. Thus, the

---

[1] Centre for Biomedical Materials Applications and Technology (BIOMAT), Mechanical and Production Engineering Department, and [2] Department of Orthopaedic Surgery, National University of Singapore, 10 Kent Ridge Crescent 119260, Singapore

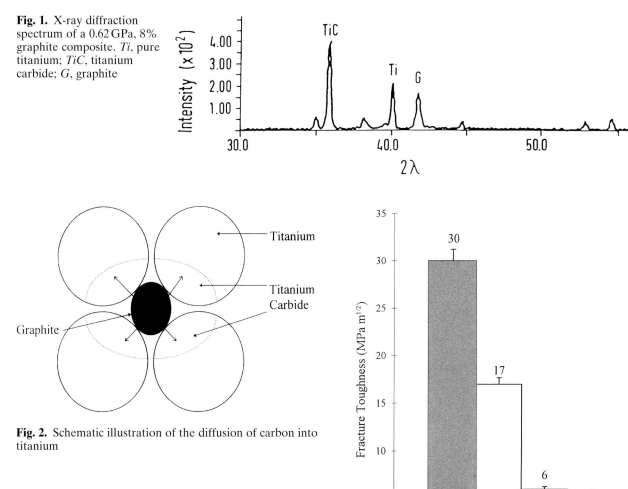

Fig. 1. X-ray diffraction spectrum of a 0.62 GPa, 8% graphite composite. *Ti*, pure titanium; *TiC*, titanium carbide; *G*, graphite

Fig. 2. Schematic illustration of the diffusion of carbon into titanium

Fig. 3. Comparison of the frature toughness of the titanium–graphite composites with 4% graphite (*dark gray column*) and 8% graphite (*white column*) to alumina (*mid-gray column*) and zirconia (*black column*)

amount of titanium carbide and graphite can be controlled by the sintering temperature, time, compaction pressure, and graphite composition. By varying these parameters, highly versatile titanium–graphite composite biomaterials with various amounts of the secondary phases can be fabricated. The fracture toughness of the composite (17–$30\,MPa\cdot m^{0.5}$) is at least double that of the commonly used bioceramics, such as alumina (2–$4\,MPa\cdot m^{0.5}$) and zirconia (6–$8\,MPa\cdot m^{0.5}$), because of the strength provided by the major titanium phase (Fig. 3).

The fracture of porous materials occurs through the failure of material ligaments arising from localized shear regions caused by deforming pores. In the fracture of titanium–8% graphite composites, both brittle titanium carbide in titanium–graphite ligaments and ductile pure titanium ligaments fail. Catastrophic failure is avoided by the plasticity and crack arrest properties conveyed by the extensive presence of ductile pure titanium [5]. A marked improvement in the wear performance of the composite compared to sintered titanium can be observed in Fig. 4: a threefold reduction in the weight loss due to wear was achieved. Although greater fracture toughness requires less

titanium carbide in the composite, this is at the expense of wear and frictional performance. The hard titanium carbide phases provide wear resistance by presenting obstacles to the plastic flow.

The wear performance is further enhanced by the release of free graphite that "smears" the articulating surfaces, thereby reducing the surface traction. This lubrication phenomenon is best observed in the frictional profile of the composite (Fig. 5). The profile is distinguished by a stage of high coefficient of friction that can be attributed to the dominance of hard titanium carbide during the initial stages of wear, followed by a slow transition to the graphite-smearing

S.H. Teoh et al.

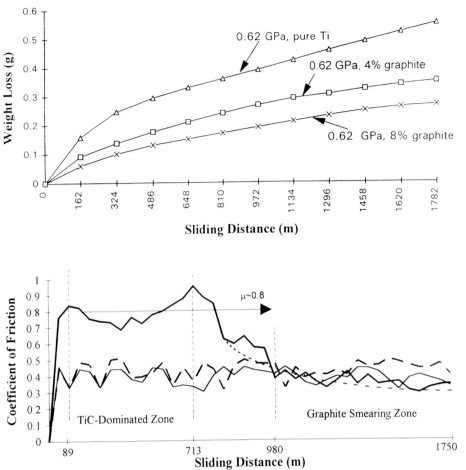

Fig. 4. Weight loss measurements of the titanium–graphite composites and the pure titanium preparation

Fig. 5. Frictional profiles of the 0.62 GPa compacted preparations: *solid line*, pure Ti; *bold line*, 8% graphite; *broken line*, 4% graphite

stage where the coefficient of friction is at least halved. A schematic representation of the phenomenon of wearing is shown in Fig. 6. Ultimately, graphite transfer from the composites to the counterface should occur and graphite–on–graphite articulation should lower the coefficient of friction of the tribosystem further. This can be seen by the decreasing trend in the coefficient of friction, over a long period, which approaches that of graphite (0.2). The free graphite in the composite, therefore, provides self-lubrication, replenishment, and protection to the abrading surfaces. The frictional profile of the titanium–4% graphite composite is also shown in Fig. 5. In these composites, the graphite composition in the initial blend was 4% by weight. In contrast to the titanium–8% graphite composites, "smearing" was not observed and the frictional profile was defined by the combination of surface traction due to pure titanium, titanium carbide, and some free graphite phases. Since the initial graphite composition was low, the amount of free graphite was too small to provide total smearing on the surface of the composite. Hence, the advantage afforded by

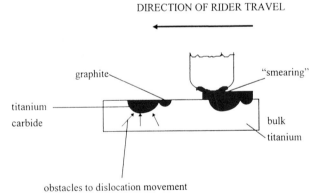

Fig. 6. Schematic illustration of the wear behavior of the composites

the release of graphite and subsequent lubrication of the composite requires that some critical amount of this constituent be included in the titanium-graphite powder blend during the manufacture of a self-lubricating composite biomaterial.

References

1. Savio JA III, Onecamp LM, Black J (1994) Size and shape of biomaterial wear debris. Clin Mater 15:101–147
2. Teoh SH, Thampuran R, Seah KWH, Goh JCH, inventer; National University of Singapore, assignee. Sintered titanium–graphite having improved wear resistance and low frictional characteristics for implant applications. Singapore patent 9501510-3. (Patent Pending)
3. Teoh SH, Thampuran R, Seah KWH, Goh JCH (1993) The effect of pore size and cholesterol–lipid on the fracture toughness of pure titanium sintered compacts. Biomaterials 14:407–412
4. Lim SC, Brunton JH (1986) The unlubricated wear of sintered iron. Wear 69:355–364
5. Teoh SH, Thampuran R, Seah KWH, Goh JCH (1997) The development of P/M titanium–graphite triphasic composites for biomedical applications. J Mater Sci Lett 16:639–641

Influence of Microporous Structures on Mural Thrombosis and Endothelialization at Blood-Contacting Surfaces

Takafumi Okoshi[1], Giorgio Soldani[2], Moses Goddard[3], and Pierre M Galletti[3]

Summary. The influence of microporous structures in the walls of small-diameter arterial prostheses was investigated with the aim of minimizing thrombosis and enhancing endothelialization of blood-contacting surfaces. Six types of spongy polyurethane–polydimethylsiloxane grafts (PUG), 1.5-mm in an internal diameter and 1.5–2 cm in length, were implanted end-to-end in the infrarenal aorta of 66 adult rats. Some had a continuous inner skin and a hydraulic permeability (HP) of $0\,ml/min/cm^2$ at the standard transmural pressure of 120mmHg (PUG-S-0). Some had a discontinuous inner skin with some isolated windows connecting penetrating micropores though the graft wall and a mean HP ranging from 11 (PUG-S-11) to 37 (PUG-S-37) or 58 (PUG-S-58) ml/min/cm^2. The rest had a microporous inner surface with penetrating micropores through the graft wall and a mean HP of 2.7 (PUG-2.7) or 39 (PUG-39) ml/min/cm^2. PUG which had a HP of less than 2.7ml/min/cm^2 showed poor patency. PUG with a HP of more than 11ml/min/cm^2 had acceptable patency, but endothelialization was limited to their anastomoses. In contrast, the patent PUG-S-37 and PUG-S-58 were largely endothelialized and all but one of the patent PUG-39 implants were completely endothelialized. In conclusion, penetrating micropores through the graft wall appear to inhibit critical mural thrombosis. A microporous inner surface seems to be superior to a skinned inner surface in achieving a high degree of endothelialization.

Key words: Polyurethane–polydimethylsiloxane — Spray phase-inversion technique — Penetrating micropores — Microporous structure — Endothelialization

Introduction

Blood-contacting surfaces for cardiovascular devices have mainly been made of smooth, nonthrombogenic surface materials [1,2]. However, mural thrombosis and thromboembolism are not completely avoided [3].

Based on observation of the rat abdominal aorta replacement model with small-diameter vascular grafts, we recently suggested that materials with a microporous surface and wall structure may be superior to smooth surfaces for inhibiting mural thrombosis and enhancing endothelialization at blood contacting surfaces [4,5]. The present paper reports further investigation of that hypothesis.

Materials and Methods

Preparation

Polyurethane–polydimethylsiloxane (Cardiothane 51, Kontron Instruments, Everett, MA, USA) vascular grafts with an internal diameter of 1.5mm and a wall thickness of 0.45mm were fabricated by a spray, phase-inversion technique described elsewhere [6] and according to well-established material-processing principles [7].

Six types of spongy vascular grafts with a continuous inner skin, a discontinuous inner skin featuring windows of varying sizes and amounts, or a totally microporous inner surface, were prepared. Their hydraulic permeability was characterized by measuring the volume of degassed distilled water collected during the first minute by filtration through the graft wall under the standard transmural pressure of 120mmHg.

The grafts with a continuous inner skin (identified as PUG-S-0) had a hydraulic permeability (HP) of $0\,ml/min/cm^2$. Three types of grafts with a discontinuous inner skin and varying density of isolated windows showed mean HP of 11, 37, or 58ml/min/cm^2 (identified as PUG-S-11, PUG-S-37, and PUG-S-58, respectively). The other two types had a microporous inner surface and an average HP of 2.7 or 39ml/min/cm^2 (identified as PUG-2.7 and PUG-39). Thus, the graft types with a discontinuous inner skin and a microporous inner surface had penetrating micropores though the graft wall. PUG stands for polyurethane graft, S means that a skin layer is formed at the inner surface, and the numbers indicate the values of hydraulic permeabilities. The material structures were

[1] Division of Cardiovascular Surgery, Second Department of Surgery, Teikyo University School of Medicine, 2-11-1 Kaga, Itabashi-ku, Tokyo 173, Japan
[2] Istituto di Fisiologia Clinica del CNR, Via Savi No. 8, 56100 Pisa, Italy
[3] Artificial Organ Laboratory, Brown University, Providence, RI 02912, USA

characterized by scanning electron microscopy (SEM, Hitachi, S-2700 or HS-800 Tokyo, Japan).

Implantation

Twelve PUG-S-0, 6 PUG-S-11, 4 PUG-S-37, 4 PUG-S-58, 23 PUG-2.7, and 17 PUG-39, 1.5–2 cm in length, were implanted by the same surgeon end-to-end in the infrarenal aorta of 66 male Sprague-Dawley rats weighing 250–350 g. Pentobarbital sodium intraperitoneal anesthesia and standard microsurgical techniques were employed. Two segments of the aorta, at the level of the left renal vein for the proximal anastomosis and proximal to the iliac bifurcation for the distal anastomosis, were separately dissected. In each case, the longest possible graft which could be accommodated anatomically and surgically was implanted. The bypassed segment of the native aorta was ligated, divided at both stumps, and left behind the implanted graft. Six to seven 10-0 nylon sutures were needed for each anastomosis. No antithrombogenic agent was administered pre- or postoperatively.

Retrieval

Specimens were retrieved between 2 h and 3 months after implantation. Under deep intraperitoneal pentobarbital anesthesia, the rat cardiovascular system was perfused through the left ventricle and simultaneously drained from the right atrium, first with 300–400 ml of heparinized saline and then with 150–200 ml of fixative (3% (w/v) paraformaldehyde + 2.5% (w/v) glutaraldehyde). Thereafter, the graft specimen was resected together with the surrounding tissues and margins of the native aorta at both ends. The graft was opened longitudinally, carefully examined, and photographed.

Study of Specimens

For light microscopy, the specimens were embedded in resin (Historesin, Reichert-Jung Optische Werke, Vienna, Austria), sectioned by a microtome (Microtome 2050 Supercut, Reichert-Jung Optische Werke), and stained with hematoxylin and eosin. Samples for SEM were dehydrated in graded alcohols (50%–100%), critical-point dried with CO_2, sputter-coated with gold and palladium, and examined with a Hitachi S-2700 or HS-800 SEM.

Statistical Analysis

The Fisher test was used to determine the significance of differences in patency between the PUG-2.7 group and PUG-39 group. Differences were considered significant if the P value was less than 0.05.

Results

In PUG-S-0 grafts with a continuous inner skin (2.2 μm in thickness), the wall section was compact and the outer surface showed a filamentous appearance with interfiber intervals ranging from 70 to 130 μm. PUG-S-11 had an inner skin (6.7 μm in thickness) with isolated pores ranging from 10 to 60 μm. The graft wall was open and the outer surface features were similar to those of PUG-S-0. PUG-S-37 had an inner skin (6.5 μm in thickness) with isolated pores measuring 10 to 80 μm in their largest dimension. The graft wall was open and the outer surface features were the same as those of PUG-S-0. PUG-S-58 had an inner skin (6.6 μm in thickness) with isolated pores measuring 10 to 50 μm. The structure of the graft wall was open and the outer surface displayed features similar to those of PUG-S-0. In the microporous surface grafts, the inner surface of PUG-2.7 showed pores measuring 30 to 70 μm in their largest dimension. The graft wall and the outer surface features were the same as those of PUG-S-0. PUG-39 showed a filamentous inner surface with interfiber spaces ranging from 90 to 130 μm. The structure of the graft wall was widely open and the outer surface displayed features similar to those of PUG-S-0.

All six types of grafts displayed good surgical handling properties and suturability. After the aortic clamp was released and blood started passing through the graft, no blood leakage was recognized through the wall of PUG-S-0. In PUG-S-11, however, a few to several reddish spots appeared on the external surface, spread, and fused with each other. Eventually, the entire external surface looked red and blood oozed for a few minutes. The polymer wall of PUG-2.7 showed a reddish tint, and occasional red spots were observed on the external surface. In contrast, blood oozed through the entire wall of PUG-S-37, PUG-S-58, and PUG-39 immediately after release of the aortic clamp; oozing continued for several minutes and the grafts looked uniformly red.

With regard to patency, in the skinned surface graft group, 2 out of 3 PUG-S-0 retrieved at 1–3 days were patent. However, all eight grafts of that type retrieved at 1 to 2 weeks were occluded. The sole graft retrieved at 3 months was also occluded with an organized tissue, which suggested that the occlusion had occurred at an early stage. In contrast, the patency of PUG-S-11 was 80% (4/5) at 3 months (one graft was acutely thrombo-occluded at 2 h after implantation). The overall patency rate, thus, was 67% (4/6) up to 3 months, below that of PUG-S-37 or PUG-S-58. The patency of PUG-S-37 and PUG-S-58 was 100% (4/4) and 75% (3/4) at 3 months, respectively. Thus PUG with a HP of more than 11 ml/min/cm^2 showed a better patency than less permeable grafts. In the

Table 1. Patency of polyurethane–polydimethylsiloxane small-diameter vascular grafts

	Within 3 days	1–2 Weeks	3 Months
Skinned inner surface grafts			
PUG-S-0	67% (2/3)	0% (0/8)	0% (0/1)
PUG-S-11	0% (0/1)	—	80% (4/5)
PUG-S-37	—	—	100% (4/4)
PUG-S-58	—	—	75% (3/4)
Microporous inner surface grafts			
PUG-2.7	—	73% (8/11)	8% (1/12)
PUG-39	—	—	76% (13/17)

microporous surface grafts, the patency was 73% (8/11) at 1 to 2 weeks and 8% (1/12) at 3 months for PUG-2.7, but 76% (13/17) at 3 months for PUG-39. The 3-month-patency rate of PUG-39 was significantly higher than that of PUG-2.7 ($P < 0.001$). Thus, in both graft types with skinned or microporous inner surface morphology, grafts with a higher hydraulic permeability exhibited better patency (Table 1).

In the patent specimens of PUG-S-0 retrieved in the first few days after implantation, a thick red thrombus layer, or a relatively thick mosaic of multiple tiny red thrombi in a proteinaceous layer of fibrin networks was observed. In the patent PUG-S-11 at 3 months, the grafts displayed endothelialization limited to 1–2 mm from the proximal and distal anastomoses. The graft inner surface was covered with a relatively thin proteinaceous layer and scattered tiny red thrombi. In contrast, the patent PUG-S-37 and PUG-S-58 were largely endothelialized with minimal neointimal hyperplasia. In PUG-2.7 at 2 weeks, endothelialization was limited to 2–3 mm from either the proximal or the distal anastomosis. Relatively thick red thrombi or proteinaceous layers covered the rest of the graft inner surface. At 3 months, the sole patent PUG-2.7 showed neointimal hyperplasia and incomplete endothelialization. Host cell migration within the graft wall was limited. On the other hand, all but one of the patent PUG-39 showed a thin, glistening, and transparent neointima with complete endothelialization. In all patent grafts at 3 months, except for PUG-2.7, numerous host cells had migrated and newly formed capillaries were identified in the voids of the graft wall, which appeared moderately to highly cellular. Thick mural thrombus, anastomotic hyperplasia, or aneurysm formation was not observed in the patent grafts with higher HP, namely PUG-39, PUG-S-37, or PUG-S-58. Mural thrombosis was least in the higher HP grafts (PUG-39, and then PUG-S-37 or PUG-S-58), followed by middle HP grafts (PUG-S-11) and lower HP grafts (PUG-2.7, and PUG-S-0) in this order.

Discussion

After graft implantation, serum proteins and thrombi attached to the inner surface and within the graft wall coexist in various proportions. This complex of serum protein and thrombus is referred to as the protein–thrombus (P–T) complex. Grafts do not occlude if the P–T complex remains thin and firmly attached on the inner surface, in part because it includes cell-adhesive proteins and favors endothelial cell adhesion. Under this hypothesis, grafts are expected to show excellent patency and endothelialization as long as the P–T complex is thin and stable.

Regardless of inner surface morphology, almost all PUG which had a HP of less than $2.7\,\text{ml/min/cm}^2$ were occluded. On the other hand, PUG and a HP of more than $11\,\text{ml/min/cm}^2$ had acceptable patency, which means that P–T complex development did not reach a critical level for occlusion. In PUG-S-11, it appears that the P–T complex was relatively thin but unstable, resulting in acceptable patency but endothelialization limited to the anastomoses. In contrast, the P–T complex was thin and stable in the PUG-S-37, PUG-S-58, and PUG-39, leading to a good patency and a high degree of endothelialization with minimal neointimal hyperplasia.

In a spongy, maze-like structure, some channels reach the outer surface of the graft while others are dead-end voids within the graft wall. Penetrating micropores starting from micropores of microporous inner surface or windows of discontinuous-skinned inner surface form microchannels which reach the outside of the graft. The density of penetrating micropores is grossly reflected by the hydraulic permeability in vitro or the blood permeability upon implantation. A continuous inner skin totally shields this maze-like structure from the blood stream, while isolated windows in the inner skin open a passageway for blood to invade the wall.

It seems that a high density of penetrating micropores prevents the P–T complex from developing to a critical level for occlusion in the acute and early stage of implantation. Further investigation is needed to establish the physical and biological mechanisms by which penetrating micropores control the thickness of mural thrombus.

With regard to the stability of the mural thrombus, P–T complexes in the continuous-skinned surface grafts cannot meet those formed within the graft wall from the outside, whereas those attaching to discontinuous-skinned or microporous inner surface grafts do connect, and appear to be more stable under the shear stress associated with the blood stream. Anchoring is best in microporous grafts, and may complement high wall porosity to explain the higher patency of vascular grafts which combine a microporous inner surface with a high hydraulic permeability.

In developing artificial organs with blood-contacting surfaces, most of the attention has been paid to chemical factors such as material composition, surface modification, and local anticoagulation. This study suggests that physical and structural factors such as material resilience and microgeometry may also contribute to reducing mural thrombosis. A combination of chemical and physical factors may be needed to achieve the best blood-contacting surfaces for cardiovascular devices.

References

1. Gibbons DF (1992) Cardiac assist devices. In: Hastings GW (ed) Cardiovascular biomaterials. Springer, London, pp 185–194
2. Kambic HE (1988) Polyurethane small artery substitute. ASAIO Trans 34:1047–1050
3. Frazier OH, Rose EA, Macmanus Q, Burton NA, Lefrak EA, Poirier VL, Dasse KA (1992) Multicenter clinical evaluation of the HeartMate 1000 IP left ventricular assist device. Ann Thorac Surg 53:1080–1090
4. Okoshi T, Goddard M, Galletti PM, Soldani G (1991) In vivo evaluation of porous versus skinned polyurethane–polydimethylsiloxane small diameter vascular grafts. ASAIO Trans 37:480–481
5. Okoshi T, Soldani G, Goddard M, Galletti PM (1993) Very small-diameter polyurethane vascular prostheses with rapid endothelialization for coronary artery bypass grafting. J Thorac Cardiovasc Surg 105:791–795
6. Soldani G, Panol G, Sasken F, Goddard MB, Galletti PM (1992) Small-diameter polyurethane–polydimethylsiloxane vascular prostheses made by a spraying, phase-inversion process. J Mater Sci Mater Med 3:106–113
7. Strathman H (1985) Production of microporous media by phase inversion processes. In: Lloyd DR (ed) Material science of synthetic membranes. American Chemical Society, Washington DC, pp 165–195

Discussion

Dr. Nosé:

Nosé, Baylor. I would like to ask a question to Dr. Okoshi. It's an excellent study. If my memory is correct, when I was in Cleveland, my former colleague Dr. Murabayashi did a similar microporous polyurethane graft study, and his study indicated it was patent, but in the porous structure there is a calcium deposition which took place. What is your experience of your graft and calcification?

Dr. Okoshi:

In this series, we have up to 3-month implants, and we haven't seen such a calcification. And also another group did a similar experiment. They followed up to 10 months and they told me no calcification was observed.

Dr. Kataoka:

I would also like to ask a question to Dr. Okoshi. I'm very impressed with the results, and could you comment on why you get such nice endothelialization by making a continuous microporous structure?

Dr. Okoshi:

Yes. Based on the experiments, my hypothesis is as follows: the microporous structure induces formation of a smooth surface layer of fibrin network. This layer contains a certain amount of albumin which is not involved in blood coagulation. The surface naturally biolized with host albumin maintained the patency of the graft with minimal thrombus formation and also accelerates endothelialization partly because the fibrin network also contains cell adhesive serum proteins.

Dr. Kataoka:

Could you measure the absorption of cell adhesive proteins like vitronectine on your surface?

Dr. Okoshi:

This is my hypothesis, but unfortunately we don't have a specimen of a short-time implant, so this is still under investigation.

Dr. Nojiri:

Dr. Ito, I have one question. Have we ever done a gas permeability study on your surface?

Dr. Ito:

The membrane showed unique characteristics as hydrogel. That is to say, it possessed high water content.

Dr. Nojiri:

Gas permeability — I'm asking about gas permeability.

Dr. Ito:

Yes. Such membranes with high water content can be expected to show fairly high oxygen permeability. But we have not tried it yet.

Dr. Galleti:

I have a question along the same line. If I understand correctly, your membranes were cast, so they were flat. Is it possible to make hollow fibers with this material?

Dr. Ito:

We have tried membrane fabrication of the BH(X) series. From the testing results, we found that a smooth, pinhole-free membrane is obtained by solvent casting onto a porous polypropylene membrane.

Dr. Galleti:

But can you fabricate it in the form of tubes?

Dr. Ito:

Yes. I have not tried it yet, but our group is making progress with it.

Part IV
Ventricular Assist Devices

The HeartMate Left Ventricular Assist System: Looking into the Future

Victor L. Poirier

Summary. The HeartMate left ventricular assist system (LVAS) is now in worldwide use in more than 100 clinical centers. To date, more than 700 implants have been completed, primarily to support patients as a bridge to a biologic heart transplant. Patients have been successfully supported for up to 546 days with a pneumatic-powered device and up to 503 days with an electrically-driven system. These implants have demonstrated the feasibility of this technology. The time has now come to evaluate these systems for permanent use in the nontransplant category. Patients in this category will tend to be older than the average age of 50 previously evaluated in the bridge category. Analysis of our database indicates that patients in the 61–70-year age group ($n = 103$) did as well as patients in the overall group of 13–70 years of age ($n = 591$). Of interest, the 61–70-year age group that received devices did significantly better than the equivalent control patients: 60% transplant rate vs 13%. In the future, patients will be supported for longer and longer periods of time. We will need to develop systems that are smaller, more reliable, quieter, more efficient, and less costly. In addition, portable systems will be of paramount importance to support future patients and to expand the use of this technology. Two clinical trials are being carried out in the USA to demonstrate the safety and effectiveness of our portable pneumatic driver and our portable electric system as a bridge to transplant. A third clinical trial is being carried out to evaluate our electric system as a permanent system in patients who do not qualify for a transplant. The trial consists of studying 65 LVAS patients and 65 randomized control patients receiving the best medical therapy available. All three studies are designed to discharge patients into the home environment.

Key words: Left ventricular assist system/device — Permanent — Nontransplant — HeartMate — Elderly

Introduction

As early as the 1940s, the US government recognized that cardiovascular disease among Americans was a serious problem. At that time, cardiovascular disease was the number one killer of Americans. In fact, cardiovascular disease has been the number one killer of Americans in every year since 1900 except one — 1918.

Recognizing that the government would have to spearhead a national effort to conduct research and development on the cause and treatments of cardiovascular disease, President Harry S. Truman signed into law on June 16, 1948, the National Heart Act that created the National Heart Institute, a new institute within the National Institute of Health [1]. This was the beginning of our national effort to develop technology that would alleviate the debilitating effects of heart disease. Thermo Cardiosystems began its involvement in this area in 1966 when it received a contract to develop a mechanical heart. Continued research through the years led to the design of the HeartMate blood pump now in commercial use. Initially, the design of this device was established in 1975. From that point, 10 years of testing was carried out with more than 120 large animal implants conducted before permission was obtained from the FDA for clinical evaluation.

In 1985, a clinical trial was initiated with the pneumatic HeartMate device as a bridge to transplant [2]. After 9 years of testing, the device was finally approved for commercial sale as a bridge to transplantation [3]. Since that time, two additional clinical trials in the bridge-to-transplant category have been started, one for a portable pneumatic driver and another using the HeartMate electric version of the device for bridge-to-transplant candidates.

In looking at future needs, it is obvious that these systems will be needed for nontransplant candidates. To fulfill that need, we have initiated a randomized trial to evaluate the HeartMate electric system as an alternative to medical treatment. The trial will consist of 65 patients receiving a device and 65 patients receiving the best medical therapy. It is estimated that 3 years will be needed to complete the study to prove that the HeartMate device is safe and effective for this application.

Much work is left to be done. We must develop smaller, more efficient, and more reliable systems for support of the left, right, or total circulation as well as devices to support the pediatric and geriatric population.

Thermo Cardiosystems Inc., PO Box 2697, 470 Wildwood Street, Woburn, MA 01888-2697, USA

Materials and Methods

The HeartMate blood pump now being used clinically is a pusher-plate type of device [4] as shown in Fig. 1. It has a discoid shape and is fabricated from titanium with 6% aluminum and 4% vanadium. The pump body is 11.2 cm in diameter and 4 cm thick. The inlet conduit consists of a 19-mm diameter inlet tube connected to a 25-mm porcine xenograft valve. The pump body has a stroke volume of 83 ml and the pump can produce flows in excess of 10 l/min. The pumping chamber consists of a polyether polyurethane diaphragm bonded to a rigid piston. The outlet conduit consists of a 25-mm diameter porcine xenograft valve attached to a 20-mm polyester conduit.

All blood-contacting surfaces are textured. Metal components are textured with titanium spheres bonded to the substrate, while the polyurethane surface is textured by extruding filaments from the base membrane [5].

The pneumatic version of the blood pump can be powered with either a hospital-based console or a portable driver. Both drivers provide a pneumatic pulse to the blood pump to pressurize the pump chamber to expel blood in a controlled fashion. Both devices are also fully instrumented to provide information on stroke volume, flow, and beat rate as well as programmed to alarm whenever an unsafe condition exists. The main difference between the two power sources is that the portable system is designed to allow patients to leave the hospital and live at home. This system is now under clinical trials to establish its safety in the hospital and in the home environment. This battery-operated system is 25 cm high, 35 cm, long, and 15 cm wide, and weighs less than 7.3 kg.

The electric HeartMate system consists of an implantable blood pump and driver coupled with an electrical vent line to an external console and battery pack. Support hardware consists of a bedside battery charger and power unit, as well as an auxiliary digital display unit that can be used in the operating room or intensive care unit (ICU), or under other nonambulatory conditions.

As shown in Fig. 2, the electromechanical driver consists of an electronically commutated low-speed torque motor that drives the pusher-plate through a pair of nested helical came. The torque motor itself consists of a stationary copper wave-wound stator, a rotating magnet assembly, and an electronic commutator.

The motor operates at physiological speeds, with one motor revolution corresponding to one pump ejection cycle. As the magnet assembly of the torque motor rotates, two diametrically opposed ball-bearing cam followers bear against nested helical cams. These face cams are fixed to the pusher plate and serve to convert the rotary motion of the pump to the linear motion of the pusher plate.

The weight of the combined pump, torque motor, and energy converter is 908 g and the displacement is 460 cm^3. The conduits weigh an additional 161 g and the displacement is 174 cm^3. This includes all protective housing, cables, tubes, and connectors.

The HeartMate left ventricular assist system (LVAS) is implanted in either the peritoneal cavity or in a surgically-created pocket in the preperitoneal position. A percutaneous line that penetrates the body carries the electrical lead as well as a conduit to permit air transfer to and from the motor chamber. Air transfer is required to maintain the pressure in this cavity at

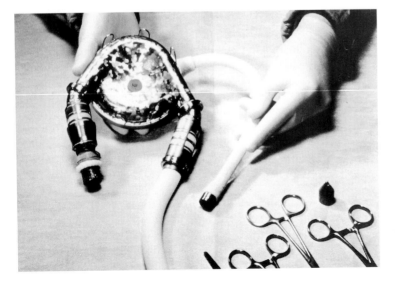

Fig. 1. The implantable HeartMate blood pump with capacity to produce more than 10 l·min^{-1} of blood flow

Fig. 2. Cross-section of the HeartMate left ventricular assist device

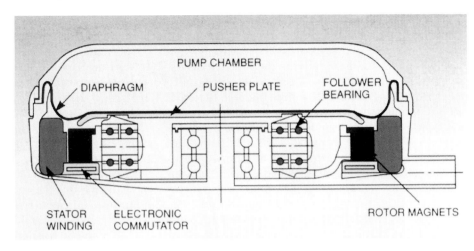

atmospheric conditions. For every beat, a volume of air equivalent to the volume of blood pumped must be accommodated.

The vented electric system is operated by a portable control system which is worn by the patients as shown in Fig. 3. It is designed to be as small as possible so that it can be conveniently clipped onto a belt. Its dimensions are $6.2 \times 7.6 \times 1.9$ cm with a total weight with attached cables and connectors of 275 g. Permanently mounted to the housing are two leads that connect to a pair of batteries via a positive acting, push-type sealed connector. Power is derived from either one of two batteries, to provide redundancy.

The control system is designed to provide power conditioning to the motor, rate control, documentation of operating parameters, diagnostic information, basal level default capability, as well as a sophisticated alarm system to provide the patient with a warning on malfunction.

Two emergency systems are provided to the patients. First, because the pump can be driven pneumatically, a portable hand-pump is provided to every patient in the event of a malfunction. The hand-pump can be attached quickly to the vent line exiting the patient. Pumping can then be restored with pneumatic energy to flows nearly equivalent to that with electrical actuation. The operation of the hand-pump can be carried out for extended durations without undue strain on the operator. Pneumatic operation can also be carried out by attaching the patient's vent line to the standard pneumatic clinical console.

Results

The HeartMate LVAS has been implanted in more than 700 patients thus far. Two basic configurations have been utilized: the first is a pneumatic driver and

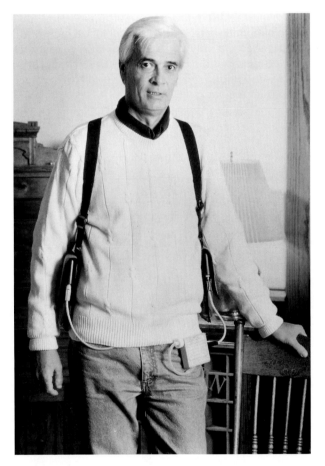

Fig. 3. Patient with the HeartMate electric system implanted illustrating the small electronic controller and battery packs

the second, an electric driver. The majority of implants have been carried out as a bridge to support patients waiting for biologic heart transplants. In looking into the future, it is clear that these devices will need to address the nontransplant candidates. These patients tend to be somewhat older than bridge patients who are, on the average, 50 years old. The HeartMate database was evaluated to determine the outcome of patients being supported over the age of 50 to try to predict future performance of this system in the older patient population.

Of the 700 patients supported, more than 100 are ongoing. These were eliminated from this analysis, leaving 591 patients on devices and 48 control patients for a total of 639 patients that had a definitive outcome. Figure 4 illustrates the distribution of patients as a function of age, type of device, and controls. The pneumatic precommercial patients were those patients included in the clinical study carried out between 1985 and 1994. The pneumatic postcommercial patients are those patients that received a device after US Food and Drug Administration (FDA) approval in 1994.

In reviewing this figure, it is important to realize that all the patients received the identical blood pump with the driver as the only variance. This figure illustrates that the distribution of patients between the entire patient population, the 51–60, and 61–70-year age group is consistent.

Of the 591 patients who received devices, 63% were idiopathic while 35% were ischemic. As shown in Fig. 5, the tendency in the older patient population was toward an increase in the ischemic category. There was no significant difference between the 51–60-year age group and the 61–70-year age group.

Approximately 85% of patients who received a HeartMate LVAS were men, and this ratio did not change significantly as a function of age. This is not to be unexpected in that up to this point these patients were transplant candidates and reflect the distribution of patients on the transplant list. In looking at nontransplant candidates in the older patient population, one may expect this trend to change.

One of the interesting outcomes of this analysis was that the average implant duration was remarkably similar for all patient categories. Figure 6 illustrates the trend. The older population in the 61–70-year age group did not require longer periods of support before transplant, as one may have thought. In addition, as shown in Fig. 7 the percentage of patients that were transplanted in the 61–70-year age group was not significantly different from the percentage transplanted in the entire population. This is an interesting outcome

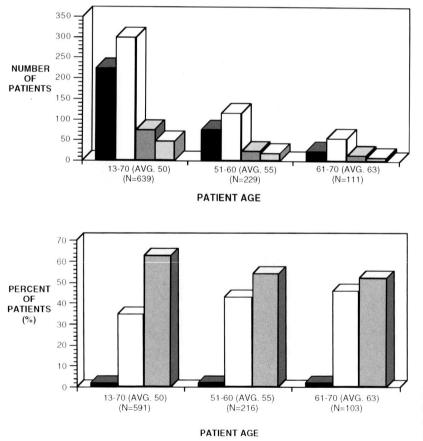

Fig. 4. Patient distribution by age and device vs controls (*pale gray bars*). Precommercial patients (pneumatic control, *black bars*) are between 1985 and 1994. Postcommercial patients are from 1994 to present: pneumatic (*white bars*) and electric (*dark gray bars*)

Fig. 5. Distribution of patients by indication: myocardial infarction (*black bars*); ischemia (*white bars*); idiopathic (*gray bars*)

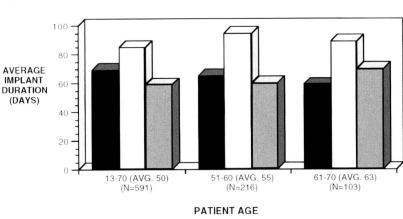

Fig. 6. Distribution of patients by age and implant duration. *Bars* as in Fig. 4

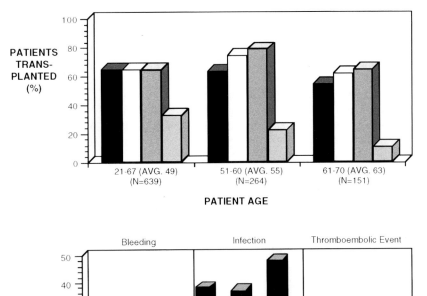

Fig. 7. Distribution of patients by age and percent transplanted. *Bars* as in Fig. 4

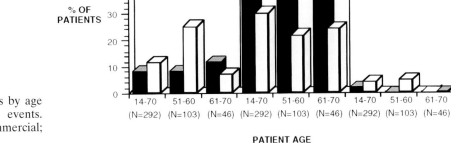

Fig. 8. Distribution of patients by age and device-related adverse events. *Black bars*, pneumatic precommercial; *white bars*, electric

when considering how the control patients fared over the same age group. As can be seen, the 61–70-year age group of control patients did poorly compared to the entire population.

Device-related adverse events that were evaluated, i.e., bleeding, infection, and thromboembolic events are shown in Fig. 8. In the bleeding category, it is not clear why bleeding was more pronounced in the 51–60-year age group with electric systems. Other than

this anomaly, bleeding was similar in all age categories. In the infection category, infections tended to increase with age with the pneumatic device and decrease with the electric device. It is not clear why this trend exists. Device-related thromboembolic events were low in all cases and were not considered significant. Of the 46 patients in the 60–70-year age group, none experienced any device-related thromboembolic events.

Discussion

We as a society have made significant progress in the development of mechanical technology to support the failing circulation in humans. We have demonstrated feasibility and safety in the bridge-to-transplant category and now must look forward to the next step in this evolutionary process. We need to develop systems that are smaller and more reliable in order to address the younger patient population, and we need to look at different concepts, such as high-speed rotary pumps as well as biologically powered devices. We also need to address the feasibility of using these systems in an older patient population that cannot benefit from transplants.

We are addressing all of these needs as we look into the future. We have analyzed our database and established that patients more than 60 years of age can do well on these devices, at least in the short term. Now, our challenge is to study how these older patients will do in the long term and, to this end, we have begun a clinical trial to evaluate these patients.

The primary objective of this multicenter randomized clinical trial is to evaluate the safety and efficacy (in terms of survival and quality of life) of left ventricular assist systems in NYHA class IV heart failure patients who are not considered candidates for cardiac transplantation. The primary endpoints will be mortality from all causes and quality of life. The secondary objectives are:

1. To compare the effect of LVAS and medical therapy on cardiovascular mortality in patients with end-stage heart failure.
2. To compare the functional capacity in the LVAS group, before and after implantation, with the medically treated group.
3. To compare the incidence of adverse events between the LVAS and control groups.
4. To compare the quality of life between the LVAS and control groups.

Study Summary

This study will be a randomized, nonblinded, controlled trial. The trial will be a parallel study with random assignment of the eligible patients to treatment with a HeartMate VE-LVAS or to the control group who continue to receive medical therapy. The minimum follow-up will be two years. It is estimated that 65–75 patients per treatment group will be required for this study.

A clinical coordinate center (CCC) will determine the eligibility of potential study candidates. After eligibility criteria have been met and informed consent is obtained, the CCC will randomly assign patients to either the LVAS or control group. For patients assigned to the VE-LVAS group, the implant surgery will be performed within 24 hours of randomization. The control group of patients will continue receiving maximal medical therapy.

The VE LVAS patients will receive routine care and rehabilitation until they are an NYHA class I or II. After the patient has completed a training program, the patients will be discharged from the hospital. Both patient groups will be followed every two weeks by alternating phone calls and clinic visits.

The study will involve detailed measurement for hemodynamic function, functional capacity, adverse events, such as bleeding and infection, and survival rates. These measurements are required for the patient's clinical management, as well as for the purposes of the study. In addition, the study will involve measuring the health-related quality of life. These measurements are preferences of patients for balancing length of life with quality of life. These measurements are conducted only for the purpose of the study, but will provide valuable input to future clinical management of these patients. All patients will be followed for at least two years after randomization. The trial will involve questionnaires to measure quality of life and patient preferences.

What is clear is that we are only at the beginning of a new era of mechanical circulatory support. Our goals must be set high to arrive at systems that can truly make a difference in the future. We must achieve success and arrive at systems that are smaller, more efficient, more reliable, quieter, and less costly than we now have, and we must have systems that can effectively be used for the younger as well as the older population.

References

1. Poirier V (1993) The quest for a solution; we must continue. We must push forward. The 16th Hastings Lecture. ASAIO J 39:853–863
2. Dasse K, Frazier OH, Lesniak J, Myers T, Burnett C, Poirier V (1992) Clinical responses to ventricular assistance versus transplantation in a series of bridge to transplant patients. ASAIO J 38:M622–M626
3. Frazier OH, Rose E, Macmanus Q, Burton N, Lefrak E, Poirier V, Dasse K (1992) Multicenter clinical evaluation of the HeartMate 1000 IP left ventricular device. Ann Thorac Surg 53:1080–1090
4. Poirier V (1995) The TCI HeartMate blood pump. In: Lewis T, Graham T (eds) Mechanical circulatory support. Edward Arnold, London, pp 229–236
5. Dasse K, Menconi M, Lian J, Stein G, McGee M, Poirier V, Frazier O (1990) Characterization of TCI's textured blood-contacting material following long-term clinical LVAD support. Cardiovas Sci Technol 1:218–220

Discussion

Dr. Jarvik:
Two questions. How many patients do you have that are out longer than 1 year, and, of those, what is the incidence of either infections or device-related complications in the patients over 1 year?

Mr. Poirier:
I'll have to give you the number from the top of my head. For over 1 year, probably 30–40 patients, something like that. The thromboembolic complications don't seem to vary much at all with time. I mean, there were some thought initially that as these devices got older and older in patients the thromboembolic rates would go up. We don't see that at all. What we do see is that infection becomes a problem. Usually exit site infection becomes a problem that's running at 20%–25%.

Dr. Jarvik:
And then other, other kinds of things like graft bleeding or mechanical failures. What's the percent in the over 1 year of those?

Mr. Poirier:
There have been a variety of things that we've seen as we learn. We've seen some outflow graft failure as a result of kinking caused by the pump migrating. We implant the pump and it fits very well and the grafts are all lined up very well, but, with time, you do see some migration, especially with the electrics and if it migrates and forms a little kink in the graft that kink will rub and tend to abrade away. We have seen that, so we're looking at changing the graft materials. We're using the DeBakey graft, which we started using in 1975, which was the best graft available at that time, but there are a lot of different grafts now that we're going to be looking at.

Dr. Jarvik:
So would you say it is something like 70% of patients over a year are free of any complications or is that too many. Is it 50%?

Mr. Poirier:
Eventually they all get complications, so it's hard for me to answer that. I mean, eventually everybody will die on this device because it wears out. Eventually this device will break because it's a mechanical device, so I can't answer that.

Dr. Jarvik:
But it's a very important issue whether it's going to be 1 year, 2 years, 5 years, 10 years, so we all wonder about that.

Mr. Poirier:
Yes, we do too, and we need to learn about that, and we need to push and keep going further and further. That's the only way we're going to learn, and we need to address the problems as they come up because there will be problems. I mean, it's naive to think there won't be problems; there will be, and it takes time to find them.

Dr. Reul:
I have actually two short questions. Maybe I missed your definition of the control group, but what was that?

Mr. Poirier:
In our clinical trial we had control patients that met the exact same entrance criteria as the device patients, and then they were followed to see what happened to them. They did not receive devices for one reason or another. We collected data on these patients, and then made the comparison between the two groups.

Dr. Reul:
And then the second question. There is always the argument for electric systems that the patients are much more mobile and that has an influence on the outcome of the results. But, according to your last slide, it doesn't make any difference if you use a pneumatic or electric system.

Mr. Poirier:
That's right. You would think that living at home and going back to work would produce more complications, but that hasn't been borne out. The electrics and pneumatics both do well.

Dr. Harasaki:
Harasaki, Cleveland. I always enjoy your presentation. I was just wondering, but do you think your system is ready for permanent usage in humans as it is, or do you have to wait for the totally implantable system?

Dr Portner:
You cannot look at it in isolation. It is too early to compare to transplantation as a therapy. Clearly, one has to consider the alternatives. The only alternative for most patients is continuing medical therapy with a poor quality of life. So, the answer is, I suppose, a qualified "yes," it is ready. Clearly, all of those in this field need to continue to make improvements to reduce the complications that are known. In fact, the system is already being used as a definitive theory.

Dr. Harasaki:
I'm just wondering, but may I extend this same question to Mr. Poirier?

Mr. Poirier:
I certainly think they are ready. I think, if you look at these patients, the alternative is death. We have to learn. The only way we're going to learn is by doing it, and we have to gain more and more experience. I think we're ready to do that, and I know we don't have perfect systems, I know we're going to have problems, and things are going to break, things are going to wear out. We're going to find complications that we don't know, but how else can we get there? We have to start, and I think we're ready. I really do. So, I'm in total favor of moving ahead and to take care of the problems as they come up.

Dr. Portner:
We have somewhat of a dilemma and I'm not quite sure how to address it. The lay population sets a much higher standard for devices than either drugs or surgical technique. Failure or side effects of a drug or of a surgical technique is more accepted than complications and failure of mechanical devices or devices in general. That is something all of us face. We need to do a better job of educating the public that nothing is perfect and one has to look at the alternatives. We have surely not done an adequate job of communicating that message. While we need to continue to improve these systems, I certainly think that they are now at the stage where definitive or long-term use is a perfectly reasonable thing to do.

Dr. Minami:
Right heart failure after implantation of the left heart assist device is sometimes a very serious problem. Do you have some number of the worldwide implantation experience? How many patients had right heart assist device after implantation of Novacor?

Dr. Portner:
I don't remember the exact number now, but 3 or 4 years ago it was between 15% and 20%. It's actually been going down. I think today the total experience is approximately 10%. I suspect that this is a consequence of intraoperative coagulopathy and bleeding leading to the use of blood products which produce a transient increase in pulmonary vascular resistance. Perhaps Dr. Kormos will expand on this. And, with the increasing use of Aprotinin, bleeding has significantly diminished. Long-term, these implants are going to be done on a much more elective basis, and under those circumstances right heart failure will be relatively infrequent.

Dr. Portner:
I'd just like to offer a comment rather than a question. I enjoyed your presentation, as I always do, Bob, but at the risk of being somewhat heretical, I would suggest there is at least one significant advantage the mechanical device has over heart transplantation. With heart transplantation there is clearly a limit to the long-term prognosis. In fact, if you look at the transplant registry, the average increase in life expectancy is about 7 years, and the only therapy following the eventual failure of heart transplantation due to vasculopathy is repeat transplantation. Today that is no longer an option, whereas a mechanical device can be replaced when it reaches the end of its useful life, just as a pacemaker or a heart valve is replaced. So with the mechanical therapeutic alternative, life extension can be substantially longer than might be expected for heart transplantation. Seven years for a 60-year-old is very different than 7 years for a 19-year-old.

Dr. Kormos:
Yes, I didn't really get into that strategy, but, you know, in my mind I can see what you're getting at and I can see a strategy where cardiac transplantation, the bridge concept will still exist, but the bridge concept will now be over a period of 10 years or even perhaps longer, depending on how often you have to replace components. But I see a place for the use of these devices, perhaps before cardiac transplantation, only in an extended period. And I think what we're going to end up doing is reserving cardiac transplantation for a very select group of patients or at some point in the patient's course of heart failure, but not as, say, the first step.

Dr. Portner:
In that scenario you might reach the conclusion that heart transplantation might in fact be reserved for older patients rather than for younger ones, whereas the currently perceived wisdom would suggest it's exactly the other way around.

Dr. Min:
Min from Seoul, Korea. I have one question, that if you are looking for permanent usage or for long-term or recovery of the natural heart, are you still going to use LV cannulation or are you going to move back to atrial cannulation?

Dr. Kormos:
To atrial?

Dr. Min:
Yes.

Dr. Kormos:
No, I think that the data is pretty clear that the risks of native heart thromboembolism increase with atrial cannulation. I think that ventricular cannulation is probably the method of choice.

Dr. Min:
But if you are looking for recovery of natural heart . . .

Dr. Kormos:
Well, you know, we're talking about devices that are currently available. I think that you have to keep in mind that the new crop of devices are much smaller and the axial flow systems that are being developed are going to be very small and these things can be removed very easily from the apex. I know Mr. Westerby is going to cover some of this, but I think we will be able to remove these pumps much more easily than we can today, and the apex can be closed and we won't have so much difficulty with ventricular cannulation techniques.

The Jarvik 2000 Oxford System. Prospects for the Future

Stephen Westaby[1], Takahiro Katsumata[1], and Robert K. Jarvik[2]

Summary. The existing Thermo Cardiosystems (TCI) Heartmate and Novacor left ventricular assist devices (LVADs) are well proven in the context of a bridge to transplantation but are unsuitable for small adults and children. Recently, chronic offloading of the left ventricle has resulted in an element of myocardial recovery in some patients with dilated cardiomyopathy and viral myocarditis. Whilst bridging to recovery is of increasing interest, the operation to remove these large devices, leaving the patient's own heart in situ, is difficult. We have designed a new system for prolonged left ventricular support based on the Jarvik 2000 axial flow impeller pump. In order to overcome driveline problems, we have employed a skull-mounted carbon pedestal with proven resistance to infection in a long-standing artificial hearing device. We have implanted the Jarvik 2000 Oxford System in 17 sheep for periods up to 198 days. We have demonstrated mechanical reliability and the ability to provide flow up to 10 l/min at speeds of up to 18000 rpm without haemolysis. The power requirement is between 7 and 10 watts and the device is silent. The device has been successfully explanted in a model of bridge to recovery. The Jarvik 2000 Oxford System has the potential for use as a permanent LVAD or for bridge to transplantation or recovery in adults and children.

Key words: Jarvik 2000 Oxford System — Artificial heart — Ventricular assist device — Heart failure — Transplantation

Introduction

In an increasingly elderly population, heart failure consumes enormous health care resources. Meanwhile, the surgical treatment of heart failure has reached a watershed. Cardiac transplantation markedly improves quality of life but outcome is limited by chronic immunosuppression, opportunistic infection, and the development of allograft coronary artery disease, which requires retransplantation in 40% of patients by six years [1]. With a severely restricted donor pool and 5-year mortality of 40%, conventional transplantation now fails to address the problem. There is little scientific evidence to suggest cardiac xenotransplantation as a realistic alternative. Also, in the absence of an alternative treatment, transplantation discards some poorly functioning but potentially recoverable hearts, particularly in dilated cardiomyopathy, viral myocarditis, or protozoal infections. Skeletal muscle myoplasty may prevent further cardiac dilatation but provides little in the way of increased stroke volume or cardiac output [2].

The clinical role of mechanical blood pumps began in the postcardiotomy setting and extended into bridge to transplantation. Data from the United Network for Organ Sharing (USA) have shown that a male with type O blood group, weighing more than 90.7 kg, will wait a mean of 595 days for a donor heart [3]. Increasing experience has shown the Thermo Cardiosystems (TCI) and Novacor electric pusher plate devices to function for prolonged periods without blood damage or risk of infection [4,5]. These devices are now used for bridges to transplantation in the community and have greatly improved the outcome in patients with multisystem failure [6]. The encouraging patient release programme with the TCI left ventricular assist device (LVAD) in the United States has led to permanent TCI implants for nontransplant candidates in Europe. Meanwhile, the critical shortage of donor hearts has resulted in prolonged left ventricular support and the crucial finding that in some patients the myocardium shows the propensity to recover [6]. Bridging to myocardial recovery by mechanical offloading now offers a new approach to the treatment of heart failure.

Evidence for Left Ventricular Recovery

Chronic left ventricular failure results in adaptive remodelling of the myocardium with alterations in the geometry of the left ventricle, orientation of cardiac myocytes, and disturbances in the biochemical function of the cellular organelles. The neurohormonal changes in heart failure (increased levels of angiotensin and norepinephrine) lead to hypertrophy and changes in the extracellular matrix

---

[1] Oxford Heart Centre, Oxford Radcliffe Hospital, The John Radcliffe, Headington, Oxford, OX3 9DU, UK
[2] Jarvik Research, New York, USA

by modifying the phenotypic characteristics of the myocyte and fibroblast. Left ventricular dilatation is a maladaptive response, which increases wall stress and imparts a mechanical disadvantage to the myofibrils. This is reflected in a shift of the end-diastolic pressure–volume relationship towards larger volumes [7]. Until recently, the structural changes of end-stage cardiomyopathy had been considered irreversible. Now, both angiotensin converting enzyme inhibitors and nitroglycerin have been shown to attenuate left ventricular enlargement after myocardial infarction, suggesting that reduction in wall stress may allow remodelling [8]. Chronic beta blockade also reduces ventricular mass and may normalise left ventricular shape [9]. In some patients, myocardial offloading by drug therapy has resulted in decreased norepinephrine levels, an index of the severity of heart failure.

Whilst drugs provide modest reductions in ventricular filling pressure and volume, mechanical blood pumps can provide complete offloading and the capacity to rest the heart whilst the patient remains active. Historically, maximal reduction in the workload of the dilated left ventricle by prolonged bed rest achieved a modest degree of left ventricular recovery in congestive heart failure [10].

Recently, at the time of cardiac transplantation, following prolonged mechanical support, it was observed that the hearts of patients with end-stage idiopathic cardiomyopathy had reverted towards normal size and weight [11]. In many patients the indices of left ventricular function approached normal values by the time a donor organ became available. This stimulated studies of left ventricular recovery at two major transplant centres — The Columbia Presbyterian Medical Centre, and The Texas Heart Institute [6,11]. The Columbia study documented substantial reversal of severe ventricular dilatation in idiopathic cardiomyopathy accompanied by normalisation of fibre-orientation and regression of myocyte hypertrophy [6]. End-diastolic pressure–volume relationships were shifted towards much lower volumes, similar to those obtained in normal hearts. Frazier et al. studied patients who had been supported for more than 30 days (mean 137 days, range 31-505 days), 17 with idiopathic cardiomyopathy and 14 with ischaemic cardiomyopathy [11]. Radiographic and echocardiographic documentation of cardiothoracic ratio and left ventricular end-diastolic volume and ejection fraction showed dramatic reductions in heart size and left ventricular mass, particularly in cardiomyopathy patients. With the device switched off, the cardiac index increased from 1.96 ± 0.52 to $2.93 \pm 0.73 \, \mathrm{l \cdot min^{-1} \cdot m^{-2}}$ ($P < 0.0001$). Pulmonary capillary wedge pressure decreased from 24.18 ± 6.27 to $14.48 \pm 3.01 \, \mathrm{mmHg}$ ($P <$

0.0001) and pulmonary vascular resistance fell from 3.34 ± 2.0 to 2.51 ± 0.88 Wood units ($P < 0.05$). Histological studies of the left ventricle showed a marked reduction in myocytolysis, whilst calcium uptake and binding studies of isolated sarcoplasmic reticulum vesicles showed deranged calcium metabolism to have normalised. Our own studies in cardiomyopathy patients suggest that recovery begins much sooner than anticipated, though changes in ventricular morphology do not necessarily imply sustainable improvement in left ventricular function. Nevertheless, LVAD removal without transplantation has been performed by Hetzer's group in Germany (R. Hetzer, personal communication), in Japan (T. Nakatani, personal communication), and in the UK (Oxford). In Berlin, recovery has been sustained for periods of up to 14 months in four dilated cardiomyopathy patients who were supported for 160, 244, 331, and 347 days. Functional recovery appears to have remained unchanged since LVAD removal. The same group have already used a miniaturised extracorporeal biventricular support (BIVAD) system (Berlin Heart) in two infants of 4 and 5 years with acute myocarditis. Both were admitted in cardiogenic shock and BIVAD implantation was performed under conditions of cardiopulmonary resuscitation. After support for 25 and 31 days respectively, the ejection fraction increased from less than 15% to 55% and 65%. After explantation of the device this improvement was sustained.

There are two requirements for bridging to myocardial recovery. Firstly, some reliable biochemical markers are needed to indicate sustainable ventricular recovery. The Berlin group have used disappearance from the serum of the autoantibody against the β_1 adrenergic receptor, hypothesising that presence of the autoantibody indicates an immune process which produces cardiac dilatation and functional impairment. The Texas group suggest normalisation of norepinephrine levels, and Frazier has recently combined LVAD removal with surgical left ventricular volume reduction instead of transplantation (O.H. Frazier, personal communication). The second requirement is a user-friendly device which can be removed easily or simply switched off. Whilst the TCI Heartmate and Novacor LVADs have an excellent record for mechanical reliability in the bridge-to-transplant setting, both are large, obtrusive devices, implanted in the abdomen with stiff percutaneous powerlines. They are unsuitable for smaller adults and children and the operation to remove the LVAD whilst leaving a functional heart in situ is technically difficult. Efforts are therefore directed towards the design of a less obtrusive blood pump for widespread use in the various settings of acute and chronic left ventricular failure.

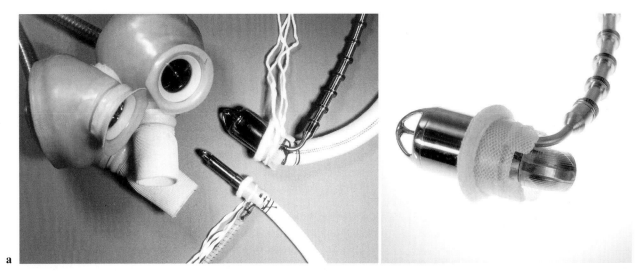

Fig. 1. a Adult (*upper right*) and prototype paediatric (*lower right*) Jarvik 2000 blood pumps compared with the Jarvik 7 total artificial heart (*upper left*). **b** Jarvik 2000 with apical sewing cuff

The Jarvik 2000 Oxford System

We are currently developing a system based on the Jarvik 2000 axial flow impeller pump that is inserted through a sewing cuff into the apex of the left ventricle (Figs. 1, 2). The adult model measures 2.5 cm in diameter by 5.5 cm in length. The weight is 85 g and the displacement volume 25 ml. The paediatric device measures 1.4 cm in diameter by 5 cm in length and is one-fifth the size of the larger model. The weight is 18 g and the displacement volume 5 ml. The electromagnetic pump consists of a rotor with impeller blades encased in a titanium shell and supported at each end by tiny blood-immersed ceramic bearings less than 1 mm in diameter (Fig. 3). Power is delivered by a fine percutaneous wire and regulated by a pulse width modulated, brushless, direct current motor controller to determine motor speed. An impervious Dacron graft conveys blood from the left ventricle to the descending thoracic aorta (Fig. 4). In order to overcome the problem of driveline infection, the fine electric cable is transmitted through a pyrolite carbon button, which in patients will be secured to the skull (Fig. 5). The combination of immobility and highly vascular scalp skin is known to resist infection in a percutaneous system for artificial hearing. In vitro studies, using a water-glycerol test solution to simulate blood viscosity, show the adult device to provide up to 10 l/min flow. At normal operating speeds of 9000–16000 rpm, flow rates between 3 and 6 l/min are obtained at a mean aortic pressure of 80 mmHg with a power requirement of 4–10 W. The device is silent to the unassisted ear but can be heard with a stethoscope. The critical feature of the Jarvik 2000 design is that a high flow stream of blood washes the tiny bearings

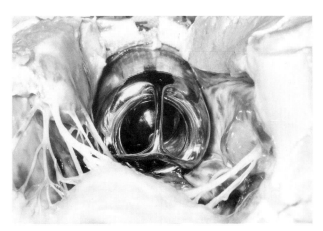

Fig. 2. Inflow of the Jarvik 2000 device aligned with the mitral orifice

continuously and prevents thrombus formation. The rotor is the sole moving part of the device, supported at each end by tiny blood-immersed ceramic bearings 1 mm in diameter. The impeller is powered by electromagnetic fields across the motor air gap, through which the blood flows. All blood-contacting surfaces are titanium. Because the bearings are so small, the surface rubbing speed, even at 20000 rpm, is very low and there is virtually no wear. A system for human use has evolved during the course of animal experiments (Fig. 6). The principal objective of these experiments was to address the safety, durability, and potential for thromboembolism or haemolysis. Sixteen adult and one paediatric device (Fig. 7) have been implanted into Welsh mule sheep of between 80 and 90 kg.

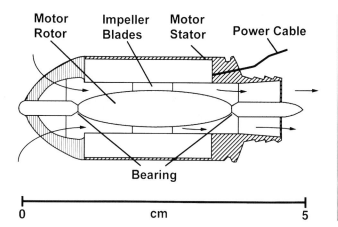

Fig. 3. Section through the blood pump

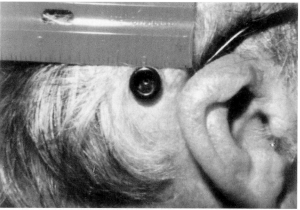

Fig. 5. Carbon button used successfully for 18 years in artificial hearing technology

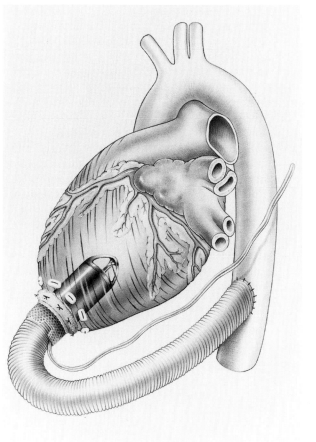

Fig. 4. Jarvik 2000 implanted into the left ventricular apex with a 16-mm Dacron graft transmitting blood to the descending thoracic aorta

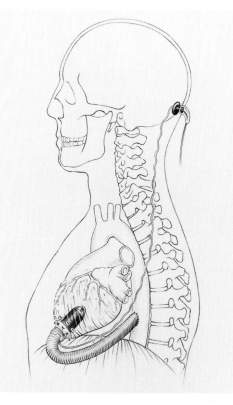

Fig. 6. The proposed Jarvik 2000 Oxford System with percutaneous power transmitted through the scalp skin via the carbon button

Method for Surgical Implantation of the Jarvik 2000 Oxford System

The surgical methods employed for implantation in the sheep are applicable to the human with the exception that patients with heart failure will be supported by cardiopulmonary bypass. Left thoracotomy is performed to provide access to the left ventricular apex without excessive cardiac displacement. The power cable with the Dacron velour-covered carbon pedestal is brought through the ribs and tunnelled under the skin to an exit point at the base of the neck. For patients, the carbon button will be fixed to the external table of the skull, whilst in the sheep this was brought through the soft subcutaneous tissues. The electric lead is attached to the external controller and batteries or mains supply attached to a vest (Fig. 8). The 16-mm Dacron graft attached to the outflow of the Jarvik 2000 device is then anastomosed to a descending thoracic aortotomy using a side clamp. The pericardium is then opened widely and suspended by sutures from the wound edges. Access to the left ventricular apex is improved by placing a swab behind the heart. The silicone-reinforced Dacron sewing cuff is then sutured around the pointed left ventricular apex using between 12 and 15 teflon pledgetted mattress sutures. In the sheep model, the excisional left ventriculotomy is performed with a cork-bore type coring knife whilst the heart continues to support the circulation. This ma-

noeuvre causes considerable left ventricular irritability and is therefore preceded by lidocaine infiltration into the apical muscle and intravenous administration of bretylium and amiodarone. Blood loss through the open apex is controlled by digital pressure and rapid insertion of the pump through the sewing cuff and into the left ventricle. Uncrossmatched blood transfusion from donor sheep is used if required.

The device is then secured in the correct position by tying down umbilical tape pursestring ties integral with the sewing ring. The saline-filled outflow graft is vented to remove residual air before the pump is switched on. Systemic heparinisation is used during pump insertion but reversed at the end of the procedure. The capacity of the pump to capture all the pulmonary venous return through the mitral valve and prevent opening of the aortic valve is tested by turning the device off and then progressively increasing the pump speed (up to 10 l/min) until the arterial pressure wave disappears. This occurs at between 12 000 and 18 000 rpm, at which point the mean arterial pressure is between 80 and 90 mmHg. There was no adverse reaction in the animals when blood flow changed from pulsatile to nonpulsatile. During the course of the animal experiments each device was maintained at a continuous speed of 10 000 rpm, providing an average flow rate of 5–6 l/min. At this flow, the arterial pulse pressure remained at about 20 mmHg and correlated with changes in pump current. Natural ventricular contraction provides a differential pressure load on the pump and the torque load on the motor varies with pulse pressure. This variation in preload corresponding to native heart function provides pulsatile flow. When the device is turned off, graft flow reverses but the functional aortic insufficiency is well tolerated by the animals.

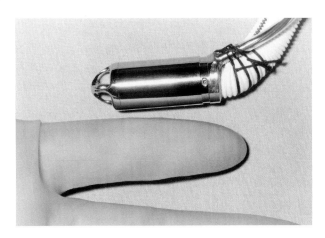

Fig. 7. The paediatric model against the terminal phalanges of the 5th finger

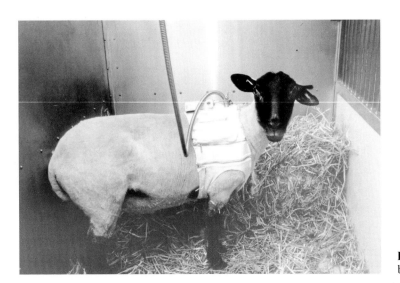

Fig. 8. Sheep with vest to carry controller and batteries

Postoperatively, aspirin, 300 mg daily, and warfarin, 20 mg daily, were used in an attempt to achieve anticoagulation. Because of the sheep's rumen it proved impossible to achieve an International Normalised Ratio of greater than 1.5:1. The animals were consequently not anticoagulated. Despite this, we have not experienced primary thrombosis of the device or thromboembolism with the pump running. On occasions when interruption in electrical power resulted in suspected thrombosis, thrombolysis with streptokinase, together with temporary heparinisation, resulted in normal pump function by electrical and auscultatory parameters. The sheep heart is thick walled with a small ventricular cavity and the adult Jarvik 2000 device completely fills the body of the ventricle. Consequently, it is important to align the inflow of the pump with the mitral valve orifice. The presence of the device did not provoke dysrhythmia and at post mortem examination there was no endothelial overgrowth of the inflow. Table 1 shows indices of haemolysis preoperatively and at 1, 4, 8, and 28 weeks. Minor elevations of lactate dehydrogenase and free haemoglobin between 1 and 4 weeks after operation probably resulted from the sequelae of blood transfusion and drug administration during surgery. When the device was dismantled at autopsy, a small ring of thrombus was found at the bearings site but in the form of a tiny torus that could not break free and embolise because it was retained by the bearing shaft which passed through the centre. Autopsy studies of the brain and kidney showed no evidence of thromboembolism.

These experiments have established mechanical reliability with freedom from haemolysis and thrombosis up to seven months in an animal model where reliable anticoagulation is virtually impossible. Lack of perceptible noise is also a great advantage in comparison to existing pusher plate LVADs. The smaller paediatric device continues to function satisfactorily, twenty weeks after implantation and with the capacity to pump 3 l/min; this model has potential for use in infants with heart failure or in myocardial infarction patients with cardiogenic shock.

Clinical Potential for the Jarvik 2000 Oxford System

Our aim is to produce a realistic temporary or permanent substitute for the left ventricle, suitable for use in all age groups with both acute and chronic heart failure. In contrast to electric pusher plate LVADs, the compact axial flow impeller pump is easily implantable and unobtrusive. The intraventricular position conveys distinct advantages. The device is practically encapsulated by the native myocardium so that infection is unlikely. There is no inflow graft at risk from thrombus formation and no prosthetic heart valve subject to deterioration. Energy requirements are less than pusher plate pumps and an infection-resistant percutaneous electric cable has the advantage of simplicity and reliability. None of the animals with a percutaneous carbon pedestal suffered drive line infection, even though the skin was freely mobile at the exit site. There are a number of potential uses for this device, including permanent left ventricular support, bridge to cardiac transplantation, and bridge to left ventricular recovery. Given the incontrovertible shortage of transplant donors, the prospect of realistic, permanent mechanical circulatory support or circulatory support as a therapeutic option is compelling. This is the first device suitable for infants and small children where viral myocarditis and miscellaneous cardiomyopathies have the potential for recovery, thus avoiding the considerable morbidity and mortality of transplantation in this age group. Besides long-term support, the Jarvik 2000 device is suitable for postcardiotomy left ventricular failure or the treatment of acute myocardial infarction with cardiogenic shock. In this setting, the infant device could be used to provide up to 3 l/min blood flow to offload the failing ventricle, perhaps in combination with myocardial revascularisation in the acute phase.

With the static situation in both donor availability and results of cardiac transplantation, new initiatives are needed to address an ever-increasing population with severe heart failure and greater expectation for treatment. Currently, the Jarvik 2000 Oxford System

Table 1. Indices of haemolysis

	Before operation	1 week	4 weeks	8 weeks	28 weeks
	($n = 17$)	($n = 11$)	($n = 8$)	($n = 4$)	($n = 1$)
Hb (g/dl)	13.6 (1.1)	10.8 (2.1)	12.3 (0.7)	11.8 (1.2)	11.1
Pl-Hb (mg/dl)	7.4 (3.6)	14.1 (6.8)	7.8 (3.2)	8.2 (4.1)	5.0
LDH (u/l)	579 (91)	941 (267)	699 (122)	701 (70)	642
Cr (µmol/l)	113 (11)	92 (15)	98 (4)	100 (14)	89

Data are mean values (SD in parentheses).
Hb, haemoglobin; Pl-Hb, plasma free haemoglobin; LDH, lactate dehydrogenase; Cr, creatinine.

offers potential in this area, particularly pending the development of a fully implantable system with transcutaneous power currently under development at The Texas Heart Institute. The potential for compact, user-friendly, axial flow impeller blood pumps is recognised by other groups as reflected by the NASA/DeBakey and NIMBUS/Pittsburgh programmes. It is only a matter of time before this type of technology provides a long-term substitute for the left ventricle. Such devices can then be used electively and earlier than transplantation, which requires a dead donor, with the view to preventing multisystem organ failure. Undoubtedly, the recent findings of the beneficial effects of chromic left ventricular offloading offer the most exciting prospects for the treatment of advanced heart failure in the future.

References

1. Kaye MP (1993) The registry of the International Society for Heart and Lung Transplantation: tenth official report — 1993. J Heart Lung Transplant 12:541–548
2. Bellotti G, Moraes A, Bocchi E, Arie S, Medeiros C, Moreira LH, Jatene A, Pileggi F (1993) Late effects of cardiomyoplasty on left ventricular mechanics and diastolic filling. Circulation 88II:304–308
3. United Network for Organ Sharing (UNOS) (1991) UNOS update 7(May):2
4. McCarthy PM (1995) Heartmate implantable left ventricular assist device: bridge to transplantation and future applications. Ann Thorac Surg 59:846–851
5. McCarthy PM, Portner PM, Tobler HG, Starnes VA, Ramasamy N, Oyez PE (1991) Clinical experience with the Novacor ventricular assist system. J Thorac Cardiovasc Surg 102:578–587
6. Frazier OH, Rose EA, McCarthy P, Burton NA, Tector A, Levin H, Kayne HL, Poirier VL, Dasse KA (1995) Improved mortality and rehabilitation of transplant candidates treated with a long term implantable left ventricular assist system. Ann Surg 222:327–338
7. Burkhoff D, Flaherty JT, Yve DT, Herskowitz A, Oikawa RY, Sugiura S, Firanz MR, Baumgartner WA, Schaefer J, Reitz BA (1988) In vitro studies of isolated supported human hearts. Heart Vessels 4:185–196
8. Pfeffer MA, Lamas G, Vaughan D, Parisi A, Braunwald E (1988) Effect of captopril on progressive ventricular dilatation after anterior myocardial infarction. N Engl J Med 319:80–86
9. Hall S, Cigassoa C, Marcouz L, Hatfield B, Peters A, Grayburn PA, Eichorn EJ (1994) Regression of hypertrophy and alteration in left ventricular geometry in patients with congestive heart failure treated with beta-adrenergic blockade (abstract). Circulation 90(Suppl I):543
10. Burch GE, DePasquale NP (1968) On resting the human heart. Am J Med 44:165–169
11. Frazier OH, Benedict CR, Radovancevic B (1996) Improved left ventricular function after chronic left ventricular unloading. Ann Thorac Surg 62:675–682

Discussion

Dr. Olsen:

Don Olsen, University of Utah. I'm a little confused. Most of the data and information on the artificial ear pedestal is a clean pyrolitic carbon fixed to the skull. What is the rationale for covering it with dacron velour?

Mr. Westaby:

This was for the sheep implants where the device goes not into the sheep skull but into the subcutaneous tissues. For the human, we will not use dacron velour against the skull. It will be the pure carbon pedestal.

Dr. Olsen:

Thanks for clearing up my confusion there. Secondly, I would caution you that the amount of lanolin produced from the skin of the sheep is very beneficial and very antibacterial. And it's rare, in our experience with percutaneous leads, that we have infections in sheep over chronic periods of time. Thank you.

Dr. Vasku:

You expect a recovery of the heart with this device, yes?

Mr. Westaby:

Yes.

Dr. Vasku:

And what do you think about combination of this kind of recovery with pharmacological support? Do you think that it would be accelerated, the recovery of the myocardium?

Mr. Westaby:

I think it could be. I think the exciting thing about this very small device is you can foresee it being available for widespread use. And I think, instead of transplantation, long-term implant of this device with medical treatment may well lead to recovery. And we have to remember that medical treatment is improving constantly as well, so the combination of a small LVAD with medical treatment, especially when it's used earlier, may well prevent end-stage heart failure. And that's the way I think it will go.

Dr. Nakatani:

Nakatani from National Cardiovascular Center, Osaka, Japan. I also have some clinical experiences of recovery of the heart. I think that, just as you mentioned, if we can put a device to the patient before his heart deteriorates too much, and if we give enough support to the heart which is in end-stage but not in the last stage, we may give a chance for recovery to the heart. And a flow of 2 to 3 liters per minute may be enough. Of course, at that time, I am always anxious to get a better device, which means it is easy to remove, and also has no risk of complications such as infection. If such kind of device, as you mentioned, has become available, I think this concept, the long-term support of the end-staged heart, becomes one of the options of the therapies. I strongly agree with you on your concept. And tomorrow I will present our clinical experiences. Thank you.

Dr. Wolner:

Steve, I congratulate you on your enthusiasm, but perhaps it seems to me that you are a little bit short in this business. I have heard in the last 20 years, I'm sure, at least ten such speeches with enthusiasm that in 5 years we will have a total artificial heart; 5 years later we will have a completely implantable system, and so on. But, we should be fair, and there is no discussion that at the moment — and there is work of 10 years or longer with all these rotary pumps — at the moment we don't have any rotary pump which works, let's say, safe in regards of FDA, as an example, longer than 6 months. That's number one.

Number two, your statements for recovery of myocardium with recovery after the use of the Novacor system. That's right, that there are some data in very few cases with mild myocarditis. But when you look on the huge majority of patients in which we have real experience, I mean, bridged patients and so on, you see no recovery, as in patients with ischemic or idiopathic cardiomyopathies when you look on the data of Drs. Poirier or Portner. What I want say here is, be cautious. And I like you and your enthusiasm; however, we have not real data for this. You should confess this.

Mr. Westaby:
I think this is an important first step because there is another area that is particularly strong in Oxford that will contribute to this that hasn't been mentioned. And that is genetic engineering. And I think in the next 5 to 10 years genetic manipulation may help to promote the recovery process. So I think this, again, is step number one. I think, I find the potential for bridge to recovery very exciting. I fully agree with you I am very enthusiastic about it. There is little data, but I think we are on the first rung of the ladder and I think, as my friend the last speaker said, in 5 years' time things are moving so rapidly that we may be able to be a little more optimistic about the whole thing. But thank you for listening and thank you for your comments.

Part V
Clinical Application

Clinical Application 1
Clinical Application 2
Muscle Pumps

Ventricular Assist Systems: Clinical Application

O.H. Frazier

Summary. The ideal therapy for chronic end-stage heart failure must be reliable, cost effective, easy to implement and maintain, and capable of providing a physiologic level of circulatory support. The therapy most likely to have these characteristics within the next 10 years will probably be one more of the ventricular assist systems. Systems currently used primarily as intermediate or long-term bridges to transplantation include the HeartMate implantable left ventricular assist system (Thermo Cardiosystems, Woburn, MA) and the Novacor left ventricular assist system (Baxter Healthcare, Novacor Division, Oakland, CA). These devices not only support the circulation but may also enable a patient's ventricle to recover before transplantation. Many patients who receive these devices become self-sufficient and can resume their normal activities. As experience accumulates, the future for heart failure patients may include long-term implantation of one of these systems as an alternative to transplantation. In fact, the US Food and Drug Administration has approved a clinical trial for use of the vented electric HeartMate as an alternative to transplantation. It may also one day be possible to implant such a system, rest the heart, and then remove the system when the patient's heart has adequately recovered. The future may also bring clinical application of smaller assist systems now being tested experimentally. The J-2000 (Jarvik Research, New York, NY), for example, is a valveless, miniaturized, intraventricular, axial-flow left ventricular assist system with blood-immersed bearings, currently under investigation at the Texas Heart Institute. The device, which is powered transcutaneously, is implanted within the left ventricle, and ongoing experimental results are promising.

Introduction

At present, heart transplantation is the preferred surgical therapy for patients with chronic end-stage heart failure. Because of a shortage of donor organs, however, as many as 20% of patients on the waiting list die before they can undergo transplantation [1,2]. In addition, patients who do undergo transplantation (particularly younger patients) may encounter problems such as chronic rejection, infection, immunoplegia, and graft atherosclerosis. Thus, alternative methods of treating these patients must be found.

The ideal therapy for chronic end-stage heart failure must be reliable, cost effective, easy to implement and maintain, and capable of providing a physiologic level of circulatory support. One possible alternative to replacing the heart with a donor organ is replacing it with a total artificial heart (TAH). Modern technology, however, has not yet been able to overcome all of the problems associated with TAH implantation, including infection, thrombus formation, and limited patient mobility [3].

The available therapy that is most likely to have the required characteristics of an alternative to heart transplantation is the left ventricular assist system (LVAS). Presently, there are several such devices on the market. Two of these devices, the HeartMate (Thermo Cardiosystems, Woburn, MA, USA) and the Novacor (Baxter Healthcare, Novacor Division, Oakland, CA, USA), are pulsatile systems primarily used for intermediate or long-term bridges to transplantation.

A number of smaller assist devices are also being tested in animal models, among them the Jarvik 2000 (Jarvik Research, New York, NY, USA). The Jarvik 2000 is a valveless, miniaturized, intraventricular, axial-flow left ventricular assist system with blood-immersed bearings. Such axial flow pumps will not require a compliance chamber and will be completely implantable.

Description of Devices

Novacor

The Novacor LVAS is a pulsatile assist system with an implantable blood pump (Fig. 1) [4,5]. The pump consists of a seamless polyurethane pump sac compressed by dual pusher plates. The pump is powered by an internal solenoid that converts electrical energy from the console to mechanical energy. This energy is then used to compress the pusher plates and pressurize the pump sac for blood ejection. A 21-mm bioprosthetic

Departments of Cardiothoracic Surgery and Cardiovascular Surgical Research, Texas Heart Institute at St. Luke's Episcopal Hospital, Houston, TX 77225-0345, USA

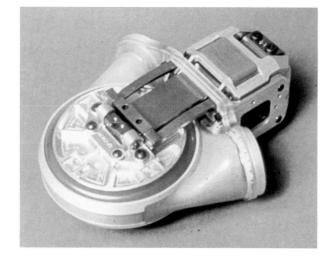

Fig. 1. The Novacor left ventricular assist system

valve is used to maintain unidirectional flow in both the inflow and outflow conduits.

An external drive console monitors the system and is capable of producing a stroke volume of up to 70 ml. Information about pump parameters is transmitted to the console by transducers within the pump. This information is displayed on the console, along with electrocardiographic signals and blood pressure.

The Novacor can operate in three different modes: the synchronized mode, the fill-to-empty mode, and the fixed-rate mode. In the synchronized mode, cardiac unloading is maximized: the pump fills with cardiac systole and ejects with cardiac diastole. In the fill-to-empty mode, pump output is maximized: the pump rate adjusts according to the pump's filling rate. Finally, in the fixed-rate mode, the pump is set at a constant rate: the device pumps asynchronously to the heart. Use of this last mode is rare.

A wearable version of the Novacor is now available [6,7]. This system can be powered by batteries (which last up to 12 hours) without using a console, although patients may use a monitor while at rest. The implantable pump remains unchanged from the console-powered model. The blood pump of the wearable Novacor, however, is controlled by a compact controller and powered by rechargeable packs which can support the pump for up to 7 hours. The controller and power packs may be worn on the patient's belt or in a portable "camera bag." This version of the Novacor results in increased patient mobility, thus improving the patient's quality of life.

HeartMate

The HeartMate Implantable Pneumatic (IP) and Vented Electric (VE) LVASs are pulsatile blood

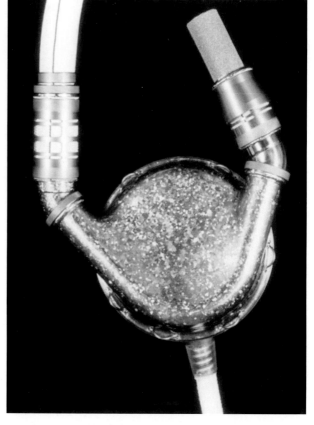

Fig. 2. The HeartMate left ventricular assist system

pumps used to support left ventricular function in patients with end-stage heart failure (Fig. 2) [4]. At present, they are used primarily to bridge patients to transplantation. The IP- and VE-LVASs have identical, portable blood pumps. The main difference between the two systems is their method of pump actuation: the IP-LVAS receives its power from a portable external drive console, while the VE-LVAS receives its power through a percutaneous electric lead, which is attached to a lightweight, rechargeable battery pack. The patient wears this battery pack in a shoulder holster, allowing almost unlimited mobility. The IP-LVAS has a maximum blood flow of 12 l/min, while the VE-LVAS has a maximum blood flow of 10 l/min. The maximum stroke volume of both systems is 85 ml.

A ridged outer housing made of titanium surrounds a flexible polyurethane diaphragm to form the HeartMate blood pump. To reduce the risk of thrombus formation, all blood-contacting surfaces are textured. Sintered titanium spheres cover the outer housing and polyurethane fibrils texture the diaphragm. The textured surface interacts with fibrin and cellular components in the blood in such a way that a pseudointimal lining develops, protecting the patient from thromboembolic complications and reducing the need for anticoagulants.

The IP-LVAS receives power from a microprocessor-based console, which is connected to the pump by a 6-foot (1.8-m) cable. This device can be operated in the automatic, external synchronous, and fixed-rate modes. In the automatic mode, pump flow is maximized by adjusting the rate of flow according to the filling status of the pump. In the external synchronous mode, the pump systole occurs with the patient's R wave. Finally, in the fixed-rate mode, the device pumps at a rate set by the operator.

In the past, a patient whose circulation was supported by an IP-LVAS could not leave the hospital while waiting for transplantation. Today, however, a new and more portable console is available. The console weighs only 8.5 kg and can be carried with a shoulder strap or pulled on wheels. Thus, patients with this new console are more mobile and should be able to return home to await transplant.

The VE-LVAS receives its power from an internal motor located inside the pump. An electrical line connects the motor to a battery pack and an external console. The VE-LVAS can also be operated in the fixed-rate or automatic modes, but not in the external synchronous mode. The patient can control the mode of the device through a system controller, which also alerts the patient to any abnormal operating conditions. The portability of the VE-LVAS allows patients who fulfill certain criteria to leave the hospital while waiting for transplantation where the equipment can be operated and maintained by the patient or a companion.

Patient Selection

The Novacor and HeartMate are used primarily for bridging patients to transplantation [4,8]. Thus, patients who receive one of these devices must eventually be able to undergo cardiac transplantation. This does not mean, however, that patients must fulfill all the transplantation criteria at the time of implant. Some conditions, such as pulmonary edema, acute renal insufficiency, and minor infections can be more easily resolved if the patient is supported by a mechanical assist device [9]. Certain conditions, however, preclude patients from receiving mechanical circulatory support [10] (Table 1).

The Food and Drug Administration's criteria for the clinical trials of the HeartMate VE-LVAS are listed in Table 2. To be bridged to transplantation with an LVAS, the patient must be near death or in danger of irreversible end-organ dysfunction. Mechanical support, however, should be considered if a patient demonstrates progressive hepatic, renal, or pulmonary

Table 1. Exclusion criteria for mechanical circulatory support

Severe coagulation disorders
Renal failure requiring hemodialysis
Irreversible cerebrovascular accident
Unacceptable psychosocial history
Severe right heart failure
Irreversible hepatic dysfunction
Age greater than 70 years
Unresolved pulmonary emboli
Respiratory insufficiency requiring intubation
Systemic life-threatening illness other than heart disease

Table 2. Patient inclusion criteria for clinical trials of the HeartMate vented electric left ventricular assist system

Approved candidate for cardiac transplantation
Circulation supported by inotropic drugs
Circulation supported by IABP (if possible)
LAP or PCWP ≥20 mmHg with cardiac index $\leq 2.0 \cdot \mathrm{l} \cdot \mathrm{min}^{-1} \cdot \mathrm{m}^{-2}$ or systolic blood pressure ≤80 mmHg

IABP, intra-aortic balloon pump; LAP, left atrial pressure; PCWP, pulmonary capillary wedge pressure.

dysfunction [9]. There have been cases in which such support was delayed because the patient was hemodynamically stable, yet later the patient developed conditions (including end-organ dysfunction) that precluded him or her from LVAS implantation and cardiac transplantation [8]. It is difficult to determine when end-organ dysfunction is irreversible; however, mechanical support can improve end-organ function if the device is implanted before the onset of irreversible organ failure [11].

Complications

Bleeding

Bleeding is one of the most common early complications occurring after LVAS implantation [12–15]. Among the risk factors for bleeding are prolonged cardiopulmonary bypass times during implant, extensive surgical dissection, preoperative hepatic congestion and failure, multiple cannulation sites, and interaction of the platelets with device biomaterial [5,16]. Because 22%–73% of cases of bleeding require reoperation, careful attention must be paid to the hematological status of the patient [17,18].

Right Ventricular Failure

Right ventricular failure is one of the most common causes of death in patients supported by an LVAS [12–

15]. Patients who require right ventricular support after implantation of the LVAS have a higher mortality rate than do those who require only left ventricular support [19,20]. Unfortunately, the need for temporary support of the right ventricle cannot be predicted before transplantation [21].

Infection

Infection is another common complication in patients supported by the Novacor and HeartMate LVASs [12–15]. Patients supported by mechanical devices like the Novacor and HeartMate are not at as great a risk for mediastinal infections as patients supported by artificial hearts because assist devices are not positioned orthotopically [11]. Because the device is percutaneous, however, infection in patients supported for prolonged periods with these devices is almost inevitable. Most infections occur at the driveline site and may be easily resolved [22]. Because these patients undergo immunosuppressive therapy after transplantation, however, each infection must be treated aggressively.

Thromboembolic Complications

Thromboembolic complications have always been a danger in patients supported for prolonged periods by a mechanical assist device. Patients supported by the HeartMate, however, only require aspirin and dipyridamole because of a unique feature: textured blood-contacting surfaces that promote the formation of a lining of neointimal tissue consisting of fibrin and collagen [23–26]. Another feature of the HeartMate that helps prevent the formation of thrombus is a shortened inlet graft. Thus far, there has been no formation of pannus on properly positioned inlet grafts [10].

End-organ Failure

End-organ failure remains a serious complication in patients supported by implantable assist systems; however, if mechanical support is instituted before the onset of irreversible organ failure, prolonged support can actually help ailing organs to recover [11]. Thus, patients with organ failure may be physically rehabilitated, making them better candidates for transplantation.

Results

The early survival rates of patients bridged to transplantation with an LVAS are comparable to those of patients undergoing transplantation with only conventional therapy [28–30]. Sixty percent of patients sup-

ported with the Novacor have undergone successful transplantation, and 82% of those supported for over 30 days were long-term survivors [31]. Seventy-one percent of HeartMate IP-LVAS patients have undergone successful transplantation, and 65% have survived longer than 60 days [14]. Because of these good results, the FDA approved the HeartMate IP-LVAS for commercial use in 1994. Clinical trials of the VE-LVAS are also underway: thus far, results are comparable to those of the IP-LVAS.

These good results are largely due to the physical rehabilitation effected by support with an LVAS. During LVAS support, end-organ and ventricular function is allowed to normalize, allowing the patient to return to everyday activities [32,33]. Thus, patients supported with an LVAS are in better physical condition to undergo the trauma of heart transplantation.

The Future of Mechanical Circulatory Support

The future of mechanical circulatory support is here. Already we have progressed to the point where patients may leave the hospital while supported by an assist device. Because of the portability of the HeartMate VE-LVAS, patients who meet the requirements of the patient release protocol can take day trips, live at home, or even return to work. This return to everyday activities allows the patient to become emotionally, as well as physically, rehabilitated.

The HeartMate has begun to fulfill its original goal: to function as a long-term alternative to cardiac transplantation. At Columbia University, the Cleveland Clinic, and the Texas Heart Institute, surgeons have begun implanting the HeartMate in patients, not as a temporary bridge to transplantation, but as a "permanent" device. In the future, such therapy may help those patients who are not eligible for transplantation.

The LVAS also has the potential to be used as a "bridge to recovery." Since clinical trials began in 1986, we have significant improvements in end-organ and ventricular function in patients supported for prolonged periods with the HeartMate. In a recent retrospective study at the Texas Heart Institute, clinical, histological, and biochemical parameters were examined and shown to normalize in HeartMate patients supported for longer than 30 days [34]. Thus, it may be possible to remove the device after a certain degree of ventricular recovery, bypassing the need for cardiac transplantation. The device has already been removed from several patients in Germany and Japan without transplantation. The initial results have been good, suggesting need for further study to determine how effective this therapy is and which patients may benefit from it.

New, smaller assist devices are also being investigated. At the Texas Heart Institute, animal studies have begun on the Jarvik-2000 (Jarvik Research, New York, NY, USA), an intraventricular axial flow pump [35]. The device is considerably smaller (25 mm diameter, 25 cm^3, 85 g) than pulsatile devices, yet is able to provide over 12 l/min of flow. The Jarvik 2000 does not require valves, nor does it require a compliance chamber (a significant obstacle to complete implantability of the pulsatile pumps). There was some concern that the high speed of the device (10000 rotations per minute) might cause severe hemolysis; this has not proved to be the case. The pump appears to cause only minimal hemolysis, at a level comparable to that of the pulsatile pumps.

Thus far, results of the animal studies have been good. The pump has functioned up to 195 days in a calf, with no physiologic complications. If this device proves to be effective clinically, it would offer several advantages over the pulsatile pumps. First, because of its small size, it can be implanted in children and small adults. Second, axial flow pumps may be completely implanted without requiring a compliance chamber. Third, insertion of the device is much less invasive than insertion of a pulsatile pump, reducing the risk of infection and surgical complications.

Conclusion

Mechanical circulatory support is a safe and effective method of supporting the circulation of patients waiting for transplantation. Patients supported with these devices have as good a chance of survival and a better quality of life than patients treated by conventional methods before transplant. This technology has the potential to help millions of patients with chronic heart failure live long, healthy lives.

References

1. Schuler S, Parnt R, Warnecke H, Matheis G, Hetzer R. (1988) Extended donor criteria for heart transplantation. J Heart Transplant 7:326–330
2. Copeland JG, Emery RW, Levinson MM, Copeland J, McAleer MJ, Riley JE (1985) The role of mechanical support and transplantation in treatment of patients with end-stage cardiomyopathy. Circulation 72(Suppl II): 7–12
3. Barker LE, DeVries WC (1993) Total artificial heart. In: Quaal S (ed) Cardiac mechanical assistance beyond balloon pumping. Mosby Year Book, St. Louis, Mo USA, pp 167–180
4. Frazier OH, Short HD, Wampler RK, Noon GP, Myers TJ, Parnis SM, Coleman CL, Macris MP (1996) Mechanical circulatory support in the transplant population. In: Frazier OH (ed) Support and replacement of the failing heart. Lippincott-Raven, Philadelphia, PA, USA
5. Shinn JA, Oyer PE (1993) Novacor ventricular assist system. In: Quaal SJ (ed) Cardiac mechanical assistance beyond balloon pumping. Mosby Year Book, St. Louis, MO, USA, pp 99–115
6. Loisance D, Deleuze PH, Mazzucotelli JP, Abe Y, LeBesnerais P, Dubois-Rande JL (1994) The initial experience with the wearable Baxter Novacor ventricular assist system. J Thorac Cardiovasc Surg 108:176–177
7. Miller PJ, Billich TJ, LaForge DH, Lee J, Naegeli A, Ramasamy N, Jassawalla JS, Portner PM (1994) Initial clinical experience with a wearable controller for the Novacor left ventricular assist system. ASAIO J 40:M465–M470
8. Reedy JE, Swartz MT, Termuhlen DF, Pennington DG, McBride LR, Miller LW, Ruzevich SA (1990) Bridge to heart transplantation: importance of patient selection. J Heart Transplant 9:473–480
9. Pennington DG, Swartz MT (1995) Mechanical circulatory support: patient and device selection. In: Lewis T, Graham TR (eds) Mechanical circulatory support. Edward Arnold, London, p 159–168
10. Frazier OH (1997) Long-term mechanical circulatory support. In: Edmunds LH (ed) Cardiac surgery in the adult. McGraw-Hill, New York, 1477–1490
11. Burnett CM, Duncan JM, Frazier OH, Sweeney MS, Vega JD, Radovancevic B (1993) Improved multiorgan function after prolonged univentricular support. Ann Thorac Surg 55:65–71
12. Shinn JA (1991) Novacor left ventricular assist system. AACN Clinical Issues 2:575–586
13. Korfer R, El-Banayosy A, Posival H, Minami K, Korner MM, Arusoglu L, Breymann T, Kizner L, Seifert D, Kortke H, et al. (1995) Mechanical circulatory support: the Bad Oeynhausen experience. Ann Thorac Surg 59:S56–62
14. Frazier OH, Rose EA, McCarthy P, Burton NA, Tector A, Levin H, Kayne HL, Poirier VL, Dasse KA (1995) Improved mortality and rehabilitation of transplant candidates treated with a long-term implantable left ventricular assist system. Ann Surg 222:327–336
15. Mehta SM, Aufiero TX, Pae WE, Jr., Miller CA, Pierce WS (1995) Combined registry for the clinical use of mechanical ventricular assist pumps and the total artificial heart in conjunction with heart transplantation: sixth official report — 1994. J Heart Lung Transplant 14:585–593
16. Farrar DJ, Lawson JH, Litwak P, Cederwall G (1990) Thoratec VAD system as a bridge to heart transplantation. J Heart Lung Transplant 9:415–422
17. Pennington DG, Kanter KR, McBride LR, Kaiser GC, Barner HB, Miller LW, Naunheim KS, Fiore AC, Willman V (1988) Seven years' experience with the Pierce–Donachy ventricular assist device. J Thorac Cardiovasc Surg 96:901–911
18. Reedy JE, Ruzevich SA, Noedel NR, Vitale LJ, Merkle EJ (1990) Nursing care of the ambulatory patient with a mechanical assist device. J Heart Transplant 9:97–105
19. Portner PM, Oyer PE, Pennington DG, Baumgartner WA, Griffith BP, Frist WR, Magilligan DJ Jr., Noon GP, Ramasamy N, Miller PJ, et al. (1989) Implantable electrical left ventricular assist system: bridge to transplantation and the future. Ann Thorac Surg 47:142–150
20. Frazier OH, Rose EA, Macmanus Q, Burton NA, Lefrak EA, Poirier VL, Dasse KA (1992) Multicenter

clinical evaluation of the HeartMate 1000 IP left ventricular assist device. Ann Thorac Surg 53:1080–1090

21. Kormos RL, Borovetz HS. Gasior T, Antaki JF, Armitage JM, Pristas JM, Hardesty RL, Griffith BP (1990) Experience with univentricular support in mortally ill cardiac transplant candidates. Ann Thorac Surg 49:261–271

22. Pennington DG (1996) Extended support with permanent systems: percutaneous versus totally implantable. Ann Thorac Surg 61:403–406

23. Frazier OH, Duncan JM, Radovancevic B, Vega JD, Baldwin RT, Burnett CM, Lonquist JL (1992) Successful bridge to heart transplantation with a new left ventricular assist device. J Heart Lung Transplant 11:530–537

24. Frazier OH, Baldwin RT, Eskin SJ, Duncan JM (1993) Immunochemical identification of human endothelial cells on the lining of a ventricular assist device. Tex Heart Inst J 20:78–82

25. Graham TR, Dasse K, Coumbe A, Salih V, Marrinan MT, Frazier OH, Lewis CT (1990) Neointimal development on textured biomaterial surfaces during clinical use of an implantable left ventricular assist device. Eur J Cardiothorac Surg 4:182–190

26. Dasse KA, Chapman SD, Sherman CN, Levine AH, Frazier OH (1987) Clinical experience with textured blood contacting surfaces in ventricular assist devices. ASAIO Trans 33:418–425

27. Pennington DG, McBride LR, Peigh LS, Peigh PS, Miller LW, Swartz MT (1994) Eight years' experience with bridging to cardiac transplantation. J Thorac Cardiovasc Surg 107:472–480

28. Reedy JE, Pennington DG, Miller LW, McBride LR, Lohmann DP, Noedel NR, Swartz MT (1992) Status I

heart transplant patients — conventional vs ventricular assist device support. J Heart Lung Transplant 11:246–252

29. Birovljev S, Radovancevic B, Burnett CM, Vega JD, Bennink G, Lonquist JL, Duncan JM, Frazier OH (1992) Heart transplantation after mechanical circulatory support: four years' experience. J Heart Lung Transplant 11:240–245

30. Pifarre R, Sullivan H, Montoya, Montoya A, Bakhos M, Grieco J, Foy BK, Blakeman B, Costanzo-Nordin MR, Altergott R, Lonchyna V, et al. (1992) Comparison of results after heart transplantation: mechanically supported versus nonsupported patients. J Heart Lung Transplant 11:235–239

31. Pennington DG, Portner PM, Swartz MT (1995) Clinical experience with the Novacor left ventricular assist system. In: Lewis T, Graham TR (eds) Mechanical circulatory support. Edward Arnold, London, UK, pp 225–228

32. Myers TJ, Dasse KA, Macris MP, Poirier VL, Cloy MJ, Frazier OH (1994) Use of a left ventricular assist device in an outpatient setting. ASAIO J 40:M471–M475.

33. Levin HR, Chen JM, Oz MC, Catanese KA, Krum H, Goldsmith RL, Packer M, Rose EA (1994) Potential of left ventricular assist devices as outpatient therapy while awaiting transplantation. Ann Thorac Surg 58:1515–1520

34. Frazier OH, Benedict CR, Radovancevic B, Bick RJ, Capek P, Springer WE, Macris MP, Delgado R, Buja (1996) Improved left ventricular function after chronic left ventricular unloading. Ann Thorac Surg 62:675–681

35. Frazier OH (1996) Cardiac devices. Transplant Proc 28:2039–2041

Discussion

Dr. Furukawa:
Two quick questions. Did you, in that last case, do a mitral valve annuloplasty with . . .

Dr. Frazier:
No. There was 3+ mitral regurgitation at the start. We just did what Batista says, sewed the valves together.

Dr. Furukawa:
Some surgeons have advocated using a posterior mitral ring in that part of the procedure. The other question I had was have you tried to rest the myocardium in the patient with ischemic cardiomyopathy after "revascularization"?

Dr. Frazier:
I think that's also a possibility. The one patient at Columbia that is a long-term survivor with LVAD removal is such a patient. It's a different pathology and a different physiology and I don't think it is going to be as uniformly successful as I hope resting dilated idiopathic myopathies will be.

International Paediatric Ventricular Assist Device Registry

Richard J. Mullaly, Andrew D. Cochrane, Christian P. Brizard, Stephen B. Horton, Eve B. O'Connor, Clarke A. Thuys, and Tom R. Karl

Summary. Previous work suggests that in the paediatric population the use of a ventricular assist device (VAD) — that is, extracorporeal life support (ECLS) without the use of an oxygenator — might be the most suitable therapy in selected patients who cannot be weaned from cardiopulmonary bypass or who are in end-stage cardiac failure and are candidates to be "bridged" to transplantation. Despite this, potential VAD candidates in this age group are often supported on extracorporeal membrane oxygenation (ECMO), with outcomes recognised to be less than optimal. One reason for the use of ECMO rather than a VAD is the lack of published data on paediatric VADs compared with the vast amount of data and the general acceptance of ECMO as a therapy. Although there are a variety of data registries relating to cardiac surgery and ECLS, to date there is none solely dedicated to analysis of data regarding the use of VADs in the paediatric population. We have recently announced the commencement of the *International Paediatric VAD Registry*. The registry will examine and report on patient variables, methods equipment, and outcome of the use of VADs in infants and children. It is expected that the combined data from many institutions (who may perform very few VAD procedures individually) should provide a powerful database form which trends will become apparent, and from which new and better methods may be developed. This paper describes the registry and our proposal to introduce an optional electronic reporting system using e-mail and the internet (World Wide Web) to minimise paperwork. Information will be available on-line (WWW) as we receive it, and annual reports will be available to participants. The information from the registry will be presented at international cardiac meetings and submitted for journal publications.

Key words: Ventricular assist device — Extracorporeal membrane oxygenation — Paediatric — Registry

Introduction

The use of mechanical circulatory assist devices has become a widely accepted treatment modality for patients with reversible cardiac dysfunction, or those with irreversible cardiac damage who are supported until a suitable donor heart becomes available for transplantation [1]. In contrast to the expanding use of ventricular assist devices (VADs) in the support of adult patients, little progress has been made in the paediatric sphere. Although there is an array of devices available for adult cardiac support, there are still few systems suitable for paediatric ventricular assistance, and published papers in this area [2–4], indicate that the centrifugal pump is the device most commonly used. The increasingly favourable outcome in adult mechanical assist generates many publications and reviews, and this exposure has a positive influence on the decision to use this type of therapy. In contrast, despite a few encouraging reports [2–5] the use of VADs in children remains very limited in comparison to the use of extracorporeal membrane oxygenation (ECMO).

Many authors cite technical difficulties, especially in the use of ventricular assistance in the neonatal group [2,5,6], as a reason for preference for ECMO. Others question the suitability of patients with certain anatomic conditions for isolated ventricular support, and elect total cardiopulmonary support in the form of ECMO [4,5].

Part of the reason for this might be that many centers have limited experience with VADs, but a larger experience with ECMO in noncardiac patients. Others will utilise ECMO in patients who may satisfy a previously published stepwise testing procedure for deciding on the suitability of either VAD or ECMO [4]. Prompted by the knowledge that many paediatric cardiac surgical centres utilise ventricular assistance for less than five cases per year, we investigated the level of support for the establishment of a database for paediatric VAD usage — the International Paediatric VAD Registry.

We contacted over 100 centres in the United States and asked for their recommendations on our proposal for an international registry. There was significant support for the concept of a registry detailing pooled data on patient demographics, indications, techniques, equipment, management, complications, and outcomes.

The notion of a registry is not new. The combined registry for the Clinical Use of Mechanical Ventricular Assist Pumps and the Total Artificial Heart — now

Department of Cardiac Surgery, Royal Children's Hospital, Flemington Road, Melbourne, VIC 3052, Australia

managed through Summit Medical Systems (Minneapolis, MN, USA) [7] — has existed for many years, providing valuable pooled information relating to cardiac support systems used in adults. While this registry can theoretically be used by those institutions supporting their paediatric patients on VADs, the registry is clearly set up to take information and provide data on procedures performed in the adult population.

The extracorporeal life support organisation (ELSO) database is a registry designed to collect data on patients undergoing ECMO. This database stores information on the use of ECMO in the pure respiratory group, as well as ECMO used to support patients requiring circulatory support, both paediatric and adults, but only if their mechanical circulatory support system incorporates an oxygenator. It provides neither access to, nor information on, patients utilising a ventricular assistance system *without* an oxygenator. In short, we believe there is clearly a group of paediatric patients receiving mechanical circulatory support for which data are not available.

Materials and Methods

The International Paediatric VAD Registry will collect information on all patients, ages newborn to 16 years, undergoing mechanical cardiac assistance *without an oxygenator*. Previously published data [2–4,8,9] indicate that most patients requiring mechanical cardiac assistance (either VAD or ECMO) will have had operations on cardiopulmonary bypass, while others will be medical patients suffering from reversible myocarditis or sepsis. A smaller group will be supported as a bridge to transplant.

Data for the registry will come from centres worldwide, which will submit information in one of two ways, either by hardcopy or by e-mail. Our department will supply forms to institutions wishing to submit data in the traditional written format, to be either posted or faxed to us. These data forms will be either mailed to the prospective registering centres or respondents (supplied on disk for subsequent printing

and completion by hand) or e-mailed to the registering centres for subsequent printing and completion. Eventually, the blank data form will be available on the internet as part of a WWW site. Institutions wishing to submit data will be able to download forms from the Web, and complete these by hand and either mail or fax them to our centre.

Other groups may choose to submit their data electronically. This will be expeditiously achieved utilising forms sent to them by e-mail or downloaded by them from the International Paediatric VAD Registry Website. The form, once completed on an individual's PC, can be sent via return e-mail or lodged back onto the Website. It is hoped that the electronic method will be the most efficient, and avoid paper, copies, filing, and lost data.

Results

Information will be continuously available on-line on the Website as it is received and analysed. In this way, the International Paediatric VAD Registry will be different from presently existing registries in that participants and nonparticipants alike will be able to view information at any time, and not need to wait for periodic publications or presentations at scientific meetings. The format that the information will take will provide for the anonymous reporting of data and individual centres and respondents will not be identifiable by those seeking to view or download data.

We aim to make an annual report available (both in hard copy and via e-mail) to all groups who participate. We feel that the full potential of the registry will be realised when centres that have a limited annual experience of perhaps 0–5 procedures per year will be able to review continuously updated data including not only their own contribution but those of all reporting groups, providing a combined experience of somewhere between 50 and 150 patients annually.

Our most recent results (Table 1) note that to July 1996, 88 patients have received circulatory support at the Royal Children's Hospital (RCH) using either a

Table 1. Royal Children's Hospital circulatory support (1989–July 1996)

	VAD	ECMO	VAD and ECMO	Total
Number of patients	41	39	8	88
Number of patients weaned [transplanted] (proportion, CL)	32 [0][a] (0.78; 0.62–0.89)	18 [1][a] (0.49; 0.32–0.65)	1 [2] (0.38; 0.09–0.76)	54 [3]
Number of patients discharged (proportion, CL)	21[b] (0.51; 0.35–0.67)	18[b] (0.46; 0.30–0.62)	0	39

VAD, ventricular assist device; ECMO, extracorporeal membrane oxygenation; CL, confidence limit.
[a] $P = 0.01$.
[b] $P = 0.66$.

Table 2. Recently published results from centres using VAD as a form of mechanical circulatory assist

Authors	Year	Number of patients on VAD	Number of patients weaned	Number of patients discharged	Device(s)
Scheinin et al. [2]	1994	9	7 (77%)	5 (55%)	CP; HP
Hausdorf and Loebe [17]	1994	8	8* (100%)	6 (75%)	BH
Costa et al. [3]	1995	13	10 (76%)	7 (53%)	CP; RP
Ishino et al. [5]	1995	14	10** (71%)	6 (43%)	BH

CP, centrifugal pump; HP, Hemopump; RP, roller pump; BH, Berlin heart.
*All patients transplanted; **8/10 patients were transplanted.

VAD ($n = 41$), ECMO ($n = 39$), or both ($n = 8$). The number (proportion) of patients weaned from the VAD was 32 (0.78) and 21 (0.51) survived to discharge. The number (proportion) of patients weaned from ECMO was 19 (0.49). One of the 19 ECMO patients was transplanted while on ECMO. Of these 19 patients, 18 (0.46) survived to discharge. One of the combined VAD and ECMO group was weaned and a further two were transplanted while on extracorporeal life support (ECLS), but none of these patients survived to be discharged from hospital. There was a significant difference ($P = 0.01$) in weaning probability between the VAD and ECMO groups; however, at discharge this was not the case ($P = 0.66$). The proportion of patients in these two groups surviving to discharge was 0.49.

Recent results from other centres suggest that between one and two thousand children die after cardiac surgery in the United States annually [6]. There will be an additional group of children who die of low cardiac output not related to cardiac surgery, during episodes of acute myocarditis or sepsis. Data also suggest that between 160 and 200 patients annually are placed onto mechanical assist devices worldwide [6,10]. Despite this, there are relatively few publications dealing with VAD use in the paediatric group. An extensive search of recent literature has revealed the results presented in Table 2, which indicate good survival figures in the patients in whom treatment is being attempted (although it must be remembered that not every unit publishes their results).

Discussion

The use of VADs would appear to have greater acceptance as a method of ECLS in adults than in children. Often cited reasons are the relative technical ease of placing a VAD in adults, that relatively fewer contraindications to the use of VADs exist, and that heart transplantation (HTx) is a realistic option in the adult group. It could be suggested that as the overall experience in adults is greater, this in itself, coupled with the aforementioned reasons, makes the use of a VAD more likely in the adult group.

By contrast, ventricular assistance is less well accepted as a treatment modality in the paediatric group. Reasons cited include technical difficulty (patient size related) [5,8,11], unsuitable anatomy [5,6,12], less possibility of HTx [4,6], congenital pathology with a generally accepted poor outlook (independent of the need for ECLS) [13], and lack of experience [11]. This latter point has greater relevance when one notes the wide acceptance of ECMO, which is available in many larger tertiary paediatric institutions that are staffed by personnel with extensive ECMO experience in noncardiac situations [10,11,14]. In these centres ECMO is nearly always chosen over VAD for ECLS. Others cite the lack of suitable VAD equipment for small patients as a reason to elect to use ECMO [5,8,12].

By contrast, in advocating the use of VADs, other authors report their favourable experience relating to the absence of size-related difficulty [3,4], the use of VADs in postcardiotomy patients with univentricular heart (UVH) anatomy and shunt-dependent circulation [15], and the successful bridging of patients using newer devices [5]. Not surprisingly, those centres publishing favourable outcomes in patients on VADs have much more experience and could be said to be further advanced on the learning curve. Their experience and moderately successful outcomes suggests that the use of VAD in children *should* be successful. Indeed, if the population of children weaned in our own series could be sustained past hospital discharge, then the use of VAD might be viewed as having a better outcome than ECMO, which is clearly the preferred current mode of ECLS in children.

Other factors suggest that the use of VAD could in fact be superior to ECMO as a form of ECLS in selected children. It would be fair to say that the comparatively simpler VAD system, without the need for an oxygenator or heat exchanger, might provide fewer circuit complications and less bleeding due to reduced surface activation and clotting factor consumption. Further studies (and indeed a response to the International Paediatric VAD Registry) may provide answers in these areas.

While the cost of maintaining a patient on VAD is not inconsequential, the necessity for an oxygenator and heat-exchanger and the extra nursing staff required for ECMO increase the cost of ECLS markedly. Our costs for an ECMO are four times those for a patient on VAD, on a per-day basis [13]. Others, too, note the expense of ECMO[8,9,14] and so there exist many reasons to support patients who are candidates for ventricular assistance without an oxygenator, with a VAD rather than on ECMO. Of course these patients must fulfill the appropriate criteria as already outlined.

The International Paediatric VAD Registry

The registry will be centred at the Royal Children's Hospital, Melbourne, Australia, and will accept data on all procedures which commenced after January 1, 1996.

The initial sections of the registry relate to *institution* and *patient details*. As some institutions will achieve better results with increasing experience with VADs, the registry asks reporting centres for the chronological order of each patient in the particular institution's total VAD experience. It is well recognised that the anatomy and pathology affecting these patients is particularly varied. Therefore, we have elected not to use prompts or defined and closed categories with respect to the cardiac diagnosis. We ask for descriptive but brief *complete cardiac diagnosis* in order of significance. We will categorise and possibly provide prompts relating to different types of anatomy and pathology after the registry has been running for some time and if responses indicate definite patterns.

VADs can be used for three main categories of patients [4]:

1. Patients supported with a VAD following cardiac surgery in whom recovery is expected. These patients might be unweanable from cardiopulmonary bypass (CPB), *or* weanable from CPB, but subsequently unsupportable on medical therapy due to low cardiac output.
2. Patients who have low cardiac output not related to surgery. This group will include those with myocarditis or sepsis, in whom recovery is expected.
3. Patients who fall into either of these groups, but in whom recovery is not expected. These patients are the bridge-to-transplant group.

The existence of these groups sets the format for the registry questions relating to *indications* and *operative data*.

1. VAD in Postoperative Patients

In this group of patients, the actual operative procedure may influence VAD outcome and so operative details are required. One known risk factor for poor outcome in ECLS is the presence of residual defects [8], which may be associated with various types of surgery. An indication of the prevalence of residual defects in VAD patients and its correlation with type of surgical procedure would be useful in predicting the need for VAD in certain types of cases. Other operative data include effect of previous sternotomy, whether the patient could be weaned from cardiopulmonary bypass (and for how long), and whether the patient left the operating room. The effects of these events on the need for (and the ultimate success of) VAD will be useful. Integral in these inquiries is the length of time that the patient was on cardiopulmonary bypass and possibly more importantly the duration of myocardial ischaemia. We also are interested in the type of cardioplegia solution, and the method of its administration.

2. VAD in Nonsurgical Patients

Patient reaction to low cardiac output is varied and may lead to multiorgan system failure. It is known that multiorgan system failure will affect the outcome and it has been cited as a possible contraindication [13] to the use of VADs. In contrast, others have used ECMO as a bridge to transplant in patients suffering from multiorgan system failure [14]. The registry asks for information relating to acid-base status immediately prior to the institution of the VAD as a marker for the response to low cardiac output, with patient outcome. If there are certain pH values below which survival is rare, it would be useful to know what the limits might be. The same can be said of the patient requirements for inotropic support for which data are also requested.

Data suggest [9,10] that the implementation of ECLS during cardiac arrest may be worthwhile. Details regarding the use of VADs in cardiac arrest, especially the pre-VAD duration of cardiopulmonary resuscitation (CPR), will be of interest. This may provide further data as to the advisability of using a VAD during a cardiac arrest situation.

3. VAD as a Bridge to Transplant

It would appear that in the paediatric group the use of VADs when recovery is unlikely — that is as a bridge to transplant (BTT) — is seen by some as inadvisable due to the scarcity of paediatric heart donors, and the nonambulatory nature of patients supported with current paediatric VAD equipment [4,6]. Others do not support the concept that "bridging" children is inadvisable, and suggest that when well-functioning donor and retrieval networks exist, in which supported patients are unlikely to wait for more than 10 days before receiving a transplant, then ECMO as a BTT has better than expected results [9,10]. Further data relating to BTT and its outcome will be valuable in evaluation and decision making for paediatric patients in the end stage of their cardiac dysfunction. The registry asks whether the patient received a transplant while on VAD and whether the patient needed a VAD after the transplant.

A variety of *equipment* and *devices* are noted to have been used in paediatric VAD procedures. The registry looks at the VAD categories — left, right, or bi-ventricular assist devices (LVAD, RVAD, or BiBAD) — and then of the devices which may be used — pneumatic, roller, centrifugal, electrical, and "totally artificial/implantable" pumps. There are at least thirteen commercial entities represented in the five pump types, and all are noted in the registry. The need for ECMO either before or after VAD, and/or the use of an intra-aortic balloon pump, is also noted in the section looking at devices.

The use of heparin bonding in VAD circuits is currently the subject of much discussion and research [3,8,10,11,16]. There have been reports noting the appearance of thrombus in the circuit when using Carmeda heparin bonding [3]. Details of the use and outcome of heparin-bonded circuits are sought for the registry under "devices."

The sites of cannulation are listed, as are the sizes of the cannulae used at these sites. This is particularly important as cannulation for the use of LVAD in the small patient can be a technical challenge, and has been a major issue in deciding to employ ECMO rather than VAD. It is possible that the choice of cannulation sites might affect outcome, and the registry seeks an indication of this.

The *management* of the patient plays an integral part in the outcome. The section of the registry dealing with this aspect seeks to identify strategies employed in the particularly important areas of anticoagulation and haemostasis monitoring. Blood cell damage, indicated by increasing serum free haemoglobin and decreasing platelet levels, is noted. All of these can adversely affect patient outcome, and might be associated with identifiable increases in morbidity or mortality. Pooled data will assist in identifying these trends.

There is evidence to suggest that the requirement for haemofiltration is associated with increased mortality in patients having ECMO for myocardial dysfunction [2,6]. It is possible that haemodialysis and peritoneal dialysis may also be associated with poor outcome and the influence of each of these will be investigated.

The degree of support required is possibly a determinant of outcome, and the *target* VAD flows including the *highest* VAD flow and lowest flow during weaning are requested items of information for the registry.

A variety of *patient complications* have been associated with ECLS including amongst others: generation of thrombus [5], cerebral [5,6], haemorrhage [6,10,16], sepsis [6,10,16], and renal failure [6]. We seek brief details of any patient complications, as they relate to cerebral, ECG, pulmonary, renal, haemorrhagic, sepsis, and metabolic complications. Once again, trends in these areas are quite likely to be noteworthy. Also of interest is the patient's requirements for blood and blood components during the ventricular assist.

As mentioned previously, the literature contains reports of haemostasic complications occuring in association with the use of heparin-bonded circuits. A section of the registry centred on mechanical circuit complications focuses on this. The categories of major complications incorporated in the registry relate to device malfunction and cessation of function, device or circuit rupture, thrombus or air in the circuit, and malposition of the cannulae.

The final section relates to *outcome* and looks at time on VAD, intensive care unit and hospital stay, and survival to hospital discharge. The primary cause(s) of death is also sought. Finally, permanent sequelae following the use of VAD are investigated including cerebral, cardiac, pulmonary, renal, and others.

It has been communicated to us that one failing of the current existing registries is their unchanging and rigid format for data collection. With this in mind, the format described here will be continually monitored for trends which would indicate that we should alter or change the questions in the registry, particularly in the areas relating to devices, mechanical complications, and patient complications. New technology and varying responses will determine the extent to which the data entry content of the registry will change.

The data collection form is based on the Excel spreadsheet and can be filled in either by hand or on the respondent's computer. There are 9 sheets or 13 pages with between 50 to a maximum of 100 responses required to complete the registry entry. This will vary depending on the patient's hospital course, complications, and outcome. It is expected that the registry will take a maximum of 10 minutes to complete.

In reply to an initial Royal children's Hospital survey querying the support for such a registry, many of the respondents indicated their willingness to use the electronic data transfer as a faster and "cleaner" method of data transfer. Naturally, many institutions will choose to fill in the data forms by hand and mail them and this will be acceptable to us. The electronic data transfer method will be achieved using any commonly available e-mail system and currently tests are under way to ensure that the data is transferred 100% of the time and with 100% accuracy.

It is proposed that both the data collection and processed data will be handled using the internet (with a World Wide Web site) and the International Paediatric VAD Registry home page will enable data collected by ourselves to be pooled, with the displayed data updated weekly. We hope that this will provide instant on-line information relating to techniques, devices, indications, and outcomes to those interested in VADs or critically contemplating the use of a VAD. By way of example, the registry may be accessed by groups who may choose to view data, in order to gain a better picture as to their next step in the surgical treatment of an unweanable CBP patient, while actually resting or weaning the patient on cardiopulmonary bypass. As we move towards the 21st century, the time is upon us when we can avail ourselves of this technology and this is why we have aggressively pursued the electronic nature of the International Paediatric VAD Registry.

It is proposed that the pooled and analysed data will be published in the international literature at either 6 or 12 monthly intervals, and submitted for presentation at selected international meetings.

References

1. Körfer R, El-Banayosy A, Posival H, Minami K, Kizner L, Arusoglu L, Körner MM (1996) Mechanical circulatory support with the Thoratec assist device in patients with postcardiotomy cardiogenic shock. Ann Thorac Surg 61:314–316
2. Scheinin SA, Radovancevic B, Parnis SM, Ott DA, Bricker JT, Towbin JA, Abou-Awdi NL, Frazier OH (1994) Mechanical circulatory support in children. European J Card Thor Surg 8(10):537–540
3. Costa RJ, Chard RB, Nunn GR, Cartmill TB (1995) Ventricular assist devices in pediatric cardiac surgery. Ann Thorac Surg 60(6, Suppl):S536–S538
4. Karl TR (1994) Extracoporeal circulatory support in infants and children. Semin Thorac Cardiovasc Surg 6(3):154–160
5. Ishino K (1996) (Personal communication)
6. Pennington GD, Swartz MT (1993) Circulatory support in infants and children. Ann Thorac Surg. 55:233–237
7. Mehta SM, Aufiero TX, Pae WE, Miller CA, Pierce WS (1995) Combined registry for the clinical use of mechanical ventricular assist pumps and the total artificial heart in conjunction with heart transplantation: Sixth official report, 1994. J Heart Lung Transplant 14:585–593
8. Black MD, Coles JG, Williams WG, Rebeyka IM, Trusler GA, Bohn B, Gruenwald C, Freedom RM (1995) Determinants of success in pediatric cardiac patients undergoing extracorporeal membrane oxygenation. Ann Thorac Surg 60:133–138
9. Dalton HJ, Siewers RD, Fuhrman BP, del Nido P, Thompson AE, Shaver MG, Dowhy M (1993) Extracorporeal membrane oxygenation for cardiac rescue in children with severe myocardial dysfunction. Crit Care Med 21:1020–1028
10. del Nido TJ (1996) Extracorporeal membrane oxygenation for cardiac support in children. Ann Thorac Surg 61:336–339
11. Pennington DG (1994) Commentary on circulatory support in infants and children. Semin Thorac Cardiovasc Surg 6(3):161–162
12. Matsuda H, Taenaka Y, Ohkubo N, Ohtani M, Nishigaki K, Ohtake S, Miura T, Taenaka N, Takano H, Hirose H, Kawashima Y (1988) Use of a paracorporeal ventricular assist device for postoperative cardiogenic shock in two children with complex cardiac lesions. Artif Organs 12(5):423–430
13. Karl TR (1997) Mechanical circulatory support at the Royal Children's Hospital. In: Hetzer R, Henning E, Loebe M (eds) Proceedings of the Mechanical Circulatory Support symposium. Springer, Berlin, pp 7–20
14. Farmer DL, Cullen ML, Philippart AI, Rector FE, Klein MD (1995) Extracorporeal membrane oxygenation as salvage in pediatric surgical emergencies. J Pediatr Surg 30:345–348
15. Karl TR, Sano S, Horton SB, Mee RBB (1991) Centrifugal pump left heart assist in paediatric cardiac operations. J Thorac Cardiovasc Surg 102:624–630
16. Von Segesser LK (1996) Heparin-bonded surfaces in extracorporeal membrane oxygenation for cardiac support. Ann Thorac Surg 61:330–335
17. Hausdorf G, Loebe M (1994) Treatment of low cardiac output syndrome in new born infants and children. Z Kardiol 83(Suppl 2):91–100

Discussion

Dr.Frazier:
Thank you. Let me ask you one question. What sort of VAD did you use, Dr. Mullaly?

Mr.Mullaly:
Firstly, I should suggest my degree is in science. I'm a perfusionist.

Dr.Frazier:
Well, I think it's a very important aspect. We're in an area now in which recording our experience is important.

Mr.Mullaly:
Those results were all obtained with the Biomedicus system. The Biomedicus system has been the device of choice from 1989 to the present, although I would suggest that the Berlin Heart and the Medos device would be devices which we would be looking hard at, to see if we can afford them.

The UCLA Experience with Assist Devices as a Bridge to Transplantation in End-Stage Heart Failure

Masaki Nonoyama, Hillel Laks, Davis C. Drinkwater Jr., Ron Brauner, Shelly Ruzevich, and Jon A. Kobashigawa

Summary. Our experience consisted of 16 patients with end-stage heart failure who needed assist devices as a bridge to transplantation before June, 1996. There were 14 males and two females; aged 15–59 (mean 49.0 ± 2.5) years. Thirteen had ischemic cardiomyopathy; three had idiopathic dilated cardiomyopathy (one was associated with muscular dystrophy). Four types of assist devices were included in this study: 16 Bio-Medicus centrifugal pumps [seven for unilateral left ventricular assist devices (LVAD), six for biventricular assist devices (BVAD), and three for right ventricular assist devices (RVAD) combined with other pumps], four Abiomed pumps (left side), one Novacor pump (left side), and one HeartMate pump (left side). The period of support ranged from 0 to 75 days (mean 10.8 ± 4.5 days). Nine patients had an intra-aortic balloon pump inserted in conjunction with the assist devices. Complications during the support period included bleeding that required reopening of the sternotomy ($n = 6$), infection ($n = 4$), neurologic disorders ($n = 2$), renal failure ($n = 1$), and respiratory failure ($n = 5$). Ten patients had cardiac transplantation and six died awaiting a donor heart. One patient was weaned from the LVAD, but died before transplant. Causes of deaths before transplant were right heart failure ($n = 3$), neurological disorder ($n = 2$), and respiratory/renal failure ($n = 1$). After transplantation, there were two early and one late mortalities. The mean survival period was 28.3 ± 11.4 months. In conclusion, assist devices may allow for a substantial number of patients with end-stage cardiac failure to receive transplants. Early ventricular assist device implantation and appropriate right ventricular support may reduce patient mortality and improve transplantation outcome.

Key words: Assist device — Heart transplantation — Complications

Introduction

At present cardiac transplant is considered as the best therapeutic option for end-stage heart failure patients. However, owing to the shortage of donors, approximately 20%–30% of listed patients die while waiting for a donor heart to become available [1,2]. After the first success in 1978 [3], mechanical circulatory support

University of California Los Angeles, School of Medicine, Department of Cardiothoracic Surgery and Department of Cardiology, 10833 Le Conte Avenue, 62-151 Center of Health Science, Los Angeles, CA 90024, USA

has been developed and is commercially available as a bridge to transplantation. Although it can be life saving, there continues to be a high mortality and morbidity.

Since the middle of the 1980s, the University of California Los Angeles (UCLA) has become a major referral center for heart transplantation, performing 654 cardiac transplants, 584 for adult and 70 for pediatric patients, between 1984 and June 1996. During this period, 16 patients had an assist device implanted as a bridge to transplantation. In this paper, we report our experience with the use of assist devices in patients with acute cardiac failure.

Methods

Between 1984 and June 1996, 16 patients underwent placement of assist devices and were listed as cardiac transplant candidates. Table 1 presents descriptive characteristics of these patients. There were 14 males and two females; age ranging from 15 to 59 (mean 49.0 ± 2.5) years. Thirteen (81.3%) had ischemic cardiomyopathy, two (12.5%) had idiopathic dilated cardiomyopathy, and one (6.3%) had cardiomyopathy associated with muscular dystrophy (not Duchenne type).

Reasons for the necessity for assist devices were inability to wean from cardiopulmonary bypass after open heart surgery ($n = 10$), cardiogenic shock or cardiac arrest ($n = 3$), and ventricular failure ($n = 3$). In all cases, the original procedure prior to ventricular assist device (VAD) implantation was a coronary artery bypass grafting (CABG), with three of these being emergent operations, and one being a combined CABG, left ventricular aneurysmectomy and aortic valve replacement.

Six patients were placed on biventricular assist devices (BVAD) and 10 had unilateral left ventricular assist devices (LVAD). Four types of assist devices were implanted:

1. Sixteen Bio-Medicus (Medtronic, Ninneapolis, MN, USA) centrifugal pumps of which seven were used for unilateral LVAD, six for BVAD (in three

Table 1. Characteristics of patients

Patient number	Diagnosis	Age (years)	Sex	BSA (m^2)	LVAD Type and duration (days)		RVAD[a] Duration (days)	Heart transplant
1	Ischemic	56	M	2.04	Bio-Medicus	2	—	Yes
2	Ischemic	55	M	NA	Bio-Medicus	10	10	Yes
3	Ischemic	54	M	2.06	Bio-Medicus	4	—	Yes
4	Ischemic	49	M	NA	Bio-Mediucs	8	4	No
5	Idiopathic	59	M	1.89	Novacor	23	6	Yes
6	Ischeimc	48	M	2.04	Bio-Medicus	6	6	Yes
7	Ischemic	54	F	1.72	Bio-Medicus	0	—	No
8	Ischemic	55	M	1.92	Abiomed	6	—	Yes
9	Idiopathic[b]	15	M	1.71	Bio-Medicus	2	—	Yes
10	Ischemic	54	M	2.04	Abiomed	8	—	Yes
11	Ischemic	45	M	2.09	Bio-Medicus	13	—	No
12	Ischemic	48	M	1.90	Abiomed	7	7	No
13	Ischemic	47	F	1.55	Abiomed	6	—	Yes
14	Ischemic	49	M	2.31	Bio-Medicus	1	—	No
15	Idiopathic	43	M	2.03	HeartMate	75	5	Yes
16	Ischemic	53	M	2.00	Bio-Medicus	2	—	No

BSA, body surface area; LVAD, left ventricular assist device; RVAD, right ventricular assist device; M, male; F, female.
[a] Bio-Medicus was used in all patients for RVAD.
[b] Associated with muscular dystrophy.

patients), and three for RVAD (combined with other LVAD)

2. Four Abiomed (Danvers, MA, USA) devices for LVAD

3. One HeartMate (Woburn, MA, USA) device for LVAD

4. One Novacor (Baxter, Oakland, CA, USA) device for LVAD

Nine patients had an intra-aortic balloon pump (IABP) inserted in conjunction with the assist devices.

Seven patients received the assist devices in other hospitals and were then transferred to UCLA hospital for orthotopic heart trnasplantation. One patient was transferred on extracorporeal membrane oxygenation (ECMO) and an assist device was implanted at UCLA. One patient was placed on ECMO after resuscitation, and a BVAD was implanted the next day because of ventricular failure.

VAD implantation was considered in patients with hemodynamic impairments. The following criteria were used: cardiac index <2.0l/min with IABP and pharmacological support, systemic vascular resistance >2100 dyne·s^{-1}·cm^{-5}, left atrial pressure >20mmHg, urine output <20cm^3·h^{-1} with optimal preload, and maximum pharmacological and hemodynamic support including IABP.

Patients were not considered candidates for VAD support when the duration of shock with multiple organ failure exceeded 12h or additional coexisting factors such as chronic renal failure, cancer, severe hepatic disease, or blood dyscrasia were present. Also,

excluded were patients with active infection (e.g., draining abscess) and symptomatic cerebrovascular disease.

During the support period, heparin sulfate infusion was continued and activated clotting time was maintained between 150 and 200s. Antibiotics were used intravenously as long as assist devices were implanted.

Postoperative complications were defined as follows:

1. Bleeding: requiring resternotomy for hemostasis
2. Renal failure: necessitating dialysis
3. Infection: with positive culture growth
4. Respiratory failure: mechanical ventilation for more than 7 days after the last operation (including hemostasis procedures)
5. Thromboembolism: identification of embolus by either computed tomography or postmortem examination
6. Thrombus: presence of thrombus within the device at the time of explantation
7. Hemolysis: serum hemoglobin level greater than 40mg/dl on 2 consecutive days
8. Device malfunction: mechanical malfunction of the control console or other components, necessitating device replacement

Data were analyzed with the Statview Statistical Software package (Brian Power, Calabasas, CA, USA). All data were expressed as mean ± standard error. Fisher's exact test was used to determine significance for discrete variables. A P value less than 0.05 was considered significant.

Results

The period of support ranged from 0 to 75 days (mean 10.8 ± 4.5 days). Six patients needed biventricular support and two of them could be weaned from the RVAD during the awaiting time. One patient could be weaned off the assist device (LVAD) and had an IABP reinserted during the awaiting period. However, he developed respiratory and renal failure and died before the transplant.

The pump flow rate was 5.6 ± 0.3 l/min for LVAD and 4.8 ± 0.3 l/min for RVAD. There was no significant difference in flow rates between survival and nonsurvival patients for both left and right sides.

There was only one patient in the survivor group who had normal renal function during the first 24h after an assist device implantation. All patients had liver dysfunction during the initial period. Renal and hepatic function, and hematological data in survivor and nonsurvivor patients were compared on the first and the last 24h of the support period (Table 2). There was no significant difference in renal function, hepatic function, or hematological data between survivor and nonsurvivor patients.

Complications after implantation included bleeding ($n = 6$), infection ($n = 4$), intracranial hemorrhage ($n = 2$), renal failure ($n = 1$), and respiratory failure ($n = 5$). One patient had an episode of seizures 4 days after removal of the LVAD. In addition, one patient had ischemic spinal cord injury causing paraplegia after the transplantation procedure.

Six patients died before transplantation. The causes of deaths before transplant are listed in Table 3. Three of the six nonsurviving patients died because of right ventricular failure. Two other patients died of cerebral bleeding, previously mentioned.

Among the ten transplanted patients, there were two early and one late mortalities (Table 3). One patient had sudden cardiac arrest several hours after the transplant operation, and was placed on ECMO. He died on postoperative day 2 owing to multiple organ failure. One patient died because of tamponade caused by aortic rupture. The cause of one late death was allograft coronary artery disease. The survival period after cardiac transplantation ranged from 0 to 113 months (mean 28.3 ± 11.4 months).

Discussion

Following increasing demand for assist devices as a bridge to transplant, recent studies have reported encouraging results with high survival rates [4–8]. The posttransplant survival rate was reported to be equal to or better [6] than in patients who did not require mechanical support prior to transplant.

A documented benefit of prolonged circulatory support as a bridge to transplantation is the ability to improve patients' nutritional and physiologic function prior to the transplantation procedure [9,10]. In our experience, there was no significant change in renal or hepatic function in patients supported for an average

Table 2. Laboratory data during supporting period

		After implantation	Before removal	P value
Renal function				
BUN	Survivor	33.3 ± 6.1	26.1 ± 3.0	0.155
(mg/dl)	Nonsurvivor	36.8 ± 5.6	43.2 ± 10.1	
Creatinin	Survivor	1.69 ± 0.37	1.36 ± 0.19	0.255
(mg/dl)	Nonsurvivor	1.61 ± 0.20	2.36 ± 0.56	
Liver function				
GOT	Survivor	526.0 ± 231.4	59.0 ± 28.3	0.237
(IU/l)	Nonsurvivor	75.7 ± 22.4	97.0 ± 27.5	
GPT	Survivor	142.0 ± 101.4	24.0 ± 5.0	0.759
(IU/l)	Nonsurvivor	104.7 ± 39.4	109.0 ± 32.5	
Total Bilirubin	Survivor	2.8 ± 0.6	3.4 ± 1.3	0.501
(mg/dl)	Nonsurvivor	3.8 ± 1.5	6.2 ± 3.2	
Hematology				
WBC	Survivor	14.44 ± 1.22	13.14 ± 1.18	0.065
($\times 10^3$/mm^3)	Nonsurvivor	7.45 ± 1.20	10.13 ± 0.96	
Platelets	Survivor	107.7 ± 11.0	144.2 ± 35.6	0.963
($\times 10^3$/mm^3)	Nonsurvivor	105.8 ± 14.2	149.0 ± 45.8	

BUN, blood urea nitrogen; GOT, glutamic oxaloacetic transaminase; GPT, glutamic pyruvic transaminase; WBC, white blood cells.

Table 3. Causes of death before and after transplant

	Patient Number	Causes of death
Before transplant	4	Sepsis, brain death
	7	Right heart failure
	11[a]	Renal and respiratory failure
	12	Brain death, gastrointestinal bleeding
	14	Right heart failure
	16	Right heart failure, coagulopathy, bleeding, acute renal failure
After transplant	2	Transplant coronary artery disease
	3	Pneumonia, tamponade owing to aortic rupture
	9[b]	Multiple organ failure

[a] After removing LVAD.
[b] Cardiac arrest on postoperative day 1 and placed on extracorporeal membrane oxygenation.

Table 4. Characteristics of devices

	Bio-Medicus	Abiomed	Novacor, HeartMate
Power	Centrifugal	Pneumatic	Electrical or pneumatic
Implanted	No	No	Yes
Weanable?	Yes	Yes	Yes
Left and right?	Both	Both	Left
Expected duration	Short term	Intermediate	Long term
Advantages	Low cost	Mobility	Higher heart rates possible
	Easy to insert	Easy to monitor	Implantable
			Mobility
Disadvantages	Limited mobility	Rate cannot exceed 120 bpm	Piece of left ventricle removed
	Increased thrombosis		Only left-sided
	Anticoagulation required		

of 10.8 days; therefore, longer support duration may be considered. This is further supported by early posttransplant deaths in two patients who were transplanted 2 and 4 days after LVAD implantation while still recovering from the initial surgery. However, six patients in our series died before receiving a donor heart.

Selection of the appropriate device is an important consideration. We based our device selection on the advantages and disadvantages of these devices as listed in Table 4. Pulsatile assist devices have been reported to decrease the required inotrope dose and improve end-organ function [11]. Furthermore, the survival rate in patients with Abiomed devices was reported to be lower than in patients with Novacor or Thoratec devices [6]. We chose the device according to the expected duration of support, required flow and rate, need for right ventricular support, and desired mobility.

It is also important whether the patient will require BVAD or only LVAD. Patients with severe right ven-

tricular failure, nonresponsive to drug therapy, cannot be expected to improve without RVAD. After placing the LVAD, an assessment of right ventricular function is made using clinical and hemodynamic criteria: a high central venous pressure in the presence of normal left atrial pressure and no preexisting pulmonary vascular disease. Clinical impression obtained by visualization and the effect of pharmacological support (e.g., inotropes) is also used to estimate the need for RVAD. Three nonsurvivors in our series may have been helped by RVAD.

The incidence of postimplant complications is consistently high in most studies [4–6,12]. Thromboembolic events, resulting in central nervous system deficits, infections, and bleeding were among the most serious problems. In our experience, two patients with neurological complications in our nonsurviving group had prior cardiac arrest episodes and were resuscitated. There was one patient who had a neurologic complication after the transplant procedure (ischemic spinal cord injury).

Recently, we have used vancomycine, 2mg per day, throughout the mechanical circulatory support period. Furthermore, we attempted early extubation when possible, total parenteral nutrition, and physical therapy as soon as possible after the implantation procedure.

In conclusion, assist devices allow for a substantial number of patients with end-stage cardiac failure to receive transplants. Early ventricular assist device implantation and appropriate right ventricular support may reduce patient mortality and improve trnasplantation outcome.

References

1. Copeland JG, Emery RW, Levinsen MM, Copeland J, McAleen MJ, Riley JE (1985) The role of mechanical support and transplantation in treatment of patients with end-stage cardiomyopathy. Circulation 72(Suppl II):II–7
2. Annual report of the US Scientific Registry for Organ Transplantation and the Organ Procurement and Transplantation Network–1990. Es 8-9, US Department of Health and Human Services, Washington DC, USA
3. Reemtsma K, Dursin R, Edie R, Bregman D, Dobello W, Hardy M (1978) Cardiac transplantation for patients requiring mechanical circulatory support. N Engl J Med 298:670–671
4. Pennington DG, McBridge LR, Peigh PS, Miller LW, Swartz MT (1994) Eight years' experience with bridging to cardiac transplantation. J Thorac Cardiovasc Surg 107:472–481
5. Sapirstein JS, Pae WE Jr, Aufiero TX, Boehmer JP, Pierce WS (1995) Long-term left ventricular assist device use before transplantation. ASAIO J 41:M530–M534
6. Koerfer R, El-Banayosy A, Posival H, Minami K, Koerner MM, Arusoglu L, Breymann T, Kizner L, Seifert D, Koertke H, Fey O (1995) Mechanical circulatory support: The Bad Oeynhausen experience. Ann Thorac Surg 59:S56–63
7. McCarthy PM (1995) HeartMate implantable left ventricular assist device: Bridge to transplantation and future applications. Ann Thorac Surg 59:46–51
8. Griffith BP, Kormos RL, Nastala CJ, Winowich S, Pristas JM (1996) Results of extended bridge to transplantation: Window into the future of permanent ventricular assist devices. Ann Thorac Surg 60:396–398
9. Burton NA, Lefrak EA, Macmanus Q, Hill A, Marino JA, Spein AM, Akl DF, Albus RA, Massimiano PS (1993) A reliable bridge to cardiac transplantation: the TCI left ventricular assist device. Ann Thorac Surg 55:1425–1431
10. Frazier OH, Duncan KM, Radovancevic B, Vega JD, Baldwin RT, Burnett CM, Lonquist JL (1992) Successful bridge to heart transplantation with a new left ventricular assist device. J Heart Lung Transplant 11:530–537
11. Minami K, Koerner MM, Vyska K, Kleesiek K, Knobl H, Koerfer R (1990) Effects of pulsatile perfusion on plasma catecholamine levels an hemodynamics during and after cardiac operations with cardiopulmonary bypass. J Thorac Cardiovasc Surg 99:82–91
12. Holman WL, Murrah CP, Ferguson ER, Bourge RC, McGiffin DC, Kirklin JK (1996) Infections during extended circulatory support: University of Alabama at Birmingham experience 1989 to 1994. Ann Thorac Surg 61:366–371

Medically Unresponsive Pulmonary Hypertension: Heterotopic Cardiac Transplant Versus Mechanical Support

R.M. Adamson[1], W.P. Dembitsky[1], B.E. Jaski[1], P.O. Daily[1], R. Moreno[1], J.C. Kim[1], J. Sono[2], T. Akasaka[2], P.M. Hoagland[1], and J.B. Gordon[1]

Summary. End-stage congestive heart failure with unresponsive pulmonary hypertension presents a unique clinical dilemma. Heterotopic graft placement is associated with decreased long-term survival and orthotopic transplantation carries high operative mortality. We report on a patient with unresponsive pulmonary hypertension who was mechanically supported with a HeartMate left ventricular assist device (LVAD). Immediately before LVAD insertion, the pulmonary artery pressure (PAP) was 74/28 mmHg with a transpulmonary gradient (TPG) of 28 mmHg, and a pulmonary vascular resistance (PVR) of 6.6 Wood units despite prolonged dobutamine, milrinone, and prostaglandin E_1 infusions. After 10 weeks on the LVAD, these parameters were: PAP 28/15 mmHg, TPG 15 mmHg, and PVR 2.8 Wood units. The patient subsequently underwent an uneventful orthotopic heart transplant. At 1 year after transplantation, PAP remains low at 34/14, TPG at 8, and PVR at 1.5 Wood units. An LVAD bridge to orthotopic cardiac transplantation should be considered in selected patients with unresponsive pulmonary hypertension. However, several weeks may be needed for normalization of pressure and resistance.

Key words: Pulmonary hypertension — Cardiac transplant — Mechanical support — Left ventricular assist device

Introduction

Pulmonary artery (PA) hypertension was identified early in the history of cardiac transplantation as a determinant of transplant candidacy and predictor of operative risk [1]. It has been associated with immediate donor organ failure [2], higher operative mortality [3], and decreased long-term survival [4,5]. A 1992 position statement from the American Heart Association Committee on Cardiac Transplantation states that the absolute level of pulmonary vascular resistance that will produce right heart failure is unknown, but in most centers patients with pulmonary vascular resistance of more than 4–6 Wood units are not accepted as candidates for transplantation [6].

For patients excluded from orthotopic transplant candidacy, heterotopic cardiac transplantation has been the procedure of choice. Heterotopic transplantation has several disadvantages including: atelectasis, native heart arrhythmias and angina, necessity for chronic Coumadin therapy, and decreased long-term survival when compared to orthotopic recipients [7]. The decision regarding orthotopic or heterotopic candidacy is further complicated by the fact that most patients have normalization of PA pressures and pulmonary vascular resistance (PVR) after orthotopic [8] as well as heterotopic transplantation [9,10], although this is not always the case [11].

The patient presented here developed fixed, medically unresponsive, pulmonary artery hypertension during inotropic support while awaiting organ availability. A Thermo Cardiosystems (TCI; Woburn, MA, USA) HeartMate pneumatic left ventricular assist device (LVAD) was placed to assess the patient's PA responsiveness and to determine orthotopic transplant candidacy.

Materials and Methods

A 41-year-old man with a congenitally bicuspid aortic valve with insufficiency developed congestive heart failure and became dobutamine-dependent in January 1994. He was listed for transplant in April. The initial PA pressure during dobutamine infusion and sodium nitroprusside challenge was 54/23 mmHg with a transpulmonary gradient (TPG) of 19 mmHg and a PVR of 3.9 Wood units. This degree of pulmonary hypertension placed the patient in an increased but acceptable risk category for an orthotopic transplant. An adequate donor organ did not become available and the patient's condition deteriorated, necessitating the addition of milrinone to his dobutamine regimen. His PA hypertension worsened and became unresponsive to prostaglandin E_1 (PGE_1). With a PA pressure of 74/28 mmHg, TPG of 28 mmHg, and PVR of 6.6 Wood units, the authors felt he was no longer an acceptable orthotopic transplant candidate.

After obtaining informed consent, a pneumatic HeartMate LVAD was inserted and the patient's

[1] Sharp Memorial Hospital, 8010 Frost Street, San Diego, CA 92123, USA
[2] Kobe City General Hospital, 4-6 Minatojima-Nakamachi, Chuo-ku, Kobe, Hyogo 650, Japan

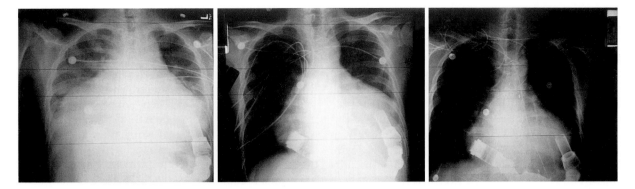

Fig. 1. Chest radiographs showing decreasing cardiac size during left ventricular support with a Thermo Cardiosystems HeartMate

Table 1. Pulmonary arterial pressures and resistances

Time	Medications	PAP	TPG	PVR	CO
Listing	Dob, SNP	54/23	19	3.9	4.9
Pre-LVAD	Dob, mil, PGE₁	74/28	28	6.6	4.2
Post-LVAD	Dob, mil, PGE₁, is	48/22	16	3.2	5.0
4 Weeks post-LVAD	None	70/25	25	3.4	7.4
10 Weeks post-LVAD	None	28/15	15	2.3	6.5
	During exercise	71/27	24	2.9	8.3
Before transplant	None	26/13	12	3.2	3.8
After transplant	Dop, is	38/18	7	1	7.0
11 Days	None	55/23	18	1.8	10.0
3 Month	None	20/12	12	2.2	5.5
6 Months	None	32/14	15	2.9	5.2
1 Year	None	35/15	12	2.7	4.4

PAP, pulmonary artery pressure (mmHg); TPG, transpulmonary gradient (mmHg); PVR, pulmonary vascular resistance (mmHg·l⁻¹·min⁻¹); CO, cardiac output (l/min); dob, dobutamine HCL; SNP, sodium nitroprusside; mil, milrinone; dop, dopamine; is, Isuprel; PGE₁, prostaglandin E₁; LVAD, left ventricular assist device.

native aortic valve was replaced. A porcine valve was used in an effort to reduce the risk of thromboembolism and avoid the need for anticoagulation postoperatively.

The pulmonary artery pressure declined immediately after LVAD insertion during isoproterenol and PGE₁ infusions, but returned to its previously elevated state when the drugs were discontinued (see Table 1). At two weeks after LVAD insertion, the PVR had fallen to 3.4 Wood units, but the PA pressure remained elevated at 70/25 mmHg with a TPG of 25 mmHg. By 10 weeks after LVAD insertion, the patient's PAP had improved to 28/15 mmHg, with a TPG of 15 mmHg, and PVR of 2.8 Wood units. Although pulmonary hypertension returned with exercise (PA of 71/27 mmHg and TPG of 24 mmHg) the PVR remained low (2.9 Wood units). Subsequent to

LVAD insertion, the patient cleared a methicillin-resistant *Staphylococcus aureus* (MRSA) pneumonia and was functionally rehabilitated. There was a marked decrease in cardiac size during this interval (Fig. 1).

After almost 3 months of LVAD support, a graft became available and the patient underwent an uneventful orthotopic transplant. At one hour after orthotopic transplantation, the PAP was 38/18, with a TPG of 7 and a PVR of 1 Wood unit during isoproterenol and dopamine infusions. At 11 days after transplantation, the PAP was 55/23 mmHg without inotropic support. The TPG was 18 mmHg, but the PVR remained low at 1.8 Wood units. At one year after transplantation the PA pressure continued to improve; PA was 32/14, TPG was 15, and PVR was 2.9 Wood units. Table 1 depicts the changes in PA pressure measurements and resistance calculations over time.

At the time of transplantation it was observed that the porcine aortic valve was thrombosed. The patient had been anticoagulated with Coumadin for one month after LVAD insertion and then received one aspirin per day until transplantation. The patient did not have evidence of peripheral embolization or cerebral vascular accident and had adequate native ventricular ejection through the LVAD after the device was turned off and before initiating cardiopulmonary bypass. During the 18 months of post-transplant follow up the patient demonstrated persistent mild elevation of pulmonary artery pressures and the potential for vasoconstriction.

Discussion

Pulmonary hypertension is a major determinant of transplant candidacy and predictor of operative risk. Severe and unresponsive pulmonary hypertension is a contraindication to orthotopic cardiac transplantation. The clinical difficulty comes in distinguishing truly unresponsive from medically refractory cases with pulmonary hypertension. Without normalizing the left atrial pressure and cardiac output, which is generally impossible with inotropic medications alone, the ultimate reactivity of the pulmonary circulation is unknown.

The majority of cardiac transplant recipients have reactive pulmonary hypertension. Griepp et al. [1] and more recently Bhatia et al. [8] demonstrated prompt return to near-normal pressures and resistance after orthotopic heart transplantation. Kawaguchi et al. [10] also demonstrated similar decreases in pressures in patients with severe pulmonary hypertension after heterotopic transplantation.

Although there is disagreement in the literature as to which indicator of pulmonary hypertension most accurately predicts graft failure: TPG, PVR, or PVR index [2], it is generally agreed that PA hypertension — defined as PA systolic 50 mmHg, mean PA 30 mmHg, TPG 15, and a PVR 2.5 Wood units — presents increased risk both immediately after transplant and long-term. It is also agreed that patients with an unresponsive PVR greater than 4–6 Wood units present at least a relative contraindication to orthotopic transplantation [6].

Several conditions appear associated with fixed pulmonary hypertension. In patients with congenital heart disease and left-to-right shunts, unresponsive pulmonary hypertension develops and is associated with anatomic pulmonary artery changes. Patients with advanced anatomic changes are generally unresponsive to vasodilator therapy or reductions in left heart filling pressures. Chronic pulmonary emboli, cor pulmonale, and primary pulmonary hypertension are also relatively unresponsive to vasodilators and reductions in left heart filling pressures. This group of patients is unlikely to improve with mechanical support.

The case we presented demonstrates that pulmonary hypertension of recent onset, unresponsive to multiple inotropic agents and PGE_1, can respond to LVAD support. It is interesting to note that PVR calculations normalized prior to actual reduction in measured PA pressures. It took 10 weeks with low pulmonary capillary wedge pressures (4–15 mmHg) and normal cardiac outputs (5–8 l/min) for pressure normalization. Even then, exercise-induced pulmonary vasoconstriction was capable of rapidly elevating pulmonary artery pressures to their pre-LVAD states.

Conclusion

Mechanical LVAD support of refractory congestive heart failure associated with unresponsive pulmonary hypertension allowed discontinuation of inotropic medications, resolution of an MRSA pneumonia, and increased recipient activity and reconditioning. The resultant improvement in pulmonary hemodynamics contributed to an uncomplicated orthotopic cardiac transplant and long-term survival.

References

1. Griepp RB, Stinson EB, Dong ED, Clark DA, Shumway NE (1971) Determinants of operative risk in human heart transplantation. Am J Surg 122:192–196
2. Addonizio LJ, Gersony WM, Robbins RC, Drusine RE, Smith CR, Reison, DS, Reemtsma K, Rose EA (1987) Elevated pulmonary vascular resistance and cardiac transplantation. Circulation 76 (Suppl V):V52–55
3. Constard-Jäckle A, Hill I, Schroeder JS, Fowler MB (1991) The influence of preoperative patient characteristics on early and late survival following cardiac transplantation. Circulation 84 (Suppl IH):IEII-329–337
4. Erickson KW, Costanzo-Nordin MR, O'Sullivan JE, Johnson MR, Zucker MJ, Pifarré R, Lawless MR, Robinson JA, Scanlon PJ (1990) Influence of preoperative transpulmonary gradient on late mortality after orthotopic heart transplantation. J Heart Transplant 9:526–537
5. Kirklin JK, Naftel DC, Kirklin JW, Blackstone EH, White-Williams C, Bourge RC (1988) Pulmonary vascular resistance and the risk of heart transplantation. J Heart Transplant 7:331–336
6. O'Connell JB, Bourge RC, Costanzo-Nordin MR, Driscoll DJ, Morgan JP, Rose EA, Uretsky BF (1992) Cardiac transplantation: recipient selection, donor procurement, and medical follow-up. A statement for health professionals from the Committee on Cardiac

Transplantation of the Council on Clinical Cardiology, American Heart Association. Circulation 86:1061–1079

7. Cooper DKC, Lanza RP (1984) Advantages and disadvantages of heterotopic transplantation. In: Cooper OKC, Ranza RP (eds) Heart transplantation, MTP Press, Lamcaster, pp 305–319

8. Bhatia SJS, Kirshenbaum JM, Shemin RJ, Cohn LH, Collins JJ, DeSesa VJ, Young PJ, Mudge GH, St. John Sutton MG (1987) Time course of resolution of pulmonary hypertension and right ventricular remodeling after orthotopic cardiac transplantation. Circulation 76:819–826

9. Villanueva FS, Murali S, Uretsky BF, Reddy PS, Griffith BP, Hardesty RL, Kormos RL (1989) Resolution of severe pulmonary hypertension after heterotopic cardiac transplantation. J Am Coll Cardid 14:1239–1243

10. Kawaguchi A, Gandjbakhch I, Pavie A, Bors V, Muneretto C, Leger P, Mesteri T, Piazza T, Cabrol A, Desruennes M, Cabrol C (1989) Cardiac transplant recipients with preoperative pulmonary hypertension: evolution of pulmonary hemodynamics and surgical options. Circulation 80 (Suppl III):90–96

11. Shumway SJ, Baughman KL, Traill TA, Cameron DE, Fonger JD, Gardner TJ, Achuff SC, Reitz BA, Baumgartner WA (1989) Persistent pulmonary hypertension after heterotopic heart transplantation: A case report. J Heart Transplant 8:387–390

First Experience of Novacor Implant at the Heart Institute of Japan

Mitsuhiro Hachida[1], Satoshi Saito[1], Shinichirou Kihara[1], Masaya Kitamura[1], Hironobu Hoshi[1], Hitoshi Koyanagi[1], and Kazutomo Minami[2]

Summary. The Novacor left ventricular assist device has been used as a bridge to heart transplantation worldwide. However, because no heart transplant has been carried out recently in Japan, temporary circulatory assists using implantable devices have not been performed. Despite the obstacles in using such devices for long-term support, we nevertheless implanted a Novacor left ventricular assist device (LVAD) (wearable type) in a patient with dilated cardiomyopathy, for lifesaving purposes. The patient was a 29-year-old wan. He had general fatigue and dyspnea in April 1990. He was diagnosed with dilated cardiomyopathy by endomyocardial biopsy. The chest roentgenogram showed cardiomegaly with a cardiothoracic ratio of 64%, and echocardiography showed severely reduced wall motion of the left ventricle with a fraction shortening of 0.03. His hemodynamic condition rapidly deteriorated, and a Novacor implant was performed on March 11, 1996. After the implantation, the patient was ectubated on day 3 and rapidly recovered after the implantation. The pump output consistently was over 5 l/min. No complications such as bleeding or thromboembolic episodes were seen. We believe that the wider application of Novacor implantation will be a significant break-through in the treatment of patients with severely deteriorated cardiomyopathy in Japan.

Key words: Heart transplantation — Novacor LVAD — Cardiomyopathy — Artificial heart

Introduction

The electrically powered implantable Novacor left ventricular assist device (LVAD; Baxter, Tokyo, Japan) is one of the most reliable and technically advanced systems of circulatory assist at present [1–5]. In Japan, no heart transplantation has been performed since 1968. Therefore, chronic circulatory assist using an implantable device such as the Novacor LVAD would be naturally the first alternative treatment for the patient with severe cardiac failure due to cardiomyopathy. However, to succeed with this treatment without the back-up of transplantation, adequate patient selection, minimum operative risk, and fewer postoperative complications are essential.

In this repost, we demonstrate our surgical modifications and the first experience of Novacor implantation at the Heart Institute of Japan.

Patient

A 29-year-old man presented with a 2-year history of progressive heart failure. At presentation, his height was 173 cm and body weight 67 kg; his New York Heart Association (NYHA) status was grade 4. On his admission, echocardiography and myocardial biopsy were performed, and he was diagnosed with end-stage dilated cardiomyopathy. Treatment with digoxin, diuretics, and an acetylcholine esterase (ACE) inhibitor was not effective and his clinical status progressively deteriorated. The chest roentgenogram showed cardiomegaly with a cardiothoracic ratio of 64%, and echocardiography showed severely reduced wall motion of the left ventricle with a fraction shortening of 0.03. The left ventricular diastolic dimension was 72 mm and its systolic dimension was 70 mm. Cardiac catheterization data was as follows: right atrial pressure 12 mmHg, right ventricular pressure 9–46 mmHg (end-diastolic pressure 12 mmHg), pulmonary arterial (PA) pressure 31–48 mmHg (mean 38 mmHg), PA wedge pressure 31 mmHg, and cardiac output 3.19 l/min (cardiac index $1.731 \cdot min^{-1} \cdot m^{-2}$). Without using a mechanical circulatory assist, it would have been impossible to prolong his life. The patient and his family completely understood the indications for assist devices, the prognosis and quality of life with the Novacor LVAD, the risk and possible complications, and the social difficulties of heart transplantation in Japan.

Implant Technique

Cutaneous incision was carried out from the jugular notch to 2 cm below the umbilicus. After median sternotomy and a longitudinal pericardial incision, the anterior fascia of the left recuts muscle of the abdomen was incised close to the linea alba, and a pump

[1] Department of Cardiovascular Surgery, The Heart Institute of Japan, Tokyo Women's Medical College, 8-1 Kawada-cho, Shinjuku-ku, Tokyo 162, Japan
[2] Department of Cardiovascular Surgery, Bad Oeynhausen Heart Center, Bochum University, 4970 Bad Oeynhausen, Germany

pocket was tailored between the posterior aspect of the muscle and the deep layer of the fascia, large enough to accommodate the pump. The ideal position of the inflow conduit in relation to the cardiac apex was tested, and the anterior diaphragmatic fibers were largely divided to the lower ribs without opening the left pleura to the peritoneum. With this approach, the pump pocket could freely communicate with the pericardial cavity and all the bleeding sites could easily be controlled. The pump was assembled and the electrical cable was tunneled to the inferior right abdominal area, 5 cm above the anterior-superior iliac process.

The patient was fully heparinized and cardiopulmonary bypass was instituted. With bicaval cannulations in place, the foramen ovale was closed through the incision of right atrium. Under moderate hypothermia at 27°C, ventricular fibrillation was induced. The apex of the myocardium was resected with a cutter and the inside of the left ventricular cavity was carefully inspected, visually verifying the position of the septum and the papillary muscles. Four U-stitches of Ethibond 0 (Ethicon, Somerville, NJ, USA) reinforced with Teflon pledgets were made through the ventricular myocardium in the apex at cardinal points. Similarly, another eight stitches were then used to complete the circumference (Fig. 1). All 12 stitches were passed through the apical Teflon ring and tied, except for the four cardinal ones, which were left untied. Then, the inflow conduit was smoothly inserted in the wide apical hole, and the apical ring purse string tied. The four cardinal stitches were passed through the skirt of the apical cannula and firmly tied. The inflow cannula was passed through the diaphragm after the pump was connected to the cannula in the abdominal pocket. The cable was passed through the edge of the right rectus muscle and connected to the controller.

Proper passage for the outflow conduit was created in the submuscular layer of the right recuts muscle. The body temperature was increased and the heartbeat was reinitiated. After the conduit was cut to the proper length, it was anastomosed to the side-clamped ascending aorta. The left ventricular venting catheter was removed and tied. A small hole was made in the graft for removing air, and the distal side of this hole was clamped. In this way, air from the left ventricle and the device was evacuated from this hole with ventricular beating (Fig. 2). After the aortic anastomosis was completed, the proximal side of the air hole was clamped and the side-clamp was released. Removal of air from the aortic root was completed through the air hole (Fig. 3). The complete removal of air was achieved passively by releasing the clamp on the outflow conduit and actively with single strokes, paying attention to avoid excess tension on the aortic suture line. Extracorporeal circulation was then stopped and the Novacor was activated. The postoperative hemodynamic parameters were remarkably stable. This patient was extubated on day 3 and complete anticoagulation therapy with coumadin and aspirin was started from day 2. The blood bilirubin level was elevated from day 2 and all examination data reached normal levels by day 14. The patient returned home 3 months after the implantation. At present, his quality of life is markedly improved, and he is awaiting transplantation (Fig. 4).

Discussion

In Japan, neigher the concept of brain death nor the practice of organ transplantation from brain-dead donors has been accepted. Organ donation from brain-dead donors has been a controversial issue in Japan

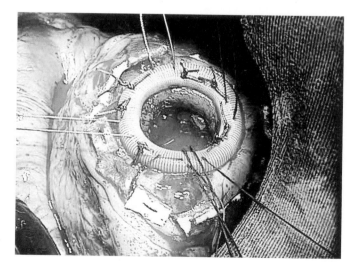

Fig. 1. Resection of the apex of the myocardium and inflow cannula insertion

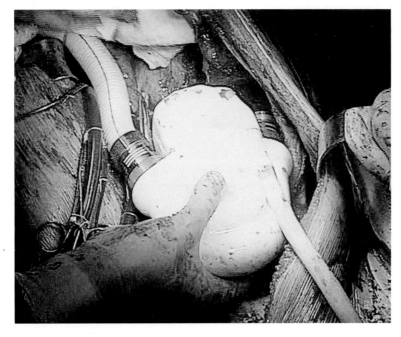

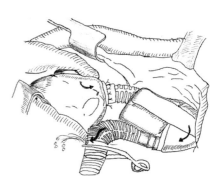

Fig. 2. Removal of air during outflow conduit anastomosis

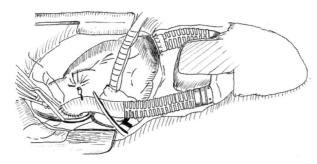

Fig. 3. Method for removing air from outflow conduit

for many years. Under such circumstances, patients do not have the option of receiving a heart transplant. Circulatory assist using implantable devices such as the Novacor left ventricular assist device (LVAD) should be stressed for use in those patients indicated for transplantation in Japan. From this point of view, this completely successful implantation of a Novacor LVAD can be seen as a new horizon for patients with end-stage cardiac failure in Japan.

A preequisite for successful assistance is the need for precise surgical technique in implantation, to avoid air embolism, bleeding, malpositioning, and infectious complications. There are several pitfalls: some risk of inaccuracy in the insertion of the apical conduit in the contracting myocardium, considerable difficulty in ret-

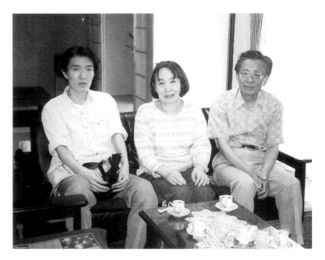

Fig. 4. The patient (*left*), shown at home with his family, has markedly improved quality of life after the Novacor implantation

rograde removal of air from the system, and the existence of a potential bleeding site away from direct control at the level of the apical cannulation and the diaphragmatic tunnel. The implantation of an LVAD is a major operation, performed on very frail patients with hemodynamic, coagulative, hepatic, renal, and cerebral problems. Therefore, we slightly modified the technique presented by Pennington et al. [6] in an attempt to minimize these problems.

Our implant method is presented here in the hope of minimizing major complications usually encoutered in LVAD implantation: bleeding, embolism, and conduit obstruction to malposition. It has been controversial whether it is preferable to use ventricular fibrillation or to induce cardiac arrest by employing cardioplegia. Vigano et al. [7] reported that aortic cross-clamping is of great advantage for removing the thrombi in the ventricle and avoiding partial obstructions due to the papillary muscle. However, the major criticism of this approach is the potential damage to the right ventricle during cardioplegic arrest [8]. In the present case, the duration of ventricular fibrillation was approximately 60 min, and the removal of air was much easier after the ventricular fibrillation. Moreover, we found that damage to the right ventricle was negligible, because there was no ischemic time during the surgery.

Removal of air from the device is the most important part of this surgery. In our case, continuous removal was achieved from the hole made at the outflow conduit during anastomosis of the outflow conduit to the aorta. It was very effective in eliminating residual bullae inside the pump and ventricle.

Transesophageal echocardiography during the operation allowed verification of the integrity of the interatrial septum, the presence of thrombi, the position of the apical conduit, and postoperative right ventricular function.

In conclusion, the implantation of the Novacor LVAD can safely be achieved using this technical method. We believe that this completely successful Novacor implantation represents a significant break-through in the treatment of patients with severely deteriorated cardiomyopathy in Japan.

Acknowledgments. The authors would like to thank Mr. Kazuhide Ichikawa and Mr. Frank Beering (Baxter Limited), for their technical assistance in the implantation. Also, we would like to thank for Ms. Marimi Mizuno for preparation of this manuscript.

References

1. Oyer PE, Stinson EB, Portner PM, Rean AK, Shumway NE (1980) Development of a totally implantable electrically actuated left ventricular assist system. Am J Surg 140:17–24
2. Portner PM, Oyer PE, Pennington DG (1989) Implantable electrical left ventricular assist system. Bridge to transplantation and the future. Ann Thorac Surg 47:142–150
3. Portner PM, Baumgartner WA, Cabrol C (1993) Internal pulsatile circulatory support. Ann Thorac Surg 55:261–265
4. McCarthy PM, Portner PM, Tobler HG (1991) Clinical experience with the Novacor ventricular assist system. J Thorac Cardiovasc Surg 102:578–587
5. Loisance DY, Deleuze PH, Mazzucotelli P, Besnerais PL, Dubois-Rande JL (1994) Clinical implantation of the wearable Baxter novacor ventricular assist system. Ann Thorac Surg 58:551–554
6. Pennington DG, McBride LR, Swartz MT (1994) Implantation technique for the Novacor left ventricular assist system. J Thorac Cardiovasc Surg 108:604–608
7. Vigano M, Martinelli L, Minzioni G, Rinaldi M, Pagani F (1996) Modified method for Novacor left ventricular assist device implantation. Ann Thorac Surg 61:23–35
8. Kormos RL, Gasior T, Antaki J (1989) Evaluation of right ventricular function during clinical left ventricular assistance. ASAIO Trans 35:547–550

Application of Wearable Novacor Left Ventricular Assist System for Patients with End-Stage Cardiomyopathy: Osaka Experience

Takafumi Masai, Keishi Kadoba, Yuji Miyamoto, Yoshiki Sawa, Hajime Ichikawa, Yasushi Kagizaki, and Hikaru Matsuda

Summary. The wearable Novacor left ventricular assist system (LVAS) has been reported to be an effective supporting device providing advantages in patient quality of life. We recently ecperienced two cases of the implantation. One of them was the first case in Japan. Patient 1 was a 43-year-old male with dilated cardiomyopathy, in severe heart failure even with intra-aortic balloon pump (IABP) support and high doses of catecholamines. His cardiac index and pulmonary capillary wedge pressure before the implantation were $2.01 \cdot min^{-1} \cdot m^{-2}$ and 18mmHg, respectively. Patient 2 was a 55-year-old male with hypertrophied cardiomyopathy of dilated phase. He had been supported with the Toyobo-NCVC extracorporeal LVAS for 93 days; this was then replaced by the Novacor system in order to improve his activity in daily life. In both patients, flow rates ranging from 4 to 6l/min were achieved with stable hemodynamics. Patient 1 developed strokes twice, with residual mild left hemiplegia. His neurological deficit has been compensated on the Novacor assist for 168 days. Patient 2 has been supported for 131 days now and is able to take a walk out of the hospital. Even under the situation in which heart transplantation is not a readily available option, the Novacor LVAS has a significant role in the management of patients with end-stage cardiomyopathy.

Key words: Wearable Novacor left ventricular assist system — Cardiomyopathy — Quality of life

Introduction

There has been considerable progress in the application of left ventricular assist systems (LVASs) to the treatment of profound heart failure including postcardiotomy heart failure, and for use as a bridge to heart transplantation [1–3]. In particular, implantable LVASs have been actively utilized in patients waiting for heart transplantation, with excellent clinical results for long-term assist [4–9]. Recent advances of technology in assist devices have allowed the modification of implantable LVAS to develop a wearable system, so that long-term mechanical support has become compatible with better patient outcome and quality of life

[8,9]. In Japan, where heart transplantation is not yet being performed and the bridge use is not currently feasible, a supporting device reliable for an extended duration with favorable quality of life seems to be necessary to salvage patients with a chronically failing heart. In this report, we describe our initial experience with the implantation of the wearable Novacor LVAS (Baxter, Novacor Division, Oakland, CA, USA (Fig. 1) in two patients with end-stage cardiomyopathy; one of them is the first case in Japan.

Patient 1

The patient was a 43-year-old male who was diagnosed with idiopathic dilated cardiomyopathy in January 1995. One year later, his hemodynamics deteriorated rapidly, requiring the placement of an intra-aortic balloon pump (IABP). Although he could be weaned from the IABP after 18 days' support, chronic inotropic support was necessary to maintain his circulation. He was judged to require the LVAS support and was transferred to our hospital in February 1996.

The cardiothoracic ratio (CTR) was 61% in the admission chest X-ray. Echocardiography demonstrated severe left ventricular (LV) dilatation [diastolic diameter/systolic diameter (Dd/Ds): 69mm/60mm] with depressed wall motion (ejection fraction 25%) (Fig. 2). The pulmonary capillary wedge pressure was 18mmHg and the cardiac index was $2.01 \cdot min^{-1} \cdot m^{-2}$ under maximal inotropic support with both dopamine and dobutamine.

With consent, he underwent the implantation of the wearable Novacor LVAS of February 14, 1996. There were no technical problems during the operation. His body surface area (BSA) was $1.8m^2$ and the pump was easily placed in the preperitoneal space. Although inotropes, prostaglandin E_1, and the inhalation of nitric oxide (NO) were required to support the right ventricle, cardiopulmonary bypass could be weaned without any difficulties with an LVAS flow rate of 6.0l/min and 12mmHg of right atrial pressure. His hemodynamics were markedly improved with the Novacor LVAS, with flow rates ranging from 4.5 to 6.0l/min. He developed convulsion on the first

First Department of Surgery, Osaka University Medical School, 2-2 Yamadaoka, Suita, Osaka 565, Japan

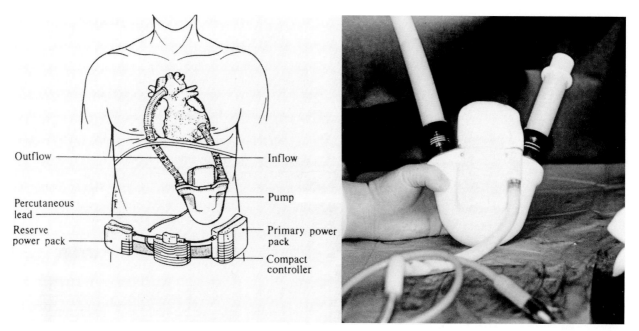

Fig. 1. The wearable Novacor left ventricular assist system (LVAS)

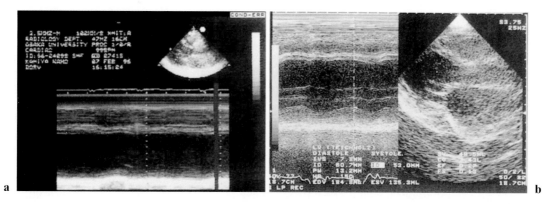

Fig. 2. Echocardiography on admission: **a** Patient 1. Left ventricular diastolic diameter (Dd) 69 mm, systolic diameter (Ds) 60 mm, fractional shortening (FS) 12%, ejection fraction (EF) 25%. **b** Patient 2. Dd 61 mm, Ds 53 mm, FS 13%, EF 27%

postoperative day resulting in mild left hemiplegia which had been compensated on the Novacor assist. However, he suffered a second stroke on the 56th postoperative day. As for anticoagulant management, as soon as the patient was able to take an oral diet on the 30th postoperative day, warfarin was started, combined with low-dose administration of aspirin, to maintain the prothrombin time at an international normalized ratio of 1.6–2.7. The patient has now been in rehabilitation to recover from his neurological complications, on the support for 168 days.

Patient 2

The patient was a 55-year-old male with hypertrophied cardiomyopathy. He had complained of general fatigue since 1991. In July 1995, he developed severe heart failure requiring an IABP. As he could not be weaned from the IABP for 3 months, he transferred to our hospital on IABP in October 1996 to wait for heart transplantation.

On chest X-ray, the CTR was 62%. Echocardiography demonstrated severe LV dilatation (Dd/Ds:

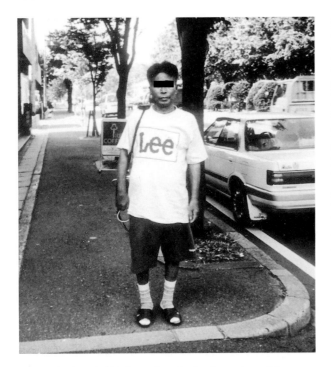

Fig. 3. Patient 2, 113 days after the implantation of the wearable Novacor LVAS, showing the ambulatory condition of the patient carrying the controller, main battery, and reserve battery held in a wide belt with pockets around the waist (concealed by the shirt). The belt-holder is suspended from the shoulder. The main battery can provide power up to 4–5 h and the reserve battery for 1 h. These are connected to the controller and then to the device through a transcutaneous lead

61 mm/53 mm) with depressed wall motion (ejection fraction 27%) (Fig. 2). The pulmonary capillary wedge pressure was 24 mmHg and the cardiac index was $2.3 l \cdot min^{-1} \cdot m^{-2}$ under IABP support.

After the transportation to our hospital, the patient was able to be weaned from the IABP; however, 45 days later, heart failure progressed rapidly, resulting in the deterioration of vital organ functions. Therefore, percutaneous cardiopulmonary support (PCPS) was started as well as the reinsertion of the IABP. Two days after the start of PCPS, a Toyobo extracorporeal LVAS (Toyobo, Osaka, Japan) was implanted for long-term support. The patient regained his spirits with excellent hemodynamic recovery with the support of the Toyobo LVAS. In hepatic function, the total bilirubin level was elevated from 2.4 mg/dl (before LVAS) to 21 mg/dl (on the 9th postoperative day), necessitating plasma exchange, however, the bilirubin level normalized by the 30th postoperative day.

Even with support for three months with the Toyobo LVAS, the patient's cardiac function did not recover. Therefore, 93 days after the implantation of the Toyobo LVAS, it was replaced by a wearable Novacor LVAS in order to improve his activity in daily life and to minimize the possible risk in longer support. His BSA was $1.6 m^2$ and the pump seemed a little large to place in the preperitoneal space. Cardiopulmonary bypass could be weaned without any difficulties with the aid of prostaglandin E_1 and NO inhalation for temporary right ventricular failure. Postoperative hemodynamics were stable with the Novacor assist (flow rates ranging from 4.0 to 5.5 l/min). Seven days after the implantation of the Novacor, he developed mechanical ileus, probably in relation to a previous abdominal operation, for about 2 months. Now, 131 days after implantation, the patient has become fully ambulatory and can take a walk out of the hospital with the support (Fig. 3).

His left ventricle was shown by chest X-ray and echocardiography to be adequately decompressed by LV drainage with the Novacor LVAS. In contrast, satisfactory LV unloading was not obtained by the left atrial drainage with the Toyobo LVAS prior to Novacor implantation (Fig. 4).

Discussion

The ventricular assist system has been a well-accepted therapeutic option to bridge patients to heart transplantation in the United States and European countries [3–9]. The implantable LVAS, in particular, has been reported to be extremely reliable for long-term support and to provide a high degree of mobility and quality of life for patients during the waiting period [4–8]. Recently, the development of the wearable system has allowed an even higher quality of life to these patients [8,9]. Some patients with an LVAS have received approval to leave the hospital, and clinical trial of the permanent use of the wearable implantable LVAS is proposed for patients considered inappropriate candidates for heart transplantation [7–9].

In Japan, heart transplantation is still in the process of negotiation because of the complicated ethical issues concerning brain death. In this complex situation, we have applied the Toyobo extracorporeal pneumatic left ventricular assist system in patients deteriorating in condition during the waiting period for possible heart transplantation [10,11]. In our series, thrombus formation, the durability of the pump, systemic infection, and patient quality of life were serious problems for durations of support longer than 6 months. A reliable long-term supporting device which also provides favorable quality of life is expected to salvage these patients in Japan.

Fig. 4. Chest X-ray and echocardiography before and after the Novacor implantation in patient 2: **a** after 78 days' support with the Toyobo LVAS prior to the Novacor implantation; **b** after 117 days' support with the Novacor LVAS

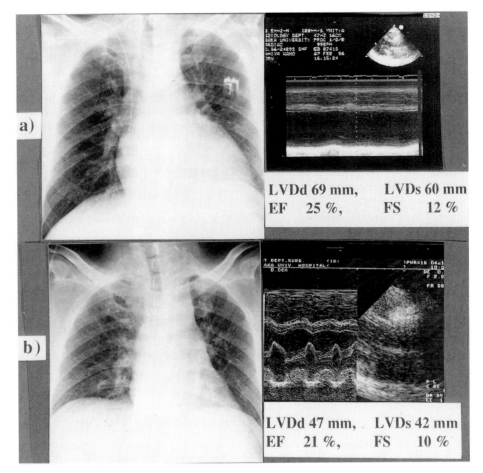

LVDd 69 mm, LVDs 60 mm
EF 25 %, FS 12 %

LVDd 47 mm, LVDs 42 mm
EF 21 %, FS 10 %

The novacor LVAS has been widely utilized for bridging to heart transplantation, with excellent clinical results, including long-term reliabiliy [4,5,7]. Since 1993, the large external console of the Novacor LVAS has been modified to provide a wearable belt containing a compact controller, battery, and back-up battery, so that patients have a higher degree of mobility and quality of life during the waiting period (Fig. 1) [9]. In both patients reported here, the wearable Novacor has been providing satisfactory and consistent hemodynamic support without any mechanical trouble for 168 and 131 days, respectively. Patient 2 has become fully ambulatory and been trained to manage his own power supply, to change batteries, and to recharge batteries for out-of-hospital walks on his own. His mental status also has been considerably improved by the extension of mobility. In this patient, the wearable Novacor seems to have provided psychological as well as physical rehabilitation.

Some authors report that thromboembolic complications remain of concern during support with the Novacor LVAS [5,7,9]. In patient 1, the cause of the second stroke appears to be device-related, in spite of the oral anticoagulation with both warfarin and aspirin and with favorable pump output (4–4.5 l/min). A suspected reason for this thromboembolic event is an association with the gradual increase of prothrombin time to an international normalized ration of 1.6, accompanied by the improvement of the patient's general condition. Precautionary anticoagulation seems to be important, especially when a patient has been recovering metabolically with the support with the Novacor system.

Right ventricular function has been reported as one of the important factors in determining the outcome of LVAS patients [3–9]. If right ventricular function is in question, we prefer to use a device capable of providing biventricular support. From our experience, the need for biventricular support is a negative prognostic indicator [2], but its importance in the experience of others has been difficult to assess. Recently, we have used the inhalation of NO for temporary right ventricular failure at the time of LVAS insertion, to reduce the right ventricular afterload [10,11]. In our two patients supported with the Novacor, the inhalation of NO was effective for obtaining adequate LVAS flow rates.

Another issue related to the Novacor LVAS is that the pump size is too large for Japanese patients with small body size. In patient 2, there were some difficulties in creating a preperitoneal pocket of appropriate size for the placement of the pump. Efforts to further reduce size and weight are expected to facilitate use in smaller patients.

In summary, the wearable Novacor LVAS has been applied in two patients with end-stage cardiomyopathy, for 168 days and 131 days, respectively. In both patients, complete hemodynamic stability was obtained, and in one patient, the wearable Novacor allowed excellent physical and psychosocial rehabilitation. Even where heart transplantation is unavailable, the Novacor LVAS has a significant role in the management of patients with end-stage cardiomyopathy.

References

1. Pae WE, Miller CA, Matthews Y, Pierce WS (1992) Ventricular assist devices for postcardiotomy cardiogenic shock. J Thorac Cardiovasc Surg 104:541–543
2. Miyamoto Y, Nakano S, Kaneko M, Matsuwaka R, Satoh H, Matsuda H (1993) Analysis of complications affecting survival after employment of ventricular assist system (VAS) using pneumatic and centrifugal pumps. In: Akutsu T, Koyanagi H (eds) Heart replacement. Artificial heart 4, Springer, Tokyo, pp 237–243
3. Pennington DB, McBride LR, Peigh PS, Miller LW, Swartz MT (1994) Eight years' experience with bridging to cardiac transplantation. J Thorac Cardiovasc Surg 107:472–481
4. Portner PM, Oyer PH, Pennington DG, Baumgartner WA, Griffith BP, Frist WR, Magilligan DJ, Noon GP, Ramasamy N, Miller PJ, Jassawalla JS (1989) Implantable electrical left ventricular assist system: bridge to transplantation and the future. Ann Thorac Surg 47:142–150
5. McCarthy PM, Portner PM, Tobler HG, Starnes VA, Ramasamy N, Oyer PE (1991) Clinical experience with the Novacor ventricular assist system. J Thorac Cardiovasc Surg 102:578–587
6. Frazier OH, Rose EA, Macmanus Q, Burton NA, Lefrak EA, Poirier VL, Dasse KA (1992) Multicenter clinical evaluation of the Heartmate 1000IP left ventricular assist device. Ann Thorac Surg 53:1080–1090
7. Kormos RL, Murali S, Amanda Dew M, Armitage JM, Hardesty RL, Borovetz HS, Griffith BP (1994) Chronic mechanical circulatory support: rehabilitation, low morbidity, and superior survival. Ann Thorac Surg 57:51–58
8. McCarthy PM (1995) HeartMate implantable left ventricular assist device: bridge to transplantation and future applications. Ann Thorac Surg 59:S46–S51
9. Vetter HO, Kaulbach HG, Schmitz C, Forst A, Uberfuhr P, Kreuzer E, Pfeiffer M, Brenner P, Dewald O, Richart B (1995) Experience with the Nocavor left ventricular assist system as a bridge to cardiac transplantation, including the new wearable system. J Thorac Cardiovasc Surg 109:74–80
10. Matsuda H, Masai T, Kadoba K, Myamoto Y, Kaneko M, Matsuwaka R, Shimazaki Y (1995) Clinical experience in assisted circulation using left ventricular assist system for patients with chronic heart failure. In: Sezai Y, Shiono M, Barron JP (Eds) Progress in the artificial heart, Axel Springer Japan, Tokyo, pp 25–30
11. Masai T, Shimazaki Y, Kadoba K, Miyamoto Y, Sawa Y, Yagura A, Matsuda H, Satoh M, Kashiwabara S (1995) Clinical experience with long-term use of Toyobo left ventricular assist system. ASAIO Trans 41:M522–M525

Discussion

Dr. Frazier:
We have a few minutes for questions. Are there any questions from the floor?

Dr. Nakatani:
I just want to confirm: Was LVAS connected from the left atrium to the ascending aorta in this same patient?

Dr. Ichikawa:
Yes.

Dr. Jarvik:
I would just like to ask Dr. Moreno-Cabral what the mechanism of reduction of pulmonary hypertension is in your opinion after long-term support.

Dr. Moreno-Cabral:
I think it was left ventricular unloading. Early on, when we put the device, the patient also had an occult pulmonary infection that was also a contributing factor of pulmonary hypertension at that time. But I think it was basically just lowering of left atrial pressure with the assist device and the improvement of congestive failure and related inflammatory response that over time decreased the pulmonary hypertension.

Dr. Mussivand:
The question I have is related to the VAD-related infection cases. Did you do analysis to see if the infections were related to the type of device, and, if yes, did you also check your rate of infection compared to other centers that use such devices?

Dr. Furukawa:
The devices that we used were the Thoratec and the TCI Heartmate. Yes, the infection rate was extremely high during the period that I discussed. The problems were mostly related to urosepsis or catheter. These patients all had indwelling silicon-coated catheters for dopamine, dobutamine, inotropic support, and we left them in. And one of the patients developed cholecystitis post-VAD insertion, and that related to the bacteremia. Since that time, we've instituted a

more aggressive therapy in terms of removal of all foreign materials besides the ventricular assist device, and we have implanted over thirteen of them without any bacteremias. We have had, still, some difficulty in keeping the outlet site of the drive line clean, but they are usually local infections and have not had systemic problems from that.

Dr. Meyns:
Dr. Moreno, do you suggest that we have to put patients with PGE-resistant pulmonary hypoertension on a long-term LVAD?

Dr. Moreno:
This is a difficult problem. In our case, the difference compared to many other patients with pulmonary hypertension is that it was of recent onset. When the patient first came to us, his pulmonary pressures were moderately elevated. We saw this developing over time, so it is not the same as a patient with a congenital anomaly with chronic pulmonary hypertension or a patient with chronic pulmonary embolism. So, one has to be quite selective on choosing which patient may benefit from left ventricular assist under these circumstances.

Mr. Westaby:
Do any members of the panel or the chairman know of any case where *Candida* has been successfully cleared from an LVAD?

Dr. Frazier:
Not without removing the LVAD.

Mr. Westaby:
So, nobody has kept an LVAD with *Candida*, Bob, as far as you know?

Dr. Minami:
May I answer that: Dr. Loisance in France has one case. He removed a valve without using extracorporeal circulation. He changed a valve of Novacor. That is, I think, the first one in the last year, and we had also such a problem but there was no infection there. This was only thromboembolism on the valve.

Dr. Moreno:
In our experience we had two patients that had *Candida*. One had a fungus ball in the inflow valve, and that patient was transplanted and survived for three months. She eventually died of a combination of rejection and infection. The second patient died prior to transplant. We could never clear the device of *Candida*, and two months later he died. We found *Candida* inside the chambers of the device.

Dr. Harasaki:
I would like to ask this question to Dr. Masai and Dr. Hachida: Would you please comment on the size of the Novacor device to the Japanese population. Do you feel that it is a little bit too big or there is no problem in fitting it to the Japanese population?

Dr. Hachida:
In my opinion, there is no problem for the Japanese patient if the body surface area is more than 1.5 or 1.6.

Dr. Masai:
The second patient we experienced was $1.6\,m^2$ in body surface area. I think it is a little small for this large pump.

Dr. Frazier:
Do you have any comments about it?

Dr. Portner:
Yes, I want to make a couple of comments. The smallest recipient of a Novacor system has actually been about 44 kg — one of Prof. Loisance's patients — and the pump extended from one lateral wall to the other, but the patient tolerated it very well and was successfully transplanted after about 6 months. Also, the patient in whom Prof. Loisance replaced the valves actually had an *Aspergillus* fungal infection. There have been a number of Novacor patients who have had fungal infections, primarily *Candida*, who have gone on to successful transplantation. But, as you said, removal of the device was ultimately necessary.

Dr. Frazier:
Well, there is a size limitation to these two implantable devices although you can shoehorn them in. The TCI pump has been placed in an 8-year-old by the Germans, but it's not desirable and I think we need better devices for the smaller patient. Certainly, I think that that patient in UCLA who had the 10-cm ventricle would have been a good case for removal of the device followed by muscle resection. Such patients are going to benefit from that technology. It's a great pleasure to see so much advance in this technology being made in Japan. I think it's going to be a great contricution for all of us.

Ventricular Circulatory Support with the Abiomed System as a Bridge to Heart Transplantation

Eduardo Castells, José María Calbet, Emilio Saura, M. Carmen Octavio de Toledo, Carles Fontanillas, Miguel Benito, Jorge Granados, Nicolás Manito, Alberto Miralles, Jaime Roca, and Catalina Rullan

Summary. The Abiomed system was initially designed as a mechanical support for postcardiotomy failure, but it has been also used as a bridge to heart transplantation. We review our experience with this system since November 1992 in 10 patients. The mean age was 46 years. Nine were men. The underlying cardiac disease was ischemic cardiomyopathy in 8, dilated cardiomyopathy in 1, and acute myocarditis in 1. The cardiogenic shock was due to an acute myocardial infarction in 7 (one after coronary bypass and another with a left ventricular rupture), end-stage cardiac insufficiency in 2 (already on the heart transplantation waiting list), and early graft failure in 1. The implantation of the system was performed without extracorporeal circulation. The type of support was biventricular in 4 and left ventricular in 6. The hemodynamic improvement was important in terms of the vital constants and cardiac output. The mean flow of the right pump was 4.6 l/min and that of the left pump, 4.4 l/min. Three (30%) died under mechanical support for a mean of 7 days, six (60%) were successfully transplanted after a mean of 3.5 days, and one (10%) was able to be weaned 7 days later. Only one (10%) died, after 2 months because of sepsis. All survivors (60%) are asymptomatic. Bleeding (50%) and thromboembolism (40%) were the most frequent complications. The Abiomed system proved to be useful in the recovery from cardiogenic shock, especially after acute myocardial infarction. It can be managed simply and the cost is limited. Of our supported patients, 60% are long-term survivors. This system can also be used as a bridge of short duration to heart transplantation.

Key words: Abiomed — Bridge to transplant — Cardiogenic shock — Acute myocardial infarction — Ventricular circulatory assistance

Introduction

The mortality from cardiogenic shock due to an acute myocardial infarction (AMI), a terminal low cardiac output in cardiomyopathy, or after a primary failure following heart transplantation, is very high. In some cases, the only chance of survival is ventricular circulatory assistance as a bridge to heart transplantation.

Although the Abiomed system was initially designed as a mechanical support for patients with postcardiotomy failure [1,2], it can also be used as a bridge of short duration to heart transplantation [3].

Material and Methods

We review our experience, since November 1992, with the Abiomed BVS-5000 (Abiomed, Danvers, MA, USA) system as a bridge to heart transplantation. It has been used in ten patients, nine men and one woman, with a mean age of 46 years, ranging from 15 to 58 years and with a mean body surface area of $1.84\,m^2$, ranging from 1.58 to $2.30\,m^2$.

The underlying cardiac disease was ischemic cardiomyopathy in eight patients (80%), dilated cardiomyopathy in one and acute giant cell myocarditis in one. The etiology of the cardiogenic shock was: (a) acute myocardial infarction (AMI) in seven patients, one of them after a triple coronary artery bypass and another in a patient in study for heart transplantation. One patient presented with a left ventricle free-wall rupture and cardiac tamponade. The ventricular tear was covered with a patch. The patient improved but one day later cardiogenic shock appeared. (b) Postcardiotomy in three patients, after primary failure of a transplant and the already mentioned triple coronary artery bypass and patch covering the ventricular rupture. (c) End-stage cardiac insufficiency in two patients, due to a dilated cardiomyopathy and myocarditis, both while on the waiting list for heart transplantation; and (d) Primary graft failure in one patient. Four patients had two causes.

All patients were in cardiogenic shock. The mean time from this diagnosis to the implant of the ventricular assist device (VAD) was 2.4 days. In the seven cases with an AMI, the mean time from its onset to implantation was 3.1 days. Nine (90%) patients had an intra-aortic balloon pump (IABP) implanted for a mean of 26 h of presupport. The only patient without an IABP was the one with primary graft failure, with a predominant right ventricular failure. Eight (80%) patients were on mechanical ventilation for an average of 42 h before the implantation of the device. Four (40%) patients experienced presupport cardiac arrest,

Ciudad Sanitaria y Universitaria de Bellvitge, Universidad de Barcelona Hospitalet, Barcelona, Spain

217

and all of the patients were undergoing inotropic support with a mean of three drugs.

The presupport hematology and blood chemistry showed an increase of leukocytes (17000/ml; ranging from 11900 to 23000) and creatinine (mean 155 mM; range 83–330 mM).

Surgical Technique

In all cases the implantation of the system was performed without extracorporeal circulation. Anesthesia was done very carefully [4]. Usually, we increased the inotropic therapy, adding or increasing the epinephrine. We used a median sternotomy. Initially, we used to heparinize the patients with about 1 mg/kg to achieve an activated clotting time (ACT) of 180–200 s [5,6]. Now, we prefer a full dose of heparin (3 mg/kg). We started cannulation by anastomosis of the arterial cannula. Air was removed from the cannula in

a retrograde fashion (from the tip in the artery), them the cannula was externalized and connected to the system. The atrial cannulation was done last. Now, we prefer the new smaller cannula (36 F), instead of the old one (46 F). Air removal was also performed in a retrograde fashion. The support was initiated using the foot pump. Fibrin glue was placed around the sutures. Then, we reduced the level of anticoagulation to give an ACT of 180–200 s, with protamine if necessary [5,6] (Figs. 1, 2). In four cases (40%) we used a biventricular support and in six patients (60%) only a left ventricular support.

Results

Hemodynamics improved significantly once on support (Table 1). The systemic and mean arterial pressure, the cardiac index, and the urinary output

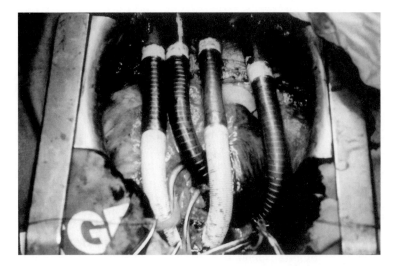

Fig. 1. Implantation of a biventricular support system. Grafts are sutured to the aorta and pulmonary artery. Atrial cannulas are implanted in the left and right atrium through double purse string sutures

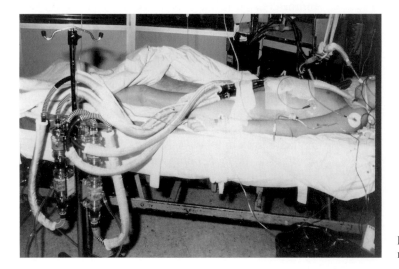

Fig. 2. The system with the blood pumps connected to the patient

Table 1. Hemodynamic improvement after support with the Abiomed system

	Presupport		Postsupport	
	Mean	Range	Mean	Range
Systolic pressure (mmHg)	66	44–81	95	75–130
Mean arterial pressure (mmHg)	51	40–69	81	75–110
Central venous pressure (mmHg)	16	9–25	13	8–35
Pulmonary arterial pressure (mmHg)	38	31–48	30	23–40
Pulmonary capillary wedge pressure (mmHg)	24	17–28	17	12–23
Cardiac index (l. $min^{-1} \cdot m^{-2}$)	1.6	1.2–2.2	2.6	2.2–2.8
Urine Output (cm^3/h)	13	0–30	60	30–1

increased until they reached normal levels. The central venous pressure, the pulmonary artery pressure, and the pulmonary wedge pressure decreased.

The management of the system once on support is quite simple. The drive console is automatic and the operator needs only to adjust the level of the blood pumps and maintain a good fluid volume to manage blood flow. Anticoagulation with heparin is maintained to give an ACT of 180–200 s. Adequate blood volume and adequate vascular resistances are necessary to obtain good hemodynamic management. In cases without right ventricular support, the inotropic therapy needs to be decreased slowly, in order to maintain acceptable right ventricular function. The pulmonary artery pressure has to be low and some specific drugs can be necessary.

In the four patients with a right ventricular pump, mean flow was 4.6 l/min, ranging from 4.2 to 5.2 l/min. Left side flows averaged 4.4 l/min in the ten patients, ranging from 3.6 to 4.8 l/min. A low pump flow (3 l/min) was observed due to compression of the venous return in two patients, to bleeding in two cases, and to tension pneumothorax in one.

The bleeding was important in relation to the quantity drained (>1.5 l) in five patients (50%). Three of them underwent reoperation. In one of these, a left atrial cannula was also displaced in order to avoid a compression of the venous return. This patient sustained an air embolism. The tension pneumothorax was drained. Only one patient could be extubated during the circulatory assistance.

The support was maintained for a mean of 4.8 days, ranging from 20 h to 12 days. All patients were on the Spanish waiting list for heart transplantation as an emergency zero (i.e., in urgent need of transplant) for at least several hours. Three patients died on support (30%), for a mean of 7 days (4–12). One, implanted for primary failure of the transplant, was the patient with an air embolism and he died on the 12th day due to coma, pneumonia, acute renal failure, sepsis, and multiorgan failure. One patient with AMI suffered a stroke and died of circulatory collapse, acute renal failure, and multiorgan failure. Another patient with

AMI was bleeding excessively and the heparin was stopped for several hours, during which time he suffered a stroke and a massive cerebral infarction. The support was stopped on the 4th day. In the first case the circulatory assistance was biventricular (25% mortality) and in the other two only left ventricular (33% mortality).

Six patients (60%) could be transplanted after a mean of 3.5 days (1–10 days) on support. We used the classical surgical technique of Lower and Shumway [7] and the myocardial protection was done with hematic cardioplegia [5,6,8].

Another patient (10%) was retired from the waiting list on the 5th day, when he started to pump spontaneously, and he was able to be weaned on the 7th day. This was the patient with an AMI and the left ventricle free-wall rupture. We observed four respiratory insufficiencies, two strokes, and one mediastinitis during the postoperative period. One patient transplanted after an AMI died during the second month due to pneumonia and sepsis.

Six patients (60%) are long-term survivors, for a mean of 29 months (2–43 months). Of these, four of seven (57%) are patients alive after an AMI, and two of two (100%) were patients in the waiting list for heart transplantation due to myocardiopathy or myocarditis. All these patients are asymptomatic, except the patient with the shortest postoperative period.

Discussion

In our experience, the Abiomed BVS-5000 system, designed primarily as a ventricular support for postcardiotomy patients, can be applied without extracorporeal circulation and produces a good hemodynamic recovery. Its management is quite simple and the cost of the device and the blood pumps is relatively low.

Used as a bridge to heart transplantation, 70% of our patients were alive the first month after support and 60% are long-term survivors, a mean of 29 months later. One of these patients recovered with the VAD, without needing a heart transplantation. Very few patients have been reported to recover without transplantation [9,10]. Nevertheless, this possibility has to be considered before putting the patient on the waiting list for transplant.

Bleeding (50%) and thromboembolism (40%) were the most frequent complications in our cases. Perhaps, the ratio of thromboembolism is higher than in other series with the same system [11]. With other left ventricular assist devices (LVAD), 47% of patients suffered from clinically evident systemic embolism [12]. In these cases, thrombus formation occurred within the LVAD and not in the native heart. The equilibrium is sometimes difficult to establish. We expect that some improvements will ameliorate the results. Now, we give a full dose of heparin (3 mg/kg) at the moment of the implantation without extracorporeal circulation, and we use a smaller atrial cannula of 36 F instead of the old one of 46 F. In this system, one of the most important foci of thrombosis seems to be the left atrial cannula. In one of our cases, a thrombus was found around this cannula at the moment of the transplant. The smaller size of the cannula can also reduce the compression of the venous return.

Patients after an AMI, the majority of our cases, seem to have an increased thrombogenicity. A high incidence of thromboembolism has been reported in patients with a VAD [13], as high as 86%. The protocol of anticoagulation can be very important, especially in such patients [14].

We believe that the treatment of choice in not very old patients with irreversible cardiogenic shock after more than 24 h of an AMI without mechanical complications is ventricular circulatory assistance as a bridge to heart transplantation, unless the patient has contraindications. Some authors [13] with a different system concluded that a recent AMI, within 6 weeks prior to LVAD implantation, is a powerful predictor of failure during bridging (83%), although this is contrary to our experience and that of others [2,9] with the Abiomed system.

The indication is still more accepted in cases of irreversible cardiogenic shock due to the end-stage of a myocardiopathy while on the waiting list. The results in cases of primary failure of a heart transplant seem worse [9].

Our results are slightly better than those reported in the worldwide registry of this system [2,9]. Over 40% of the cardiomyopathy patients we able to go home and slightly less than 40% of the AMI group are discharge survivors. These results are better than in cases after cardiotomy [15].

The most important disadvantage of this system is its inability to maintain long-term support. The longest successful bridge to transplant reported is 37 days [9].

At present, this is not an important problem in Spain, because we have the highest level of organ donation in the world and patients in emergency zero can be transplanted within a few days [16]. In conclusion, the Abiomed BVS 5000 system can also be used as a bridge of short duration to heart transplantation, with good results.

References

1. Lederman DM (1988) Technical considerations in the development of clinical system for temporary and permanent cardiac support. In: Akutsu T (ed) Artificial heart 2. Springer, Tokyo, pp 115–127
2. Shook BJ (1993) The Abiomed BVS 5000 biventricular support system. In: Ott RA, Gutfinger DE, Gazzaniga AB (eds) Cardiac surgery. State of the art reviews, vol 7(2). Hanley and Belfus, Philadelphia, pp 309–316
3. Champsaur G, Ninet J, Vigneron, Cochet P, Boissonnat P (1990) Use of the Abiomed BVS System 5000 as a bridge to cardiac transplantation J Thorac Cardiovasc Surg 100:122–128
4. Octavio de Toledo MC (1995) Asistencia circulatoria. In: Cochs J (ed) I jornadas de investigación en anestesiología y reanimación. ICS, Barcelona, pp 29–37
5. Castells E (1994) Bridge to transplant with the BVS 5000. The initial Spanish experience. In: Proceedings of the third worldwide symposium on ventricular support with the BVS 5000. Abiomed, Danvers, MA, USA, pp 31–35
6. Castells E, Calbet JM, Granados J, Manito N, Míralles A, Octavio de Toledo MC, Roca J, Rullan C, Saura E, Benito E, Casanova T, Worner F, Gausí C (1995) Ventricular circulatory assistance with the Abiomed system as a bridge to heart transplantation. Transplant Proc 27:2343–2345
7. Lower RR, Shumway NE (1960) Studies on orthotopic transplantation of the canine heart. Surg Forum 11:18
8. Maníto N, Castells E, Roca J, Míralles A, Octavio de Toledo MC, Casanovas T, Saura E, Calbet JM, Sabate X, Serrano MT, Gausi C (1995) Heart transplantation program at "Prínceps d'España" Hospital, Central University of Barcelona: the first three-year experience. Transplant Proc 27:2349–2350
9. Shook BJ (1994) Review of the Abiomed BVS 5000 worldwide registry. In: The proceedings of the third worldwide symposium on ventricular support with the BVS 5000. Abiomed, Danvers, MA, USA, pp 1–4
10. Piccione W, Djuric M, Da Valle MJ, March RJ (1994) Successful postmyocardial infarction support with the Abiomed BVS 5000. In: Circulatory support 94. Society of Thoracic Surgeons, Pittsburgh, pp 31–32
11. McBride LR (1994) Bridging to cardiac transplantation with external ventricular assist devices. In: Loop FD (ed) Seminars in thoracic and cardiovascular surgery 6. Saunders, Philadelphia, pp 169–173
12. Schmid C, Nabavi DG, Georgiadis D, Hammel D, Deng M, Weyaud M, Scheld HH (1996) Systemic embolization during Novacor LVAD support. J Heart Lung Transplant 15:S87
13. Boehmer JP, Pae WE, Aufiero TX, Davis D, Pierce WS (1995) Acute myocardial infarction within 6 weeks be-

fore LVAD implantation predicts an unsuccessful bridge to heart transplantation. Circulation 92:I–49

14. Copeland JG, Szefner J (1995) Anticoagulants and artificial heart. In: Lewis T, Graham TR (eds): Mechanical circulatory support. Arnold, London, pp 306–311

15. Guyton RA, Schonberger JPAM, Everts PAM, Kimble G, Gray LA, Gieldchinsky I, Raess DH, Vlahakes GJ, Woolley SR, Gangahar DM, Soltanzadeh H, Piccione WJ, Vaughn CC, Boonstra PW, Buckley MJ (1993) Postcardiotomy shock: clinical evaluation of the BVS 5000 biventricular support system. Ann Thorac Surg 56:346–356

16. Organización Nacional de Trasplantes (1996) Memoria ONT 1995. Rev Esp Trasp 5:9–16

Discussion

Dr. Minami:
Congratulations for the good results in your series. If I understand correctly, you lost one patient on the 12th postop day with air embolism. What happened? Can you explain that?

Dr. Castells:
We had compression of the right atrium and then when we were removing the left atrial cannula some aspiration was performed and air passed through the system to the patient.

Dr. Minami:
Oh, yes. Thank you.

Dr. Kormos:
Were you able to mobilize these patients out of bed or did they pretty much, all of them, stay in their bed during the support period?

Dr. Castells:
No, the period was very short and except in one occasion the patients were also on mechanical ventilation.

Dr. Minami:
One of the disadvantages of this system is heat loss because of the long tube between the ventricle and the patient. How can you manage that? We have experienced in former times the patient's temperature decreases down to 30 degrees, and sometimes we have to be afraid of having fibrillation, therefore, how do you manage the heat loss?

Dr. Castells:
We only put some material around the tubes, covering them. We really didn't have problems with the temperature of the patients.

Bridging to Cardiac Transplantation with the Thoratec Ventricular Assist Device in Australia

Hiroshi Niinami[1], Julian A. Smith[2], Marc Rabinov[2], Peter J. Bergin[2], Meroula Richardson[2], Robert F. Salamonsen[2], Franklin L. Rosenfeldt[2], and Donald S. Esmore[2]

Summary. Mechanical support devices are being used with increasing frequency in patients with cardiac failure refractory to medical therapy and intra-aortic balloon pump counterpulsation. Since July 1990, the Thoratec left ventricular assist device (LVAD) has been implanted as a bridge to cardiac transplantation in 21 patients (16 men, mean age 43 years) with cardiogenic shock. The underlying cardiac diseases were dilated cardiomyopathy ($n = 11$), ischemic heart disease ($n = 5$), allograft rejection ($n = 2$), restrictive cardiomyopathy ($n = 1$), toxic cardiomyopathy ($n = 1$), and hypertrophic cardiomyopathy ($n = 1$). The mean cardiac index at the time of LVAD insertion was $1.61 \cdot \min^{-1} \cdot m^{-2}$; this improved to $2.91 \cdot \min^{-1} \cdot m^{-2}$ within several hours. Aggressive management of the right side of the circulation with inotropes, pulmonary vasodilators, and inhaled nitric oxide resulted in a need for additional right ventricular assistance (RVAD) in only 2 patients (10%). The mean duration of LVAD support was 45 days, with four patients being supported and fully mobilized within the hospital for more than 90 days. Major device-related morbidity included acute renal failure ($n = 7$), infection ($n = 7$), reoperation for bleeding ($n = 6$), and cerebral ischaemia ($n = 4$). Eight patients died prior to transplantation and 13 have been transplanted, 10 of whom are currently alive, all in New York Heart Association (NYHA) functional class I. Actuarial survival for the patients having a first time cardiac transplantation ($n = 12$; 83% at 1 year and 83% at 5 years) compares favourably with nonbridged transplant patients. The Thoratec, in LVAD configuration alone, is able to support terminally ill patients until a suitable donor organ becomes available. Chronic support for extended periods (>90 days) may serve as a prelude to the permanent implantation of LVADs.

Key words: Heart transplantation — Left ventricular assist device — Biventricular support — Bridge to transplant — Mechanical heart support — Thoratec VAD system

Introduction

The use of prosthetic hearts to assist the circulation in cardiac transplant candidates who are in imminent risk of dying before a donor organ becomes available has increased greatly over the last decade [1]. Bridging to transplantation is a two-step process requiring implantation of the assist device and subsequent orthotopic cardiac transplantation. The Thoratec ventricular assist device (VAD) was first used successfully as a bridge to transplantation in September 1984 in left ventricular assist mode (univentricular support) in the United States [2]. Also, this system was used in the first successful bridge to transplantation as a biventricular assist device in March 1985, also in the United States [3]. Since then, several articles have confirmed the efficacy of the Thoratec VAD system as a bridge to transplantation [3–5].

Since July 1990 the Thoratec VAD system has been used in 21 patients for bridge to transplantation in Australia. The purpose of this article is to summarize this experience.

Patients and Methods

Ventricular Assist Device

The Thoratec VAD system (Thoratec Laboratories, Berkeley, CA, USA) consists of prosthetic ventricles with a 65-ml stroke volume, appropriate cannulas for atrial or ventricular inflow and arterial outflow connections, and a pneumatic console [3,6,7]. The pneumatic drive console provides alternating positive and negative air pressure to empty and fill the blood pump, and has three control modes depending on the needs of the patients: asynchronous (fixed rate), volume (full-to-empty variable rate), and synchronous. The full-to-empty mode was used in most bridge cases, because it automatically adjusts beat rate and thus flow output in accordance with venous return and the needs of the body. VAD implants were performed with the aid of full cardiopulmonary bypass with moderate hypothermia (32°–34°C). Cardioplegic arrest was not used. Single venous-ascending aortic cannulation was used in all patients. For support of the left side of the heart, left ventricular apical cannulation was preferred as inflow cannulation. However, several early patients ($n = 5$) had left atrial cannulation. Ventricular device outflow is through a

[1] Department of Cardiovascular Surgery, The Heart Institute of Japan, Tokyo Women's Medical College, 8-1 Kawadacho, Shinjuku-ku, Tokyo 162, Japan
[2] Heart and Lung Transplant Service, The Alfred Healthcare Group, Commercial Road, Prahan Melbourne, Victoria, 3181, Australia

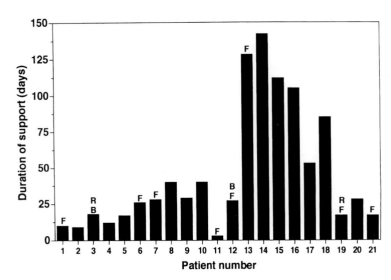

Fig. 1. Duration of support in 21 individual patients. The *vertical axis* shows duration of support and *horizontal axis* indicates patient number. Note that the trend is towards increased duration of support. *R*, bridge to retransplantation; *B*, biventricular assist; *F*, failed bridge to transplantation; all others were transplanted

polyurethane cannula attached to a preclotted 14-mm polyester graft anastomosed to the ascending aorta. For support of the right side, cannulation is from the right atrium with return blood flow to the pulmonary artery ($n = 2$). These heterotopic prosthetic ventricles are placed in a paracorporeal position on the anterior abdominal wall and are connected to the heart and great vessels with cannulas crossing the body wall.

Patient Population

Between July 1990 and January 1996 the Thoratec VAD for left-sided support only or for biventricular support was implanted in 21 patients as a bridge to cardiac transplantation. Cardiomyopathy in 14 patients (dilated in 11, restrictive in 1, toxic in 1, and hypertrophic in 1), end-stage ischemic heart disease in 5 patients, and chronic allograft rejection after heart transplantation in 2 patients were the underlying diseases when the patients were evaluated as heart transplantation candidates. There were 16 male and 5 female patients with an average age of 43 years (range 15–58 years), an average body surface area of $1.9\,\text{m}^2$ (range 1.5–$2.1\,\text{m}^2$) and an average weight of 72 kg (range 50–90 kg).

Preoperative Status

Before the implantation procedure, all patients were receiving maximal inotropic support, 14 (67%) received cardiac assistance with the intra-aortic balloon pump, 10 (48%) had pulmonary oedema, 6 (29%) were receiving mechanical ventilation, 4 (19%) had one or more cardiac arrests, 11 (52%) had renal dysfunction, and 7 (33%) had hepatic dysfunction. Despite maximal therapy, the average cardiac index was $1.6 \pm 0.41 \cdot \text{min}^{-1} \cdot \text{m}^{-2}$ with a pulmonary capillary wedge pressure of $24 \pm 8\,\text{mmHg}$. The decision to implant VADs was made when the clinical and haemodynamic status indicated that the patients would probably die before a donor heart could be located.

Statistical Analyses

Data were obtained from patient charts. The corrected chi-squared and Fisher's exact tests were used to analyze nonparametric data, and the two-sample t-test was used for parametric data. Survival results were obtained by the Kaplan-Meier product limit method and were compared with Gehan's test. Results are presented as the mean ± standard deviation. A P value of 0.05 was considered significant.

Results

Blood flow from the VAD maintained the circulation for up to 142 days until a donor heart could be located and heart transplantation performed. The haemodynamic situation was significantly improved after implantation of the VADs. The mean cardiac index, $1.6 \pm 0.41 \cdot \text{min}^{-1} \cdot \text{m}^{-2}$ before VAD implantation, rose to $2.9 \pm 0.41 \cdot \text{min}^{-1} \cdot \text{m}^{-2}$ 24h after the commencement of mechanical circulatory support ($P < 0.05$). The average pulmonary capillary wedge pressure was $24 \pm 8\,\text{mmHg}$ before operation and decreased to $12 \pm 3\,\text{mmHg}$ after operation ($P < 0.05$).

In terms of the patient mobilization on the device,

Table 1. Complications during support

Complication	Number of patients
Device malfunction or failure	Nil
Infection (systemic, respiratory, LVAD skin site)	7
Renal failure (dialysis-dependent)	7
Postimplantation haemorrhage (early and late)	6
Cerebrovascular accident: transient permanent	4 2
Hepatic failure	3
Coagulopathy	2

LVAD, left ventricular assist device.

Table 2. Causes of death during support

Mortality on the device ($n = 8$)	Number of patients
Multiorgan failure	5
Sepsis	2
Cerebrovascular accident	1

we believe they should be mobilized as soon as possible following insertion of the device. In 14 out of 21 patients, this was achieved within 10 days after operation. Intensive physiotherapy was instituted. Patients were encouraged to sit out of the bed and ambulate within the intensive care unit and hospital. Ambulation was to some extent limited by patient attachment to the large console.

Duration of Ventricular Assist Device Support

The mean duration of all bridge cases was 45 days, and the range was from 3 days to 142 days. The Thoratec VADs were used over a period of 935 patient-days. Four patients were supported for more than 90 days. The utilization of this device has been increasing since 1990, being in use 45% of the time on average and increasing to 90% of the time in 1995. There was overlap in the use of the devices in two patients for the period of 44 days. Throughout the duration of this study, patients with mechanical support devices were given the highest priority for access to donor hearts. In the early years of this study, patients were listed for cardiac transplantation shortly after implantation of the assist device. However, patients who had implantation of the device within a few weeks were not fully recovered yet. On the other hand, patients who received transplants after longer waits were fully ambulatory and exercised regularly on a stationary bicycle. In general, these patients ate well, lost oedema, and gained muscle mass by the time the transplant operation was performed. This explains the recent trend towards increased duration of support (Fig. 1).

Management of the Right Heart

Our philosophy of implantation technique was to aim for isolated left ventricular assist device (LVAD) support if it was physiologically possible. In this series, only two patients (10%) required additional right ven-

tricular assist device (RVAD) support following LVAD insertion. To minimize the additional usage of RVAD, most patients required adrenaline infusion (up to $50\,\mu g \cdot min^{-1} \cdot kg^{-1}$) for periods of 3–28 days. Several other drugs were used including isoprenaline, sodium nitroprusside, and milrinone to reduce pulmonary vascular resistance. Atrial or atrioventricular pacing was also required to augment right heart output in nine patients. Nitric oxide was used in ten patients perioperatively to minimize pulmonary vascular resistance.

Complications

In Table 1, the complications encountered during the interval of mechanical support are enumerated. The most common complication observed during the bridge period was bleeding attributed to either coagulopathy or surgical causes in nine patients. Reoperations were necessary to control this complication in six patients. The recent use of procoagulants such as aprotinin and tranexamic acid at the time of device insertion has diminished bleeding and the need for reoperation. The next major complication was infection, which occurred in seven patients and was a cause of death in two. Renal failure necessitating dialysis occurred also in seven patients. Renal function failed to improve in four patients, and four of them died. Cerebrovascular accidents occurred in six patients: four were transient, and two were permanent. One patient with severe neurological impairment died. Eight patients died prior to the transplantation. Causes of mortality on the device are listed in Table 2.

After transplantation, there was one hospital death due to graft failure and two late deaths (at 74 days and 704 days). The patient who died 704 days after transplantation was a retransplant patient. The causes of the late deaths were recurrent giant cell myocarditis and chronic rejection.

Actuarial Survival

The actuarial survival for those who underwent transplants is shown in Fig. 2, along with the survival for conventional heart transplantation according to the Registry of the International Society for Heart and Lung Transplantation [8]. Of the 13 transplanted pa-

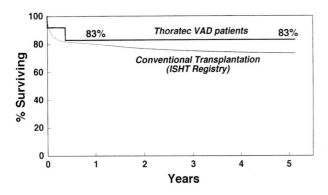

Fig. 2. The actuarial posttransplantation survival of Thoratec ventricular assist device (VAD) patients having a first time cardiac transplantation (n = 12) (83% at 1 year and 83% at 5 years; *thick line*) is comparable with that of conventional heart transplantation (*thin line*). *ISHT*, International Society for Heart and Lung Transplantation

tients, 10 remain alive, all in New York Heart Association (NYHA) functional class I, with actuarial survival of 90% at 1 year and 65% at 5 years. Excluding 1 retransplant patient, actuarial survival for the patients having a first time cardiac transplantation was 83% at 1 year and 83% at 5 years (n = 12).

Discussion

From the preceding results, it is obvious that bridging to cardiac transplantation with circulatory assist devices has been successful, with survival much better than that obtained in patients receiving the same devices for myocardial recovery [9]. These studies further demonstrate that the use of pulsatile VADs such as the Thoratec, Novacor LVAS (Baxter Healthcare, Novacor Division, Oakland, CA, USA), and Thermo Cardiosystems VADs (Thermo Cardiosystems, Woburn, MA, USA) before transplantation can provide early survival durations equal to or better than those of patients undergoing transplantation without the need for mechanical support [10]. Because of the intense competition for donor hearts, it has become necessary to support patients for several weeks to months before locating a suitable donor. The hospital survival of 92% in our series is primarily attributable to our insistence on performing transplantation only in patients whose general medical and nutritional condition was improved, and in most cases who were ambulatory with improved exercise tolerance compared with their preimplantation state.

Patient selection is one of the major problems remaining in bridging to transplantation and in the field of circulatory support devices in general. The identification of a recipient with irreversible myocardial failure but no irreversible end-organ failure is of utmost importance, and early VAD implantation is absolutely essential to sustain or to improve secondary organ function.

The frequency of the additional usage of an RVAD following insertion of an LVAD was only two patients (10%) in our series, which is considerably less than that in other centres reporting experience with Thoratec VADs for bridging to cardiac transplantation [3–5,7,10]. The reason for our low additional RVAD use was because we aimed to manage the right side of the circulation pharmacologically in the first instance rather than opt for immediate RVAD insertion. We have inserted a left VAD then used inotropic support, pulmonary vasodilators, and nitric oxide for the right ventricle and pulmonary vasculature.

Unlike the Novacor or Thermo Cardiosystems devices, the Thoratec VAD can provide either left or right ventricular support. Some Thoratec investigators implant biventricular assist devices in all patients to eliminate the potential problems of progressive right heart failure and ventricular arrhythmias associated with isolated left ventricular support. Although discrepancies among studies make it difficult to evaluate the type of support a particular patient may need, it is apparent that patients who receive biventricular support have decreased chance of survival and successful transplantation [11–13]. This increased mortality may be related to the severity of the heart failure or to the added complexity of two devices. Kormos et al. summarized the experience with univentricular support using the Novacor LVAS, regardless of whether the patient had biventricular or left ventricular failure [14]. They concluded that left ventricular support alone may be satisfactory for most chronically failing hearts. Our clinical experience was quite similar to theirs. However, we used inotropic support and other drugs to minimize pulmonary vascular resistance for extended periods (up to 28 days).

We encountered one interesting case, a patient with progressive severe biventricular failure due to viral myocarditis. Despite maximal medical therapy, the patient continued to deteriorate, and had the Thoratec LVAD inserted. He improved haemodynamically following device insertion, but his right ventricle continued to deteriorate, and finally his heart became asystolic. He survived on the LVAD alone with his right heart providing a Fontan type circuit and was successfully transplanted after more than a month in asystole. This episode reinforced our desire to bridge patients to transplantation with an LVAD alone. Further studies are needed to refine techniques for determining the need for biventricular support.

We conclude that the Thoratec LVAD can successfully support terminally ill patients until a suitable donor heart becomes available. Aggressive medical management of the right heart and the pulmonary vasculature minimizes the requirement for additional RVAD support. Support of patients for extended periods may serve as a prelude to permanent implantation of LVADs.

References

1. Hill JD (1989) Bridging to cardiac transplantation. Ann Thorac Surg 47:167–171
2. Hill JD, Farrar DJ, Hershon JJ, Compton PG, Avery GJ, Levin BS, Brent BN (1986) Use of a prosthetic ventricle as a bridge to cardiac transplantation for postinfarction cardiogenic shock. N Engl J Med 314:626–628
3. Farrar DJ, Hill JD, Gray LA Jr, Pennington DG, McBride LR, Pierce WS, Pae WE, Glenville B, Rass D (1988) Heterotopic prosthetic ventricles as a bridge to cardiac transplantation: a multicenter study in 29 patients. N Engl J Med 318:333–340
4. Farrar DJ, Lawson JH, Litwak P, Cederwall G (1990) Thoratec VAD system as a bridge to heart transplantation. J Heart Transplant 9:415–423
5. Farrar DJ, Hill JD (1993) Univentricular and biventricular Thoratec VAD support as a bridge to transplantation. Ann Thorac Surg 55:276–282
6. Pierce WS, Parr GVS, Myers JL, Pae WE Jr, Bull AP, Waldhausen JA (1981) Ventricular assist pumping in patients with cardiogenic shock after cardiac operations. N Engl J Med 305:1601–1610
7. Pennington DG, Kanter KR, McBride LR, Kaiser GC, Barner HB, Miller LW, Naunheim KS, Fiore AC, Willman V (1988) Seven years' experience with the Pierce-Donachy ventricular assist device. J Thorac Cardiovasc Surg 96:901–911
8. Kriett JM, Kaye MP (1991) The Registry of the International Society for Heart and Lung Transplantation: eighth official report — 1991. J Heart Transplant 10:491–498
9. Pennington DG, Swartz MT (1992) Assisted circulation and the mechanical heart. In: Braunwald E (ed) Heart disease. A textbook of cardiovascular medicine, 4th ed. Saunders, Philadelphia, pp 535–550
10. Pennington DG, McBride LR, Peigh PS, Miller LW, Swartz MT (1994) Eight years' experience with bridging to cardiac transplantation. J Thorac Cardiovasc Surg 107:472–481
11. Portner PM, Oyer PE, Pennington DG, Baumgartner WA, Griffith BP, Frist WR, Magilligan DJ, Noon GP, Ramasamy N, Miller PJ (1989) Implantable electrical left ventricular assist system: bridge to transplanation and the future. Ann Thorac Surg 47:142–150
12. Frazier OH, Rose EA, Macmanus Q, Burton NA, Lefrak EA, Pairier VL, Dasse KA (1992) Multicenter clinical evaluation of the HeartMate 1000 IP left ventricular assist device. Ann Thorac Surg 53:1080–1090
13. Johnson KE, Prieto M, Joyce CD, Pritzker M, Emery RW (1992) Summary of the use of the Symbion total artificial heart: a registry report. J Heart Lung Transplant 11:103–116
14. Kormos RL, Borovetz HS, Gasior T, Antaki JF, Armitage JM, Pristas JM, Hardesty RL, Griffith BP (1990) Experience with univentricular support in mortally ill cardiac transplant candidates. Ann Thorac Surg 49:261–272

Discussion

Dr. Hachida:
The complications in your institute were a little bit higher in the patients with Thoratec. The complications in some patients were overlapping in the table?

Dr. Niinami:
Yes.

Dr. Matsuda:
I thank you for a very good report. I have a question about the right ventricular support by the inotropes or others. You said that aggressive treatment for the right side of the heart is helpful to avoid the right ventricular assist device, but after revealing the results, could you tell us what are the important factors which eventually lead to right ventricle assist? What is your comment on the right ventricle ejection fraction, the right ventricle dimension or the preoperative status? Because we have to select which patients can be managed medically or by biventricular support.

Dr. Niinami:
This is a difficult issue, and it is still controversial whether to use LVAD alone or biVAD. In our series, out of 21 patients we used two additional RVAD supports after insertion of LVAD. As I mentioned in my presentation, we try not to use RVAD support. In order to do that, patients who had a sick right ventricle required lots of inotropic support. Also I believe nitric oxide helped right heart circulation a lot. Actually, our series of two patients who required RVAD support was before the introduction of nitric oxide in our center. In other words, we don't have experience with additional RVAD support since the introduction of nitric oxide. So I don't know how we can decide whether the patients needs RVAD or not. However, my impression is that once the patient gets used to the LVAD circulation even with failing right heart, the patient could tolerate it even without right heart circulation. Until that point is reached, those patients need inotropic support and nitric oxide. So I believe most patients can be managed without RVAD support.

Dr. Hachida:
I think Dr. Kormos has more experience. Do you have any further comments?

Dr. Kormos:
The only question I had, I had a couple, but I wanted to ask you, the nine patients that died: of those nine, were they all LVAD or did they also include biVAD?

Dr. Niinami:
One patient was on biVAD.

Dr. Kormos:
And the rest were LVAD? Now, of those LVAD patients that died, eight patients, how many of those had multiorgan failure before device implantation?

Dr. Niinami:
Most patients had multiple organ failure. I think that's the major reason, because we expected to recover after the insertion of VAD but we couldn't manage the multiple organ failure after the insertion of the VAD. That is the major reason why we lost the patients. But not on all patients. Like, five in eight patients.

Dr. Kormos:
See, I think there are two components here that are important. One is preop timing, and it's possible that if timing of implantation was a little sooner you may have avoided some of those. But the other issue, I think, is that using biventricular support, there are two reasons: one is because you suspect the right ventricle may not function adequately, but I think that data possibly from David Ferrar's analysis of their complete series shows that patients with multiorgan failure do better with biventricular support than with univentricular support. And that may also be a possibility, and, in the patients that you had LVAD, although you had adequate flow on LVAD, were you using a lot of inotropic support and high CVP? This sort of situation?

Dr. Niinami:
Yes, indeed. But of course not all patients. Some of the patients whose right heart was not good required lots

of inotropic support and high CVP. However, I believe LVAD support also helps pulmonary vascular resistance, so that most of the patients could be weaned from inotropic support for certain periods. We had a very interesting case in which the heart stopped completely a couple of weeks after insertion of the LVAD. This patient's ECG was flat but he could move around in the room. He was on LVAD support for a few months, then was successfully transplanted. He is alive and in very good condition now. At the time of his operation, his heart was a like a soccer ball, no contraction at all, which means his circulation was almost like Fontan circulation. I think this is also another reply to Prof. Matsuda's previous question. I believe patients who have irreversible right heart dysfunction could get through the critical period using inotropic drugs and nitric oxide, and it might be possible to maintain whole body circulation by LVAD alone. Of course not all cases, but most cases, I believe.

Dr. Minami:
Yes, it's very difficult to decide or to determine the function of the right ventricle after implantation of the left ventricular assist device. But we have also two cases out of our 55 assisted patients with Thoratec who got a right heart assist device secondly. These two patients had initially a decrease of central venous pressure and bilirubin level during one-week support with left heart assist device. But, on the second and third weeks, they got an increase in both levels again, so that we decided to implant a right heart assist device using a Thoratec pump. I think both parameters are very useful to decide or to determine the right ventricular function.

Patient Selection for Successful Outcome with the CardioWest Total Artificial Heart as a Bridge to Heart Transplantation

F.A. Arabía, J.G. Copeland, R.G. Smith, G.K. Sethi, D.A. Arzouman, A. Pavie, D. Duveau, W.J. Keon, B. Foy, M. Carrier, W. Dembitsky, J. Long, and A. Tector

Summary. The CardioWest Total Artificial Heart (TAH) is the only device in its class currently used worldwide as a bridge to heart transplantation. It is a pneumatic device that totally replaces the failing ventricles. Patient selection criteria include: patient must be a transplant candidate; cardiac index (CI) $<2.0 l \cdot min^{-1} \cdot m^{-2}$; body surface area (BSA) $>1.7 m^2$; maximal inotropic support including the use of the intra-aortic balloon pump; and evidence of biventricular failure. A total of 79 patients have received the TAH in 10 centers around the world, with the intention to bridge to heart transplantation. The patient demographics include: 73 males, 6 females; average age 45 years (range 16–63 years); average BSA $1.94 m^2$ ($n = 59$); average preoperative cardiac index (CI) $1.841 \cdot min^{-1} \cdot m^{-2}$ ($n = 43$); and average length of implantation 34 days (1–186 days). Fifty-five patients underwent heart transplantation, and 50 patients were eventually discharged home, 21 patients died on the device, and 3 patients remain on the TAH waiting to be transplanted. The overall survival of patients on the TAH is 66%, and 91% if the patient reaches transplantation. The most common cause of death while the patient is on the TAH is multiple organ failure. The survival rate with the CardioWest TAH is comparable with the survival rates of other mechanical assist devices currently available. This is the result of careful patient selection.

Key words: CardioWest Total Artificial Heart — Patient selection — Bridge to transplantation

Introduction

Heart transplantation remains the main therapeutic modality for end-stage heart disease in a selected group of patients with no other organ failure. The number of potential donors remains fairly constant throughout the world while the number of potential recipients continues to increase. There are several types of ventricular assist devices that provide temporary support if a patient deteriorates prior to the availability of a donor. There are currently four devices used worldwide with this intent. They have been classified as to their position in the body: extracorporeal (univentricular and biventricular), implanted (univentricular), and total artificial heart (TAH; biventricular). The use of a TAH was first described by DeVries et al. [1].

The CardioWest Total Artificial Heart (Fig. 1) is a direct descendent of the Jarvik TAH that was first utilized as a bridge to transplant in 1985 [2]. It is a pneumatic device that totally replaces the failing ventricles. The prosthetic ventricles are made of polyurethane and four Medtronic-Hall (Medtronic, Minneapolis, MN, USA) mechanical valves provide unidirectional flow. Blood and air are separated by a four-layer, segmented polyurethane diaphragm which retracts during diastole and is displaced forward by compressed air during systole to propel blood out of the prosthetic ventricle. The TAH can provide flows up to 10 l/min. However, it is usually used to provide flows at 6–8 l/min.

The device controller provides adjustment of the heart rate, systolic duration, and drive line pressures for each of the ventricles (Fig. 2). The TAH is operated so that there is incomplete filling but complete emptying with each stroke. The atrial pressure on each side determines ventricular filling; as atrial pressure increases, a higher stroke volume and cardiac output is obtained [3].

In 1990, the US Food and Drug Administration (FDA) withdrew permission from Symbion, Inc., the Jarvik-7 manufacturers, to continue production of the TAH. One year later, CardioWest Technologies acquired assets and technology from Symbion. In 1992 the FDA granted CardioWest Technologies, for limited clinical investigation, permission to manufacture the Jarvik-7-70, now renamed the CardioWest C-70, to undergo clinical trials as a device to bridge patients to heart transplantation. The first CardioWest was implanted in 1993 [4].

Inclusion criteria for implantation for the US centers were according to the CardioWest investigational protocol accepted by the FDA: (1) patient listed for heart transplantation and in imminent danger of dying within 48h or becoming ineligible for transplant; (2) cardiac index $<2.0 l \cdot min^{-1} \cdot m^{-2}$ with either systolic blood pressure <90 mmHg or central venous pressure >18 mmHg and/or at least 2 ino-

University of Arizona Health Sciences Center, 1501 N. Campbell Avenue, PO Box 245071, Tucson, AZ 85724, USA

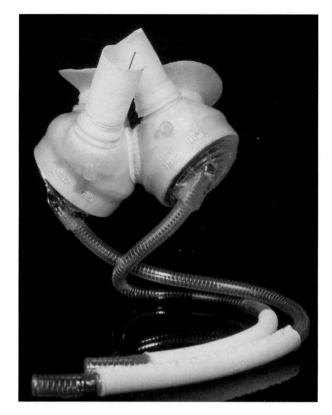

Fig. 1. The CardioWest C-70 showing both ventricles and drive lines

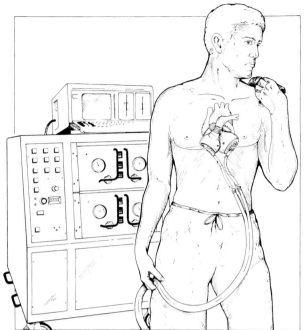

Fig 2. Drawing of the CardioWest C-70 in a patient, and the console (drive) unit

tropes: dopamine $>10\,\mu g \cdot Kg^{-1} \cdot min^{-1}$, dobutamine $> 10\,\mu g \cdot Kg^{-1} \cdot min^{-1}$, epinephrine $>0.02\,\mu g \cdot Kg^{-1} \cdot min^{-1}$, isoproterenol $>0.02\,\mu g \cdot Kg^{-1} \cdot min^{-1}$, or amrinone $>10\,\mu g^{-1} \cdot Kg^{-1} \cdot min^{-1}$; or 1 inotrope and a balloon pump; (3) pulmonary vascular resistance <8 Wood units (640 dyne $\cdot$ s $\cdot$ cm^{-2}); (4) absence of active systemic infection; (5) absence of renal or hepatic failure; (6) cytotoxic antibody level <10%; (7) absence of support devices other than the intra-aortic balloon pump. The inclusion criteria at the European centers were left up to the judgment of the investigators. This set of criteria is an extension of criteria that had been developed at earlier stages [5].

Anticoagulation was maintained in all patients. The protocols varied among the centers; however, a protocol typically consisted of low molecular weight dextran in the immediate postoperative period followed by heparin, dipyridamole, aspirin, pentoxyfylline, and ticlopidine [6]. Once the patients were hemodynamically stable and tolerating a diet, heparin was changed to warfarin.

Once a TAH had been implanted and the patients were hemodynamically stable, early ambulation was initiated. Physical rehabilitation and nutritional status assessment were done very early in an attempt to improve their physiologic status. Hepatic and renal functions were monitored (total bilirubin, creatinine) to insure preservation of these organ functions.

Morbidity with the TAH is defined as adverse events during the time of implantation. These events are defined as follows: (1) renal dysfunction: creatinine >5 mg/dl; (2) hepatic dysfunction: total bilirubin >5 mg/ dl; (3) infection: positive cultures/clinical signs of infection with negative cultures; (4) bleeding: using 8 or more units of red blood cells during surgery or at least 3 units in the first 24h post implant; (5) need for reoperation; (6) respiratory dysfunction: requiring mechanical ventilation after initial cessation of respiratory support; (7) neurologic event: stroke, seizure activity, or transient ischemic attack; (8) hemodynamic insufficiency: cardiac index $<2.01 \cdot min^{-1} \cdot m^{-2}$ or systolic blood pressure <90 mmHg for >4h; (9) hemolysis: plasma free hemoglobin >30 mg/dl; (10) fit complications: impaired TAH function due to problems with fit; (11) device malfunction; (12) peripheral thromboembolism: blood clot in the body other than the brain; (13) miscellaneous. The most common adverse event encountered was infection; however, most patients experienced some degree of renal dysfunction. The average number of adverse events was three per patient (range 0–7).

Table 1. Medical centers utilizing the CardioWest C-70 total artificial heart (TAH)

Centers	Number of patients
Europe	
La Pitie Hospital, Paris	31
Hospital of G. and R. Laennec, Nantes	10
North America	
University of Arizona, Tucson	13
Loyola University, Chicago	11
Ottawa Civic Hospital, Ottawa	5
LDS Hospital, Salt Lake City	4
Sharp Memorial Hospital, San Diego	3
University of Pittsburgh, Pittsburgh	1
Montreal Heart Institute, Montreal	1

Table 3. Preoperative characteristics of patients

	Number of patients	Mean	SD
CVP (mmHg)	32	19.5	4.33
PCWP (mmHg)	25	25	7.4
CI ($l \cdot min^{-1} \cdot m^{-2}$)	32	1.8	0.5
PVR (Wood units)	32	2.7	1.7
BSA (m^2)	32	2.05	0.15
Cr (mg/dl)	32	1.5	1
Tbili (mg/dl)	32	1.75	0.7

CVP, central venous pressure; PCWP, pulmonary capillary wedge pressure; CI, cardiac index; PVR, pulmonary vascular resistance; BSA, body surface area; Cr, creatinine; Tbili, total bilirubin.

Table 2. Etiology of patients requiring CardioWest TAH

Etiology	Number of patients	Patients transplanted Number (%)	Discharged home Number (%)
Idiopathic/dilated cardiomyopathy	37	29 (78%)	26 (70%)
Ischemic cardiomyopathy	23	16 (70%)	14 (61%)
Acute myocardial infaction	5	4 (80%)	4 (80%)
Graft failure	6	1 (17%)	1 (17%)
Post cardiopulmonary bypass	1	0	0
Valvular cardiomyopathy	3	2 (67%)	2 (67%)
Viral cardiomyopathy	1	1	1
Congenital cardiomyopathy	1	0	0
Myocarditis	1	1	1
Sarcoid	1	1	1

Patient Population

Seventy-nine patients underwent placement of the CardioWest TAH between January 1993 and August 1996 in 10 centers worldwide. There were 73 males and 6 females with an average age of 45 years (range 16–63 years); 41 implants were performed in the European centers and 38 in the North American centers (Table 1). Idiopathic/dilated cardiomyopathy was diagnosed in 47% of the patients, ischemic cardiomyopathy in 29%, graft failure in 7.6%, and acute myocardial infarction in 6.3%. Post cardiopulmonary bypass, valvular cardiomyopathy, viral cardiomyopathy, congenital cardiomyopathy, acute myocarditis, and sarcoid accounted for the remaining 10% (Table 2).

Preoperative hemodynamic and physiologic parameters were obtained in 32 patients prior to the implantation of the TAH. The average body surface area (BSA) was $1.94\,m^2$ ($n = 59$), the average central venous pressure (CVP) was 18mmHg, and the pulmonary capillary wedge pressure (PCWP) was 26.3mmHg ($n = 25$). The average pulmonary vascular resistance (PVR) was 3.0 Wood units and the average cardiac index (CI) was $1.81 \cdot min^{-1} \cdot m^{-2}$. Renal and hepatic function were established by preoperative creatinine (Cr) and total bilirubin (Tbili) which averaged 1.8 mg/dl each (Table 3). No significant technical difficulties were encountered during implantation.

Postoperatively, an attempt was always made for early extubation and ambulation as early as possible. Some of these patients were severely debilitated and in multiple organ failure. In some cases, organ function recovered and the nutritional status was improved, as well as their level of activity. Once the patients were stable, some were transferred out of the intensive care unit to a less critical unit. The patients were required to stay in the hospital; however, small excursions were allowed.

The average length of implantation was 34 days (range 0–186) in all centers and 43 days in the North American centers. A total of 21 patients died while on the device. The average length of stay for this group of patients was 19 days (range 0–86 days). Data are available in only 18 out of the 21 patients. Multiple organ failure was the most common cause of death and it affected 15 patients (84%). The other 3 patients died of hemorrhage from the pulmonary artery, sepsis, and tamponade, respectively.

Fifty-five patients (72%) were bridged to heart transplantation and 3 patients remain on the TAH waiting to be transplanted. Fifty patients are alive today and 5 died after transplant: 2 died of multiple organ failure, 2 of acute rejection, and one of a still unknown cause.

The most common complication encountered was the presence of renal dysfunction that was encountered in 38% of the patients. This followed by infection that was encountered in 37% of the patients. Patients with multiple organ failure developed renal and hepatic dysfunction.

Discussion

The patients who required placement of the CardioWest TAH were critically ill and not expected to survive more than 1–2 days. They experienced a compromised cardiac index ($1.841 \cdot min^{-1} \cdot m^{-2}$), with elevated central venous pressure (18 mmHg) and elevated pulmonary capillary wedge pressure (26.3 mmHg). They also manifested some degree of end-organ dysfunction as shown by an elevated serum creatinine and total bilirubin. The only alternative for these patients was heart transplantation; however, the lack of donors dictated the urgent need to bridge with a TAH. Intraoperatively, the major risks are bleeding, fit complication, and the need for re-exploration. The summary of adverse effects shows that although the

incidence of bleeding was 33%, reoperation was required in only 27%. Also important is the incidence of fit complications, which was minimal at 4%. Fit complications may become more significant if patients are selected with BSA < 1.7 m². If a patient is selected with a smaller BSA, then it is recommended that the recipient must have significant cardiomegaly to provide the necessary space. Another dimension that may be helpful in small patients is the distance between the anterior surface of the vertebral bodies and the undersurface of the sternum which should be > 10 cm. Fit complications may manifest by compression of the inferior vena cava by the right atrial cuff. Transesophageal echocardiography has become very helpful intraoperatively to evaluate inferior vena cava compression. None of the patients died because of these complications.

Postoperative infections were the most common adverse events; however, this definition covers from simple infections to infections of the TAH. One patient died of multiple organ failure and sepsis from mediastinitis. Device malfunction occurred in only one patient when one of the drive lines was transiently and accidentally kinked. This did not result in the death of the patient. Hemolysis did not appear to be significant, and when the levels were over 30 mg/dl it was only transient. Thromboembolic events, either peripheral or with neurologic sequelae, were never a cause of death.

Multiple organ failure, which usually manifested itself as renal dysfunction associated with hepatic and respiratory dysfunction, was the most common cause of death. These patients are usually already at risk for organ failure as they present already with manifestations of poor organ perfusion. Patients who did not survive the bridging to transplantation usually died in the earlier postoperative period (19 days vs 34 days). Currently, results with the CardioWest TAH are very encouraging. Once a patient is bridged and reaches transplantation, the overall chance of the patient surviving is 91% as compared with the Symbion Jarvik survival of 55% [7–9].

In summary, patient selection for the CardioWest TAH is essential to provide the best outcome. The patients must be waiting for heart transplantation. The group of patients with evidence of biventricular failure without irreversible organ damage, who deteriorate without the availability of a donor, are those who must benefit the most. It is important to consider placement of a TAH as soon as knowledge about the patient becomes available and not to wait until the patient has deteriorated to the point where end-organ damage is evident. Currently, results with the CardioWest TAH as a bridge to heart transplantation are comparable to those with other assist devices available with the intention of bridging (Table 4) [10]. Proper patient

Table 4. Ventricular assist device success rates[a]

Device	Discharged home
Novacor console	90%
Novacor wearable	92%
TCI pneumatic	89%
TCI electric	89%
Thoratec LVAD	93%
Thoratec BIVAD	81%
CardioWest	92%

LVAD, left ventricular assist device; BIVAD, biventricular assist device.
[a] Success rates defined as number of patients who reached transplantation and were discharged home.

selection is essential for a good outcome. The patient requiring a TAH must be a transplant candidate, of adequate size, with evidence of biventricular failure, minimal evidence of end-organ damage, and a very limited life expectancy.

References

1. DeVries WC, Anderson JL, Joyce GL, Anderson FL, Ammond EH, Jarvik RK, Kolff WJ (1984) Clinical use of the total artificial heart. N Engl J Med 310:273–278
2. Copeland JG, Levinson MM, Smith R, Icenogle TB, Vaughn C, Cheng K, Ott R, Emery RW (1986) The total artificial heart as a bridge to heart transplantation. A report of two cases. JAMA 256:2991–2995
3. Arabía FA, Copeland JG, Larson DF, Smith RG, Cleavinger MR (1993) Circulatory assist devices: Applications for ventricular recovery or bridge to transplant. In: Gravlee GP, Davis RF, Utley JR (eds) Cardiopulmonary bypass: principles and practice. Williams and Wilkins, Baltimore, pp 693–712
4. Copeland JG, Smith RG, Cleavinger MR (1995) Development and clinical use of the total artificial heart: a review of the current status of the CardioWest C-70 TAH (Jarvik-7). In: Lewis T, Graham T (eds) Mechanical circulatory support. Edward Arnold, London, pp 186–198
5. Copeland JG, Smith RG, Cleavinger MR, Icenogle TB, Sethi GK, Rosado LJ (1991) Bridge to transplantation indictions for Symbion TAH, Symbion AVAD, and Novacor LVAS. In: Akutsu T, Koyanagi H (eds) Artificial heart 3. Springer, Tokyo, pp 303–308
6. Szefner J, Cabrol C (1993) Control and treatment of hemostasis in patients with a total artificial heart: the experience of La Pitie. In: Pifarre R (ed) Anticoagulation, hemostasis, and blood preservation in cardiovascular surgery. Hanley and Belfus, Philadelphia, pp 237–264
7. Joyce LD, Johnson KE, Cabrol C, Griffith BP, Copeland JG, DeVries WC, Keon WJ, Wolner E, Frazier OH, Bucherl ES, Semb B, Akalin H, Aris A, Carmichael MJ, Cooley D, Dembitsky W, English T, Halbrook, Hetzer R, Herbert Y, Keon WJ, Loisance D, Noon G, Pennington G, Peterson A, Phillips SJ, Pierce WS, Unger F, Pifarre R, Tector A (1988) Nine-year experience with the clinical use of total artificial hearts as cardiac support devices. ASAIO Trans 34:703–707
8. Copeland JG, Smith RG, Cleavinger MR, Icenogle TB, Sethi GK, Rosado LJ (1991) Bridge to transplantation indications for Symbion TAH, Symbion AVAD, and Novacor LVAS. In: Akutsu T, Koyanagi H (eds) Artificial heart 3. Springer, Tokyo, pp 303–308
9. Copeland JG, Pavie A, Duveau D, Keon WJ, Masters R, Pifarre R, Smith RG, Arabía FA (1996) Bridge to transplantation with the CardioWest total artificial heart: the international experience 1993 to 1995. J Heart and Lung Transplant 15:94–99
10. Arabía FA, Smith RG, Rose DS, Arzouman DA, Sethi GK, Copeland JG (1996) Success rates of long-term circulatory assist devices used currently for bridge to heart transplantation. ASAIO J 42:M542–M546

Bridge for Transplantation with the Symbion and Cardiowest Total Artificial Heart: The Pitie Experience

Alain Pavie, Philippe Leger, Jacques Szefner, Patrick Nataf, Valeria Bors, Rama Akhtar, Elisabeth Vaissier, Jean Pierre Levasseur, and Iradj Gandjbakhch

Summary. Since April 1986, 92 patients have received a pneumatic total artificial heart, Jarvik-7: 62 a Symbion model, and 30 a Cardiowest model. The duration of support ranged from less than 1 day to 603 days (mean duration 23 ± 64). The indications were acute shock (41 cases) or chronic deterioration on the transplant waiting list (51 cases). The etiology was mainly idiopathic and ischemic cardiomyopathy. With the help of our scoring system, we divided our patients into three groups: (1) Chronic Implantation group, represented by two females staying on the device for 6 and 19 months, respectively; (2) a Rescue group of 35 patients characterized by high-risk indications: graft failure, rejection, postcardiotomy patient, postpartum cardiomyopathy, and reoperation for valvular and congenital conditions. In addition, the dilated and ischemic cardiomyopathy patients operated on in very bad condition with a score over 6 were included in this group; and (3) a Low Risk Indication group (55 patients) comprising mostly the dilated and ischemic cardiomyopathy patients with a score under 6. Due to the shortage of donors, our criteria for transplantation are very strict. Transplants should be carried out only in cases of hemodynamic stability, on an extubated patient with normal renal and liver function, without coagulation problems or infection. With such criteria, in the Rescue group, only seven patients could be transplanted and of these, three are still alive. In contrast, in the Low Risk group, 33 were transplanted (60%), and 70% of these patients were discharged. The rate has improved in the most recent cases, with 83% of the Cardiowest patients being survivors.

Key words: Total artificial heart — Bridge to transplantation — Cardiac assist

Introduction

Demikhov [1] was the first surgeon to remove dog's heart experimentally and replace it with a mechanical device, but it was not until the 1960s that Cooley et al. [2] attempted the first clinical use of a total artificial heart (TAH) as a bridge to transplantation. Fourteen years of effort and technological development made

Department of Thoracic and Cardiovascular Surgery, La Pitie Hospital, Paris, France

the first permanent implantation of the Jarvik-7 (Symbion, Salt Lake City, UT, USA) possible; by Jarvik and DeVries [3] on a patient, Barney Clark, who lived 112 days. The first five implantations were performed as a permanent circulatory support. Due to complications, the US Food and Drug Administration (FDA) allowed testing thereafter only as a bridge to heart transplantation. Three years later, the first successful use of a Jarvik-7 TAH as a bridge procedure was achieved (August 1985) by Copeland et al. [4]. After this success, many implantations were performed worldwide.

We performed our first case at La Pitie Hospital in April 1986 [5], with a Jarvik TAH from Symbion Other European teams, notably in England, France, Spain, Sweden, and Turkey, also developed a program of Jarvik TAH implantation. During the same period, some teams developed their own TAH and performed implantation (Berlin Heart, Brno, Ellipsoid Heart) [6,7]. Recently, the FDA banned the use of the Symbion Jarvik TAH in the United States and consequently the number of implantations has decreased. However, in Europe, this device was still used by some teams.

More recently, Copeland and the University of Tucson, Arizona team restarted in 1992, using a new FDA-approved device manufactured by the company Cardiowest (Richmond, Canada). Cardiowest is now able to ship some devices to Europe. The opportunity to continue using the Cardiowest TAH allows one to expand the spectrum of indications for some patients requiring a TAH due to a specific situation. The development of a new electric implantable left ventricular assist device (LVAD) does not allow the treatment of all patients. About one-third of the patients whose conditions qualify them for bridging to transplant also require a right ventricular support. The actual status of transplantation programs, with a slight decrease of donors, has reinforced the need to transplant only the patients with a maximal chance of success, in order to avoid graft loss. The Symbion Jarvik and Cardiowest TAHs allowed us to reach this goal. In this article, we would like to report the La Pitie Hospital experience with the pneumatic artificial heart.

Materials

From April 1986 to July 1996, at La Pitie Hospital, 92 patients received a pneumatic TAH, Jarvik-7: 62 a Symbion model and 30 a Cardiowest. The group consisted of 78 males and 14 females, aged from 15 to 60 years (mean age 40 ± 12). Sixty-two Symbion TAHs (22 with the 100 cm^3 model and 40 with the smaller 70-cm^3 model) were implanted from April 1986 to September 1992. Since October 1992, 30 Cardiowests have been implanted using the same surgical technique that we have already described [8]. The duration of support ranged from 1 to 603 days (mean duration 24 ± 64). The total duration on support was 2164 days. The indications for implantation were acute shock (41 cases), or chronic deterioration on the transplant waiting list (51 cases), due to idiopathic and ischemic cardiomyopathy. There were also other indications, summarized in Fig. 1.

With the help of our scoring system, developed on our first 37 cases by univariate and multivariate analyses [9–11] (Table 1), it is possible to divide our patients into three groups:

1. **Chronic Implantation** group, represented by two females staying on the device for 6 and 19 months, respectively. These two women had dilated cardiomyopathy, but they developed antibodies. It was possible to transplant the first patient after 6 months, when we found a crossmatch-negative donor. Unfortunately, she died 2 days later from acute vascular rejection. The second patient had higher levels of antibodies, it was impossible to find a compatible graft even after plasmapheresis. She died after 603 days from a brain hemorrhage.

2. **Rescue** group: 35 patients characterized by high-risk indications: graft failure in 5, rejection in 6, postcardiotomy in 3, postpartum cardiomyopathy ($n = 4$), and reoperation for valvular and congenital conditions, especially when an associated repair was needed before device implantation ($n = 4$). With these etiologies, we included also the high-risk dilated and ischemic cardiomyopathy patients in particularly bad preoperative status with a score of over 6 ($n = 13$).

3. The **Low Risk Indication** group (55 patients): comprising all the dilated and ischemic cardiomyopathy patients with a score under 6.

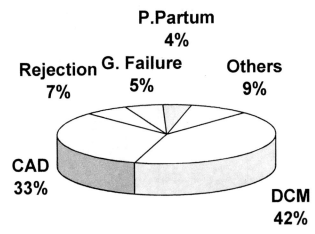

Fig. 1. Etiology of cardiac failure. *CAD*, ischemic cardiomyopathy; *DCM*, dilated cardiomyopathy; *P. Partum*, postpartum cardiomyopathy; *G. Failure*, graft failure

Device Description and Surgical Technique

Jarvik Ventricle

The Symbion Jarvik ventricle is an air-driven, intracorporeal, diaphragm ventricle coated with polyurethane urea. Two Medtronic valves are placed in the outflow and inflow orifices. Two different sizes are available: small (Jarvik 7, 70 cm^3) and large (Jarvik 7, 100 cm^3). The Cardiowest model presents very few modifications; only a small size is available (70 cm^3).

Drive Unit Control

The Utah heart drive controller has several functions. Two parameters should be preset before starting the support: heart rate (range between 0 and 199 beats/

Table 1. Preoperative score table

	Preoperative score			
	1	2	3	4
Indication			Graft failure after cardiopulmonary bypass	Rejection Rejection
Body surface area (m^2)	<1.8		<1.73	
Height (cm)		<175	<170	
Weight (kg)		<60		
Bilirubin (μM)		>24		
Age (years)	>40			

min); and systole duration (from 0% to 99%). Each unit comes with one active drive system and a second security back-up system. The activation pressure can be regulated between 0 and 300 mmHg, and a negative pressure can be used in case of poor ventricle filling (0 to 20 mmHg). A computer system (COMDU) is connected to the Utah drive system, allowing continuous measurement of the cardiac output from each ventricle, depending on the air coming out from the ventricle during diastole. Tendency curves are also displayed on the monitor of the computer.

Surgical Technique

Through a median sternotomy [8], the pericardium was opened from the ascending aorta to the diaphragm. First, the ventricular drivelines were tunneled through two separate skin incisions in the left upper quadrant of the abdomen as far as the pericardial cavity. Once the drivelines were in position, both ventricles were carefully checked (Fig. 2). Cardiopulmonary bypass was established using two right-angle caval cannulae inserted anteriorly and an arterial cannula placed in the ascending aorta.

The heart excision was carefully carried out in order to facilitate subsequent cardiac transplantation. The pulmonary artery and the aorta were transected just above their respective valves. The right and left ventricles were transected 2–3 cm distal to the atrioventricular groove. The coronary sinus ostium

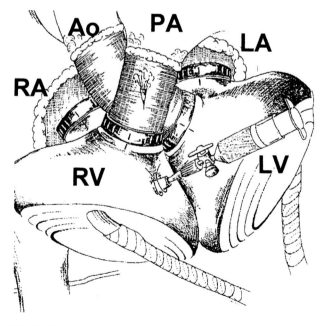

Fig. 2. Surgical implantation of total artificial heart. *Ao*, ascending aorta; *PA*, pulmonary artery; *LA*, left atrium; *RA*, right atrium; *RV*, right ventricle; *LV*, left ventricle

and the venous coronary sinus were closed to avoid bleeding.

The anastomosis between the atrial cuffs and the atrioventricular remnants was started at the cephalic portion of the septum: a double anastomosis with a simple running suture joining both cuffs to the septum remnant. Then, each cuff was sutured to its respective right and left free ventricular wall. The aortic and pulmonary grafts (7 cm long) were sutured end-to-end to their respective vessels. In Europe, before final testing of the suture, it is possible to supplement an anastomosis with fibrin glue or gelatin resorcin formol adhesive, "the French glue." This technique allows a reduction in postoperative bleeding. The artificial ventricles were attached to their respective cuffs and after air-purging, support was started, with the left ventricle being the first to be activated.

Coagulation Control

Anticoagulation regimens vary from hospital to hospital. We have developed a special approach based on a general idea: the complex cardiac assist and blood interface requires a systematic and personalized approach to avoid thromboembolic complications [12], with control of platelet function, thrombin formation pathways, and fibrinolytic status. If a pathological fibrinolytic state was found, aprotinin was given until normalization. Small doses of heparin were used to control coagulation balance. Platelet stabilization is probably essential due to the presence of mechanical valves, extensive exposure of blood to foreign materials, and localized blood turbulence. Dipyridamole in large doses was given to stabilize platelet activity and very small doses of aspirin to lower aggregation. With this approach it was possible to control all biological bleeding and not a single thromboembolic incident occurred in this series. Reoperation for control of hemorrhage was for surgical reasons.

Results

Excluding the chronic patients already discussed, we still need to analyze two different risk categories of patients: the Rescue group and the Low Risk group. It is also interesting to compare the initial period from April 1986 to September 1992, corresponding with the first 60 Symbion patients, and the second phase, with the Cardiowest implantation, from October 1992 to July 1996.

The most frequent postoperative complications were renal failure and infection (Table 2). Among them, mediastinitis was very rare (one patient). Some infection of the drive lines occurred, but the majority consisted of septicemia and pulmonary infection. The main causes of death (Table 3) were multiple organ failure in 25 or untreatable sepsis in 10 patients. Due to the shortage of donors, our criteria for transplantation are very strict. Transplants should be undertaken only in cases of hemodynamic stability, on an extubated patient with normal renal and liver function, without coagulation problems or infection. With such criteria in the Rescue risk group (Fig. 3), only seven patients could be transplanted. Three of these are still alive. In contrast, in the Low Risk group (34 Symbion and 21 Cardiowest), 33 were transplanted (60%), and 70% of these patients were discharged. The survival rate has improved in the most recent cases, 83% of the Cardiowest transplanted patients being survivors. In the period before September 1992, with the Symbion patients, Rescue group indications represented 42% of the indications. During the period since October 1992, with the Cardiowest model, only 30% of all cases have had high-risk indications.

Table 2. Frequency of postoperative complications

Postoperative complication	Number (percentage)
Infection	22 (24%)
Renal failure	41 (44%)
Reoperation for bleeding	15 (16%)
Reoperation to reposition device	2 (2.2%)
Stress-induced gastric ulcer	2 (2.2%)

Table 3. Causes of death while on total artificial heart

Cause of death	Number of patients
Multiple organ failure	25
Sepsis	10
Pulmonary cause	5
Hemorrhage	2
Related to the device	3
Others	5

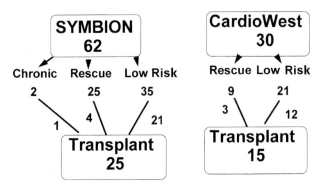

Fig. 3. Outcome of 92 patients: Symbion versus Cardiowest

Discussion

Today, many aspects of patient selection for a cardiac transplant are more clearly defined than at the beginning of the study, even if certain problems still exist. It has been well demonstrated that clinical results depend essentially on the preimplantation status of the patients. At the beginning of our study, due to the absence of criteria for implantation, we included a wide range of indications. This attitude was also explained by the large number of donors available during this period. The decision on device implantation was always taken at a late stage.

In the following situations, we have implanted TAH in patients who would qualify today as high risk [13]. Primary graft failure occurred due to poor myocardial conservation and due to high pulmonary vascular resistance, a condition that practically no longer exists due to the progress made in myocardial preservation techniques. Graft failure in the latter situation usually arises following a poor evaluation of the recipient. A high pulmonary vascular resistance will not be improved.

Chronic rejection is an especially difficult situation. The decision is often made too late after an initial trial of immunosuppressive therapy — high-dose steroids and monoclonal antibody — exposing the patient to a major infection risk during the reoperation. However, it is with this group of patients that the psychological and emotional problems are maximal for the team. The use of a TAH after cardiotomy may well be regarded as a contraindication even if we can be completely certain that the myocardium has been totally destroyed. The prolongation of cardiopulmonary bypass (CPB) needed for the implantation further compromises an already grave clinical state.

We have also included patients with previous multiple valvular replacements, with cachexia (first patient of the series), or with complex congenital diseases having already undergone multiple surgical procedures. The previous palliative operations sometimes completely exclude the use of another external cardiac assist device or LVAD, but they being candidates for TAH implantation, we are obliged to perform complex surgical repair on the vena cava or pulmonary bifurcation. The increased duration of CPB is deleterious to particularly ill patients. For example, one of four patients required a reconstruction of the superior vena cava and the pulmonary bifurcation due to a previous intervention for single ventricle: Glenn and Blalock anastomoses. A CPB of more than 6 hours' duration was probably one of the main causes of death under the device. The postpartum cardiomyopathies also qualify as a high-risk group, taking into account the acute nature of the failure occurring in a particular situation where immunological phenomena play an essential role.

Like many teams, we have developed a preoperative score, on our first 37 patients [9,10] (Table 1); this was later improved [11]. Kawaguchi had selected some preoperative factors among our first Jarvik 7 patients, including high-risk indications: rejection, postoperative failure, mode of decompensation, patient's size, bilirubin above 24µM, and dialysis (Table 1). In the first series, the successful bridge cases had an average score of 1.3 versus the failed cases with a score of 6.6.

It also seems important to include in this Rescue group, the dilated or ischemic cardiomyopathies with a severe deterioration in their preoperative status. Thirteen patients had a score over 6, corresponding to their particularly severe status.

In the initial phase of using the Symbion Jarvik TAH, Rescue indications represented 42% of the indications (25 patients); more recently, with the Cardiowest since October 1992, only 30% (9 patients) had high-risk indications. Even if such cases are today a contraindication, ethical, psychological, and social arguments explain the decision to use the device in these remaining cases. Unfortunately, the experience acquired did not allow us to improve the results in this group.

In contrast, the elective group is represented by patients with lower risk with a preoperative score under 6. In spite of this better preoperative status, the follow-up is not without complications. The most frequent complications under the device, as in other series of cardiac assist, are renal failure and infection. It is important to note that mediastinitis is very rare in this series (one case), as in the study of Lonchyna et al. [14], in contrast to a previous report [15]. Nevertheless, infection and multiple organ failure remain the main causes of death, postoperatively. With our strict transplantation criteria, only 60% of the patients in this group were transplanted; similar percentages were transplanted in another registry and with other devices [16,17]. The mortality after transplantation was due to many causes, but none were directly related to the TAH. Among the more recent patients with a Cardiowest, 83% of the transplanted patients are alive; these results are similar to those with the new electric implantable systems [13,17,18].

Conclusion

The Jarvik-7 TAHs, Symbion or Cardiowest, remain probably the best systems to achieve total circulatory support in a case of severe biventricular failure. With strict selection criteria, this system allows the support of patients in good condition, to await transplantation.

The infectious risk, especially of mediastinitis, is very low. No thromboembolic events occur with a careful and particular coagulation approach.

A strict selection of elective indications is absolutely necessary, even though it is not always possible to exclude high-risk patients for affective, social, or psychological reasons. During the last 3 years of using the Cardiowest TAH, 60% of patients were transplanted and 83% of these are still alive and well. If we accept the tendency of each team to use a specific device, the opportunity to use a total artificial heart allowed us to expand the indications for some patients in a particular clinical situation where the other devices cannot be used, such as aortic insufficiency, massive thrombosis of a left ventricular aneurysm, a previous aortic or mitral prosthesis, or a postinfarction septal defect. While waiting for the completely implantable electric TAH, the pneumatic TAH has already proven that it can provide long-term support for a patient with a satisfactory rate of success.

References

1. Demikhov VP (1947) Experimental transplantation of vital organs. Haig B (translator). Consultants Bureau, New York, p 212
2. Cooley DA, Liotta D, Hallman GL, Bloodwell RD, Leachman RD, Milam JD (1969) Orthotopic cardiac prosthesis for two-staged cardiac replacement. Am J Cardiol 24:723–730
3. Jarvik RK, DeVries WC (1986) Clinical use of total artificial heart. J Heart Transplant 5:184–195
4. Copeland JG, Emery WR, Levinson MM (1985) The role of mechanical support and transplantation in treatment of patients with end-stage cardiomyopathy. Circulation 72 (Suppl II):7–12
5. Cabrol C, Gandjbakhch I, Pavie A, Bors V, Mestiri T, Cabrol A, Leger Ph, Levasseur JP, Vaissier E, Szefner J, Auriol A, Aupetit B, Solis E (1988) Total artificial heart as a bridge for transplantation: La Pitie 1986 to 1987. J Heart Transplant 7:12–17
6. Viazis P (1990) The Berlin pneumatic device. In: Pavie A (ed) Medical indications and system choice. European concerted action "Heart" proceedings. Paris, pp 35–36
7. Unger F, Genelin A, Hager J, et al (1984) Functional heart replacement with non-pulsatile assist devices. In: Assisted circulation 2. Springer Berlin, p 163
8. Solis E, Muneretto C, Cabrol C (1988) Total artificial heart. In: Cooper DK, Novitzky D (eds) The transplantation and replacement of thoracic organs. Kluwer Academic, Boston, pp 57, 431–444
9. Kawaguchi AT, Gandjbakhch I, Pavie A, Muneretto C, Solis E. Bors V, Leger P, Vaissier E, Levasseur JP, Szefner J, (1990) Factors affecting survival in total artificial heart recipients before transplantation. Circulation 82 (Suppl IV):322–327
10. Kawaguchi AT, Cabrol C, Gandjbakhch I, Pavie A, Bors V, Muneretto C (1991) Preoperative risk analysis

in patients receiving Jarvik-7 artificial heart as bridge to transplantation. Eur J Cardiothorac Surg 5:509–514

11. Kawaguchi AT, Cabrol C, Pavie A, Leger P, Bors V, Takahashi N, Gandjbackhch I (1992) Survival prediction in staged heart transplantation using Jarvik-7 artificial heart. Circulation 86 (Suppl II):11-311–11-315

12. Szefner J, Cabrol C (1993) Control and treatment of hemostasis in patients with a total artificial heart: the experience of La Pitie. In: Pifarre R (ed) Anti-coagulation, hemostasis, and blood preservation in Cardiovascular surgery. Hanley and Belfus, Philadelphia

13. Pavie A, Leger P, Regan M, Nataf P, Bors V, Szefner J, Cabrol C, Gandjbakhch I (1995) Clinical experience with a total artificial heart as a bridge for transplantation: the Pitie experience. J Card Surg 10:552–558

14. Lonchyna V, Pifarre R, Sullivan H, Montoya A, Bakhos M, Grieco J, Foy B, Blakeman B, Attergott R, Calandra D (1992) Successful use of the total artificial heart as a bridge to transplantation with no mediastinitis. J Heart Lung Transplant 11:803–811

15. Johnson KE, Prieto M, Joyce LD, Pritzker M, Emery RW (1992) Summary of the clinical use of the Symbion total artificial heart: a registry report. J Heart Lung Transplant 11:104–116

16. Griffith BP, Kormos RL, Hardesty RL, Armitage JM, Dummer JS (1988) The artificial heart: Infection related morbidity and its effect on transplantation. Ann Thorac Surg 45:409–414

17. Oaks TE, Pae WE, Miller CA, Pierce WS (1990) Combined registry for the clinical use of mechanical ventricular assist pumps and the total artificial heart in conjunction with heart transplantation: fifth official report. J Heart Transplant 10:621–625

18. Copeland JG, Pavie A, Duveau D, Keon WJ, Masters R, Pifarre R, Smith RG, Arabia FA (1996) Bridge to transplantation with the CardioWest total artificial heart: the international experience 1993 to 1995. J Heart Lung Transplant 15:94–99

Discussion

Dr. Wolner:

First, I disagree that an aortic prosthesis is an absolute contraindication for the implantation of a total artificial heart, because we have one patient, he is now 2 or 3 months on the Novacor device, which had before an artificial, Smeloff-Cutter valve in aortic position, and we switched during implantation to a bioprosthesis without any problems. But I have a question: You have such a huge experience with both systems, total artificial heart and left heart assist devices, in which cases do you recommend from your experience the CardioWest system, and in which cases, let's say, the Thoratec or something else, and in which the Novacor or the TCI?

Dr. Pavie:

I totally agree with you for the first comment, but if you have the total artificial heart it is easiest to remove all the valves and you avoid some complication. For your final comment, for example, last year, the number of indications in bridge to transplant had decreased, probably due to the cardiologists' evolution with medical treatment like you said yesterday, and we have performed four implantations this year. Two were performed with Novacor and two with CardioWest. The two first cases with Novacor were always ischemic cardiomyopathy and in each case, it seemed to us that the right ventricle was correct. In one case I performed coronary graft on the right coronary and the two patients stayed on the device 2 and 3 months, we're transplanting and they are alive. So, two of the cases where we used the CardioWest were referred too late. It's clear. In all the presentations we said you have to implant early with the device, and so on. But very often the surgeons don't decide. It depends on the cardiologist, when the patient is referred, and sometimes we have a patient who is referred too late. And when you have really biventricular failure with degradation of renal and liver function, we have two solutions: to do nothing or to use a device where we are more confident in case of biventricular failure. It is for these reasons that we continue to use total artificial hearts in such cases. For external biventricular assist we only use it in very small-size people where it is difficult to use a Novacor or a total

artificial heart. And in the very good indication in the young patient for recovery.

Dr. Nosé:

You experienced both types of device, Symbion and CardioWest. With Symbion, everybody experienced a high rate of infection; now, infection disappeared. What is the difference? Is the device different? Can you tell us what is the reason of the disappearing infection?

Dr. Pavie:

I apologize, because Dr. Kormos is the chairman of this session. Since the beginning we have not the same experience as Pittsburgh. Unfortunately, in classical surgery, we are not probably the best team and we have some mediastinitis for classical surgery, but with Symbion and today with CardioWest we have only one case of mediastinitis. It's true that some patients died on the device with multiple organ failure, and in such cases, we have always a positive blood culture and so on, but we never had local infection. We sometimes had local infection on the drive line but it's never a problem with the total artificial heart.

Dr. Kormos:

I think when we went back and looked at the reasons for infection rates in the early Symbion series that we had, it's very clear that infection rates were related to two variables. One was length of stay in hospital before implantation. The second was number of days of intraaortic balloon before implantation. Very often, the same organism, which was found at the time of post-transplant death was present preop from the skin or from line cultures, and so I think, when we look back at our own series, it was a reluctance to move early with the device, as opposed to any particular device-related problem.

Dr. Jarvik:

I just would like to comment. To my understanding, there is virtually no difference between the Symbion and CardioWest device, and I think your experience in Paris is a superb example of the learning curve that the whole field is going through. So, I think we have to learn to understand that everybody working in this field is gaining by this interaction, is doing better, it's coming together, and now we even see teams having very good success with their first use of any number of these devices. I think the whole field has advanced, and that's part of the reason why the early complications are going away, not just the device, because it's the same device.

Dr. Hachida:
Yes, we have a little bit more time, so can anybody tell us the current status of the CardioWest in the United States? Dr. Watson, can you tell us the current status of CardioWest ? Oh, Dr. Olsen.

Dr. Olsen:
I apologize for the University of Arizona people not presenting. Had I known, I would have brought some slides and occupied this valuable time. The device is being used. There have been 15 cases this year. We have the fourth case at the LDS hospital in Salt Lake currently ongoing. All have done well on the device. We implanted 26 patients around the world last year and we have not experienced device failures. We have not experienced permanent thromboembolic episodes with permanent residual effects from the central nervous system, and I think all of the people are presently quite pleased with the use of the device.

The Effect of Cardiomyoplasty on Coronary Blood Flow and Diastolic Dimension of the Left Ventricle

M. Okada, Y. Toyoda, T. Mukai, M.A. Kashem, and T. Tsukube

Key words: Dynamic cardiomyoplasty — Latissimus dorsi — Coronary blood flow — Diastolic dimension — Dog

Introduction

Since the development of cardiac surgery and myocardial protection, open heart surgery has been carried out for severely ill patients with heart disease. Some of these patients need mechanical circulatory assistance. Intra-aortic balloon pumping (IABP), V–A bypass, and artificial assist devices have been used according to the severity of heart failure, and satisfactory results have been obtained.

In Japan, however, surgeons have not had the option of performing heart transplantation since 1968. Therefore, we have attempted dynamic cardiomyoplasty (DCMP), using the latissimus dorsi muscle, for cardiac failure [1,2]. However, problems were encountered such as disturbance of the coronary blood flow and diastolic dimension of the left ventricle due to the wrapping of muscle around the failing heart. In this study, the hemodynamic performance of the left ventricle and coronary blood flow after dynamic cardiomyoplasty were investigated to clarify these problems.

Materials and Methods

Fifteen mongrel dogs of either sex weighing 12–18 kg were used for this study. General anesthesia was induced in all animals by ketamine hydrochloride (5 mg/kg) and thiamylal sodium (30 mg/kg) followed by intravenous pentobarbital sodium (25 mg/kg) before endotracheal intubation. Respiration was managed using a respirator (MA-1, Acoma, Tokyo, Japan) and intermittent administration of pentobarbital sodium. The left latissimus dorsi muscle flap (LDMF) was mobilized by dissecting the surrounding attachments from the costal, vertebral, and iliac insertions, preserving carefully the thoracodorsal neurovascular

Kobe University School of Medicine, Department of Surgery, Division II, 7-5-2 Kusunoki-cho, Chuo-ku, Kobe, Hyogo 650, Japan

bundles. The LDMF was then wrapped around the heart in a clockwise fashion (Fig. 1).

Two unipolar pacing electrodes (Model 6500, Medtronic, MN, USA) were implanted into the LDMF: one around the thoracodorsal bundle and the other 6–8 cm away. The pacemaker wires were connected to an external R wave synchronous stimulator (Model BC-03, Fukuda Denshi, Tokyo, Japan) to stimulate the LDMF. The pacemaker protocols were as follows: pacemaker mode, DDD; trained pulse, 50 Hz; synchronous ratio, 2:1 or 3:1; synchronous delay, 10–100 m.s; pulse duration, 100–150 m.s; pulse amplitude, 2–9.9 V; and cardiac sensitivity, 0.5–1.5 V. the synchronization mode applied was 2:1 when the heart rate was less than 100 beats/min and 3:1 when the heart rate was less than 200 beats/min. A Doppler ultrasonic catheter (DC-201, Miller, TX, USA) for the measurement of coronary flow velocity (Cardiometrics, CA, USA) was inserted into the left main trunk through a Judkins catheter (5F) via the femoral artery. Instantaneous measurement of the coronary arterial blood flow velocity was obtained using fast Fourier transformation analysis after inducing acute heart failure by multiple ligation of the branches of the left anterior descending artery, or chronic heart failure by propranolol injection (2 mg/kg).

Measurements of the hemodynamic parameters and coronary blood flow were carried out after stimulation of the LDMF. Also, right and left heart catheterizations were performed in the stimulated and unstimulated phases during cardiac cycles [2–7]. Statistical analyses were performed with a statistical program. All values were expressed as the mean ± standard error. Differences were considered significant when the P value was <0.05.

Results

Hemodynamic Changes in the Acute Heart Failure Phase

Aortic pressure (AoP), left ventricular pressure (LVP), and descending aortic flow were all increased

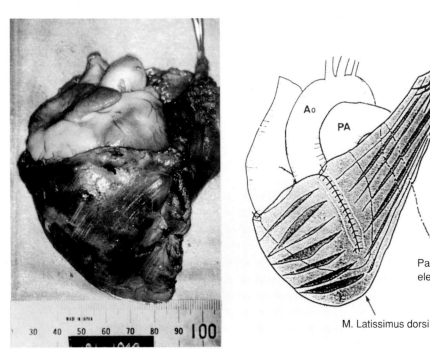

Fig. 1. Photograph and schematic illustration of cardiomyoplasty. Ao, aorta; PA, pulmonary artery. Scale bar 1 mm

Table 1a. Hemodynamic changes with dynamic cardiomyoplasty (acute phase)

	DCMP off	DCMP on	% Change	P-Value
Aop (mmHg)				
Systolic	81.0 ± 3.4	93.8 ± 4.1	15.8 ± 1.5	<0.005
Diastolic	49.7 ± 1.3	53.4 ± 1.4	8.6 ± 2.3	<0.01
(Mean)	59.9 ± 2.0	69.6 ± 2.3	16.4 ± 1.3	<0.005
LVP (mmHg)				
Systolic	84.6 ± 3.8	97.1 ± 3.4	15.6 ± 2.1	<0.005
Diastolic	8.4 ± 0.6	7.9 ± 0.3	−4.0 ± 4.3	NS
Descending aorta flow				
(ml/beat)	5.3 ± 0.6	8.9 ± 1.4	67.5 ± 5.3	<0.005

DCMP, dynamic cardiomyoplasty; AoP, aortic pressure; LVP, left ventricular pressure; TVi, total velocity integral; SF, systolic fraction; DF, diastolic fraction.

Table 1b. Coronary blood flow with dynamic cardiomyoplasty (acute phase)

	DCMP off	DCMP on	% Change	P-Value
Systolic				
Peak velocity (sm/s)	20.8 ± 1.3	25.9 ± 1.5	26.9 ± 6.5	<0.005
TVi (cm)	2.1 ± 0.3	2.5 ± 0.3	20.9 ± 4.8	<0.005
% SF (%)	20.3 ± 2.4	22.0 ± 3.1	8.3 ± 4.9	NS
Diastolic				
Peak velocity (cm/s)	33.5 ± 3.4	34.8 ± 3.6	4.0 ± 1.6	<0.05
TVi (cm)	8.5 ± 0.8	9.4 ± 1.0	10.0 ± 4.6	<0.05
% DF (%)	79.7 ± 2.4	78.0 ± 3.1	−2.1 ± 1.4	NS

in the acute phase by dynamic cardiomyoplasty (Table 1a). Concurrently, a significant increase of coronary arterial blood flow was recognized in both systolic and diastolic phases of the cardiac cycle (Table 1b). The enhancement of coronary blood flow velocity was associated with an increase in mean aortic pressure from 59.9 ± 2.0 mmHg to 69.6 ± 2.3 mmHg. Thus, the improved systolic coronary blood flow velocity was related to the increase in aortic pressure and cardiac output. Also, an increase in diastolic aortic pressure of 8.6% ± 2.3% increased the coronary perfusion pressure. Total velocity integrals (TVi) were increased markedly during systole, but less in diastole. Furthermore, an increase in the % systolic fraction (SF) as well as a decrease in the % diastolic fraction (DF) were also confirmed.

Hemodynamic Changes in the Chronic Heart Failure Phase

Chronic heart failure was produced by the infusion of propranolol (2mg/kg) 6–12 months after DCMP. Subsequently, the aortic systolic and diastolic pressures fell to 61.5 ± 2.1mmHg and 47.7 ± 1.8mmHg, respectively. LVP was depressed to 91.3 ± 1.9mmHg. After the initiation of DCMP, the aortic pressure increased by 36.3% ± 2.2%, and the LV systolic pressure rose by 8.7% ± 0.9%. Concurrently, the cardiac output (CO) increased from 1.0 ± 0.0 to 1.3 ± 0.4 (26.6% ± 5.1%) and the ejection fraction (EF) increased from 45.6 ± 1.1 to 55.4 ± 1.5 (20.1% ± 1.5%) (Table 2a).

These improvements in hemodynamic parameters were due to the augmentation of cardiac function during systolic and diastolic assistance. In the chronic phase with cardiac assistance, coronary blood flow during systole and diastole was markedly increased. The peak velocity of coronary arterial blood flow rose by 29.1% ± 5.7% in systole and 12.2% ± 3.8% in diastole. The total velocity integral showed an increase of 21.9% ± 9.1% (Table 2b). Thus, coronary arterial blood flow increased with DCMP even in the chronic phase during cardiac assistance (Fig. 2).

Diastolic Dimension of the Left Ventricle

Another purpose of this study was to clarify whether adhesion between the epicardium and the LDMF impairs the diastolic dimension of the left ventricle (LVDd). In both acute and chronic phases after dynamic cardiomyoplasty, the diastolic limitation of the left ventricle by compression of the LDMF was evaluated by echocardiography.

No impairment of the diastolic dimension (Dd) of the left ventricle could be observed, using either echocardiography or left ventriculography. On

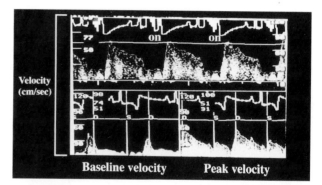

Fig. 2. Coronary blood flow velocity with dynamic cardiomyoplasty

Table 2a. Hemodynamic changes with dynamic cardiomyoplasty (chronic phase)

	DCMP off	DCMP on	% Change	P-Value
AoP (mmHg)				
Systolic	61.5 ± 2.1	83.7 ± 2.2	36.3 ± 2.2	<0.005
Diastolic	47.7 ± 1.8	49.7 ± 1.4	4.4 ± 1.3	<0.05
(Mean)	52.2 ± 1.9	61.3 ± 1.5	17.9 ± 2.6	<0.005
LVP (mmHg)				
Systolic	91.3 ± 1.9	99.1 ± 1.8	8.7 ± 0.9	<0.005
CO (l/min)	1.0 ± 0.0	1.3 ± 0.4	26.6 ± 5.1	<0.005
EF (%)	45.6 ± 1.1	55.4 ± 1.5	20.1 ± 1.5	<0.005

CO, cardiac output; EF, ejection fraction.

Table 2b. Coronary blood flow with dynamic cardiomyoplasty (chronic phase)

	DCMP off	DCMP on	% Change	P-Value
Peak velocity (cm/s)				
Systolic	12.0 ± 0.3	15.5 ± 0.7	29.1 ± 5.7	<0.05
Diastolic	20.4 ± 2.8	22.9 ± 3.5	12.2 ± 3.8	0.05
Total velocity integral				
(Systolic + diastolic)	3.8 ± 0.9	4.4 ± 0.96	21.9 ± 9.1	<0.05

Table 3. Effect of dynamic cardiomyoplasty on left ventricular systolic and diastolic function

Hemodynamic results

DEMP	AoP (mmHg)	LVSP (mmHg)	LVEDP (mmHg)
Off	74.1 ± 4.1	73.0 ± 5.8	5.3 ± 1.6
On	84.9 ± 3.2	83.2 ± 8.6	2.8 ± 1.5
P	<0.05	<0.05	NS

Echocardiographie results

DCMP	Dd (mm)	Ds (mm)	% FS	A/E ratio
Off	44.5 ± 0.7	33.8 ± 1.0	24.0 ± 2.4	0.85 ± 0.09
On	44.5 ± 0.7	27.6 ± 1.2	38.0 ± 2.6	0.90 ± 0.06
P	NS	<0.01	<0.01	NS

LVSP, left ventricular systolic pressure; LVEDP, left ventricular end-diastolic pressure; Dd, diastolic dimension; Ds, systolic dimension; FS, fractional shortening; A/E, atrial kick/early filling.

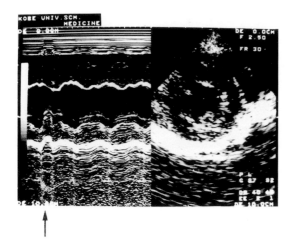

Fig. 3. Echocardiogram of the left ventricle with dynamic cardiomyoplasty. *Arrow*, dynamic cardiomyoplasty (DCMP)

echocardiograms there was no change in the LVDd even with dynamic cardiomyoplasty (44.5 ± 0.7mm, DCMP on or off, Table 3; Fig. 3).

Discussion

Since the report of Carpentier and Chachquies in 1985 [8], dynamic cardiomyoplasty has been carried out on 500 patients with dilated and ischemic cardiomyopathy in many medical centers throughout the world [9–12]. Precise clinical data have been reported for 356 patients. The overall mortality rate in patients classified as New York Heart Association (NYHA) III was 16% and as NYHA IV, 36%. The rate of survival

for longer than 1 year was 70% in NYHA III and 40% in NYHA IV patients. In general, the results obtained have been satisfactory. However, none of these reports has described precisely the effects of dynamic cardiomyoplasty on coronary arterial blood flow and the diastolic dimension of the left ventricle.

In this study, the problem of constrictive pericarditis due to adhesion between the epicardium and the skeletal muscle flap was clarified experimentally. No such impairment was observed. This appears to be the first report in the world on this subject.

Kantrowitz was one of the pioneers who attempted to induce an increase in cardiac output by stimulating a diaphragmatic muscle flap wrapped around the failing heart. Since then, many experimental studies have been carried out in various places. These studies show hemodynamic improvement due to the dynamic cardioplasty. However, no precise data on the coronary blood flow or the diastolic dimension of the left ventricle have been reported. In this study, an increase in the coronary blood flow was evident, and there was no impairment of the diastolic dimension of the left ventricle, in spite of the presence of adhesion.

These results could be due to an increase in both the LVP and the cardiac output, together with a decrease in the LVedp. The contractility of the adhesive muscle flap was shown to reflect the improvements in the hemodynamic parameters. The strong adhesion between the myocardium and the skeletal muscle was evident histologically. This tight adhesion strengthens the contractility of the failing heart. Moreover, we have continued the electrical stimulation for several weeks to achieve durable long-term contractility of the LDMF.

These data indicate the possibility of clinical application of DCMP in the severely ill patient for whom coronary artery bypass grafting and heart transplantation cannot be carried out. However, before clinical application, there are some further problems to be solved, such as the preconditioning of the skeletal muscle to prevent muscle fatigue, and the probability of impairment of the coronary flow in the long-term. Further experimental studies are needed in the near future on these aspects.

References

1. Okada M, Tsukube T, Mukai T, Kashem MA (1995) Role of dynamic cardiomyoplasty for pump failure. Artif Organs Today 4:183–189
2. Tsukube T, Okada M, Mukai T, Kashem MA (1994) Effect of dynamic cardiomyoplasty on coronary blood flow. J Thorac Cardiovasc Surg 108:609–615
3. Sibley D, Millar H, Hartley C, Whitlow P (1986) Subselective measurement of coronary blood flow velocity

using a steerable Doppler catheter. J Am Coll Cardiol 8:1332–1340

4. Serruys PW, Mario CD, Meneveau N, Jaegere PD, Feyter PJD, Emanuelsson H (1993) Intra-coronary pressure and flow velocity with sensor-tip guide wire: a new methodologic approach for assessment of coronary hemodynamics before and after coronary interventions. Am J Cardiol 71:41D–53D

5. Chilian W, Layne S (1990) Ultrasonic measurement of coronary blood flow. Springer, Tokyo, pp 55–72

6. Doucette JW, Corl PD, Payne HM, Flynn AE, Goto M, Nassi M, Segal J (1992) Validation of a Doppler guide wire for intravascular measurement of coronary artery flow velocity. Circulation 85:1899–1911

7. Okada M, Mukai T, Tsukube T (1993) Dynamic cardiomyoplasty as a circulatory assist. Cardiac pacing and electrophysiology today, Simul International, Tokyo, pp 513–519

8. Carpentier A, Chachquies J (1985) Myocardial substitution with a stimulated muscle: first successful clinical case (letter). Lancet I:1267

9. Kantrowitz A, McKinnon W (1959) The experimental use of the diaphragm as an auxillary myocardium. Surg Forum 9:266–268

10. Olsson R, Bunger R, Spaan J (1991) Coronary circulation: the heart and cardiovascular system, 2nd edn. Raven, New York, pp 1393–1425

11. Nakamura K, Glenn W (1964) Graft of diaphragm as a functioning substitute for myocardium: an experimental study. J Surg Res 4:435–439

12. Jatene AD, Moreira LFP, Stolf NAG, Bocci EA, Seferian P Jr, Fernandes PMP, Abensur H (1991) Left ventricular function changes after cardiomyoplasty in patients with dilated cardiomyopathy. J Thorac Cardiovasc Surg 102:132–139

What Is the Ideal Frequency for Skeletal Muscle Ventricle Electrical Stimulation?

Susumu Isoda[1], Robert L. Hammond[2], Huiping Lu[2], Nakajima Hidehiro[2], Henry L. Walters[2], and Larry W. Stephenson[2]

Summary. Cardiac assist using skeletal muscle as an energy source has been utilized as a surgical therapy for heart failure. Although the long-term efficacy of the procedure has been proven, chronic muscle degeneration after several years of electrical stimulation has been reported. Stimulating frequencies around 30 Hz might be higher than is ideal, producing muscular degeneration because of long-term imbalances of energy demand and supply. Using seven skeletal muscle ventricles made of electrically conditioned latissimus dorsi muscle, a 10-min fatigue test was performed with burst frequencies of 20, 33, and 50 Hz, while monitoring stroke work. A frequency of 50 Hz produced initial high performance; however, within two minutes there was serious fatigue resulting in less total energy output than that obtained with 33 Hz stimulation. Although 33 Hz produced a higher total energy output than 20 Hz stimulation, there was greater fatigue with 33 Hz than with 20 Hz stimulation. This suggest a greater imbalance of energy demand and supply during the 33 Hz stimulation. The ideal frequency of stimulation for canine skeletal muscle for cardiac assist may be less than 33 Hz.

Key words: Cardiac assist — Skeletal muscle — Frequency — Fatigue

Introduction

In the field of skeletal muscle powered cardiac assist — including cardiomyoplasty [1,2], aortomyoplasty [3], and skeletal muscle ventricles (SMVs) [4,5] — the type of electrical impulse is essential in maximizing power output. High-frequency stimulation results in higher force [6], which is followed by rapid fatigue wherein the muscle must pay an energy debt. Long-term maximal energy output of skeletal muscle should be regulated by energy input. Although clinical and experimental successes have been reported with skeletal-muscle-powered cardiac assist, degeneration of the muscle tissue after years of electrical stimulation may occur [7–9]. Since excessive contractile demand or imbalance of the energy supply and demand seems to cause fatigue and muscle damage, it is probable that pulse frequencies used for cardiomyoplasty (30 Hz) or SMVs (33 Hz) might be higher than optimal to preserve muscle tissue. There may be a conflict between the goals of higher muscle energy output and longer muscle preservation in the field of cardiac assist with skeletal muscle. We tried to determine the relationship between energy output and the frequency of the intermittent burst electrical stimulation using the SMV. This model enables us to analyze the power output easily.

Materials and Methods

Construction of Skeletal Muscle Ventricles (SMVs)

Seven mongrel dogs (mean 17.9 ± 1.0 kg) were studied. All operations were performed in accordance with the "Guide for the care and use of laboratory animals" (NIH publication No. 85-23, revised 1985). Anesthesia was induced with intravenous thiamylal (12–18 mg/kg) and maintained by inhalation of isoflurane (1%–2%). The left latissimus dorsi muscle (LDM) was dissected preserving the neuromuscular bundle. A bipolar nerve cuff electrode (model 4080; Medtronic, Minneapolis, MN, USA) was placed around the thoracodorsal nerve. The elevated LDM flap was wrapped approximately twice around a polypropylene mandrel with a volume of 20 ml. The muscle was secured to a sewing ring at the base of the mandrel. SMVs were placed within the thoracic cavity, following a partial resection of the left third rib. The electrode was connected to a neurostimulator (Itrel, Model 7421, Medtronic), which was implanted under the left rectus abdominis muscle. The wound was closed in layers and the dog was allowed to recover. SMVs were left without electrical stimulation for three weeks to allow vascular recovery [10]. After the vascular healing period, the stimulator was activated to deliver 2 Hz continuous stimulation. Each pulse had a 210-microsecond duration and 2-V amplitude. Electrical stimulation was continued for six weeks in order to transform the muscle into a fatigue-resistant form [11].

[1] First Department of Surgery, Yokohama City University, School of Medicine, 3-9 Fuku-ura, Kanazawa-ku, Yokohama, Kanagawa 236 Japan
[2] Division of Cardiothoracic Surgery, Wayne State University, Detroit, MI, USA

Measurements

During a second procedure, animals were anesthetized in the same manner as for the first surgery. The left thoracotomy was made removing a left fourth rib. Electrical stimulation was stopped, the mandrel was removed from the SMV, and the orifice of the SMV was exposed and connected to a mock circulation system as previously described [12], which allowed dynamic contraction of the SMVs with preload and afterload to be 40 mmHg and 80 mmHg, respectively. The parameters of the SMV electrical stimulation were as follows: duty cycle = 312 ms on, 695 ms off; voltage 3 V; pulse width 210 μs. Prior to the fatigue test, the performance at each frequency was measured for 10 s to obtain initial values. A fatigue test was performed for 10 min at 60 contractions/min with a burst stimulation at 20, 33, and 50 Hz, consecutively, each followed by a 20-min rest period. The SMV pressure and stroke volume were measured every 2 min for 10 s.

Data Collection and Analysis

The analogue signals were monitored and recorded with a Gould ES 1000B display and recorder (Gould Instruments, Cleveland, OH, USA). The parameters were also digitally sampled using real-time data acquisition software (AT-Codas; Dataq Instruments, Akron, OH, USA) and stored on a personal computer (model 386-20; Northgate Computer Systems, Plymouth, MN, USA). Stored data was analyzed using data playback software (Windaq; Dataq Instruments). All data are expressed as the mean ± standard error of the mean. The statistical significance of differences between values was calculated using the paired Student's t-test (Sigmaplot, Jandel Scientific, Corte Madera, CA, USA). A P value of less than 0.05 was considered significant.

Results

The initial stroke work at 50 Hz was significantly higher than that at 33 Hz, and the initial stroke work at 33 Hz was also significantly greater than that at 20 Hz. At the end of a 10-min fatigue test, the stroke work at all stimulation frequencies was significantly lower than the initial values. The higher frequencies caused a greater percentage (Fig. 1) and absolute decrease in stroke work. At 50 Hz the 60.4% decrease in stroke work was significantly higher than the 37% decrease at 33 Hz or the 25.2% decrease at 20 Hz. The difference in stoke work between the 20 Hz and 33 Hz stimulation was also significant. A fatigue test at 50 Hz demonstrated a steep decrease in stroke work during the

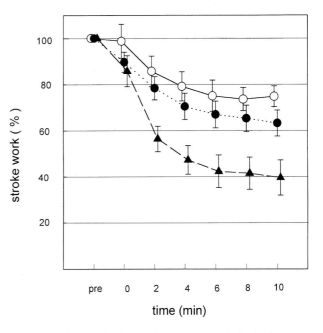

Fig. 1. Stroke work change during fatigue tests. Values are expressed as percent of initial stroke work values. *Error bars* represent standard error of the mean. *Open circles* 20 Hz, *closed circles* 33 Hz, *triangles* 50 Hz

initial 2 min. This was also significantly lower than the stroke work at 33 Hz at 4 min and afterward. The stroke work at 33 Hz was significantly higher than the value at 20 Hz throughout the duration of the fatigue test (data not shown). At 50 Hz, the value of total generated external work during the fatigue test was lower than that at 33 Hz, but the difference did not reach statistical significance ($P = 0.054$). At 20 Hz, the total generated external work was significantly lower than that at 33 Hz.

Discussion

Imbalance of energy supply and demand seems to cause muscle fatigue and finally results in the degeneration of muscle tissue. Energy supply and blood perfusion play a significant role in the process. Since perfusion of the distal part of latissimus dorsi muscle is impaired with ligation of the perforating blood vessels when the flap is elevated [7,10], ischemia is a likely etiology for muscle degeneration. On the other hand, energy demand is primarily controlled by the pattern of electrical stimulation which determines the stroke work at a given preload and afterload. During supramaximal stimulation, adjustable parameters are burst frequency, burst duration, and duty cycle per minute.

Global fatty degeneration of latissimus dorsi muscle 2 to 4 years after cardiomyoplasty [8] suggests that the frequency of electrical stimulation (burst frequency 30 Hz, duration 185 ms, maximum contraction frequency 100 beats per minute) is too high. Fatty degeneration of tissue during long-term studies in the circulation can also occur with SMVs [9] where the muscle the muscle is stimulated with a burst frequency of 33 Hz and a duration of 185 ms (or 30%–45% of the duration of one cardiac cycle) synchronized to every other cardiac contraction.

In summary, although 50 Hz burst stimulation produced greater stroke work initially, the fatigue was rapid with this intense level of burst stimulation. Eventually, the stroke work was less than that for 33 Hz stimulation. Hennig and Lømo [13] reported that the physiological burst frequency of the slow skeletal muscle of rats was from 18 to 21 Hz, for a duration of 5–8 hours daily. Electrically conditioned skeletal muscle has characteristics similar to slow skeletal muscle [14]. Therefore, the frequency of 20 Hz may, in the long run, be ideal, although there is lower initial stroke work and even less stroke work at the end of the 10-min fatigue test when compared with 33 Hz. The stimulation at 20 Hz is probably associated with a lower energy demand and a better energy supply/demand ratio. The ideal frequency to stimulate skeletal muscle for cardiac assist is still unknown, but is likely between 33 Hz and 20 Hz.

References

1. Carpentier A, Chachques JC, Acar C, Relland J, Mihaileanu S, Bensasson D, Kieffer JP, Guibourt P, Tournay D, Roussin I, Grandjean PA (1993) Dynamic cardiomyoplasty at seven years. J Thorac Cardiovasc Surg 106:42–54
2. Moreira LFP, Stolf NAG, Bocchi EA, Bacal F, Pego-Fernandes PM, Abensur H, Meneghetti JC, Jatene AD (1995) Clinical and left ventricular function outcomes up to five years after dynamic cardiomyoplasty. J Thorac Cardiovasc Surg 109:353–363
3. Chachques JC, Haab F, Cron C, Fischer EC, Grandjean P, Bruneval P, Acar C, Jebara VA, Fontaliran F, Carpentier AF (1994) Long-term effects of aortomyoplasty. Ann Thorac Surg 58:128–134
4. Mocek FW, Anderson DR, Pochettino A, Hammond RL, Spanta AD, Ruggiero R, Thomas GA, Lu H, Fietsam R, Nakajima H, Nakajima HO, Krakovsky A, Hooper TL, Niinami H, Colson M, Levine S, Salmons S, Stephenson LW (1992) Skeletal muscle ventricles in circulation long-term: one hundred ninety-one to eight hundred thirty-six days. J Heart Lung Transplant 11:S334–S340
5. Isoda S, Thomas GA, Nakajima H, Lu H, Hammond RL, Nakajima HO, Walters HL III, Stephenson LW (1996) Skeletal muscle ventricle: Frontiers in 1995. Artif Organs 20:114–119
6. Chiu RCJ, Kochamba G, Walsh G, Dewar M, Desrosiers C, Dionisopoulos T, Brady P, Ianuzzo D (1989) Biochemical and functional correlates of myocardium-like transformed skeletal muscle as a power source for cardiac assist devices. J Cardiac Surg 4:171–179
7. Kratz JM, Johnson WS, Mukherjee R, Hu J, Crawford FA, Spinale FG (1994) The relationship between latissimus dorsi skeletal muscle structure and contractile function after cardiomyoplasty. J Thorac Cardiovasc Surg 107:868–878
8. Kalil-Filho R, Bocchi E, Weiss RG, Rosemberg L, Bacal F, Moreira LFP, Stolf NAG, Magalhaes AAC, Bellotti G, Jatene A, Pileggi F (1994) Magnetic resonance imaging evaluation of chronic changes in latissimus dorsi cardiomyoplasty. Circulation 90(2): II-102–II-106
9. Nakajima H, Nakajima HO, Thomas GA, Hammond RL, Mocek FW, Fietsam R, Pochettino A, Lu H, Spanta AD, Isoda S, Stephenson LW (1994) Chronic morphologic changes of skeletal muscle ventricles in circulation. Ann Thorac Surg 57:912–920
10. Isoda S, Yano Y, Jin Y, Walters HL III, Kondo J, Matsumoto A (1995) The influence of a delay on latissimus dorsi muscle flap blood flow. Ann Thorac Surg 59:632–638
11. Mannion JD, Bitto T, Hammond RL, Rubinstein N, Stephenson LW (1986) Histochemical and fatigue characteristics of conditioned latissimus dorsi muscle. Circ Res 58:298–304
12. Bridges CR, Clark BJ III, Hammond RL, Stephenson LW (1991) Skeletal muscle bioenergetics during frequency-dependent fatigue. Am J Physiol 260 (Cell Physiol 29):C643–C651
13. Hennig R, Lømo T (1985) Firing pattern of motor units in normal rats. Nature 314:164–166
14. Pette D, Vrbova G (1992) Adaptation of mammalian skeletal muscle fibers to chronic electrical stimulation. Rev Physiol Biochem Pharmacol 120:115–202

Muscle Blood Pump Driven by Roller Screw Linear Actuator

Masamichi Nogawa[1], Yasushi Sasaki[1], Miyuki Asano[1], Genta Chikazawa[2], Hiroshi Nishida[2], Hitoshi Koyanagi[2], and Setsuo Takatani[1]

Key words: Roller screw linear actuator — Muscle-driven — Ventricular assist device — Blood pump

Introduction

In patients with severe heart failure, the ventricular assist devices (VAD) have proved their usefulness for temporary bridging to heart transplantation and for more permanent usage [1,2]. Patients implanted with the mechanical devices can go home and return to work while waiting for heart transplantation. The currently available mechanical circulatory assist devices, Novacor (Division of Baxter Health Care, Oakland, CA, USA) and TCI (Thermo Cardio Systems, Woburn, MA, USA), both use an external power source, chemical batteries. The skin transformer is used to deliver transcutaneously electrical power inside the body. The external batteries usually last from 7 to 8h before needing to be recharged. As an alternative, biological energy sources such as skeletal muscle power have been also investigated since the 1950s. In 1958, Kantrowitz wrapped the diaphragm around the left ventricle to assist its contraction [3,4]. Although he could not demonstrate adequate performance in assisting the left ventricle, he was successful in augmenting the diastolic pressure by wrapping the diaphragm around the descending aorta as a counterpulsator. In 1973, Kusaba from the Kantrowitz lab was successful in demonstrating left heart assistance by using a burst-signal stimulator. However, the study was stopped after 3h due to fatigue of the muscle. In the 1980s, Stephenson's and Chiu's groups demonstrated that the skeletal muscle can be transformed into fatigue-resistant muscle through proper training [5,6]. Latissimus dorsi (LD) muscles have been used in cardiomyoplasty in a total of 78 patients during 1985–1990, demonstrating potential application in New York Heart Association functional class III patients [7]. Besides the cardiomyoplasty application, the LD muscle has been used to construct a ventricle with built-in valves and to actuate an artificial ventricle inserted beneath the LD as a counter-pulsator [8,9]. However, wrapping of the LD muscle around the heart or insertion of the ventricle beneath the LD muscle resulted in inefficient utilization of the muscle power. Since the muscle contracts in a linear direction, a linear-pull energy converter can provide better utilization of its power. In 1992, Farrar et al. developed a hydraulic linear-pull energy converter and demonstrated its potential application in left heart assistance [10].

In this study, a roller screw linear actuator, together with a computerized evaluation system, has been developed to translate the muscle pull-force for actuation of a left ventricular assist device. This paper summarizes the evaluation of the computerized roller screw linear muscle translation system with human arm muscle and untrained canine latissimus dorsi (LD) muscle.

Muscle-Driven VAD with a Roller Screw Linear Actuator

The design specifications of the muscle-driven VAD are: (1) pump flow of 3–4l/min against 100mmHg afterload, (2) muscle stroke length of 3–5cm, (3) power requirement of 3–5 W, and (4) actuator efficiency greater than 45%. To meet these design specifications, a double-chamber VAD with a roller screw actuator driven by the left and right LD muscles has been designed. A schematic diagram of the VAD is shown in Fig. 1 [11]. The VAD consists of two chambers sandwiching a roller screw linear actuator. Alternate stimulation of the left and right LD muscle will eject one chamber into a common outflow port, while filling the other chamber through a common inflow port. Bilateral alternate stimulation of the LD muscles allows (1) reversal of the roller screw movement, (2) preloading of the unstimulated side muscle, and (3) doubling of the pump flow. The stroke volume of each chamber is designed to be $35cm^3$, with a stroke length of 7mm. The roller screw actuator translates the muscle pull force through winding and unwinding of the cable around the spool attached at each end of the

[1] Yamagata University, Biomedical Systems Engineering, 4-3-16 Joh-nan, Yonezawa, Yamagata 992, Japan
[2] Tokyo Women's Medical College, Cardiovascular Surgery, 8-1 Kawada-cho, Shinjuku-ku, Tokyo 162, Japan

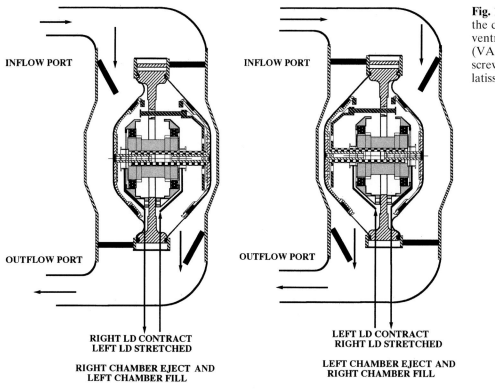

Fig. 1. Schematic diagram of the double chamber ventricular assist device (VAD) driven by the roller screw linear actuator. *LD*, latissimus dorsi (muscle)

INFLOW PORT

INFLOW PORT

OUTFLOW PORT

OUTFLOW PORT

**RIGHT LD CONTRACT
LEFT LD STRETCHED**

**RIGHT CHAMBER EJECT AND
LEFT CHAMBER FILL**

**LEFT LD CONTRACT
RIGHT LD STRETCHED**

**LEFT CHAMBER EJECT AND
RIGHT CHAMBER FILL**

roller screw nut. Turning of the nut through pulling the cable will result in the linear motion of the screw. The contraction of the LD muscle, for example, the left side, will turn the roller screw nut to advance the screw in one direction, while winding the cable on the other side around the other spool. Theoretically, stimulation of the left and right LD muscles alternately at a rate of 50 bpm will result in a pump flow of 3.5 l/min ($35 \, \text{cm}^3 \times$ 2 chambers ×50 bpm), meeting the design requirement. The anatomical placement of the VAD is shown in Fig. 2.

Evaluation with Human Arm Muscle

Initially, the performance of the roller screw actuator was studied with pull exerted by human arm muscle. Figure 3 shows the experimental setup used for this study. The weight was attached to the roller screw to simulate the left pump load. The force developed by the arm muscle and the roller screw displacement were continuously monitored using a load cell and Hall-effect sensor, respectively. The weight simulating the pump load was varied from 5 to 10 kg. The study was conducted at simulated pump rates of 30, 40, 50, and 60 bpm. All the data were digitized and analyzed using a personal computer.

Figure 4 shows the input power, output power, and actuator efficiency as the weight was varied from 5 to

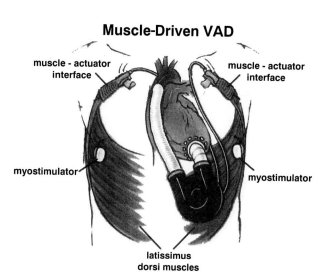

Muscle-Driven VAD

muscle - actuator interface

muscle - actuator interface

myostimulator

myostimulator

latissimus dorsi muscles

Fig. 2. Anatomical placement of the VAD driven by the latissimus dorsi muscles

10 kg. The input (PI) and output (PO) power of the system were computed as

$$PI = \frac{1}{T} \int F_m \cdot v_m \, dt$$

$$PO = \frac{1}{T} \int W \cdot v_w \, dt$$

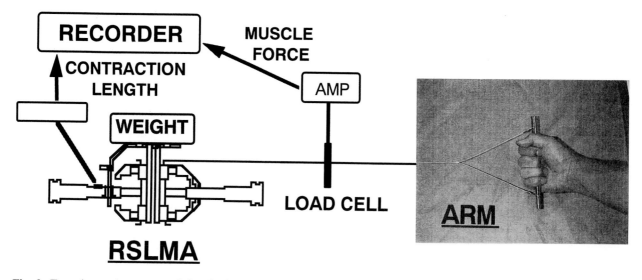

Fig. 3. Experimental set-up used for the human arm muscle study. *AMP*, amplifer; *RSLMA*, roller screw linear muscle actuator

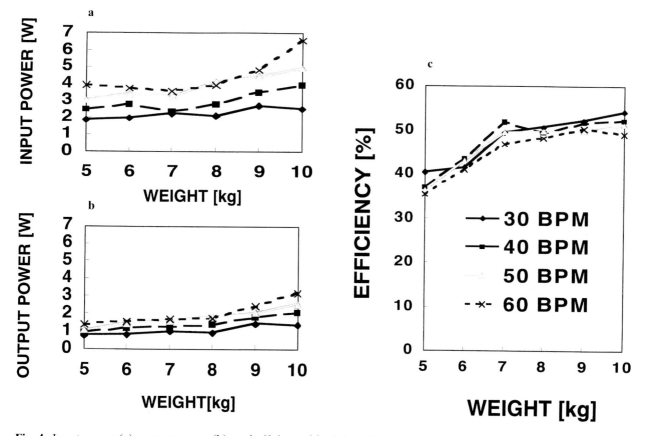

Fig. 4. Input power (**a**), output power (**b**), and efficiency (**c**) of the roller screw actuator in the human arm muscle study

where F_m and W are the muscle force and weight; V_m and V_w are the velocity of the muscle contraction and of the weight movement; and T is the time required to move one full stroke. From these values, the efficiency of the actuator, η, was colculated as $\eta = \dfrac{PO}{PI} \times 100$. According to the results shown in Fig. 4, the actuator efficiency was greater than 50% for weights above

7 kg. Following this study, the double-chamber VAD was assembled and connected in a mock circulatory loop. Both left and right arms were used to actuate the double-chamber VAD. The pump rate vs pump flow is shown in Fig. 5, indicating a flow of 3–4 l/min with a pump rate of 50 bpm.

Untrained Canine Muscle Study

Under anesthesia, a left thorax skin incision was performed to free the left latissimus dorsi muscle of mongrel dogs (weight 15–20 kg). The thoracodorsal attachment of the LD muscle was kept intact, while freeing the distal end from the vertebral region, allowing the muscle to contract toward the thoracodorsal region. Gore-tex velour was sutured to the free end of the muscle to attach the actuator cable. One of the intramuscular stimulating electrodes was placed around the thoracodorsal nerve with the other being placed distally closer to the Gore-tex velour. The muscle was stimulated at 30–60 bpm, with a burst frequency of 30–50 Hz, gate time of 0.3–0.5 s, and burst pulse duration of 0.5–1 ms . Figure 6 shows the experimental set-up for the untrained canine LD muscle study. Figure 7 shows a typical result obtained in one of the animals. The contractile force and muscle stroke length developed were sufficient to drive the VAD against the left pump afterload with the untrained muscle, However, muscle fatigue prevented a long-term study.

Discussion

The newly developed roller screw linear actuator has been evaluated using human arm muscle and untrained canine latissimus dorsi muscle. The human arm muscle study confirmed that the efficiency of the actuator was greater than 45%. Since the power requirement to pump 3–4 l/min blood against an afterload of 100 mmHg is in the range of 1 W, an actuator efficiency of 50% means that the muscle has to generate 2 W of power. According to Jacobs et al. [12], the trained LD muscle can generate 3–4 W of power; this indicates that this actuator can successfully utilize the muscle power. Secondly, the muscle stroke length of the trained LD muscle is in the range of 3–4 cm. The current system required a 6–8-cm muscle stroke length to obtain a 7-mm actuator stroke. However, the muscle stroke length can be reduced by decreasing the spool diameter. Although this will increase the instantaneous muscle force required without changing the overall power requirement, additional study using the smaller diameter spool confirmed that the muscle force requirement was within the allowable range.

In the study with the untrained canine LD muscle, it was confirmed that the properly stimulated LD muscle can generate sufficient power to actuate the left ventricular assist pump. In addition, the ex vivo study with the untrained LD muscle has allowed us to work out various technical problems such as (1) the muscle–actuator interface method, (2) the muscle stimulation protocol, and (3) the surgical procedure. The major obstacle in the untrained muscle study was the muscle

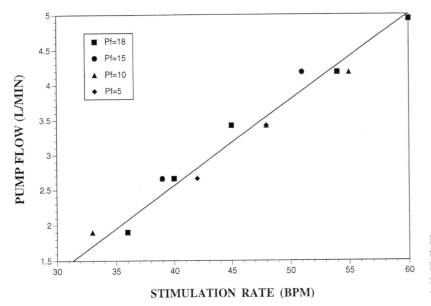

Fig. 5. Pump outflow vs pump rate of the double chamber VAD driven by the human arm muscle. *Pf*, filling pressure for the pump. Pump outflow pressure was kept at 100 mmHg

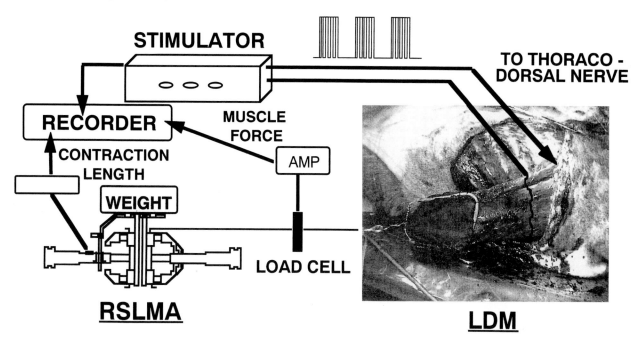

Fig. 6. Experimental setup of the untrained canine latissimus dorsi muscle (*LDM*) study

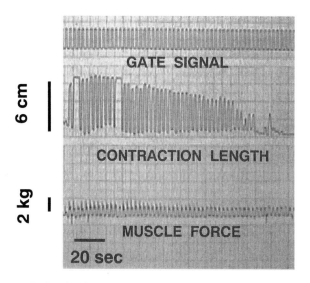

Fig. 7. Stroke length and contraction force of the canine latissimus dorsi muscle

fatigue. During the next phase of this study, therefore, we will work with trained LD muscle in the ex vivo setup, followed by chronic implantation of the VAD.

Acknowledgment. This study was partially supported by a grant-in-aid from the Japan Research Promotion Society for Cardiovascular Diseases, 8-1 Kawada-cho, Shinjuku-ku, Tokyo, Japan.

References

1. Prista JM, Stephen W, Nastala CJ, Gifford J, Conner EA, Brovetz HS, Griffity BP, Portner PN, Kormos RL (1995) Protocol for releasing Novacor left ventricular assist system patients out-of-hospital. ASAIOJ 41(3): M539–M543
2. Cloy MJ, Myers TJ, Stutts LA, Kacris MP, Frazier OH (1995) Hospital charges for conventional therapy vs left ventricular assist system therapy in heart transplant patients. ASAIOJ 41(3):M535–538
3. Kantrowitz A, Kantrowitz A (1953) Surgery 34:678
4. Kantrowitz A (1960) Functioning autogenous muscle used experimentally as an auxiliary ventricle. ASAIO Trans 6:305
5. Chiu RCJ, Walsh GL, Dewar ML, De Simon JH, Khalafalla AS, Ianuzzo D (1987) Implantable extraaortic balloon assist powered by transformed, fatigue-resistant skeletal muscle. J Thorac Cardiovasc Surg 94:694–701
6. Mannion JD, Bitto T, Hammond R, Rubinstein NA, Stephenson LW (1986) Histochemical fatigue characteristics of conditioned canine latissimus dorsi muscle. Circ Res 58:298–304
7. Chiu RCJ (1994) Using skeletal muscle for cardiac assistance. Sci Am Sci Med 1(5):68–77
8. Pochettino A, Mocek F, Lu H, Hammond RL, Spanta AD, Hooper TL, Niinami H, Ruggiero R, Colson M, Stephenson LW (1992) Skeletal muscle ventricles with improved thrombo-resistance: 28 weeks in circulation. Ann Thorac Surg 53:1025–1032
9. Novoa R, Jacobs G, Sakakibara N, Chen JF, Davies C, Cosgrove DM, Golding LR, Nosé Y, Loop FD (1989) Muscle powered circulatory assist device for diastolic counterpulsator. ASAIO Trans 35:408–411

10. Farrar DI, Hill JD (1992) A new skeletal linear-pull energy converter as a power source for prosthetic circulatory support devices. J Heart Lung Transplant 11: S341–S350

11. Takatani S, Takami Y, Nakazawa T, Jacobs G, Nosé Y (1995) Double chamber ventricular assist device with a roller screw linear actuator driven by left and right latissimus dorsi muscles. ASAIOJ 41(3):M475–M480

12. Jacobs G, Novoa R, Davies C, Irie H, Chen J-F, Cosgrove D (1991) Power output of the goat latissimus dorsi in a linear configuration. Proceedings of Cardiovascular Science and Technology Conference, p 80

Circulatory Assistance Using Linear Skeletal Muscle Ventricle

Yukihiro Kaneko, Masahiko Ezure, Hirotaka Inaba, and Akira Furuse

Summary. We have developed a novel type of skeletal muscle ventricle (linear skeletal muscle ventricle: LSMV). The LSMV is powered by linear contraction of the latissimus dorsi muscle which is stretched by regurgitation of the highly pressurized aortic blood into the LSMV during muscle relaxation. The LSMV consists of two cylindrical bellows of different diameters joined by a connector containing a valve. The smaller bellows is connected to the left atrium with another valve, and the larger bellows is connected to the aorta. The latissimus dorsi muscle is attached to the connector so that its contraction pulls the connector to compress the larger bellows and to stretch the smaller bellows.

This study was conducted to investigate the usefulness of the LSMV by evaluating its pumping performance and hemodynamic effect. In acute-phase canine experiments, the LSMV in normal hearts generated a pump output of 199 ml/min, stroke work of 201 mJ, and power output of 137 mW, equivalent to 14.1%, 166%, and 55% of the respective normal canine left ventricular values at an average filling pressure of 4.7 mmHg. In a condition of temporary heart failure induced by propranolol and mannitol, LSMV output, stroke work, and power output were 164 ml/min, 180 mJ, and 91 mW, respectively, equivalent to 15.4%, 185%, and 62% of the respective failing left ventricular values. The LSMV not only assisted systemic circulation but also reduced the workload of the failing left ventricle. The study suggests that the LSMV represents a promising method of skeletal muscle cardiac assistance.

Key words: Skeletal muscle ventricle — Cardiomyoplasty — Assisted circulation — Heart failure

Introduction

Cardiac assistance with autologous skeletal muscle is an attractive surgical treatment for end-stage heart failure. Attempts have focused mainly on the use of the latissimus dorsi muscle (LD) because of its plasticity and bulk. In one form of skeletal muscle cardiac assistance, dynamic cardiomyoplasty (DCMP), the LD is wrapped around the heart and then electrically stimulated in synchrony with systole to augment cardiac contraction. DCMP has been performed in more than 700 patients worldwide as of 1995, and excellent symptomatic improvements have been documented [1].

Another form of skeletal muscle cardiac assistance, the skeletal muscle ventricle (SMV), has been investigated as an auxiliary blood pump driven by skeletal muscle. When the SMV is used as an atrio-aortic bypass pump, filling pressures around the physiological left atrial pressure cannot stretch the muscle adequately, because of low skeletal muscle compliance [2]. Moreover, the filling pressure may fluctuate because the position of the SMV relative to the left atrium change due to postural change of the recipient, resulting in pump output fluctuation (postural fluctuation). When the SMV is used as an aortic counterpulsator or a ventriculo-aortic bypass pump, high filling pressure, although sufficient to stretch the muscle, impedes blood perfusion to the muscle, and thereby causes chronic ischemic damage [3,4]. In addition, the aortic counterpulsator and ventriculo-aortic bypass pump cannot reduce the left ventricular volume load directly. If an applicable muscle stretch system can be developed, a high power output could be achieved with low filling pressure.

For the purpose of harnessing the high power output from the LD in an atrio-aortic bypass type SMV, we designed a new SMV — the linear skeletal muscle ventricle: LSMV — powered by linear contraction of the LD which is stretched by regurgitation of the highly pressurized aortic blood into the LSMV during muscle relaxation. To investigate the usefulness of the LSMV, we evaluated its pumping performance and hemodynamic effect by comparing the LSMV with DCMP.

Materials and Methods

The design of the LSMV has been detailed elsewhere [5]. Briefly, the LSMV consists of two cylindrical bellows of different diameters joined by a connector containing a valve (outflow valve). An additional valve is attached at the other end of the smaller bellows (inflow vale). The smaller bellows is connected to the left atrium, and the larger bellows is connected to the

Department of Cardiothoracic Surgery, Faculty of Medicine, University of Tokyo, Japan aorta. The LD is attached to the connector so that LD contraction pulls the connector towards the aortic end. When the LD contracts, the connector is pulled to compress the larger bellows and to stretch the smaller bellows, causing the outflow valve to close and the inflow valve to open. Blood is thereby drawn from the left atrium into the smaller bellows, while blood in the larger bellows is ejected to the aorta. When the LD relaxes, as blood in the aorta regurgitating into the larger bellows compresses the smaller bellows, the internal pressure in the smaller bellows increases to the level of the aortic pressure, causing the inflow valve to close and the outflow valve to open. Force placed on the connector — the difference between the products of the pressures in the two bellows multiplied by the cross-sectional areas of respective bellows — shifts the connector towards the atrial end, allowing displacement of blood from the smaller bellows to the larger bellows. This motion generates LD preload for the next contraction (Fig. 1).

The LSMVs were constructed in six mongrel dogs weighing 15–23 kg. The larger and smaller bellows — 7.5 cm in length, and 32 and 20 mm in diameter, respectively — were made of vascular grafts (Cooly low-porosity graft, Meadox Medicals, Oakland, NJ, USA). Two valve prostheses were used as the inflow and outflow valves (Fig. 1; inflow valve: 29 mm, St. Jude Medical, St. Paul, MN, USA; outflow valve: Model 2310, 12A, 27 mm, Edwards Laboratories, Santa Ana, CA, USA). A hand-made connector which contained the outflow valve was attached between the adjacent ends of each bellows. Two metal rings which hooped the other ends of the two bellows were anchored to a wooden plate to keep the total length of the LSWV constant.

Each animal was anesthetized with intravenous pentobarbital (40 mg/kg). The left LD was mobilized taking care to preserve the thoracodorsal neurovascular pedicle and the humeral insertion. Two pacing leads (6500, Medtronic, Kerkrade, Netherlands) were sutured to the LD. A left thoracotomy was made, the pericardium was opened, and a sensing lead was sutured to the left ventricle. The left front leg and the plate on which the LSMV was placed were fixed to the operating table, and the caudal tendon of the LD was sutured to the connector. Axial alignment was carefully checked to avoid kinking of each chamber. Heparin (100 U/kg) was given intravenously, and the

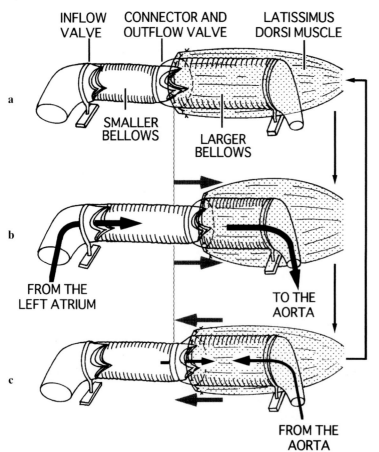

Fig. 1. Motion of the linear skeletal muscle ventricle (LSMV): **a** before contraction, **b** during contraction, and **c** during relaxation

LSMV was filled with saline containing heparin (2 U/ml). The aortic and atrial perfusion cannulas (aortic cannula: 75012 Arterial cannula, DLP, Grand Rapids, MI, USA; atrial cannula: V122-20, Stöckert Instrumente, Munich, Germany) were connected to the free ends of the larger and smaller bellows, respectively, with hand-made connectors. The LSMV was connected to the canine circulation by inserting perfusion cannulas into the descending aorta and the left atrial appendage using the standard cardiopulmonary bypass technique.

Left atrial and aortic pressures were measured by fluid-filled transducers (Cobe, Lakewood, CO, USA). Blood flows in the aortic cannula and in the ascending aorta were measured by a dual-channel Doppler flow meter (T201, Transonic Systems, Ithaca, NY, USA). The volume of blood ejected to the aorta from the LSMV during LD contraction, and the volume of blood regurgitated from the aorta to the LSMV during the preceding LD relaxation period, were defined as the LSMV stroke volume and LSMV regurgitant volume, respectively. Pacing and sensing leads were connected to an electrical stimulator (Fukuda Denshi, Tokyo, Japan) programmed to deliver burst pulses (pulse width of 0.2 ms, frequency of 33 Hz for 200 ms at 5 V) at a rate of 1:3 with the heart beat in a counterpulsatile mode. Measurements were carried out during the nine heart beats before the stimulator was switched on, and during the nine heart beats from the start of the second contraction of the LD. After these measurements, propranolol (3 mg/kg) was administered intravenously to induce temporary heart failure. Subsequently, a mannitol solution of 20% (W/V) concentration was administered to increase the left atrial pressure to 18 mmHg. Hemodynamic measurements before and during LD stimulation were repeated as just described.

Another six mongrel dogs weighing 16–23 kg underwent DCMP. General anesthesia was induced, and the left LD flap was mobilized as described earlier. A left thoracotomy was made, and the LD was introduced into the thoracic cavity through a window made at the second rib. After the pericardium was opened, the LD was wrapped around the heart in a clockwise fashion (posterior to anterior), and fixed to the pericardium. The left front leg was fixed to the operating table. Data were obtained as described with the stimulator switched off. Propranolol and mannitol solutions were then administered, and data were obtained again with the stimulator switched on and off. LSMV stroke work and left ventricular stroke work were defined by the following equations:

$$\text{LSMV stroke work (mJ)} = \{(\text{mean aortic pressure during LSMV ejection (mmHg)} - \text{mean left atrial pressure (mmHg)}) \times \text{LSMV stroke volume (ml)} -$$

$$(\text{mean aortic pressure during LSMV relaxation (mmHg)} - \text{mean left atrial pressure (mmHg)}) \times \text{LSMV regurgitant volume (ml)}\} \times 0.1333$$

$$\text{Left ventricular stroke work (mJ)} = (\text{mean systolic aortic pressure (mmHg)} - \text{mean left atrial pressure}) \times \text{cardiac stroke volume (ml)} \times 0.1333$$

Statistical analysis was performed by the paired or unpaired Student t-test, where appropriate. Significance was set at a P value of less than 0.05.

Results

The LSMV worked properly in all experiments. No mechanical failure, graft kinking, nor graft deformation was seen throughout the study. Gross inspection of the LSMV done at the end of each LSMV experiment revealed sparse clot formation inside the grafts.

Hemodynamic values are summarized in Table 1. Before heart failure induction, the left atrial pressure, aortic pressure, and stroke volume were significantly lower in the LSMV group than in the DCMP group. These differences are attributable to bleeding during LSMV construction because they disappeared as a result of propranolol and mannitol administration.

In normal heart conditions, LSMV output, LSMV stroke work, and LSMV power output were equivalent to 14.1%, 166%, and 55% of the respective normal left ventricular values before LSMV assistance. However, the left atrial pressure and systolic aortic pressure, as well as the left ventricular stroke work and left ventricular power output, remained unchanged when the LSMV was driven. The LSMV assisted systemic circulation but failed to reduce the workload of the normal left ventricle.

After heart failure induction, the LSMV output, LSMV stroke work, and LSMV power output were equivalent to 15.4%, 185%, and 62% of the respective failing left ventricular values before LSMV assistance. The left atrial pressure and systolic aortic pressure, as well as the left ventricular stroke work and power output, decreased significantly as a result of LSMV assistance. The LSMV not only assisted systemic circulation but also reduced the workload of the failing left ventricle. On the other hand, the systolic aortic pressure increased mildly, and the left atrial pressure, mean aortic pressure, stroke volume, and cardiac output remained unchanged as a result of DCMP assistance.

Discussion

The LSMV has, in theory, four beneficial characteristics as compared with the SMVs in which muscle

Table 1. Changes in hemodynamic indices and LSMV function

		Normal heart Assist (−)	Normal heart Assist (+)	Failing heart Assist (−)	Failing heart Assist (+)
Heart rate (beat/min)	LSMV	123 ± 5	123 ± 5	91 ± 3***	92 ± 4
	DCMP	120 ± 9	—	89 ± 4***	90 ± 4
Left atrial pressure (mmHg)	LSMV	4.7 ± 0.6 ⎤*	4.7 ± 0.6	18.0 ± 0.0 —**— 14.8 ± 0.6 ⎤**	
	DCMP	10.2 ± 1.5 ⎦	—	18.0 ± 0.0 18.0 ± 0.4 ⎦	
Mean AoP (mmHg)	LSMV	64.3 ± 3.7 ⎤** —**— 81.5 ± 4.4		61.0 ± 4.0 —**— 79.7 ± 2.9 ⎤**	
	DCMP	92.8 ± 7.7 ⎦	—	62.3 ± 3.7*** 63.5 ± 3.5 ⎦	
Systolic Aop (mmHg)	LSMV	86.2 ± 4.0 ⎤**	84.7 ± 5.1	82.6 ± 4.1 —**— 79.3 ± 3.9	
	DCMP	118.8 ± 8.6 ⎦	—	84.7 ± 5.7*** —*— 87.8 ± 5.3	
Cardiac output (ml/min)	LSMV	1407 ± 72	1407 ± 74	1090 ± 89***	1062 ± 85
	DCMP	1607 ± 55	—	1067 ± 90***	1115 ± 96
Left ventricular stroke work (mJ)	LSMV	126 ± 8 ⎤*	121 ± 6	103 ± 10*** —*— 97 ± 9	
	DCMP	197 ± 18 ⎦	—	107 ± 12*** 117 ± 13	
Left ventricular power output (mW)	LSMV	257 ± 15 ⎤**	247 ± 9	156 ± 15*** —*— 148 ± 13	
	DCMP	386 ± 27 ⎦	—	160 ± 12*** 175 ± 23	
AoP during LSMV ejection (mmHg)			145.3 ± 7.4		134.0 ± 4.5
AoP during LSMV regurgitation (mmHg)			69.3 ± 4.1		60.2 ± 3.5
LSMV stroke volume (ml)			14.7 ± 0.4		14.9 ± 0.9
LSMV regurgitant volume (ml)			9.8 ± 0.3		9.6 ± 0.6
LSMV output (ml/min)			199 ± 13		164 ± 17
LSMV stroke work (mJ)			201 ± 14		180 ± 17
LSMV power output (mW)			137 ± 10		91 ± 8***

LSMV, linear skeletal muscle ventricle; DCMP, dynamic cardiomyoplasty; AoP, aortic pressure.
*$P < 0.05$; **$P < 0.01$; ***$P < 0.05$ as compared with normal heart.

preload is derived from pressure in the left atrium. Firstly, the filling capacity is improved since LD contraction draws blood from the left atrium actively. Secondly, the aortic pressure provides a steady muscle preload despite postural fluctuation. Thirdly, the most appropriate muscle preload and afterload can be determined by calculation based on arterial pressure and on ventricular and outflow chamber diameters. Lastly, as LD power output correlates with LD preload, LD preload correlates with arterial pressure, and arterial pressure correlates with the degree of body activity, the LSMV may have the capability to autoregulate its power output, for instance, by increasing output in proportion to an increase in body activity.

In a normal heart, the LSMV was found to achieve stroke work that exceeded normal canine left ventricular stroke work, at a filling pressure that was lower than normal canine left atrial pressure. In conditions of heart failure, LSMV stroke volume and stroke work were found to be similar to those in the normal heart. This implies that LSMV pump function is relatively independent of the recipient's heart function, and that the LSMV can maintain steady pump function even if the recipient's heart failure worsens. The LSMV regurgitant volume was about tow-thirds of the LSMV stroke volume. Blood regurgitation into the LSMV occurred mainly during cardiac systole, and blood ejection from the LSMV occurred during cardiac diastole. This counterpulsatile action can be expected to assist the failing heart by systolic unloading and diastolic augmentation.

DCMP is currently not applied to New York Heart Association functional class 4 patients because DCMP is not effective enough [1,6]. In this study, the hemodynamic enhancement by LSMV was obviously greater than that by DCMP. This result suggests that the LSMV could be beneficial to patients for whom DCMP treatment is not.

Limitations of this study are as follows. The LDs were neither electrically preconditioned nor given vascular delay, the data were obtained immediately after muscle stimulation. Therefore, the pump performance shown here may differ from that in chronic situations. As the material used and the design of the LSMV were perhaps not optimal, there may be room for improvement in LSMV pump performance.

In conclusion, we have developed a new skeletal muscle ventricle (LSMV) in which the latissimus dorsi muscle is appropriately stretched by regurgitation of blood from the aorta. In a canine experiment, the LSMV not only assisted systemic circulation but also reduced the workload of the failing left ventricle. This study suggests that the LSMV represents a promising method of skeletal muscle cardiac assistance.

References

1. Carpenter A, Chachques JC, Acar C, Relland J, Mihaileanu S, Bensasson D, Keiffer J, Guibourt P, Tourney D, Roussin I, Grandjean PA (1993) Dynamic cardiomyoplasty at seven years. J Thorac Cardiovasc Surg 106:42–54
2. Spotnitz HM, Merker C, Malm JR (1974) Applied physiology of the canine rectus abdominis force–length curves correlated with functional charactaristics of a rectus powered "ventricle": potential for cardiac assistance. ASAIO Trans 20:747–756
3. Badylak SF, Wessale JE, Geddes LA, Tacker WA, Janas W (1992) The effect of skeletal muscle ventricle pouch pressure on muscle blood flow. ASAIO J 38:66–71
4. Gealow KK, Solien EE, Lang GR, Evanson CM, Bianco RW, Chiu RCJ, Shumway SJ (1992) Blood flow to the latissimus dorsi muscle pouch during chronic counterpulsation stimulation. J Heart Lung Transplant 11:S306–314
5. Kaneko Y, Furuse A (1996) Linear skeletal muscle ventricle: a pilot study. Artif Organs 20:156–161
6. Grandjean PA, Austin L, Chan S, Terpstra B, Bourgeois IM (1991) Dynamic cardiomyoplasty: clinical follow-up results. J Card Surg 6:S80–88

Discussion

Dr. Wolner:

We enter now into the discussion. Questions from the auditorium? The first paper, Cardiomyoplasty, who wants to ask Dr. Okada?

Dr. Suga:

Suga, Okayama, to Professor Okada You showed the increasing coronary, sort of, time integral velocity, but I interpreted it as an increase in the coronary flow. Is that OK, to begin with? Coronary flow? And I really wonder why it increases, because you put the mechanical work onto the heart and the heart is actually assisted by that, so I think cardiac work, or performance, may be considerably assisted by a heart. Then, cardiac contraction does not need the coronary flow to the extent that you showed. So, I really wonder, what is the mechanism? What is the reason or mechanism which requires the coronary flow increase?

Dr. Okada:

That's a good question. I have just a few problems in this field of the experimental studies, so I tried to check the hemodynamic changes in the left ventricle and the right ventricle. As shown in this slide, I obtained experimental data that it depends on the increase of the left ventricular pressure and decrease of the left ventricular end diastolic pressure. And, besides increase of the cardiac output, this depends on the increase of the coronary arterial blood velocity.

Dr. Wolner:

Professor Okada, I was a little bit surprised about your results in regards to the hemodynamic improvement with cardiomyoplasty. And as I know the literature, nobody before you was ever able to show such a difference and such a hemodynamic improvement in healthy animals or in animals with chronic failure. What was the trick in your experimental setup that you get such results?

Dr. Okada:

We had no such trick for this experimental study. But we had an acute phase and a chronic phase. We have compared hemodynamic change, but in chronic states there is a bigger effect of the hemodynamics than in the acute stage. It depends on the strong adhesions of the epicardium to the skeletal muscle. It's a very important factor to get enough hemodynamics. But, in the long term follow-up, I heard of some cases in which we had atrophy of the muscle, of the skeletal muscle, over the right ventricle, especially in cases without preconditioning, and 1 year later we had some terminal portion of the muscle we had atrophy. It this case it's enough hemodynamic change.

Dr. Wolner:

Other questions to Professor Okada? If not, then let's proceed to the next paper, Dr. Isoda's paper, Frequency. Dr. Isoda, can you comment a little bit, not only what is the best frequency in regards to the power, what is also, then, Dr. Stephenson's group has a lot of experience with long-term application of such pumps, what is the best frequency in regard to muscle atrophy and muscle degeneration in the long-term follow-up? Have you any results?

Dr. Isoda:

Actually, we don't know really the ideal frequency. We used 25 and 33 Hz and temporarily 50 Hz we used to present a nice pressure wave. But we think that when we see the skeletal muscle ventricles 1 year or 2 year later, as Dr. Okada said, atrophy of skeletal muscle we see, and most of the skeletal muscle tissue is replaced by the adipose tissue, so we think that our stimulation protocol is a little bit too aggressive or perfusion of the skeletal muscle is impaired by some reason. One of the reasons of the impairment of the perfusion of the skeletal muscle is the dissection of the latissimus dorsi muscle. Two-thirds of the latissimus dorsi muscle is perfused by the perforating vessels through the trunk. So when we get the latissimus dorsi muscle we already had two-thirds of the ischemic muscle, and those skeletal muscles are recovered after vascular delay but are not perfect. So we need to save the frequency of the electrical stimulation. I think, in my opinion, 20 Hz is the recommended frequency.

Dr. Kurosawa:

According your data, including ejection fraction and stroke work, in my impression, less than 20 still seems acceptable. What do you think? What's the basic reason why your recommend that between 20 and 33 is ideal?

Dr. Isoda:
Actually, in this study, we didn't check less than 20 Hz; we didn't try. So, I cannot define or decide completely but we could see the stroke work reduction hit the bottom during the fatigue test. In my opinion, that is, we could get a balance of the energy supply and demand. When the stroke work is decreasing, we still didn't get a balance of supply and demand. So, imbalance is happening, so when we see these data I feel that with at least 20 Hz we can get a balance of the energy supply and demand.

Dr. Olsen:
Dr. Isoda, is there something magical about a 2-week postsurgery recovery period before initiating myostimulation?

Dr. Isoda:
It's a similar recovery as actually we proved 3 weeks or 4 weeks later that distal latissimus dorsi muscle perfusion is dramatically improved, but it's not the same level as the proximal portion of the latissimus dorsi muscle. But 2 weeks is practically enough we are thinking, even though we proved 3 weeks or 4 weeks is needed to improve latissimus dorsi muscle perfusion because we used 2 Hz of electrical preconditioning so after 2 weeks of vascular recovery period, 2 Hz is not such aggressive stimulation, and I think it's an acceptable length of vascular healing period.

Dr. Wolner:
OK, thank you. I think we have to proceed to Dr. Mesana's paper, Dynamic Aortomyoplasty. Questions?

Dr. Meyns:
Dr. Mesana, I have to congratulate you that you've shown clinically that the aortomyoplasty increased diastolic blood pressure, but I wonder, of course, did you, in these severely sick patients, measure any change in filling pressures? Did you measure any changes in heart dimension, cardiac output, ejection fraction? Did it change anything?

Dr. Mesana:
We found an improvement, a small improvement of filling pressure, but ejection fraction, mainly, was improved in the first case. As you observed, we had four cases. One is more than 1 year after the operation. Two others died after the operation, and the last one is now 4 to 5 months, and, unfortunately, we cannot do a lot of things to him because he had preoperative and

now he has postoperatively also very severe renal insufficiency which was not dependent from the heart failure, so we were limited in investigation. We didn't do many investigations on him but we do not expect that it should be a very high improvement of that sort.

Dr. Jarvik:
Yes, you showed, I think, it was data from your fourth patient where you showed very clear pressure change with counterpulsation at 3 to 1. And then you showed the flow, Doppler flow data, on the same patient, and that indicated, as I read that slide, that there was a variation of about 200 cc per minute in flow between something like 2.8 and 3 liters a minute during the counterpulsation beat. Now, if you are counterpulsing that way, every second or third beat, and if you have no valve in the system, it would seem to me the net contribution to flow is very trivial, could not be more than perhaps a tenth of a liter augmentation, if that much. And I find it almost unbelievable that that could have had any clinical effect to improve the patient, so I'd like you to tell us what you really think the clinical effectiveness is there, and how can it be true that such a small amount of hemodynamic effectiveness could alter the course of the patient.

Dr. Mesana:
Well, we were not able to demonstrate it, of course. I think the counterpulsation was not enough on this patient. We did not see enough diastolic augmentation, and I think that probably you are right, it's not enough, that's why the patient was improved clinically but he will not be, probably, improved in the long period of time. But, the way we have to think is probably to improve the counterpulsation, I mean the length and level of counterpulsation.

Dr. Jarvik:
It would seem that prior to doing a procedure like this there should be a rationale where if it works optimally the hemodynamic effect could be enough to be worthwhile, and the whole aspect of that, the size of the muscle wrap, the size of the aorta, and the likeliness of hemodynamic effectiveness seem so small, I would wonder why that should be done at all.

Dr. Mesana:
That's your opinion.

Dr. Wolner:
Dr. Olsen.

Dr. Olsen:
Dr. Mesana, you implant the myostimulator some 1 to 2 weeks postsurgery. When do you actually start stimulating the muscle?

Dr. Mesana:
Two weeks after surgery. But we do a special simulation protocol. Every 1 week we increase the number of spikes. We don't do as we do cardiomyoplasty every 2 weeks, we do one every 1 week, so we shorten the total length of simulation protocol.

Dr. Olsen:
You showed a nice slide of your diastolic augmentation using your aortomyoplasty. However, I'm not sure you're advocating this ischemic cardiomyopathy, and you don't have any afterload reduction such as a balloon pump. I'm not quite sure if augmenting diastolic pressure will "increase" your coronary blood flow, especially if you did not do any revascularizations to the areas that are "ischemic."

Dr. Wolner:
Perhaps, Dr. Mesana, I can contribute with an historic case. I think '74 or '75, long before transplantation and all these devices, we treated a patient with ischemic cardiomyopathy at that time 6 or 8 weeks with an intraaortic balloon pump and what we have done, at that time, we implanted this balloon surgically. So we implanted him through the iliac artery via the subcutaneous skin tunnel and the patient, I remember, improved dramatically. However, after 6 weeks, we got an infection, so we had to remove the whole device and then a few weeks later the patient died, So, I think that's clear indication that long-term counterpulsation can help, and I'm wondering that this concept is not now in our armentarium. Like Dr. Jarvik, I have also from my long experience with counterpulsation some concerns that such a small and more or less no augmentation of diastolic pressure can help such patients with severe congestion, but you should try to get a much better augmentation and, I think, unloading of the left ventricle.

Dr. Mesana:
You know, surgery is not purely research, or lab, or engineering. Well, you cannot say if you just see a small counterpulsation that the operation does not work. The problem is that the muscle is revascularizing in a certain way. You do the operation and the patient's condition may change, and you cannot assume that for every patient we had always the same status of the muscle. Perhaps you can do another patient and have a very strong counterpulsation if this patient had a very simple postoperative course with no drugs and no vasoconstriction and at that time the operation works very well. And we do see this in the cardiomyoplasty, because some patients do very well after the operation. They have a very nice muscle, probably, a few weeks after the operation and it goes

well. So you cannot say: Oh, aortomyoplasty does not work because we just see this amount of percentage. It's not mathematics because you are not sure how is the muscle 2 weeks after the operations. And that's the big point with every operation that uses the skeletal muscle, that people just think muscle is like a mechanical device. It's not a mechanical device. You are sure what you have done at the operation, but after the operation there is some uncertainty. It's not engineering, it's surgery.

Dr. Olsen:
It is mathematics.

Dr. Mesana:
No.

Dr. Olsen:
It is. There is a physical amount of work that has to be done. There has to be a physical theory. It has to have adequate stroke volume; it has to augment coronary flow; it has to increase filling of the ventricle or increase ventricular performance somehow. There has to be a mathematical rationale behind it, which says that if it does what you think it will do, that effect is sufficient to be beneficial. I think that is crucial for it to be an ethical thing to do.

Dr. Isoda:
In my opinion, about the performance of the aortomyoplasty device, I can think it is similar to SMV. Maybe aortic wall can reduce some effect of the counterpulsation but I think our skeletal muscle ventricle is easy to measure its performance and you use it outside the aorta. Aortic counterpulsation you make, and, in our calculation, our SMV has a performance of one-ninth to one-third of left ventricle performance, it has. So, I assume that your aortomyoplasty has the performance of such a level. Of course, the individual patient has a different performance, but we measure and you use it, that's fine, I think. It's mathematics, I also think.

Dr. Kurosawa:
Dr. Mesana, the patient may occasionally have aortic wall sclerosis or something. If the patient has such an aortic wall change, including a sclerosis or calcification, your method is still applicable?

Dr. Mesana:
What, you shouldn't do the operation?

Dr. Kurosawa:
If the calcification or sclerosis is very severe in the region of the aortic wall, what do you think?

Dr. Mesana:
I think you must check that before the operation with the . . . that's what we did, with the scan. CT scan.

Dr. Kurosawa:
Is there any question? We have a very limited time so we would like to move to the final topics by Dr. Kaneko. Are there any questions? Yes, please.

Dr. Harasaki:
Possibly, I didn't' follow very well, but I wonder when the second valve in your system opens? There is a schematic drawing on page 49 which indicates that the smaller bellows is filled with left atrial pressure which is 18 mmHg, and then the blood should move to the large bellows against the pressure gradient.

Dr. Kaneko:
Not against the pressure gradient, because when the muscle relaxes blood in the aorta regurgitates into the larger bellows.

Dr. Harasaki:
Yes.

Dr. Kaneko:
Then, the internal pressure of the larger bellows increases and larger bellows elongates.

Dr. Harasaki:
Yes.

Dr. Kaneko:
So, the internal pressure of the smaller bellows increases.

Dr. Harasaki:
With what pressure? With what force?

Dr. Kaneko:
With the force on the connector moving to compress the smaller bellows.

Dr. Harasaki:
Is that the pressure in the larger bellows which is to be 120 mmHg, and to open the valve against this pressure?

Dr. Kaneko:
Pressure in the smaller bellows increases to the level of the aortic pressure by the compression of the connector, and the valve opens.

Dr. Harasaki:
That's what I don't understand. But the compression pressure is 120 mmHg, right?

Dr. Kaneko:
Yes.

Dr. Harasaki:
And then this blood pressure in the small bellows has to open the valve against this pressure, and then the forward blood-flow follows.

Dr. Kaneko:
Because of the difference of cross-sectional areas of the two bellows, the smaller bellows is compressed by the force of aortic blood regurgitation into the larger bellows (and pressure in the smaller bellows surpasses that in the larger bellows.)

Dr. Harasaki:
OK. Let me ask this way. You measure the flow through this ventricle, right?

Dr. Kaneko:
Yes, I measured the flow in the SMV.

Dr. Harasaki:
Where did you measure the flow?

Dr. Kaneko:
The outflow. Outflow to the aorta. I measured the flow in the tube connecting the larger bellows and the aorta.

Dr. Harasaki:
So there is a possibility that you are measuring the volume which has been regurgitating from the aorta to the large bellows.

Dr. Kaneko:
But the volume ejected to the aorta was larger than the volume regurgitated to the larger bellows, so there is forward flow from the left atrium to the aorta.

Dr. Harasaki:
How do you know?

Dr. Kaneko:
I measured.

Dr. Harasaki:
Both regurgitant flow and the forward flow?

Dr. Kaneko:
Yes.

Dr. Harasaki:
I see. OK. So when you say that the stroke output volume is 164 ml, that is a combination of these flows?

Dr. Kaneko:
The difference...the difference between the regurgitant volume and the ejected volume.

Dr. Harasaki:
I see. But I still don't understand why the valve can open against the pressure, with which the small bellow is being pressurized.

Dr. Kaneko:
But it did open. But the valve did open in the experiment, so I think I am correct.

Dr. Kurosawa:
Are there any other questions? May I ask one question? During the filling phase of the larger bellows, you mentioned two flows occurred from the aorta. One is from the aorta and the other is from the smaller one. So how about a balance of the two flows?

Dr. Kaneko:
Forward flow is one-third of the total flow — that is, regurgitant volume was two-thirds of the total ejected volume, therefore regurgitant volume was twice as large as the forward flow.

Dr. Kurosawa:
Twice.

Dr. Harasaki:
Possibly, it might be more effective if you put the second valve at the outlet of the large bellows.

Dr. Kaneko:
No, because if you put the outflow valve near the aorta you can't use the power of highly pressurized aortic blood. We have to use, in that pump, the energy of highly pressurized aortic blood regurgitating into the larger bellows. That is the source of preload for the LD muscle.

Dr. Harasaki:
It is understandable that this pump must get some preload energy, and for that the valve should not be put in the outflow position. Is this correct? If there is a valve, then you cannot get the energy, correct?

Dr. Kaneko:
Yes.

Dr. Wolner:
Of that question, I must confess that I have also difficulties to understand the system. It doesn't matter. Perhaps personal discussion will solve the problem.

Part VI
Pathophysiology

Mechanoenergetics of Natural Hearts: Contractility, Mechanical Energy, Oxygen Consumption, and Efficiency

Hiroyuki Suga[1], Hiroki Yamaguchi[1], Junichi Araki[1], Shunsuke Suzuki[1], Juichiro Shimizu[1], Hiromi Matsubara[1], Osamu Kawaguchi[2], Hitoshi Yaku[3], and Miyako Takaki[4]

Summary. This review briefly summarizes the essence of cardiac mechanoenergetic studies extensively carried out for the last three decades by the senior author Suga and his co-workers. This research began with his proposal of E_{max} (end-systolic maximum elastance) as an index of ventricular contractility on the basis of the left ventricular (LV) pressure–volume (P–V) relationship in canine hearts and its time-varying elastance model. Using this model, he proposed PVA (systolic P–V area) as a conceptually novel and sound measure of the total mechanical energy generated by LV contraction. We then experimentally found in canine hearts that PVA closely correlates with LV myocardial O_2 consumption (VO_2) at a given E_{max} and that the VO_2–PVA relation shifts up and down with increases and decreases, respectively, in E_{max}. The VO_2–PVA relation indicates the O_2 cost of PVA (its reciprocal: contractile efficiency) and separates VO_2 into the PVA-independent and PVA-dependent components. The PVA-independent VO_2-E_{max} relation indicates the O_2 cost of E_{max}. Our extensive research has indicated that this VO_2–PVA–E_{max} framework is a novel paradigm to characterize the mechanoenergetics of normal and pathological hearts in a manner entirely different from the other conventional methods. Among its various applications, this mechanoenergetic framework has already elucidated the VO_2-saving effect of cardiac mechanical assistance, proving its potential usefulness to the advancement of artificial heart research.

Key words: Heart — Ventricle — Contractility — Pressure–volume relation — Myocardial O_2 consumption

Introduction

How to characterize the mechanoenergetics of the heart has long been, and still is, one of the hot topics in cardiovascular medicine [1–6]. Mechanical contraction is a process of converting free energy of ATP into mechanical energy by crossbridge (CB) cycling which is triggered by the sarcoplasmic free Ca^{2+} in the excitation–contraction (E–C) coupling following membrane excitation. Beside CB cycling, the Ca^{2+} handling consumes a considerable amount of ATP. Membrane excitation, however, consumes a relatively small amount of ATP above basal metabolism.

Although these individual subcellular mechanisms have been much elucidated, mechanical determinants of myocardial energetics in terms of O_2 consumption or ATP have not completely been accounted for by those subcellular elementary terms. Since we have been interested in a better understanding of cardiac performance in the circulatory system, we have continued to explore cardiac mechanoenergetics from a macroscopic or systems viewpoint [1–6]. We believe that knowledge of the mechanoenergetics of natural hearts will facilitate better understanding of failing hearts, not only alone, but also under artificial mechanical assistance, as well as leading to better design of artificial hearts and assist devices.

History

In the late 1960s, Suga, the senior author of this review, scrutinized left ventricular (LV) pressure–volume (P–V) relations at end-systole, end-diastole, and other times of cardiac cycles under various loading conditions in canine hearts. First, he discovered that the P–V loops could be enveloped by a virtually straight line called the end-systolic P–V relation (ESPVR), as shown in Fig. 1. Second, he observed that the instantaneous P–V relation increased in slope during contraction (isovolumic contraction phase and ejection phase) and decreased in slope during relaxation (isovolumic relaxation phase and filling phase), and also shown in Fig. 1. When he plotted these changes in the slope [i.e., $E(t) = P(t)/V(t)$] as a function of time, he obtained mutually superimposable curves (Fig. 1). The peaks (E_{max}) of these curves correspond to the end-systolic points of the P–V loops. On the basis of these observations, he proposed a time-varying elastance model $E(t)$ of a contracting cardiac chamber by the analogy of a variable elastance (inverse capacitance) [7–9]. Third, he found that the

[1] Department of Physiology II, Okayama University Medical School, 2 Shikatacho, Okayama 700, Japan
[2] Department of Cardiothoracic Surgery, Nagoya University School of Medicine, Nagoya, Aichi, Japan
[3] Department of Surgery II, Kyoto Prefectural University of Medicine, Kyoto, Japan
[4] Department of Physiology II, Nara Medical University, Nara, Japan

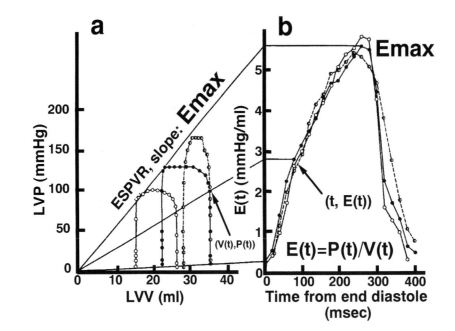

Fig. 1. Left ventricular pressure–volume (P–V) diagram and time-varying elastance. **a** left ventricular pressure (*LVP*)–volume (*LVV*) loops of three differently loaded contractions in a stable control contractile state in an in situ canine heart. The *left upper* (end-systolic) *shoulders* of these P–V loops fall on a line called *ESPVR* (end-systolic P–V relation). Isochronic P–V data points of these P–V loops also fall on different lines. The *slopes* of these isochronic P–V lines increase during contraction and decrease during relaxation. The ESPVR corresponds to the P–V line with the maximal slope (E_{max}). **b** the increases and decreases of the slope of the P–V relation with time during contraction and relaxation. $V(t)$, $P(t)$, $E(t)$; volume, pressure, and elastance at time t

linear slope of the ESPVR or E_{max} increased by positive inotropism and decreased by negative inotropism, as shown in Fig. 2. This finding qualified E_{max} as an index of contractility [7–9].

Although several circulatory system modellers by then had intuitively adopted a time-varying capacitance or elastance model of the heart, none had validated their models in a physiologically sound manner [7–9]. Suga reconfirmed the $E(t)$ model after joining the late Dr. Kiichi Sagawa at the Johns Hopkins University in the 1970s [10–14]. Although almost 30 years have passed since the proposal of the $E(t)$ model, no better model of ventricular global performance has yet been accepted.

End-Systolic P–V Relation (ESPVR) and E_{max}

Figure 2 shows a representative example of P–V loops in a control contractile state before epinephrine and an enhanced contractile state during administration of epinephrine in an in situ canine LV [12]. The left upper corners of the P–V loops under varied loading conditions in a given contractile state fall on or near a straight slant line called the ESPVR, as shown in Fig. 2a,b [12–14]. We have recognized that both ESPVR

lines intercept the volume axis virtually at the small positive dead volume V_0. The shoulders of those P–V loops fall on a steeper ESPVR in an enhanced contractile state, as shown in Fig. 2c, and on a less-steep ESPVR in a depressed contractile state (not shown). From these results, we have concluded that the slope of the ESPVR sensitively changes with inotropism. Therefore, the slope of the ESPVR quantifies the end-systolic elastance of the ventricular chamber. This finding is the basis of Suga's proposal of E_{max} as an index of ventricular contractility [7–14].

Soon after the publication of E_{max} [12,13], cardiologists started clinical application of E_{max} [15–17]. Thereafter, more investigators tested E_{max} with various results. The majority supported the utility, feasibility, and advantages of E_{max}, but some encountered difficulties and limitations with E_{max} application. These limitations include the difficulty of performing accurate ventricular volumetry, the nonlinearity of ESPVR, a negative V_0, the load-dependence of ESPVR, the difficulty in normalizing E_{max} for heart size, etc. [10,11,14]. Despite these problems, the E_{max} concept has gradually spread worldwide and is still favored conceptually as well as practically by many groups as a largely load-independent index of contractility of a cardiac chamber [11].

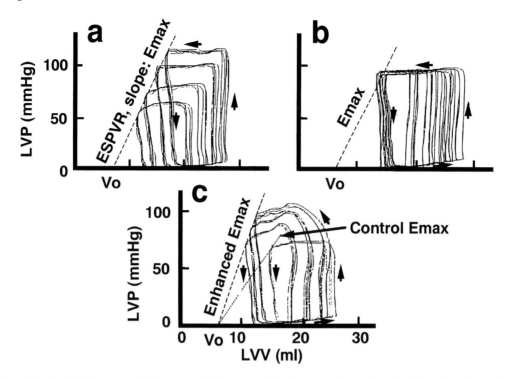

Fig. 2. Left ventricular (*LV*) pressure (*P*)-volume (*V*) loops of contractions under different conditions of both preload and afterload (**a**) and preload alone (**b**) in a stable contractile state and in an enhanced contractile state with epinephrine (**c**). *Arrows* indicate the direction of rotation of a P–V working point on P–V loops. V_o is a dead volume where peak systolic pressure is zero. E_{max} is the slope of the end-systolic P–V relation (*ESPVR*)

The E_{max} concept has also been applied to ventricular wall regions and shown to be useful for comparing end-systolic elastances between different regions with different contractilities [18].

Systolic P–V Area (PVA) and Myocardial Energetics

Using the time-varying elastance model of the ventricle, Suga proposed another innovative concept in 1976: that the total mechanical energy of ventricular contraction could be quantified as a specific area in the P–V diagram [19]. Figure 3 is a schematic illustration of the time-varying P–V relation (Fig. 3a,b) which is the basis of the time-varying elastance model of the ventricle (Fig. 3c). Figure 3d,e illustrates the specific area in the P–V diagram, "systolic P–V area," abbreviated as PVA, representing the total mechanical energy that the ventricle has generated in an isovolumic contraction (Fig. 3d) or an ejecting contraction (Fig. 3e). PVA is the sum of mechanical potential energy (PE) and external mechanical work (EW). The PVA concept is physically sound, but its physiological validity had to be examined experimentally. Suga and co-workers then hypothesized that PVA in the real ven-

tricle would somehow correlate with myocardial O_2 consumption (*VO_2*), which represents the total energy utilization of the heart under obligatorily aerobic conditions [19–21].

Suga and co-workers then tested this hypothesis extensively in the excised, cross-circulated canine heart preparation [1–6,20–32]. Its LV was connected to a custom-made volume servo pump. Its coronary flow and arteriovenous O_2 content difference were accurately and continuously measured with an electromagnetic flowmeter and a custom-made photospectrometric O_2-content difference analyzer placed in the cross-circulation tubing. VO_2 was obtained as the product of mean coronary flow and arteriovenous O_2 content difference. It was divided by heart rate to obtain VO_2 per beat in a steady state. Both VO_2 and PVA are energy quantities with equivalence of $1\,ml\,O_2 = 20\,J$ and $1\,mmHg \cdot ml = 1.33 \times 10^{-4}\,J$, where J (joule) is the SI unit of energy.

Figure 4 is a representative example of an experimentally obtained relation between LV VO_2 and PVA on a per-beat basis. Figure 4a shows data plots in isovolumic contractions at different preloads. Figure 4b shows data plots in variously preloaded and afterloaded ejecting contractions in the same canine LV in the same stable contractile state (constant E_{max}).

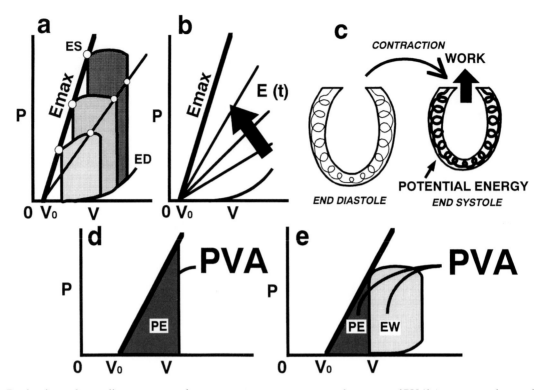

Fig. 3. Derivation of systolic pressure–volume area as a measure of total mechanical energy of ventricular contraction. Schematic illustration of three ventricular pressure (*P*)–volume (*V*) loops and their E_{max} line in a stable contractile state (**a**); time-varying elastance *E*(*t*) to simulate a family of instantaneous P–V relations (**b**); and the time-varying elastance model at end-diastole and end-systole (**c**). The

pressure–volume area (*PVA*) represents the total mechanical energy of an isovolumic contraction (**d**) and an ejecting contraction (**e**). PVA consists of the sum of potential energy (*PE*) and external work (*EW*), if any. V_0, dead volume at which end-systolic pressure is zero; *ES*, end-systole; *ED*, end-diastole

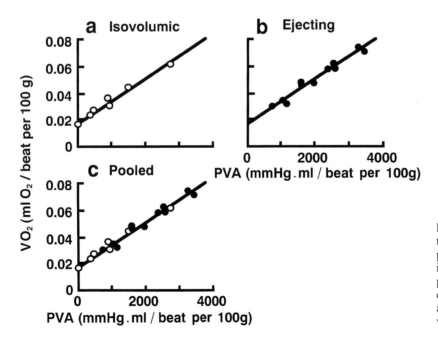

Fig. 4. Relationship between left ventricular O_2 consumption (*VO₂*) and pressure–volume area (*PVA*) of isovolumic contractions at different preloads (**a**) and ejecting contractions at different preloads and afterloads (**b**) in a stable contractile state in a canine left ventricle. **c** pools all the data in **a** and **b**

Figure 4c superimposes these two data sets. LV VO_2 linearly correlates with PVA over a wide range of preload and afterload in a stable contractile state in a given LV [3]. This has been reconfirmed by a series of studies using various types of contractions [1–6,20–32]. The empirical equation that we have obtained is $VO_2 = a \cdot PVA + b$. The $a \cdot PVA$ is the PVA-dependent fraction of VO_2 and coefficient a is the slope of the relation. The reciprocal of a may be called the "contractile efficiency" of CB cycling from PVA-dependent VO_2 to PVA when it has been obtained at a stable E_{max}. Constant b is the PVA-independent fraction of VO_2 and corresponds to the VO_2 of unloaded contraction [1–6,20–32]. It consists of basal metabolism and Ca^{2+} and Na^+ handling energy, of which Ca^{2+} handling energy is coupled to E_{max}.

Figure 5 is a representative set of experimentally obtained VO_2–PVA relations in the control state (Fig. 5a) and in an enhanced contractile state (enhanced E_{max}) with epinephrine (Fig. 5b) in the same canine LV at the same atrial pacing rate [3]. Figure 5c superimposes the data plots in Fig. 5a,b. Epinephrine enhanced E_{max} and elevated the VO_2–PVA relation in a parallel manner. Various positive inotropic agents and interventions enhanced E_{max} and simultaneously yielded similar parallel elevations of the VO_2–PVA relation [1–6,23,31]. They include isoproterenol, norepinephrine, dobutamine, denopamine, calcium, ouabain, paired pulse stimulation, and several first-generation new cardiotonic agents such as milrinone, amrinone, sulmazole, vesnarinone, DPI 201-106, pimobendam, and EMD-53998 [1–6]. Various negative inotropic agents and interventions such as

Ca^{2+}-antagonists (verapamil, nifedipine), β-blockers (propranolol, nipradilol), capsaicin, anesthetics (pentobarbital sodium, isoflurane), and low coronary perfusion (to 50mmHg) depressed E_{max} and lowered the VO_2–PVA relation in a parallel manner [1–6,23,31].

From these results, we expanded the first empirical equation to $VO_2 = a \cdot PVA + c \cdot E_{max} + d$, where $c \cdot E_{max} + d$ has replaced b. The $c \cdot E_{max}$ term is the E_{max}-dependent fraction of the PVA-independent VO_2 and d is VO_2 for basal metabolism and Na^+ handling for membrane excitation at zero PVA and E_{max} [1–6].

We interpreted the terms of the empirical equation as follows. $a \cdot PVA$ represents the energy utilization primarily for CB cycling [1–6]. $c \cdot E_{max}$ represents the energy utilization primarily for active transport of ions (mostly Ca^{2+} handling, but also Na^+, K^+, and H^+ handling) in the excitation and E–C coupling. $c \cdot E_{max}$ contains virtually no energy for residual CB cycling, if any, at zero PVA [5]. Na^+ handling for the membrane excitation is only 1% of total VO_2 [1]. However, Na^+ handling energy coupled with Na^+/Ca^{2+} exchange should be included in $c \cdot E_{max}$ and considered as part of Ca^{2+} handling energy [28–30].

We also confirmed that basal metabolic VO_2 under KCl arrest was insensitive to positive and negative inotropic agents and preload [24]. Therefore, the increases in PVA-independent VO_2 with E_{max} are primarily attributable to increases in the VO_2 component for Ca^{2+} handling in the E–C coupling. This Ca^{2+} handling seems to involve primarily the sarcoplasmic reticulum (SR) Ca^{2+} pump, and secondarily the combination of the Na^+/Ca^{2+} exchanger and the Na^+-K^+ pump.

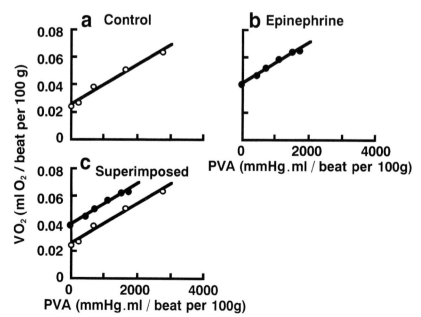

Fig. 5. Relationship between left ventricular O_2 consumption (VO_2) and pressure–volume area (PVA) of variously loaded contractions in control (**a**) and an enhanced contractile state (**b**) in a canine left ventricle. **c** superimposes all the data in **a** and **b**

Figure 6 schematically shows the VO_2–PVA relationship of variously loaded contractions in a stable control contractile state (Fig. 6a) and in three different contractile states (or E_{max} levels) (Fig. 6b). Note that the VO_2–PVA relation ascends with an increase in E_{max} and descends with a decrease in E_{max} in a parallel manner [1–6]. Figure 6c relates PVA-independent VO_2 (b) with E_{max}. Slopes a and c mean the O_2 costs of PVA and E_{max}, respectively. These costs mean O_2 costs for unit increments in PVA and E_{max}. The parallelism of the VO_2–PVA relations for different E_{max} levels means no change in the O_2 cost of PVA with E_{max} [1–6].

O_2 Cost of PVA and O_2 Cost of E_{max}

We have found that most inotropic agents shift the VO_2–PVA relation without affecting the O_2 cost of PVA (Fig. 6, slope a) [1–6]. Upward and downward shifts of the VO_2–PVA relation with E_{max} by these inotropic interventions mean a positive O_2 cost of E_{max}. Moreover, the O_2 cost of E_{max} was comparable among most positive and negative inotropic interventions [1–6]. These results are intriguing because we had ex-

pected different responses of the O_2 costs of PVA and E_{max} to different inotropic mechanisms (Ca^{2+} channel, β stimulation, cAMP, Ca^{2+} sensitivity, myosin ATPase activity, etc.) among interventions. No difference in the O_2 cost of PVA may reflect no net effect of these inotropic interventions on CB cycling kinetics, although they may affect the E–C coupling in different ways. No difference in the O_2 cost of E_{max} for different inotropic interventions seems to reflect no net effect on the relation between E_{max} and Ca^{2+} handling energy. These results are not yet predictable by integration of the analytical knowledge available at present.

There are, however, several exceptional inotropic interventions that showed an abnormal O_2 cost of E_{max} [1–6]. Cardiac cooling from 36°C to 29°C enhanced E_{max} by 70% but did not elevate the VO_2–PVA relation nor change its slope [25]. In contrast, cardiac warming from 36°C to 41°C depressed E_{max} but did not lower the VO_2–PVA relation nor change its slope [26]. These results mean that the O_2 cost of E_{max} for graded cooling and warming is virtually zero because changing E_{max} by temperature is not accompanied by any change in PVA-independent VO_2. This suggests no change in the amount of Ca^{2+} to be handled in the E–C coupling despite the positive and negative inotropism of tem-

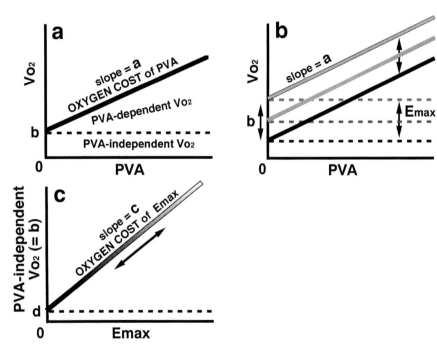

Fig. 6. VO_2–PVA-E_{max} framework. Relationship between left ventricular O_2 consumption (VO_2) and pressure–volume area (PVA) of variously loaded contractions in a stable contractile state (**a**) and in three different contractile states (E_{max}) (**b**). **c** relates the changes in PVA-independent VO_2 (b) against E_{max}. The slope (a) of the VO_2–PVA relation at a given E_{max} means the O_2 cost of PVA. The VO_2–PVA relation divides VO_2 at b into PVA-independent and PVA-dependent components of VO_2. The slope (c) of the PVA-independent VO_2–E_{max} relation means the O_2 cost of E_{max}. Its intercept (d) means basal metabolism. The *arrows* correspond to E_{max} changes

perature [25,26]. However, the O_2 cost of E_{max} was augmented at 41°C [26]. This indicates that the apparent insensitivity of PVA-independent VO_2 to warming, despite its negative inotropism, derives from a gradual increase in the O_2 cost of E_{max} by graded hyperthermia. It also suggests that the apparent insensitivity of PVA-independent VO_2 to cooling, despite its positive inotropism, derives from a gradual decrease in the O_2 cost of E_{max} by graded hypothermia (unpublished observation by A. Saeki).

Further exceptions are pathological conditions such as myocardial postischemic stunning, postacidotic stunning, and hypercapnic acidosis [28–30]. Although a very low coronary perfusion pressure (33mmHg) lowered the VO_2–PVA relation and slightly decreased its slope, this decreased slope was the result of gradually decreased E_{max} with increases in PVA because of a severely insulted coronary reserve [31]. However, stunned hearts reperfused for 1–2h following 15min normothermic global ischemia had a decreased E_{max} as well as a decreased O_2 cost of PVA, with almost no change in its elevation [28]. Although we do not know the mechanism underlying the decreased O_2 cost of PVA, this suggests the existence of a yet unknown mechanism to increase the contractile efficiency in stunned myocardium. The unchanged elevation of the VO_2–PVA relation despite the decreased E_{max}, however, indicates a considerably increased O_2 cost of E_{max}, which means O_2 is wastefully used for contractility. We speculated that this wasting reflects one or more of a decreased Ca^{2+} responsiveness of the contractile machinery, an increased Ca^{2+} futile cycling in the SR, and an increased Na^+/Ca^{2+} exchange resulting in an augmented Na^+-K^+ pumping [28–30]. No method is yet available to differentiate the contributions of these three mechanisms in beating whole hearts. Similar situations hold in acidotic hearts and postacidotic stunned hearts [29,30]. Nevertheless, the increased O_2 cost of E_{max} indicates that O_2 wasting has occurred in the Ca^{2+} handling in these pathological hearts. We have proposed that ryanodine-treated hearts may serve as a useful pathological heart model for better understanding of such abnormal cardiac mechanoenergetics [32].

Our recent study showed, intriguingly, that a short-term Ca^{2+} overloading protocol produced a failing heart without an increased O_2 cost of E_{max} [33] despite a comparable decrease in E_{max} to the stunned heart [28,30]. This failing heart looks similar in mechanoenergetics to the heart depressed by a Ca^{2+}-antagonist or a β-blocker [1–6]. This finding indicates that not all Ca^{2+}-overloaded failing hearts can be equally characterized by an increased O_2 cost of E_{max} despite their similar contractile failure.

Ca^{2+} sensitizers are expected to decrease the amount of Ca^{2+} involved in the E–C coupling for the same contractility. Therefore, a decrease in VO_2 for the same E_{max} and hence a decreased O_2 cost of E_{max} from control had been expected. However, a Ca^{2+} sensitizer, EMD53998, did not yield the expected result [34,34a]. More recently, Goto et al. reported that EMD53998 decreased the pathologically increased O_2 cost of E_{max} in canine chronic failing hearts induced by tachycardial pacing [35].

Efficiency

Cardiac efficiency is usually defined as the ratio of external mechanical work to the total energy consumption, the latter being usually VO_2. This efficiency is not constant in a given heart, but varies with loading, heart rate, and contractile conditions.

By contrast, the contractile efficiency, as the reciprocal of the O_2 cost of PVA obtained in a stable LV, indicates the efficiency of total mechanical energy from the PVA-dependent VO_2. This efficiency represents the product of the efficiency of energy conversion of CB cycling from ATP to total mechanical energy and the efficiency of energy conversion of mitochondrial oxidative phosphorylation from O_2 to ATP [1–6]. The latter is about 60% according to the P:O ratio of 3:1.

The O_2 cost of PVA is 1.7×10^{-5} ml O_2/(mmHg·ml) on average. It is approximately 2.5 (dimensionless) after both VO_2 and PVA units are expressed in the common energy unit of J (Joule). Then, its reciprocal yields a contractile efficiency of 0.4 or 40%. Dividing this efficiency by the O_2:ATP efficiency of 60%, yields 60%–70%. This is the efficiency of CB cycling from ATP to total mechanical energy. The constancy of the O_2 cost of PVA therefore means the constancy of the CB cycling efficiency, regardless of ventricular loading conditions and contractile states [1–6]. The contractile efficiency became obtainable thanks to our concept of PVA [1–6]. Contractile efficiency has also been successfully studied in human hearts using the PVA concept [36–38].

Cardiac efficiency is a variable fraction of the contractile efficiency because PVA = EW + PE. Therefore, the contractile efficiency indicates the maximum limit of cardiac efficiency [1,3].

Relevance to Artificial Heart and Cardiac Assist

We hope that the present review so far contains important fundamental information on cardiac mechanoenergetics which will be helpful to cardiac surgeons and engineers interested in artificial hearts and assist devices. We believe that the same VO_2–PVA–E_{max} framework will also hold in natural hearts assisted by artificial mechanisms, including artificial hearts. Some predictions are shown here.

Figure 7 shows four P–V diagrams of a natural heart under various loading conditions. Figure 7a shows the heart alone without any mechanical assistance. Figure 7b–d shows the same heart with the same E_{max} under three different mechanical assist conditions. Figure 7b is a case of preload assist where the ventricular preload and hence stroke volume are reduced with a parallel pump. The end-systolic P–V point falls along the same E_{max} line. The PE of PVA remains unchanged but the EW is reduced. Therefore, PVA and hence VO_2 are reduced. Figure 7c is a case of afterload assist where the ventricular afterload is reduced and hence stroke volume is increased with an aortic series pump. The end-systolic P–V point falls along the same E_{max} line. The EW may be slightly changed but the PE is markedly reduced, considerably decreasing PVA and hence VO_2.

Figure 7d is a case of dynamic cardiac compression to simulate the desired effect of cardiomyoplasty. Ventricular compression inputs mechanical energy into the contracting ventricle and serves as if E_{max} increases. The added mechanical energy could increase stroke volume against an increased afterload. Although PVA apparently increases as the result of the added energy, the PVA of the natural ventricle, and hence its VO_2, do not need to increase and remain unchanged. In any case, VO_2 is saved by the preload and afterload assists (Fig. 7b,c), or remains unchanged by the work assist (Fig. 7d). Thus, the mechanoenergetics of the natural heart under artificial assist is explicitly quantifiable by the VO_2–PVA–E_{max} framework.

Figure 8 shows actual data to show the beneficial mechanoenergetic effects of direct cardiac compression (DCC) as compared to volume loading (VOL) and enhancement of contractility with dobutamine (DOB) [39–40a]. The data show that for comparable increases in PVA by the three different methods, DCC was accompanied by the least increment in VO_2. This symbolizes the beneficial mechanoenergetic effects to be expected from ideal cardiomyoplasty. However, there seems no such report from cardiomyoplasty studies [41]. This may indicate that the cardiomyoplasty technique should be improved to convey effectively skeletal muscle work into cardiac chambers.

Ventricular fibrillation is often encountered or produced under cardiac assist. A fibrillating heart consumes considerable VO_2 for mechanical activity as well as E–C coupling, despite the lack of mechanically effective contraction. Figure 9 shows our innovative approach to the prediction of the VO_2 of a fibrillating LV using the VO_2–PVA relation [42–48]. Our theoretical consideration yielded the result that PVA under the isobaric (horizontal) line passing through a working P–V point of a fibrillating LV indicates the total mechanical energy generated by fibrillation [42]. We therefore called this area "equivalent PVA" (ePVA in Fig. 9a). Comparing VO_2–PVA data before and during ventricular fibrillation, we found that the per-min VO_2–PVA relation at varied isovolumic volumes of a fibrillating LV falls on one of the per-min VO_2–PVA relations of the same LV beating regularly at different pacing rates before fibrillation. From the matched per-min VO_2–PVA relations, we can determine the equivalent heart rate (eHR) of the fibrillating LV [44]. We have found an average eHR of 220 beats/min in normothermic canine hearts and interpreted this value to indicate the average frequency of asynchronous contraction of individual myocardial cells

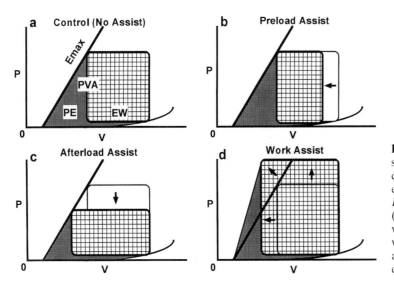

Fig. 7. Mechanoenergetic effects of cardiac assist. Pressure–volume (P–V) diagrams, mechanical potential energy (*PE, shaded area*), external work (*EW, cross-hatched area*), and *PVA* (= PE + EW) of a natural ventricle alone (**a**). The same ventricle under preload assist with a parallel pump (**b**), under afterload assist with an aortic series pump (**c**), and under work assist by cardiac compression (**d**). *Arrows* indicate affected variables

Fig. 8. Mechanoenergetics under work assist by dynamic cardiac compression (*DCC*) in comparison to those under volume loading (*VOL*) and positive inotropism of dobutamine (*DOB*). **a** the resultant shifts of the VO_2–PVA data point from control in different directions by the three interventions. **b** compares the different increments in VO_2 (ΔVO_2) for comparable increments in external work (ΔEW)

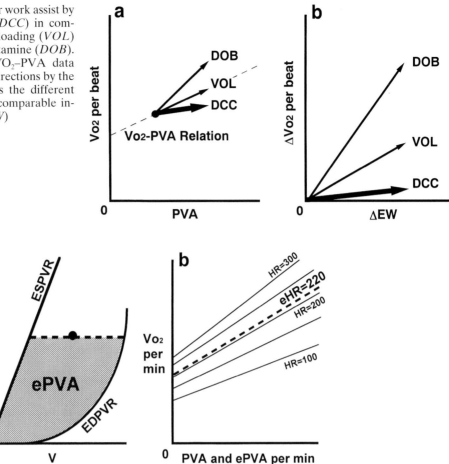

Fig. 9a,b. Concepts of equivalent PVA (*ePVA*) and equivalent heart rate (*eHR*) of a fibrillating left ventricle. ePVA represents a pressure–volume (P–V) area (*shaded*) between the end-systolic and end-diastolic P–V relations (*ESPVR* and *EDPVR*, respectively) under the imaginary isobaric (*horizontal, dashed*) P–V trajectory drawn through the fibrillating P–V data point (*solid circle*) in **a**. eHR corresponds to the heart rate of one of a family of regularly beating VO_2–PVA relations (per min) at different heart rates (*solid lines*) on which the fibrillating VO_2–ePVA relation (per min) (*dashed line*) falls in the same left ventricle. *HR*, heart rate

[44]. This mechanoenergetic knowledge may facilitate better understanding of the metabolic states of fibrillating hearts under cardiac assist.

Conclusion

The VO_2–PVA–E_{max} framework has provided an entirely new, physically and physiologically sound paradigm to characterize the mechanoenergetics of hearts under various physiological and pathological conditions, including artificial mechanical assistance to the heart. We hope that the present framework will greatly facilitate the conquering of heart diseases by various methodologies including artificial hearts and assist devices.

Acknowledgments. Partly supported by Grants-in-Aid for Scientific Research (05221224, 06213226, 06770494, 07508003, 08670052, 08770499) from the Ministry of Education, Science, Sports and Culture, a Research Grant for Cardiovascular Diseases (7C-2) from the Ministry of Health and Welfare, 1994–1996 Joint Research Grants Utilizing Scientific and Technological Potential in the Region and a 1997 Frontier Research Grant on Cardiovascular System Dynamics from the Science and Technology Agency, and a Research Grant from the Mochida Memorial Foundation, all of Japan.

References

1. Suga H (1990) Ventricular energetics. Physiol Rev 70:247–277
2. Sagawa K, Maughan WL, Suga H, Sunagawa K (1988)

Cardiac contraction and the pressure–volume relationship. Oxford University Press, New York

3. Suga H, Goto Y (1991) Cardiac oxygen costs of contractility (E_{max}) and mechanical energy (PVA): new key concepts in cardiac energetics. In: Sasayama S, Suga H (eds) Recent progress in failing heart syndrome. Springer, Tokyo, pp 61–115

4. Takaki M, Namba T, Araki J, Ishioka K, Ito H, Akashi T, Zhao LY, Zhao DD, Liu M, Fujii W, Suga H (1993) How to measure cardiac energy expenditure. In: Piper HM, Preusse CJ (eds) Ischemia-reperfusion in cardiac surgery. Kluwer Academic, Dordrecht, pp 403–419

5. Takaki M, Matsubara H, Araki J, Zhao LY, Ito H, Yasuhara S, Fujii W, Suga H (1996) Mechanoenergetics of acute failing hearts characterized by oxygen costs of mechanical energy and contractility. In: Sasayama S (ed) New horizons for failing heart syndrome. Springer, Tokyo, pp 133–164

6. Suga H, Takaki M, Matsubara H, Araki J (1996) Cardiac mechanics and energetics. In: Endoh M, Morad M, Scholz H, Niijima T (eds) Molecular and cellular mechanisms of cardiovascular regulation. Spring, Tokyo, pp 373–389

7. Suga H (1969) Analysis of left ventricular pumping by its pressure–volume coefficient (in Japanese with English abstract). Jpn J Med Electr Biol Eng 7:406–415

8. Suga H (1971) Theoretical analysis of a left-ventricular pumping model based on the systolic time-varying pressure/volume ratio. IEEE Trans Biomed Eng 18:47–55

9. Suga H (1971) Left ventricular time-varying pressure/volume ratio in systole as an index of myocardial inotropism. Jpn Heart J 12:153–160

10. Sagawa K (1978) Pressure–volume diagram revisited. Circ Res 43:677–687

11. Suga H (1994) Paul Dudley White international lecture: cardiac performance as viewed through the pressure–volume window. Jpn Heart J 35:263–280, or its abstract (1993) Circulation 88 (Suppl part 2):I-C

12. Suga H, Sagawa K, Shoukas AA (1973) Load independence of the instantaneous pressure–volume ratio of the canine left ventricle and effects of epinephrine and heart rate on the ratio. Circ Res 32:314–322

13. Suga H, Sagawa K (1974) Instantaneous pressure–volume relationships and their ratio in the excised, supported canine left ventricle. Circ Res 35:117–126

14. Suga H (1990) Cardiac mechanics and energetics — from E_{max} to PVA. Front Med Biol Eng 2:3–22

15. Weisfeldt ML, Shoukas AA, Weiss JL, Dashkoff N, Conic P, Griffith LSC, Achuff SC, Ducci H, Sagawa K (1976) E_{max} as a new contractility index in man (abstract). Circulation 54 (Suppl II):II-31

16. Sasayama S, Takahashi M, Osakada G, Hamashima H, Nishimura T, Sakurai T, Hirose K, Kawai C, Kotura H (1977) Evaluation to left ventricular function in clinical patients. Analysis of end-systolic length–tension relation and force–velocity relation (abstract). Jpn Circ J 41:778

17. Grossman W, Braunwald E, Mann T, McLaurin LP, Green LH (1977) Contractile state of the left ventricle in man as evaluated from end-systolic pressure–volume relations. Circulation 56:845–852

18. Goto Y, Suga H, Yamada O, Igarashi Y, Saito M, Hiramori K (1986) Left ventricular regional work from wall tension-area loop in the canine left ventricle. Am J Physiol 250:H151–H158

19. Suga H (1979) Total mechanical energy of a ventricle model and cardiac oxygen consumption. Am J Physiol 236:H498–H505

20. Khalafbeigui F, Suga H, Sagawa K (1979) Left ventricular systolic pressure–volume area correlates with oxygen consumption. Am J Physiol 237:H566–H789

21. Suga H, Hayashi T, Shirahata M (1981) Ventricular systolic pressure–volume area as predictor of cardiac oxygen consumption. Am J Physiol 240:H39–H44

22. Suga H, Hayashi T, Suchiro S, Hisano R, Shirahata M, Ninomiya I (1981) Equal oxygen consumption rates of isovolumic and ejecting contractions with equal systolic pressure–volume areas in canine left ventricle. Circ Res 49:1082–1091

23. Namba T, Takaki M, Araki J, Ishioka K, Suga H (1994) Energetics of the negative and positive inotropism of pentobarbitone sodium in the cane left ventricle. Cardiovasc Res 28:557–565

24. Norzawa T, Yasumura Y, Futaki S, Tanaka N, Suga H (1988) No significant increase in O_2 consumption of KCl-arrested dog heart with filling and dobutamine. Am J Physiol 255:H807–H812

25. Suga H, Goto Y, Igarashi Y, Yasumura Y, Nozawa T, Futaki S, Tanaka N (1988) Cardiac cooling increases E_{max} without affecting relation between O_2 consumption and systolic pressure–volume area in dog left ventricle. Circ Res 63:61–71

26. Saeki A, Goto Y, Hata K, Takasago T, Nishioka T, Suga H (1992) Hyperthermia increases oxygen cost of contractility in dog left ventricle. Circulation 86 (Suppl I):I-428

27. Nishoka T, Goto Y, Hata K, Takasago T, Saeki A, Suga H (1992) Mechanism of the inhibitory effect of vibration on left ventricular contractility in isolated blood perfused dog heart (abstract). J Mol Cell Cardiol 24 (Suppl I):S-66

28. Ohgoshi Y, Goto Y, Futaki S, Yaku H, Kawaguchi O, Suga H (1991) Increased oxygen cost of contractility in stunned myocardium of dog. Circ Res 69:975–988

29. Hata K, Goto Y, Kawaguchi O, Takasago T, Saeki A, Nishioka T, Suga H (1994) Hypercapnic acidosis increases oxygen cost of contractility in the dog left ventricle. Am J Physiol 266:H730–H740

30. Hata K, Takasago T, Saeki A, Nishioka T, Goto Y (1994) Stunned myocardium after rapid correction of acidosis. Increased oxygen cost of contractility and the role of the Na^+-H^+ exchange system. Circ Res 74:795–805

31. Suga H, Goto Y, Yasumura Y, Nozawa T, Futaki S, Tanaka N, Uenishi M (1988) O_2 consumption of dog heart under decreased coronary perfusion and propranolol. Am J Physiol 254:H292–H303

32. Takasago T, Goto Y, Kawaguchi O, Hata K, Saeki A, Nishioka T, Suga H (1993) Ryanodine wastes oxygen consumption for Ca^{2+} handling in the dog heart. A new pathological heart model. J Clin Invest 92:823–830

33. Araki J, Takaki M, Namba T, Mori M, Suga H (1995) Ca^{2+}-free, high-Ca^{2+} coronary perfusion suppresses contractility and excitation-contraction coupling energy. Am J Physiol 268:H1061–H1070

34. de Tombe PP, Burkhoff D, Hunter WC (1992) Effects of calcium and EMD53998 on oxygen consumption in isolated canine hearts. Circulation 86:1945–1954

34a. Takasago T, Goto Y, Kawaguchi O, Hata K, Saeki A, Taylor TW, Nishioka T, Suga H (1997) 2, 3-Butanedione monoxime suppresses excitation-contraction coupling in the canine blood-perfused left ventricle. Jpn J Physiol 47:205–215

35. Goto Y, Hata K, Takasago T, Saeki A, Nishoka T (1995) Calcium-sensitizing drug reduces oxygen cost of contractility in the failing heart, but not in the normal heart. Program and abstracts: the fifth Antwerp-La Jolla-Kyoto research conference on cardiac function. Heart failure: new insights into mechanisms and management. Kyoto, Japan, Dec 13–15, 1995

36. Kameyama T, Asanoi H, Ishizaka S, Yamanishi K, Fujita M, Sasayama S (1992) Energy conversion efficiency in human left ventricle. Circulation 85:988–996

37. Takaoka H, Takeuchi M, Yokoyama M (1992) Assessment of myocardial oxygen consumption (Vo_2) and systolic pressure–volume area (PVA) in human hearts. Eur Heart J 13 (Suppl E):85–90

38. Takaoka H, Takeuchi M, Odake M, Hayashi Y, Hata K, Mori M, Yokoyama M (1993) Comparison of hemodynamic determinants for myocardial oxygen consumption under different contractile states in human ventricle. Circulation 87:59–69

39. Kawaguchi O, Guto Y, Futaki S, Ohgoshi Y, Yaku H, Suga H (1992) Mechanical enhancement and myocardial oxygen saving by synchronized dynamic left ventricular compression. J Thorac Cardioacasc Surg 103:573–581

40. Kawaguchi O, Goto Y, Futaki S, Ohgoshi Y, Yaku H, Suga H (1994) The effects of dynamic cardiac compression on ventricular mechanics and energetics. Role of ventricular size and contractility. J Thorac Cardiocasc Surg 107:850–859

40a. Kawaguchi O, Goto Y, Ohgoshi Y, Yaku H, Murase M, Suga H (1997) Dynamic cardiac compression improves contractile efficiency of the heart. J Thorac Cardiovasc Surg 113:923–931

41. Nakajima H, Niinami H, Hooper TL, Hammond RL, Nakajima H, Lu H, Ruggiero R, Thomas GA, Mocek FW, Fietsam R, Krakovsky AA, Spanta AD, Suga H, Stephenson LW, Baciewicz FA (1994) Cardiomyoplasty: Probable mechanism of effectiveness using the pressure–volume relationship. Ann Thorac Surg 57:407–415

42. Yaku H, Goto Y, Futaki S, Ohgoshi Y, Kawaguchi O, Suga H (1991) Multicompartment model for mechanics and energetics of fibrillating heart. Am J Physiol 260:H292–H299

43. Yaku H, Goto Y, Futaki S, Ohgoshi Y, Kawaguchi O, Suga H (1991) Equivalent pressure–volume area accounts for O_2 consumption of fibrillating heart. Am J Physiol 261:H1534–H1544

44. Yaku H, Goto Y, Futaki S, Ohgoshi Y, Kawaguchi O, Hata K, Takasago T, Suga H (1991) Equivalent heart rate during ventricular fibrillation in the dog heart: mechanoenergetic analysis. Jpn J Physiol 41:945–959

45. Yaku H, Goto Y, Futaki S, Ohgoshi Y, Kawaguchi O, Suga H (1992) Ventricular fibrillation does not depress postfibrillatory contractility in blood-perfused dog heart. J Thorac Cardiovasc Surg 103:514–520

46. Yaku H, Goto Y, Futaki S, Ohgoshi Y, Kawaguchi O, Suga H (1992) Myocardial oxygen consumption of fibrillating ventricle in hypothermia. Successful account by new mechanical indexes — equivalent pressure–volume area and equivalent heart rate. J Thorac Cardiovasc Surg 104:364–373

47. Yaku H, Goto Y, Futaki S, Ohgoshi Y, Kawaguchi O, Hata K, Takasago T, Suga H (1992) Comparable efficiencies of chemomechanical energy transduction between beating and fibrillating dog hearts. Am J Physiol 262:H1734–H1743

48. Yaku H, Goto Y, Ohgoshi Y, Kawaguchi O, Oga K, Oka T, Suga H (1993) Determinants of myocardial oxygen consumption in fibrillating dog hearts. J Thorac Cardiovasc Surg 105:679–688

Discussion

Dr. Galletti:

You showed an effect of what you may call a ventricular assist system on the oxygen cost of E_{max}. Have you ever looked at the effect on the basal metabolic oxygen consumption?

Dr. Suga:

We measure the basal metabolism by arresting the heart by KCl. There is no significant difference in any case. Even if we change the temperature, the change in the basal metabolism in very small, as compared to the significant change in the total oxygen consumption. Your concern is a very important thing, but we can say that change in basal metabolism in this particular system is negligible. Thank you for your question.

Dr. Nitta:

As you know, I'm also using your E_{max} in the evaluating of cardiac assistance, I mean, left ventricular assistance. Could you give me some comments in that special situation?

Dr. Suga:

I actually, frankly speaking, don't remember the details of it, but I quickly scanned yours. I think it is useful if the measurement is correct. The measurement is very important because we have to depend on ... pressure is very easy but volume information should be very reliable, and often the volume measurement is not accurate. Then you may come to very serious misunderstanding or misconclusion. So volume measurement must be very careful. Another thing is that although I simplified the conclusion, E_{max} actually varies in a transient situation as compared to a stable situation. So when you get E_{max} from only two beats, one is ejecting, the other is isovolume, for example, then that E_{max} may not exactly be the same as the E_{max} you obtain from stable contractions. So that sort of difference has to be remembered when you do your type of research.

Treatment of Idiopathic Dilated Cardiomyopathy (Beta-Cardiomyopathy) by Insertion of a Left Ventricular Mechanical Support System

J. Müller[1], G. Wallukat[2], Y. Weng[1], M. Dandel[1], S. Spiegelsberger[1], S. Semrau[1], K. Brandes[1], M. Loebe[1], R. Meyer[1], and R. Hetzer[1]

Summary. The implantation of a mechanical cardiac support system (MCSS) is normally used in patients with end-stage heart disease who otherwise face imminent death because of worsening heart failure. We followed patients after insertion of an MCSS closely in order to assess the possibility of weaning from the MCSS. Six patients with end-stage nonischemic idiopathic dilated cardiomyopathy (IDC) underwent MCSS implantation as a bridge to transplantation. All patients were in New York Heart Association Class (NYHA) IV-D, and each had a cardiac index below 1.6 liters per minute per square meter of body surface area ($1 \cdot min^{-1} \cdot m^{-2}$), a left ventricular ejection fraction (EF) below 16%, a left ventricular internal dismeter in diastole (LVIDd) above 68mm, and all were found positive in tests for humoral anti-β_1-adrenoceptor autoantibodies (A-β_1-AAB). Echocardiography and serum processing for A-β_1-AAB were performed weekly after insertion of the assist device. Replacement fibrosis and collagen III were measured in myocardial tissue specimens taken at the time of device insertion and more than one year after device explantation. The assist device was explanted after a mean duration of support of 324 days, and the patients have been off the device for between 81 and 631 days (as of November 30, 1996). The mean level of A-β_1-AAB was 6.9 ± 0.8 laboratory units (LU) at the time of implantation. A-β_1-AAB disappeared after a mean period of 12.7 ± 4.8 weeks and remained undetectable thereafter. Concomitant to the disappearance of the A-β_1-AAB was an increase in ejection fraction from below 16% to a mean of 47% $\pm$ 3%, and a decrease in LVIDd from 72 ± 3mm to 54 ± 2mm. The mean volume density of myocardial replacement fibrosis at the time of insertion was 24%. One year after explantation, fibrosis was in the normal range with a mean of 5.5%. All patients showed a persistently stable cardiac function with an ongoing trend towards further improvement after 6.5 cumulative years without mechanical cardiac support. Cardiac function can successfully be normalized in selected patients with end-stage idiopathic dilated cardiomyopathy by MCSS application. On the assumption that A-β_1-AAB are causative for the development of IDC, the disappearance of A-β_1-AAB can be interpreted as a marker of myocyte recovery and can therefore determine the earliest moment for weaning from MCSS. A-β_1-AAB can be used as a follow-up parameter to survey patients after weaning. The normalization of myocardial fibrosis makes it most likely that the therapeutic effect of MCSS application is a lasting one.

Key words: Idiopathic dilated cardiomyopathy — Beta-cardiomyopathy — Assist device explantation — Auto-antibodies — Replacement fibrosis — Collagen III

Introduction

Idiopathic dilated cardiomyopathy (IDC) can be induced by several mechanisms in an experimental setting. This can be done through (1) high-frequency pacing (more than 240 beats per minute over a period of several weeks), (2) humoral autoantibodies directed against β_1-adrenoceptors (A-β_1-AAB), and (3) over-expression of the cardiac Gs_α protein [1–4]. It is known from clinical experience that a chronic myocarditis may also lead to the development of A-β_1-AAB and consecutively to an IDC.

The effect of A-β_1-AAB is, as far as is known today, that the β_1-adrenoceptor remains in a state of permanent activation, which leads to chronic stimulation of the myocytes with subsequent influence on intracellular energy and calcium metabolism [3,4]. Accordingly, arrhythmia is very often the first clinical symptom in the initial phase of a cardiomyopathy [5].

Idiopathic dilated cardiomyopathy whose underlying cause is A-β_1-AAB should therefore be called beta-cardiomyopathy, to differentiate this disease from that of another origin.

About 90% of the patients who receive a cardiac assist device in our institution suffer from beta-cardiomyopathy. Generally, the implantation of a mechanical assist device as a bridge to transplantation is the only means available to support patients with terminal heart failure.

An alternative to the implantation of a mechanical cardiac support system (MCSS) as a bridge to transplantation is the permanent implantation or the temporary application of a MCSS with the aim of explanting the device after natural recovery of the heart.

Up to now, the longest chronic ("permanent") implantation time of a monoventricular system worldwide is 794 days, in our institution. Although this patient generally was in good condition and could spend most of the time at home until removal of the

[1] German Heart Institute Berlin, Augustenburger Platz 1, 13353 Berlin, Germany
[2] Max Delbrück Center, Berlin, Germany

device, he nevertheless showed within the last four months with the device general signs of infection such as slight temperature, elevated white blood count, and C-reactive protein. During that time, he was admitted three times into hospital for treatment.

Furthermore, the temporary implantation of a MCSS with the aim of a myocardial recovery has proved to be of little success in a great number of patients [6–10]. The reason for this is not clear and seems to lie in a misjudgment of the ability of the myocardium to recover.

We have therefore started to develop criteria with the help of which we hope to decide under which conditions a patient with beta-cardiomyopathy can be weaned from an assist device.

Methods

Patients

In six patients with the clinical diagnosis of end-stage IDC, a left ventricular cardiac assist device was implanted. All patients were men between the age of 37 and 58 (mean: 48 ± 9 years) with a body surface area of $2.01 \pm 0.12 \, m^2$ (range $1.83–2.13 \, m^2$). At the time of implantation, all patients fulfilled the established criteria defining cardiogenic shock and required positive inotropic support by dobutamine, dopamine, and phosphodiesterase inhibitors [11]. The cardiac index was below $1.61 \cdot min^{-1} \cdot m^{-2}$, the EF below 16%, and the LVIDd above 68 mm, and it had been necessary to increase the positive inotropic support in the duration of one week.

All patients had at least a 4-year history of dilated cardiomyopathy with two or more episodes of cardiac decompensation before being admitted with cardiogenic shock. We saw patients with severe biventricular cardiac insufficiency, tachypnea, and sinus tachycardia exhibiting all the signs of a chronic low-output syndrome, most requiring oxygen via a nasal tube. Humoral A-β_1-AAB were detected in all. A left ventricular assist device was implanted on the day of admission or one day thereafter. Detailed patient-specific hemodynamic data at the time of device implantation are listed in Table 1.

Cardiac Assist Devices

Five patients received the Novacor N100 (Baxter Healthcare, Novacor Division, Oakland, CA, USA), and one patient the TCI HeartMate (Thermo Cardiosystems, Woburn, MA, USA).

The assist devices were implanted anteriorly to the fascia musculi recti abdominis posterioris in the left upper abdominal quadrant. The inflow conduit was anastomosed to the apex of the left ventricle and the outflow conduit to the ascending aorta in an end-to-side position. All implantations were performed under extracorporeal circulation [12,13].

To avoid postoperative thrombus formation, the patients with the Novacor N100 device were anticoagulated with warfarin (coumarin), aiming at a prothrombin time in the international normalized ratio of 2.5, while patients with the TCI HeartMate were orally administered 100 mg of acetylsalicylic acid and 225 mg of dipyridamole per day.

Postimplant Management

Early postoperative management of cardiac assist patients was similar to that of any critically ill patient after cardiac surgery. Invasive postoperative monitoring included a thermodilution pulmonary artery catheter and a left atrial line. Pump output, stroke volume, and pulmonary and radial arterial and central venous pressures were continuously monitored during the initial postoperative phase. In addition to the standard postsurgical care of cardiac patients, postoperative management of the assisted patients included percutaneous exit-side care and the device-specific anticoagulant regimen. All patient problems and the handling of decisions regarding mechanical assist management were under the care of a specially trained mechanical support team.

Blood Samples

During routine clinic visits immediately before implantation and once a week thereafter, samples of 10 ml of peripheral blood were drawn in a serum syringe without additives and treated in accordance with established clinical guidelines. To obtain the sera for determining A-β_1-AAB by bioassay, the blood was centrifuged at 3600 rpm.

Bioassay

An exact description of the bioassay for the A-β_1-AAB scan is published elsewhere [14,15]. The underlying principle is the registration of the stimulating effect of A-β_1-AAB on single myocytes dissociated from minced ventricles after the immunoglobulin G fraction has been isolated and the precipitates dialyzed from the sera. The incremental change of myocytal undulation in a 15-s interval was used to quantify the amount of functionally effective autoantibodies present [laboratory units (LU)].

Echocardiography

EF and LVIDd were measured by echocardiography before MCSS implantation and once a week thereafter

Table 1. Data for the weaned patients at the time of left ventricular assist device insertion (preimplant) and 3 days after explantation (postexplant)

Weaned patient	Age [years] / Sex	Body surface area [m²]	Days on device	Positive inotropic medication		Arterial blood pressure [systolic/diastolic] [mmHg]		Heart rate [beats per minute] Rhythm		Mitral valve incompetence Cardiothoracic ratio		Left ventricular internal diameter in diastole [mm]; Left ventricular ejection fraction [20]		Cardiac index [l·min⁻¹·m⁻²] Mean pulmonary artery pressure [mmHg] Mean pulmonary capillary wedge pressure [mmHg] Mean pulmonary Central venous pressure [mmHg]		Level of anti-β₁-adrenoceptor auto-antibodies [Laboratory Units (LU)]	
				Preimplant	Postexplant	Preimplant	Postexplant	Preimplant	Postexplant	Preimplant	Postexplant	Preimplant	Postexplant	Preimplant	Postexplant	Preimplant	Postexplant
1	39 / Male	2.00	160	Dobutamine, dopamine	0	95/50	115/65	128 / Sinus rhythm	76 / Sinus rhythm	Grade II / 0.67	0 / 0.48	72 / <15	53 / 50	1.5 / 36 / 28 / 21	3.1 / 18 / 6 / 9	7.2	Not detectable
2	43 / Male	2.10	243	Dobutamine, dopamine, phospho-diesterase-inhibitors	0	90/55	120/75	125 / Sinus rhythm	69 / Sinus rhythm	Grade II / 0.62	0 / 0.43	70 / 15	54 / 48	1.4 / 38 / 31 / 24	3.0 / 15 / 8 / 10	6.8	Not detectable
3	58 / Male	2.13	347	Dobutamine dopamine, phospho-diesterase-inhibitors	0	100/55	125/80	134 / Sinus rhythm	75 / Sinus rhythm	Grade II / 0.64	0 / 0.45	70 / <15	55 / 47	1.4 / 40 / 29 / 27	2.9 / 19 / 11 / 11	7.1	Not detectable
4	53 / Male	2.08	200	Dobutamine, dopamine, phospho-diesterase-inhibitors	0	105/60	110/75	115 / Sinus rhythm	80 / Sinus rhythm	Grdel I / 0.64	0 / 0.5	69 / <15	52 / 50	1.5 / 33 / 27 / 19	3.2 / 14 / 8 / 8	6.2	Not detectable
5	56 / Male	1.91	201	Dobutamine, dopamine, phospho-diesterase-inhibitors	0	105/60	110/70	120 / Sinus rhythm	70 / Sinus rhythm	Grdel I / 0.67	0 / 0.45	78 / 15	52 / 47	1.5 / 36 / 26 / 18	3.4 / 22 / 12 / 8	5.9	Not detectable
6	37 / Male	1.83	794	Dobutamine, dopamine,	0	110/65	105/80	112 / Sinus rhythm	64 / Sinus rhythm	Grdel II / 0.69	0 / 0.48	74 / <15	58 / 41	1.5 / 34 / 28 / 17	3.1 / 16 / 10 / 6	5.4	Not detectable

with the pump turned off for 4 min. All examinations were conducted by the same examiner to ensure a minimum of variability in the echocardiographic parameters.

Morphometry of Replacement Fibrosis

Myocardial full-thickness samples taken during insertion of the device and biopsy specimens taken about one year after explantation of the support system, but not at the time of device removal, were fixed in 10% formalin followed by paraffin embedding, and sectioned at 5-µm thickness. Domagk staining was used for visualization of the connective tissue and for morphometry of fibrosis. The volume fraction of fibrosis was determined using the method of Weibel [16]. A 100-point grid with an area of 400 µm was used. All points counted in tissue occupied by fibrosis were expressed as a percentage (volume density, percent) of the entire tissue sample (after subtraction of points occupied by empty area, arterioles, and veins). Interstitial tissue volume density was evaluated at a magnification of × 400 by light microscopy. It was calculated that 20 adjacent fields should be analyzed per specimen to ensure a standard error of an average of 5% or less. For assessment of collagen type III, the sections were deparaffinized, rehydrated, and treated with pepsin before immunohistochemical staining was performed with a polyclonal antibody (Quartett Immundiagnostica and Biotechnologie, Berlin, Germany) specific to human placental collagen type III. Assessment of collagen content was performed semiquantitatively on the basis of a five-grade ranking scale.

Weaning Procedure

The drive unit was programmed in an unsynchronized mode (a fixed pumping rate mode) for three consecutive weeks to test the stability of the recovered cardiac function. The fixed-rate mode leads to a dissociation in the coordination between the moment of maximum cardiac ejection and that of optimum filling of the pump, a discrepancy which tends to increase left ventricular afterload. When this occurs, synchronization between heart and pump is random, at best.

Pump Explantation

Explantation was performed by opening the pouch containing the device and ligating both inflow and outflow conduits from below the diaphragm in the patients with the Novacor system, and via a left thoracotomy to the inflow cannula in the patient with the TCI.

Statistics

All data summaries and statistical analyses were performed using SPSS for Windows 95, version 7.0. To assess the significance of the differences between individual groups, the nonparametric Mann-Whitney two-sample test was applied. Paired data were analyzed by the Wilcoxon signed rank test. A P value of less than 0.05 was considered to indicate statistical significance.

Results

The presentation of the results concentrates on the clinical progression of LVIDd, EF, volume density of replacement fibrosis, and the A-β_1-AAB levels found in the patients during mechanical support and thereafter.

The patients were weaned from the device 160, 243, 343, 200, 201, and 794 days respectively after insertion. They have been without mechanical support for 631, 547, 539, 424, 85, and 81 days (as of November 30, 1996).

All sera were tested and found positive for A-β_1-AAB with a mean value of 6.9 ± 0.8 LU (range 5.9–8.2 LU) before implantation. Following assist insertion, A-β_1-AAB decreased in all patients and finally disappeared after 12.7 ± 4.8 weeks (range 9–22 weeks), and could not be detected thereafter (Fig. 1).

The cardiothoracic ratio showed improvement from a mean value of 0.66 ± 0.03 (range 0.62–0.69) to a mean of 0.46 ± 0.03 (range 0.43–0.5) ($P < 0.05$) at the time of explantation.

Regarding cardiac function we found that the mean LVIDd decreased from 72 ± 3 mm (range 69–78 mm) to 54 ± 2 mm (range 52–58 mm) and EF rose from below 16% to a mean value of 47% ± 3% (range 41%–

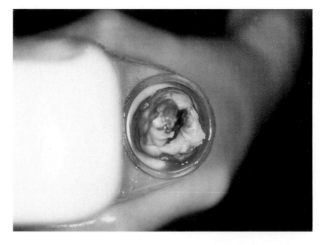

Fig. 1. The outflow valve of a Novacor N100 after 794 days of mechanical support

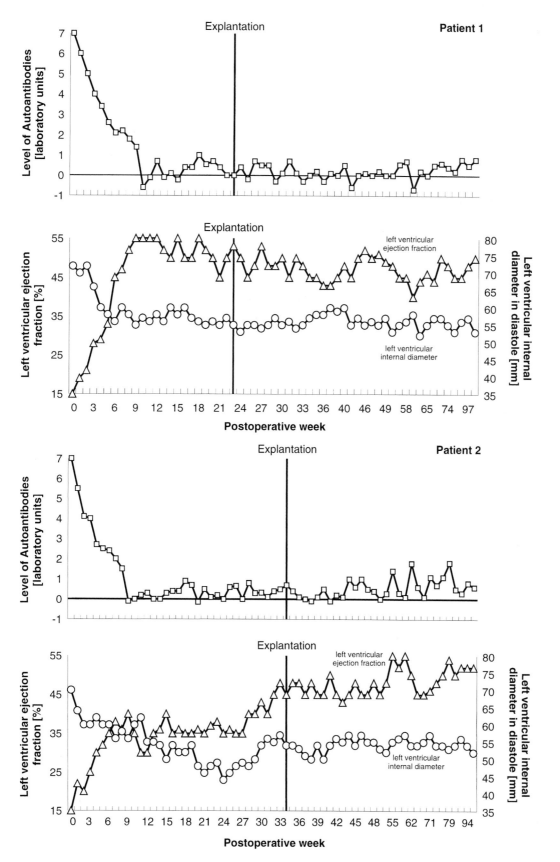

Fig. 2. The weekly progress in each individual weaned patient of left ventricular ejection fraction (*lower panels, triangles*) left ventricular internal diameter in diastole (*lower panels, circles*), and level of humoral anti-β₁-adrenoceptor autoantibodies (A-β₁-AAB; *upper panels*) from the time of insertion of the mechanical left ventricular support system up to the indicated week. Explantation is shown with a *vertical line*

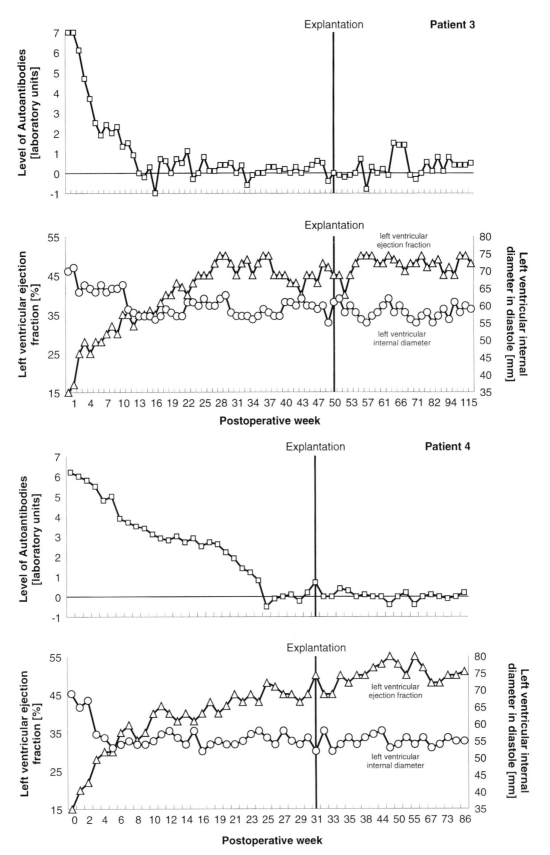

Fig. 2. *Continued.*

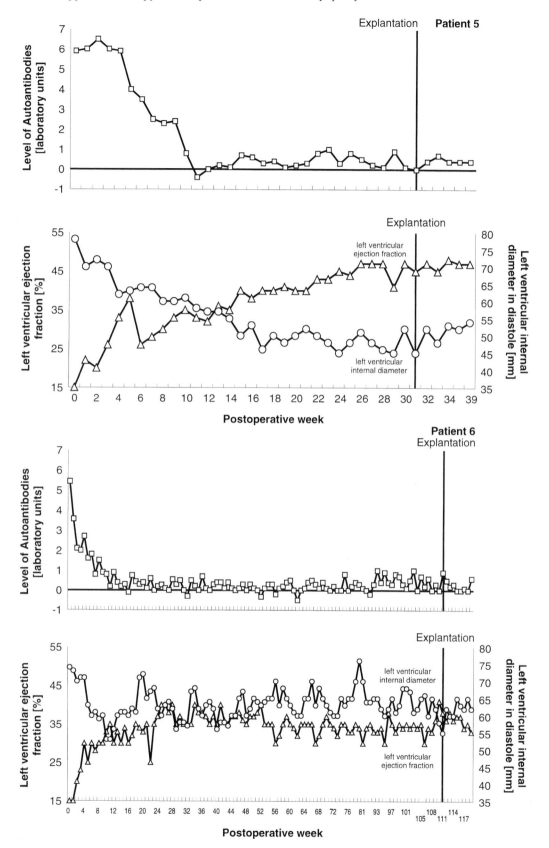

Fig. 2. *Continued.*

50%) (Fig. 2, Table 2). The individual hemodynamic and functional data of these patients at the time of insertion and three days after explantation is listed in Table 1.

A noteworthy trend in the LVIDd as compared with the progression of the EF (Fig. 2) was observed in patients 2 and 6: while EF almost continously increased during left ventricular unloading, LVIDd only decreased during the first three and six months, respectively, and thereafter increased again without any sign of increase in intraventricular volume.

The patient (6) who was supported for 794 days showed an increasing flow through the aortic valve and clinical signs of infection during his last 4 months on the device. In this patient the physiological boundaries of long-term implantation seemed to have been met (Fig. 1). However, after explantation, neither the devicecontaining pouch nor the pump chamber was contaminated.

The mean volume density of replacement fibrosis derived from myocardial full-thickness samples exhibited a mean value of 24% ± 4% (range 19%–28%) (Fig. 3). Myocardial specimens taken from the first four patients 437 ± 90 days (range 308–517 days) after pump explantation showed a mean value of 5.5% ± 2% (range 3%–8%). This difference is significant ($P < 0.05$).

Furthermore, collagen subtype III was semiquantitatively graded. All patients were highly posi-

tive at the time of insertion. One year after explantation, collagen III was no longer detectable in the histologic tissue samples of three patients. In one it was positive and in another it was just slightly positive (Table 3).

Since explantation of the assist pumps, all six patients have remained in a stable physical and circulatory condition. Invariably, they have been in NYHA class I-A. One patient has fully returned to his professional occupation, one has entered an employment retraining course, and three are permanently retired. One patient is planning to go back to his work as a

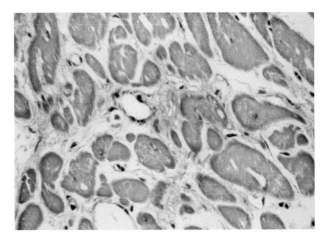

Fig. 3. Histological appearance of a myocardial tissue specimen taken at the time of device insertion from patient 2 (subsequently weaned). Replacement fibrosis is evident, and volume density was calculated at 21%. Domagk staining, × 400

Table 2. Changes of left ventricular internal diameter in diastole and left ventricular ejection fraction immediately before assist device insertion and at the time of explantation

	At time of device insertion	At time of device explantation	Statistical significance
Left ventricular internal diameter in diastole (mm)	72 ± 3	54 ± 2	$P < 0.05$
Left ventricular ejection fraction (%)	<16	47 ± 3	$P < 0.05$

Table 3. Semiquantitative identification of collagen III from myocardial tissue specimen of the weaned patients taken at time of device insertion and after one year of explantation

Weaned patient	Collagen III content	
	at the time of device insertion	one year after explant
1	++++	+
2	++++	Negative
3	++++	++
4	++++	Negative
5	++++	No data
6	++++	No data

++++, highly positive; ++, positive; +, slightly positive.

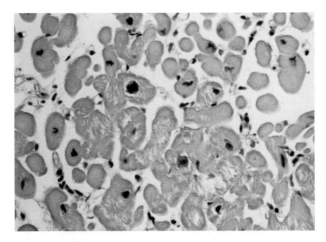

Fig. 4. Histological appearance of a myocardial tissue specimen taken one year after device explantation from the same patient as in Fig. 3. Replacement fibrosis is no longer detectable at this magnification. A volume density of 8% was calculated. Domagk staining, × 400

roofer. The follow-up echo data (LVIDd below 58mm, EF above 41% in all patients, as of November 30, 1996) demonstrate a persistently stable cardiac function with no trend towards deterioration over a period of 3–20 months. All patients have been given medication comprising of β-blockers (bisoprolole, 2.5mg per day) and angiotensin-converting enzyme inhibitors (enalapril, 10mg per day). There was no recurrence of A-β$_1$-AAB.

Discussion

It was shown that MCSS could be effectively used in selected patients with end-stage beta-cardiomyopathy, as a tool to normalize cardiac function. Through their use, the cardiac transplantation originally planned became unnecessary. Weaning patients with advanced cardiac dilation from MCSS after more than 160 days of left ventricular unloading is a new and hitherto unknown procedure of which the success could not be anticipated with certainty. A complete recovery to normal cardiac function could not be expected because of the persistent trauma through the implantation of the inflow-cannula into the left ventricular apex. However, after a cumulative observation period of more than 6 years it can now be assumed that this treatment will succeed.

This result is contrary to the expectations of many authors who considered lasting improvement of cardiac function in patients with end-stage IDC to be most unlikely, or who failed with a similar trial [6,8,17].

The decision to choose this method of treatment as opposed to carrying out the originally planned transplantation was facilitated by either the occurrence of device-related complications or by patient option, on the one hand, and the observation of functional cardiac recovery and the persistent disappearance of A-β$_1$-AAB as a sign of myocyte recovery, on the other. In view of the fact that during mid-term follow-up observation, both cardiac function and A-β$_1$-AAB levels have not pointed towards relapse, our experience with this concept, although still limited, would seem to indicate new avenues of treatment, at least for some of the patients otherwise destined for transplantation.

The idea that hearts ravaged by advanced stages of cardiac insufficiency may indeed profit from long-term unloading dates back to earlier cardiologists, who saw substantial improvements in such patients after prolonged periods of strict bed rest. However, those patients did not depend on high doses of positive inotropic medication before they began bed-rest therapy [18,19]. In the era of assist devices, there have been some rare unpublished studies of unexpectedly good heart function after longer assist periods. To our knowledge, there has been no report on planned assist explantation, not to mention accounts of successful patient progress after explantation in patients with chronic IDC. Success of this nature was achieved in patients with acute heart failure caused by ischemic heart disease, acute myocarditis, and in patients after cardiac surgery [20,21].

The detection of A-β$_1$-AAB by bioassay is based on their stimulating effect on myocytes, an effect which can be inhibited in the assay by β-blockers. This supports the hypothesis that A-β$_1$-AAB may also have a chronically stimulating effect on the heart rate of patients with a beta-cardiomyopathy, and may indeed initiate or accelerate the further course of cardiac enlargement [3,4]. This view is, in turn, supported by animal experiments, where chronic stimulation over a period of 3 weeks with abnormally high heart rates (up to 240 beats per minute) has been seen to induce dilated cardiomyopathy [1,2]. Matsui, Fu, and colleagues were able to prove for the first time a causative linkage between the effect of A-β$_1$-AAB and the development of dilated cardiomyopathy. A-β$_1$-AAB seem to act as a primary trigger of cardiac dilatation and reduction of wall thickness in their animal setting [4]. Furthermore, Iwase et al. also showed that overexpression of the cardiac Gs$_\alpha$-protein leads to cardiac enlargement, cellular necrosis, and replacement fibrosis [3].

Nevertheless, the reason why long-term left ventricular unloading leads to the disappearances of A-β$_1$-AAB remains unexplored. A similar but inverse process was observed: in an experimental setting, exercise by subjects with known autoimmune myocarditis resulted in an augmentation of autoimmunity associated with increasing cardiac dilatation [22].

The morphometric analyses of the biopsy specimens taken from patients more than one year after explantation exhibited a quasi-normal myocardial histology. Fibrosis had been reduced to normal myocardial volume density. We unfortunately did not perform a biopsy at the time of explantation. Data from the literature shows increased fibrosis at the time of transplantation compared to fibrosis at the time of insertion [7,23–26]. We therefore hypothesize that the process of fibrosis reduction may start or continue even after explantation.

One patient was on the device for 794 days. His heart showed the highest level of fibrosis within the group of weaned patients. However, even his cardiac function improved parallel to the disappearance of A-β$_1$-AAB until he reached an EF of 35%. This seemed to us to be insufficient for device removal at that time. To reach 41% he required almost a further 2 years of unloading. Therefore, we assume that the process of normalization depends on both in the first place improvement of myocyte function, and the reduction of connective tissue thereafter. This process may be additionally supported by a deactivation of the neuroendocrine axis [27].

The observation we made concerning the development of LVIDd in two single patients can probably be interpreted as structural remodeling of the ventricular geometry because of chronic unloading.

Conclusions

Weaning patients from an assist device can be performed successfully. It saves donor hearts, saves costs, and is superior to cardiac transplantation for selected patients.

Although a final statement about preoperative predictive parameters that would allow selection of patients with IDC for successful weaning from mechanical cardiac unloading cannot be made, the sustained disappearance of A-β_1-AAB gives evidence to the assumption that chronic unloading initiates a process of recovery that continues after removal of the device. This observation has been supported by the normalization of the volume density of fibrotic tissue inside the myocardium.

The clinical significance of this study should lead to further investigations as to the underlying causes of IDC and to develop new strategies of therapy.

Addendum

After termination of this report, two further patients with beta-cardiomyopathy have been successfully weaned from the device. Their cardiac function had increased from initial values of LVIDd of 75 and 72 mm, respectively, an EF <16%, and a cardiac index <1.61·min^{-1}·m^{-2}, to LVIDd values of 45 and 59 mm, EFs of 50% and 42%, and cardiac indexes of 2.9 and 2.81·min^{-1}·m^{-2}, respectively. The initially high levels of A-β_1-AAB have completely disappeared. Our cumulative experience is based on eight patients now, as of January 17, 1997.

Acknowledgment. We would like to acknowledge the support of the Berliner Sparkassenstiftung Medizin.

References

1. Spinale FG, Zellner JL, Tomita M, Crawford FA, Zile MR (1991) Relation between ventricular and myocyte remodeling with the development and regression of supraventricular tachycardia-induced cardiomyopathy. Circ Res 69(4):1058–1067
2. Spinale FG, Tomita M, Zellner JL, Cook JC, Crawford FA, Zile MR (1991) Collagen remodeling and changes in LV function during development and recovery from supraventricular tachycardia. Am J Physiol 261(2, part 2):H308–318
3. Iwase M, Uechi M, Vatner D, Asai K, Shannon R, Kudej R, Wagner T, Wight D, Patrick T, Bishop S, Ishikawa Y, Homcy C (1996) Dilated cardiomyopathy indued by cardiac Gs-alpha overexpression. Circulation 94(Suppl I): I-16
4. Matsui S, Fu MLX, Katsuda S, Hayase M, Yamaguchi N, Teraoka K, Kurihara T, Takekoshi N, Murakami E, Hoebeke J, Hjalmarson Å (1997) Peptides derived from cardiovascular G-protein-coupled receptors induce morphological cardiomyopathy changes in immunized rabbits. J Mol Cell Cardiol 29(2):641–655
5. Chiale PA, Rosenbaum MB, Elizari MV, Hjalmarson Å, Magnuson Y, Wallukat G, Hoebeke J (1995) High prevalence of antibodies against beta 1- and beta 2-adrenoceptors in patients with primary electrical cardiac abnormalities. J Am Coll Cardiol 26(4):864–869
6. Levin HR, Oz MC, Catanese KA, Rose EA, Burkhoff D (1996) Transient normalisation of systolic and diastolic function after support with a left ventricular assist device in a patient with dilated cardiomyopathy. J Heart Lung Transplant 15:840–842
7. McCarthy PM, Nakatani S, Vargo R, Kottke-Marchant K, Harasaki H, James KB, Savage RM, Thomas JD (1995) Structural and left ventricular histologic changes after implantable LVAD insertion. Ann Thorac Surg 59:613
8. Levin HR (1995) Invited commentary to: McCarthy PM, Nakatani S, Vargo R, Kottke-Marchant K, Harasaki H, James KB, Savage RM, Thomas JD (1995) Structural and left ventricular histologic changes after implantable LVAD insertion. Ann Thorac Surg 59:613
9. Levin HR, Oz MC, Chen JM, Packer M, Rose EA, Burkhoff D (1995) Reversal of chronic ventricular dilatation in patients with end-stage cardiomyopathy by prolonged mechanical unloading. Circulation 91:2717–2720
10. Frazier OH, Benedect CR, Radovancevic B, Bick RJ, Capek P, Springer WE, Macris MP, Delgado R, Buja M (1996) Improved left ventricular function after chronic left ventricular unloading. Ann Thorac Surg 62:675–682
11. Nomenclature and criteria for diagnosis of diseases of the heart and great vessels, 9th edn (1994) Dolgin M (ed). American Heart Association, Little Brown Boston, p 240
12. Pennington DG, McBride LR, Swartz MT (1994) Implantation technique for the Novacor left ventricular assist system. J Thorac Cardiovasc Surg 108:604–608
13. Radovancevic B, Frazier OH, Michael JM (1992) Implantation etchnique for the HeartMate left ventricular assist device. J Card Surg 7(3):203–207
14. Wallukat G, Wollenberger A (1987) Effects of serum gamma globulin fractions of patients with allergic asthma and dilated cardiomyopathy on chronotropic β-adrenoceptor function in cultured neonatal rat heart myocytes. Biomed Biochim Acta 46:634–639
15. Wallukat G, Wollenberger A (1988) Die kultivierte Herzmuskelzelle. Ein funktionelles Testsystem zum Nachweis von Autoantikörpern gegen den β-adrenergen Rezeptor. Acta Histochem (Suppl XXXV):145–149
16. Weibel ER, Kistler GS, Scherle WF (1966) Practical stereological methods for morphometric cytology. J Cell Biol 30:23–38
17. Tayama E, Nosé Y (1996) Can we treat dilated cardiomyopathy using a left ventricular assist device? (editorial). Artif Organs 20:197–201

18. Burch GE (1966) On resting the human heart. Am Heart J 71:422

19. Burch GE, McDonald CD, Walsh JJ (1971) The effect of prolonged bed rest on postpartal cardiomyopathy. Am Heart J 81:186–201

20. Holman WL, Bourge RC, Kirklin JK (1991) Case report: circulatory support for seventy days with resolution of acute heart failure. J Thorac Cardiovasc Surg 102 (6):932–934

21. Noon GP (1993) Clinical use of cardiac assist devices. In: Akutsu T, Koyanagi H (eds) Heart replacement. Artificial heart 4. Springer, Tokyo, pp 195–205

22. Hosenpud JD, Campbell SM, Niles NR, Lee J, Mendelson D, Hart MV (1987) Exercise induced augmentation of cellular and humoral autoimmunity associated with increased cardiac dilatation in experimental autoimmune myocarditis. Cardiovasc Res 21:217–222

23. Nakatani S, McCarthy PM, Kottke-Marchant K, Harasaki H, James KB, Savage RM, Thomas JD (1996) Left ventricular echocardiographic and histologic changes: Impact of chronic unloading by an implantable ventricular assist device. J Am Coll Cardiol 27:894–901

24. Scheinin SA, Capek P, Radovancevic B, Buncan JM, McAllister HA, Frazier OH (1992) The effect of prolonged left ventricular support on myocardial histopathology in patients with end-stage cardiomyopathy. ASAIO J 38:M271–M274

25. Kinoshita M, Takano H, Takaichi S, Taenaka Y, Nakatani T (1996) Influence of prolonged ventricular assistance on myocardial histopathology in intact heart. Ann Thorac Surg 61:640–645

26. Tomantek RJ, Cooper G (1981) Morphological changes in the mechanically unloaded myocardial cell. Anat Rec 200:271–280

27. James KB, McCarthy RM, Thomas JD, Vargo R, Hobbs RE, Sapp S, Bravo E (1995) Effect of the implantable assist ventricular device on neuroendocrine activation in heart failure. Circulation 92(Suppl II):II-191–II-195

Discussion

Dr. Frazier:
Of course this is a very important observation and those of us who have seen those patients have been very impressed by their well-being. I wonder how you obtained those collagen levels. Were they right ventricular biopsies periodically, or ...?

Dr. Müller:
Well, we examined the tissue specimens we got during insertion of the apex cannula and we did not additionally perform biopsies while the patients were on the device.

Dr. Frazier:
Right.

Dr. Müller:
However, now, about 1 year after explantation we performed biopsies of the weaned patients and found the mentioned results.

Dr. Frazier:
During support?

Dr. Müller:
No no. After explantation.

Dr. Frazier:
After explantation. OK. So it was a retrospective ...

Dr. Müller:
We did it 2 months ago, yes.

Dr. Frazier:
Yes.

Dr. Müller:
We just wanted to know whether improvement in the histology of the myocardial tissue would be detectable. We chose the replacement fibrosis and collagen subtype III.

Dr. Frazier:
Have you measured the plasma norepinephrine levels?

Dr. Müller:
No, we did not, because many groups did it, and what is to expect, there is a decrease in the level of the catecholamines.

Dr. Frazier:
Well, but it is inconsistent, too. I don't think ...

Dr. Müller:
One of my colleagues did that some years ago in patients with assist devices and found a continuous decrease after implant concomitant with clinical improvement.

Dr. Frazier:
Do you think there is a level of dilatation beyond which these patients won't improve? Do you still believe that?

Dr. Müller:
My impression is that the larger the ventricle is, the less is the chance to recover. However, you have shown, yourself, an example of a patient with 90-mm internal diameter who improved to near normal values. Another parameter may be the duration of heart insufficiency.

Dr. Frazier:
Well, they can improve. They don't necessarily recover. It is interesting that in Burch's old papers, the patients who improved were the ones with the least duration of heart failure. He reported that ten patients with idiopathic myopathies that improved had an average duration of symptoms of 14 months; in the other patients it was beyond 2 years. That is very interesting work. Thank you.

Dr. Nosé:
I was very impressed about your presentation. One question: You said you removed the autoantibodies. Is that membrane system or adsorption system for autoantibody removal?

Dr. Müller:
We removed the autoantibodies you find in the serum of the patients with dilated cardiomyopathy by

immunoadsorption as an alternative therapy to implantation of an assist device.

Dr. Nosé:
So you didn't use any active removal of autoantibodies from the patient's blood?

Dr. Müller:
Yes, we removed the autoantibodies by immunoadsorption. We did this after we realized that autoantibodies may be involved in the process of dilating the heart. It was the logical next step to remove the autoantibodies instead of implanting an assist device. But this is a different, still-ongoing study and these results are very preliminary.

Dr. Nosé:
So you intend to remove them passively.

Dr. Müller:
Yes, but not in the patients with assist devices.

Dr. Nosé:
OK.

Dr. Müller:
We did it with patients on the waiting list for transplantation.

Dr. Nosé:
So, before the device implantation?

Dr. Müller:
The study with immunoadsorption was done in different patients, not in patients with assist devices.

Dr. Nosé:
OK, I understand. Thank you very much.

Dr. Müller:
I have mentioned this study in order to show that there are eventually other possibilities of treatments of idiopathic dilated cardiomyopathy.

Dr. Nosé:
Thank you very much.

Dr. Nakatani:
Congratulations. It is a very good study. In your patient group, you said if the LV diameter is beyond 72 mm, could you anticipate that patients might not recover?

Dr. Müller:
Well, it is just an observation that all patients with ventricular enlargement of above 74 mm could not be weaned from the device.

Dr. Nakatani:
From your presentation, 72 min in LV diameter is the critical point. In the group of patients whose LV diameter was less than 72 mm, the antibody decreased; and in the other patient group, whose LV diameter was greater than 72 mm, it did not decrease. So it also means that some staging of the disease has occurred, as shown by the difference of the left ventricular diameter.

Dr. Müller:
Yes, I think those patients with considerably large hearts have much more replacement fibrosis, more scars, more collagen between the cells. That may need much more time for disappearance and for improvement as in our observation time.

Dr. Galletti:
If I follow you correctly, in your series of patients in which you follow the autoantibodies under cardiac assist, the decrease in autoantibodies could be simply an index of the reduction. On the other side, in the series in which you are using immunoadsorption it seems that removing the autoantibodies has a therapeutic effect. Tell me, to the decrease in the collagen, do you think that by the cardiac assist system, you are acting on the metabolism of figroblasts in the heart because that collagen has to be secreted by fibroblasts, so are you acting on the metabolism of fibroblasts by cardiac assist system?

Dr. Müller:
Yes, I understand your point. But I have no idea whether this is true or not. I could speculate, but I have no data for that.

Dr. Jarvik:
Are you interested in other pathologies, other than the idiopathic cardiomyopathies, that may recover following reduction in the size of the heart and, if so, what are you looking at and what other kinds of conditions do you think might be promising to be weaned after all that?

Dr. Müller:
Sorry, I didn't get your question.

Dr. Jarvik:
What other pathologies, other than idiopathic cardiomyopathies, might you think could work where, after improving the function and ejection fraction through LVAD use, you could remove the device, and if you think there are other categories like ischemic disease or anything what would your thoughts be about the reason, the mechanism why that heart would improve?

Dr. Müller:
You ask me a question which I can't answer because I don't have data for that.

Dr. Jarvik:
I'm asking hypotheses and whether you've thought about it and whether you're planning to work on it.

Dr. Müller:
I think there are many parameters which will change during cardiac support and many of these will normalize. But we have to distinguish between those which were pathologically secondary to bad hemodynamic conditions and those which are involved in the development of the disease. My feeling is that most of the parameters which are discussed in the literature are secondary parameters. However, we know from animal experiments that the mentioned autoantibodies are able to induce a dilated cardiomyopathy.

Altered Hemodynamic, Humoral, and Metabolic Conditions in Nonpulsatile Systemic Circulation

Eisuke Tatsumi, Koichi Toda, Koji Miyazaki, Yoshiyuki Taenaka, Takeshi Nakatani, Toru Masuzawa, Yuzo Baba, Yoshinari Wakisaka, Kazuhiro Eya, Takashi Nishimura, Yoshiaki Takewa, Takashi Ohno, Makoto Nakamura, Seiko Endo, Koki Takiura, Young-Sang Sohn, and Hisateru Takano

Summary. Acute-phase changes in hemodynamic, hormonal, and metabolic conditions after depulsation of systemic circulation were investigated in 25 anesthetized goats. A total left heart bypass was instituted between the left atrium and ventricle and the descending aorta with an extracorporeal circuit consisting of pulsatile and nonpulsatile blood pumps. The blood flow rate was finely controlled to maintain the minimum level that allowed total left heart bypass. In this experimental setting, the character of systemic flow was rapidly converted from pulsatile to nonpulsatile mode, and the measurements were made 5 min before and 5 min after the depulsation. Blood flow rates stayed at the rather low levels of 62.2 ± 15.3 and $62.5 \pm 15.4 \, \text{ml} \cdot \text{min}^{-1} \cdot \text{kg}^{-1}$ in the pulsatile and nonpulsatile modes, respectively. The mean aortic pressure increased from 99 ± 3 to $107 \pm 3 \, \text{mmHg}$ and norepinephrine concentration rose from 300 ± 39 to $373 \pm 53 \, \text{pg/ml}$, strongly indicating that the sympathetic tone was comparatively high in the initial stage of nonpulsatile circulation. Despite keeping oxygen delivery constant at depulsation, the total oxygen consumption dropped from 1.5 ± 0.2 to $1.0 \pm 0.1 \, \text{ml/min}$, the venous oxygen saturation increased from $78\% \pm 6\%$ to $85\% \pm 5\%$, and the serum lactate level increased from 34 ± 3 to $40 \pm 4 \, \text{mg/dl}$. Thus, the oxygen uptake became less efficient after the depulsation. We conclude that changes in hemodynamic, hormonal, and metabolic conditions occur immediately after the depulsation of systemic circulation in anesthetized goats at relatively low blood flow rates.

Key words: Nonpulsatile circulation — Artificial heart — Norepinephrine — Sympathetic nerve — Oxygen consumption

Introduction

Nonpulsatile blood circulation is observed in cardiopulmonary bypass during open heart surgery or circulatory support using continuous flow blood pumps. However, the nature of the physiologic response of mammals to nonpulsatile circulation is still a controversial issue despite previous intensive studies. While awake mammals have been proven to acclimate to chronic nonpulsatile circulation [1,2], acute-phase hemodynamic, hormonal, and metabolic changes after

systemic depulsation have not yet been fully clarified. To distinguish the subtle influence of nonpulsatile flow from artifacts which necessarily accompany experimental procedure is one of the key considerations in studying this subject.

In the present study, we investigated acute-phase changes in hemodynamic, humoral, and metabolic conditions upon the conversion of systemic flow from pulsatile circulation to nonpulsatile circulation. The experiment was performed under total left heart bypass, using a specially designed circuit that permitted rapid depulsation, to minimize the influence of bypass mode, extracorporeal circuit, and experimental time.

Materials and Methods

Twenty-five adult goats weighing from 45 to 69 kg ($55.8 \pm 6.6 \, \text{kg}$, mean $\pm$ SD) were used in the present study. Under general anesthesia with isoflurane (1%–2.5%) and nitrous oxide (30%–70%), an extracorporeal left heart bypass circuit was installed through left thoracotomy. A return cannula with a graft was sutured to the descending aorta, and two uptake cannulae were inserted into the left atrium and ventricle through the left atrial appendage and the left ventricular apex, respectively. In the circuit, pulsatile and nonpulsatile pumps were placed in parallel to permit the instantaneous conversion of flow from the pulsatile to nonpulsatile mode (Fig. 1). A pneumatic ventricular assist device developed in our institute [3] and a centrifugal pump (Bio-Pump, Biomedicus, Medtronic, Eden Prairie, MN, USA) were used as the pulsatile and nonpulsatile pumps, respectively.

After surgical preparation was completed, anesthesia was changed to continuous intravenous administration of sodium pentobarbital (5 mg/kg per h). The animal was given 3 mg/kg of heparin intravenously and put on partial left heart bypass by activating the pulsatile pump. The pumping rate was set at 90 bpm, irrespective of the animal's native heart rate. Total bypass was subsequently instituted by activating the nonpulsatile pump to collect all the blood eluted from the left atrium to the left ventricle. Thereafter, the blood flow rate (BF) was not set at any fixed level but

Department of Artificial Organs, National Cardiovascular Center Research Institute, 5-7-1 Fujishiro-dai, Suita, Osaka 565, Japan

was finely controlled to maintain the minimum level that allowed total left heart bypass, by changing the driving condition of the blood pumps. Total bypass was confirmed by the maintenance of left ventricular pressure consistently lower than the concurrent aortic pressure (AoP). Under stable pulsatile total left heart bypass, instant depulsation of systemic flow was accomplished by changing the clamping site in the circuit. In nonpulsatile circulation, all the blood was drawn from both the left atrium and ventricle by the nonpulsatile pump.

The acute-phase response to the conversion of the flow mode from pulsatile to nonpulsatile was evaluated by comparing the hemodynamics, vasoactive hormone levels, and oxygen metabolic condition 5 min before and 5 min after the depulsation. Hemodynamic parameters included the mean AoP (mAoP), right atrial pressure (RAP), BF, central venous pressure (CVP), and systemic vascular resistance (SVR). The vasoactive hormones measured in the present study were epinephrine, norepinephrine, dopamine, 6-keto prostaglandin $F_{1\alpha}$ as the end product of prostaglandin I_2, prostaglandin E_2, thromboxane B_2 as the end product of thromboxane A_2, antidiuretic hormone, plasma renin activity, angiotensin I, angiotensin II, atrial natriuretic peptide, endothelin, and nitrite/nitrate as the end products of nitric oxide. The oxygen metabolic condition was evaluated by assaying arterial blood gas, oxygen delivery (DO_2), oxygen consumption (CO_2), oxygen extraction ratio (ExO_2), mixed venous oxygen saturation (SvO_2), and serum lactate concentration.

Values are expressed as mean ± standard deviation (SD). Where appropriate, statistical differences in mean value between pulsatile and nonpulsatile circulation were assessed by the Student's paired t-test. Statistical significance was defined as $P < 0.05$.

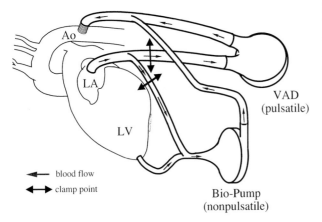

Fig. 1. Schematic drawing of left heart bypass circuit. A ventricular assist device (*VAD*) and a centrifugal pump (*Bio-Pump*) were connected in parallel in the circuit to permit rapid conversion of flow character from pulsatile to nonpulsatile mode by changing the clamping point in the circuit, as indicated by the *arrows*. *Ao*, aorta; *LA*, left atrium; *LV*, left ventricle

Results

In all the animals, the pulse pressure of more than 40 mmHg under conditions of pulsatile circulation was reduced to less than 5 mmHg with nonpulsatile circulation (Fig. 2). The mAoP significantly increased after the depulsation, from 99.1 ± 14.5 to 106.6 ± 13.3 mmHg ($P < 0.005$) (Table 1). No significant change was found

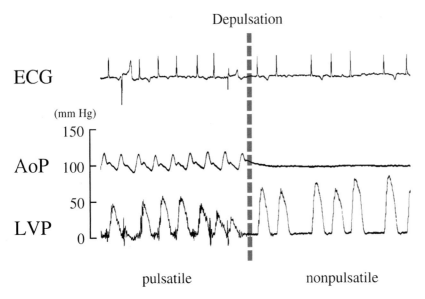

Fig. 2. Waveforms of electrocardiogram (*ECG*), aortic pressure (*AoP*), and left ventricular pressure (*LVP*). Pulsatile pumping rate was set at 90 bpm, regardless of the native heart rate. The mode of flow was rapidly converted from pulsatile to nonpulsatile. Note that the LVP was always less than the AoP, indicating that total bypass was maintained with both pulsatile and nonpulsatile circulation

Table 1. Hemodynamic parameters in pulsatile and nonpulsatile circulation

Parameter (unit)	Pulsatile (mean ± SD)	Nonpulsatile (mean ± SD)	Sample number	Paired t-test P-value
mAoP (mmHg)	99.1 ± 14.5	106.6 ± 13.3	22	0.004*
CVP (mmHg)	5.3 ± 4.2	6.2 ± 5.3	22	0.168
BF (ml·kg^{-1}·min^{-1})	62.2 ± 15.3	62.5 ± 15.4	19	0.725
SVR (dyne·s·cm^{-5})	2265 ± 591	2390 ± 527	19	0.058

mAoP, mean aortic pressure; CVP, central venous pressure; BF, systemic blood flow rate; SVR, systemic vascular resistance.
*Significant difference.

Table 2. Vasoactive hormone levels in pulsatile and nonpulsatile circulation (1)

Parameter (unit)	Pulsatile (mean ± SD)	Nonpulsatile (mean ± SD)	Sample number	Paired t-test P-value
Epinephrine (pg/ml)	84.4 ± 144.9	84.4 ± 119.1	22	0.998
Norepinephrine (pg/ml)	299.6 ± 182.3	372.9 ± 250.0	22	0.017*
Dopamine (pg/ml)	9.6 ± 7.4	11.0 ± 12.4	22	0.802
6-Keto prostaglandin $F_{1\alpha}$ (pg/ml)	496.2 ± 116.2	401.1 ± 69.8	18	0.247
Prostaglandin E_2 (pg/ml)	47.3 ± 46.8	42.5 ± 40.4	18	0.382
Thromboxane B_2 (pg/ml)	2030.9 ± 2933.7	1689.6 ± 3482.3	18	0.973

*Significant difference.

Table 3. Vasoactive hormone levels in pulsatile and nonpulsatile circulation (2)

Parameter (unit)	Pulsatile (mean ± SD)	Nonpulsatile (mean ± SD)	Sample number	Paired t-test P-value
Antidiuretic hormone (IU/l)	22.0 ± 9.0	33.0 ± 17.6	17	0.259
Plasma renin activity (ng·ml^{-1}·h^{-1})	2.42 ± 0.34	2.16 ± 0.43	21	0.197
Angiotensin I (pg/ml)	452.9 ± 61.4	477.5 ± 70.4	17	0.577
Angiotensin II (pg/ml)	39.5 ± 7.2	36.5 ± 7.0	17	0.606
Atrial natriuretic peptide (pg/ml)	165.1 ± 31.4	157.5 ± 31.6	17	0.578
Endothelin (pg/ml)	4.76 ± 0.53	4.74 ± 0.44	17	0.958
Nitrite/nitrate (μM/l)	10.6 ± 5.1	10.8 ± 5.2	17	0.269

in either the CVP or the BF. Although not statistically significant, the SVR tended to rise on the advent of nonpulsatile circulation (2390 ± 527 dyne·s·cm^{-5} with nonpulsatile vs 2265 ± 591 with pulsatile circulation, $P = 0.058$).

With regard to catecholamines, the epinephrine and dopamine levels stayed constant, whereas the norepinephrine concentration increased significantly from 299.6 ± 182.3 pg/ml before the depulsation to 372.9 ± 250.0 pg/ml after the depulsation ($P < 0.02$) (Table 2). The concentrations of prostaglandins, including 6-keto prostaglandin $F_{1\alpha}$, prostaglandin E_2, and thromboxane B_2, remained unchanged. No significant difference between pulsatile and nonpulsatile circulation was observed in the levels of antidiuretic hormone, plasma renin activity, angiotensin I, angio-

tensin II, atrial natriuretic peptide, endothelin, or nitrite/nitrate (Table 3).

The hemoglobin concentration was comparable before and after the depulsation, as shown in Table 4. No significant change was observed in arterial blood gas data, including pH, PaO_2, $PaCO_2$, HCO_3^-, and oxygen saturation. The DO_2 value stayed constant upon altering the flow character (7.43 ± 2.27 vs 7.19 ± 2.05 ml·kg^{-1}·min^{-1} in pulsatile vs nonpulsatile circulation) (Table 5). On the other hand, the VO_2 value decreased significantly, from 1.51 ± 0.76 ml·kg^{-1}·min^{-1} with pulsatile circulation to 0.99 ± 0.43 ml·kg^{-1}·min^{-1} with nonpulsatile circulation ($P < 0.02$). A significant decrease accompanying the depulsation was noted in ExO_2, the values of which were 20.1% ± 7.6% with pulsatile circulation and 14.1 ± 5.9% with nonpulsatile

Table 4. Arterial blood gas in pulsatile and nonpulsatile circulation

Parameter (unit)	Pulsatile (mean ± SD)	Nonpulsatile (mean ± SD)	Sample number	Paired t-test P-value
Hemoglobin (g/dl)	9.0 ± 2.1	8.8 ± 2.1	10	0.468
pH	7.38 ± 0.09	7.38 ± 0.10	10	0.618
PaO$_2$ (mmHg)	200.3 ± 135.6	214.3 ± 129.4	10	0.605
PaCO$_2$ (mmHg)	34.4 ± 8.0	34.4 ± 8.5	10	0.957
HCO$_3^-$ (mEq/l)	19.8 ± 2.3	19.4 ± 2.9	10	0.429
SaO$_2$ (%)	93.8 ± 10.9	94.0 ± 11.0	10	0.772

PaO$_2$, arterial oxygen partial pressure; PaCO$_2$, arterial carbon dioxide partial pressure; SaO$_2$, arterial oxygen saturation.

Table 5. Oxygen metabolic parameters in pulsatile and nonpulsatile circulation

Parameter (unit)	Pulsatile (mean ± SD)	Nonpulsatile (mean ± SD)	Sample number	Paired t-test P-value
DO$_2$ (ml·kg^{-1}·min^{-1})	7.43 ± 2.27	7.19 ± 2.05	10	0.358
VO$_2$ (ml·kg^{-1}·min^{-1})	1.51 ± 0.76	0.99 ± 0.43	10	0.014*
ExO$_2$ (%)	20.1 ± 7.6	14.1 ± 5.9	10	0.002*
SvO$_2$ (%)	78.4 ± 15.2	84.8 ± 14.4	10	0.001*
Lactate (mg/dl)	33.7 ± 11.1	40.0 ± 16.2	17	0.018*

DO$_2$, oxygen delivery; VO$_2$, oxygen consumption; ExO$_2$, oxygen extraction ratio; SvO$_2$, mixed venous blood oxygen saturation.
* Significant difference.

circulation ($P < 0.005$). A significant increase occurred in SvO$_2$, from 78.4% ± 4.8% with pulsatile circulation to 84.8% ± 4.6% with nonpulsatile circulation ($P < 0.005$). The lactate level increased significantly after the depulsation, from 33.7 ± 6.8 to 40.0 ± 15.9 mg/dl ($P < 0.02$).

Discussion

In the experimental design of this study, we intended to minimize the influence of bypass mode, circuit, and experimental time. The pulmonary circulation, which plays an important role both in autonomic nervous control through the cardiopulmonary pressor sensors and in metabolism of various vasoactive hormones including catecholamines, prostaglandins, and angiotensins, was maintained with native pulsatile flow. By employing the unique left heart bypass circuit, we could eliminate the use of an oxygenator and reduce the blood-contacting surface and priming volume of the circuit. Furthermore, the character of systemic flow could be instantaneously converted from pulsatile to nonpulsatile, and the very early adaptive response to nonpulsatile circulation could be successfully detected. However, the possible contributions of anesthesia and surgical stress were not excluded in this study, and, therefore, the results should be interpreted

within the context of the limitations of the experiment, not as general findings for nonpulsatile circulation conditions.

With respect to hemodynamic parameters, the BF ranges in the present study were 62.2 ± 15.3 and 62.5 ± 15.4 ml·min^{-1}·kg^{-1} with pulsatile and nonpulsatile circulation, respectively. While the level of BF did not change, the mAoP increased significantly and the SVR also tended to increase (though not significantly) after the depulsation. In acute experimental or clinical studies under general anesthesia and surgical intervention, higher mAoP and SVR during nonpulsatile circulation have been described by many researchers who employed relatively low flow rates, of less than 100 ml·kg^{-1}·min^{-1} [4,5]. The results of this study, made at comparatively low flow rates, appear to coincide with such findings. In contrast, others who perfused at relatively high flow rates of more than 130 ml·kg^{-1}·min^{-1} failed to observe any difference in these parameters [6,7]. Flow rate has been pointed out by several researchers as one of major factors that contribute to the inconsistent effects of nonpulsatile circulation [8]. However, the requisite flow rate in nonpulsatile circulation in the absence of anesthetic and surgical stress is still controversial. Golding et al. [1] postulated that a flow rate greater than 120 ml·kg^{-1}·min^{-1} was necessary to maintain a mammal's circulation with nonpulsatile flow, based on their long-term animal experiments in which both the systemic and the pulmonary circulation of a calf were perfused using centrifugal pumps surgically installed under the fibrillated native heart for more than 3 months. On the other hand, in our earlier study of chronic nonpulsatile circulation using goats, systemic blood flow was depulsated with the animal awake, while pulmonary circulation was maintained by native heart beating, simply by replacing the pulsatile pump in the previously installed total left heart bypass circuit with a centrifugal pump, and the animal's systemic circulation was successfully maintained with 90–130 ml·kg^{-1}·min^{-1} of nonpulsatile flow for as long as 32 days without producing any significant hemodynamic change [2,9]. Thus, the effect of nonpulsatile circulation on hemodynamic condition is very likely to be influenced by the conditions under which the study is performed.

The higher norepinephrine level with nonpulsatile than pulsatile circulation observed in the present study is consistent with the findings in the other acute-phase experimental and clinical studies [10,11]. Providing that the increase in plasma norepinephrine concentration reflects activation of the sympathetic system, the sympathetic tone must have become higher in the initial stage of nonpulsatile circulation than before the depulsation. The higher sympathetic tone in nonpulsatile circulation is in agreement with previous reports showing an increase in afferent nerve activity from carotid sinus and aortic arch baroceptors [12,13]. The increased afferent nerve activity may, in turn, inhibit the vasomotor discharge, thus resulting in increased SVR and mAoP as observed in the present study.

Prostaglandin levels have been reported to be different under conditions of pulsatile and nonpulsatile circulation [14]. In contrast, no significant change in those levels was found in this study. Since we intended to examine the very acute response after depulsation, and sampled blood after 5 min of nonpulsatile circulation, the different results may be ascribable to the duration of the absence of pulsatile flow. With respect to antidiuretic hormone and the renin–angiotensin system, as in the present study, most of the previous reports did not observe any pulsatility-dependent changes in acute experimental and clinical settings [15,16].

So far as is known, this is the first report that compares the levels of endothelin and nitric oxide, the most potent vasoconstricting and vasodilating autacoids, before and after systemic depulsation. Our results indicated that changes in these parameters in the acute phase after the flow mode conversion were imperceptible as far as the plasma concentration was concerned. Further investigation is necessary to clarify the role of these autacoids in the regulation of regional blood circulation at the time of systemic depulsation.

The present investigation manifested an unfavorable effect of nonpulsatile circulation on the metabolic condition. The decreased VO_2 and ExO_2, along with the increased SvO_2 and plasma lactate concentration, indicated that the oxygen uptake was less efficient in the initial stage of nonpulsatile circulation, and as a consequence anaerobic metabolism might have increased. Lesser oxygen uptake, denoted by lower VO_2 or lower ExO_2 and higher plasma lactate concentration, in nonpulsatile circulation has been shown by many researchers [17,18], while this finding has been dismissed in other studies [9,19]. Hickey et al. [20] pointed out that the untoward effects of nonpulsatile circulation on metabolic condition might become apparent only at low blood flow rates, of less than 100 ml·kg^{-1}·min^{-1}. The results of the present study, therefore, were in good agreement with their deduction. However, the question of whether this relationship of blood flow rate to the metabolic condition is applicable to the chronic stage of nonpulsatile circulation is still open to discussion. The results of the afore-mentioned long-term animal study, in which metabolic parameters including VO_2 and plasma lactate level were maintained at normal levels with nonpulsatile circulation at blood flow rates of 90–130 ml·kg^{-1}·min^{-1}, indicate that an awake goat without anesthetic or surgical stress may have much more versatility to adapt to nonpulsatile circulation than an anesthetized goat.

Conclusion

Hemodynamic, humoral, and metabolic conditions changed immediately after the depulsation in anesthetized goats. The elevated norepinephrine concentration and the increased mAoP and SVR implied higher activity of the sympathetic system, and the decreased VO_2 and ExO_2, along with the increased SvO_2 and plasma lactate concentration, indicated less efficient oxygen uptake, in the initial stage of nonpulsatile systemic circulation.

References

1. Golding LR, Murakami T, Harasaki H, Takatani S, Jacobs G, Yada I, Tomita K, Yozu Y, Valdes F, Fujimoto K, Nosé Y (1982) Chronic nonpulsatile blood flow. ASAIO Trans 28:81–85
2. Tatsumi E, Taenaka Y, Sakaki M, Nakatani T, Takano H (1994) Rapid conversion of systemic flow pattern from pulsatile to non-pulsatile in conscious goats. In: Niimi H, Oda M, Sawada T, Xiu R-J (eds) Progress in microcirculation research. Pergamon, Oxford, pp 463–467

3. Takano H, Nakatani T, Taenaka Y, Umezu M (1986) Development of the ventricular assist pump system: Experimental and clinical studies. In: Akutsu T (ed) Artificial Heart 1. Springer, Tokyo, pp 141–150

4. Nakayama K, Tamiya T, Yamamoto K, Izumi T, Akimoto S, Hashizume T, Iimore T, Odaka M, Yazawa C (1963) High-amplitude pulsatile pump in extracorporeal circulation with particular reference to hemodynamics. Surgery 54:798–809

5. Levy BI, Bardou A, Touchot B, Menascher P, Piwnicca A (1981) Regional blood flow during pulsatile and nonpulsatile cardiopulmonary bypass. ASAIO Trans 27:127–131

6. Wesolowski SA, Sauvage LR, Pinc RD (1955) Extracorporeal circulation: the role of the pulse in maintenance of the systemic circulation during heart–lung bypass. Surgery 37:663–682

7. Boucher JK, Rudy LW, Henly Edmunds L (1974) Organ blood flow during pulsatile cardiopulmonary bypass. J Appl Physiol 36:86–90

8. Nakamura K, Koga Y, Sekiya R, Onizuka T, Ishii K, Chiyotanda S, Shibata K (1989) The effects of pulsatile and non-pulsatile cardiopulmonary bypass on renal blood flow and function. Jpn J Surg 19:334–345

9. Taenaka Y, Tatsumi E, Nakamura H, Nakatani T, Yagura A, Sekii H, Sasaki, Akagi H, Goto M, Takano H (1990) Physiologic reactions of awake animals to an immediate switch from a pulsatile to nonpulsatile systemic circulation. ASAIO Trans 36:M541–M544

10. Minami K, Vyska K, Korfer R (1992) Role of the carotid sinus in response of integrated venous system to pulsatile and nonpulsatile perfusion. J Thorac Cardiovasc Surg 104:1639–1646

11. Minami K, Korner MM, Vyska K, Kleesiek K, Knobl H, Korfer R (1990) Effects of pulsatile perfusion on plasma catecholamine levels and hemodynamics during and after cardiac operations with cardiopulmonary bypass. J Thorac Cardiovasc Surg 99:82–91

12. Angell James JE, deBurgh Daly M (1971) Effects of graded pulsatile pressures on the reflex vasomotor responses elicited by changes of mean pressure in the perfused carotid sinus-aortic arch regions of dog. J Physiol (Lond) 214:51–64

13. Chapleau MW, Abboud FM (1989) Determination of sensitization of carotid baroreceptors by pulsatile pressure in dogs. Circ Res 65:566–577

14. Brunkwall JS, Stanley JC, Graham LM, Burkel WE, Bergqvist D (1989) Arterial 6-keto-PGF$_1$ alpha and TXB$_2$ release in ex vivo perfused canine vessels: effects of pulse rate, pulsatility, altered pressure and flow rate. Eur J Vasc Surg 3:219–225

15. Philbin DM, Levin FH, Kono K, Coggins CH, Moss J, Slater EE, Buckley M (1981) Attenuation of the stress response to cardiopulmonary bypass by the addition of pulsatile flow. Circulation 64:808–812

16. Goto M, Kudoh K, Minami S, Nukariya M, Sasaguri S, Watanabe M, Hosoda Y (1993) The renin-angiotensin-aldosterone system and hematologic changes during pulsatile and nonpulsatile cardiopulmonary bypass. Artif Organs 17:318–322

17. Dunn J, Kirsh MM, Harness J, Carroll M, Straker J, Sloan H (1984) Hemodynamic, metabolic, and hematologic effects of pulsatile cardiopulmonary bypass. J Cardiovasc Surg 25:530–536

18. Dapper F, Neppl H, Wozniak G, Strube I, Zickmann B, Hehrlein FW, Neuhof H (1992) Effects of pulsatile and nonpulsatile perfusion mode during extracorporeal circulation — a comparative clinical study. Thorac Cardiovasc Surg 40:345–351

19. Boucher JK, Rudy LW, Edmunds LH Jr (1974) Organ blood flow during pulsatile cardiopulmonary bypass. J Appl Physiol 36:86–97

20. Hickey PR, Buckley MJ, Philbin DM (1983) Pulsatile and nonpulsatile cardiopulmonary bypass: Review of a counterproductive controversy. Ann Thorac Surg 36:720–737

Discussion

Dr. Nosé:

To compare the physiology of nonpulsatile and pulsatile perfusion it is extremely important to compare the blood flow. You didn't mention anything about blood flow. What was the level?

Dr. Tatsumi:

We drove both the pulsatile and nonpulsatile blood pumps to minimize blood flow as long as total bypass was maintained. We never tried to fix the blood flow, so the blood flow was actually determined by the amount of blood coming back to the left atrium. So, in that sense, the blood flow must be influenced by right heart function. That might be affected by the venous return in response to the vascular resistance, or even the right heart function or bronchial flow. But anyway, we did not fix the blood flow.

Dr. Nosé:

During the last 15 years we repeatedly mentioned the importance of blood flow. I hope in your next study you will consider giving details of the differences in blood flow and the differences in physiology. Then I think we can assess the difference more clearly.

Dr. Tatsumi:

What you say is very true. I mentioned the blood flow itself, and, in the present work, the blood flow ranged from 2.6 to 5.2 liters per minute from that amounted to around 60 to 70 ml per kilogram per minute. In that sense our study was performed at relatively low blood-flow rates, and if we look at the previous studies, the researchers did experiments under relatively low flow rate. They tended to find a significant difference; however, if we keep the blood flow above a certain level, more than maybe 110 or 120, regardless of the acute or chronic experiments, most of the researchers failed to find any difference between the pulsatile flow and nonpulsatile flow.

Dr. Nosé:

I agree with you, but I think it is extremely important to compare different conditions with accurately measured flow.

Dr. Tatsumi:

Thank you very much for your comment.

Dr. Imachi:

In your group you have experienced long-term nonpulsatile circulation over a half-year or so. I remember that in that case almost all the data were very normalized. How do you explain the discrepancy between the current data and the chronic data?

Dr. Tatsumi:

The reason is the same as before. In our previous chronic experiment, the blood flow was maintained above 110 ml/kilogram/minute and in this study it was constantly 60 to 70 ml/kg/minute, so the blood flow rate was different. I can't say anything definitely, but maybe this difference in blood flow caused the difference in the results.

Dr. Takatani:

Why did you maintain such a low level?

Dr. Tatsumi:

As I said, we tried to minimize the flow rate. We didn't have any intention of fixing the blood-flow rate, but we just kept the 100% left heart bypass. We didn't want to overexpel the blood.

Dr. Takatani:

In your slide you said hemoglobin levels are the same and also the oxygen delivery the same between the nonpulsatile and pulsatile flows. That means flow levels should be the same, right?

Dr. Tatsumi:

Right.

Dr. Vasku:

I have some basic comments to this problem because it's a physiologic law that the cardiovascular center receives information about blood pressure, velocity of the pulse rate, and the pulse wave fluctuation as a whole. If you do a pulseless circulation you remove this information practically from the central nervous system, from the cardiovascular center, and the cardiovascular center then cannot inform by the efferent ways the periphery exactly. And I think after a long time, especially renal circulation will be compromised. What do you think about this?

Dr. Tatsumi:
Yes, that might be true. We also measured the renal sympathetic nerve activity directly in another series of experiments with the same experimental setting. We measured the sympathetic nerve activity for a very short period of time, but what we wanted to see in this experiment was the accommodation process after the depulsation. It must be very rapid, but, in a longer-term phase, we don't exactly know the result in the sympathetic activity.

Dr. Müller:
In patients after cardiac transplantation you see an increase in norepinephrine level for about half a year after operation. After that time the norepinephrine level normalized. How did you measure and in which time frame did you measure norepinephrine? Did you measure acute after switching to a nonpulsatile mode or after long-term?

Dr. Tatsumi:
We measured at 5 minutes before and 5 minutes after the flow-mode conversion. At that time we sampled the blood and measured everything.

Influence of Long-Term Support upon the Severely Failing Left Ventricle

Takeshi Nakatani, Yoshikado Sasako, Yoshio Kosakai, Keiji Kumon, Fumitaka Isobe, Kiyoharu Nakano, Junjiro Kobayashi, Kiyoyuki Eishi, Seiki Nagata, Yoshitsugu Kito, Hisateru Takano, and Yasunaru Kawashima

Summary. It is unclear how long-term support with a left ventricular assist system (LVAS) affects the severely failing left ventricle (LV). From 1994, we applied our LVAS to seven patients with profound heart failure. Of those, six patients were supported for more than 3 weeks. The etiologies of heart failure were valvular heart disease (VHD) in one, ischemic heart disease (IHD) in two, dilated phase hypertrophic cardiomyopathy (DHCM) in one, and dilated cardiomyopathy (DCM) in two. In one patient, biventricular assist was performed because of coexisting severe right heart failure. Each LVAS was installed between the left atrium and the ascending aorta and the pump was positioned paracorporeally. After stabilization of general condition, exercise was started. The natural heart size was examined and systolic heart function was evaluated by the systolic time interval (STI) under LVAS pumping by using echocardiography. This STI was calculated from the equation: ejection time divided by pre-ejection period measured from aortic valve movement. At the beginning of assistance, the STI was low (<0.7) and the LV was dilated. Four patients (1 CM, 2 IHD, 1 VHD) showed increased STI and decreased LV diastolic dimension (LVDd) during LVAS assistance and these patients were weaned from the LVAS after 26–94 days' support. The STI of these patients rose to >1 and their LVDd decreased to <70 mm. Two of them (1 CM, 1 VHD) are doing well now 2 years after LVAS removal. From these data, the cardiac function of the patient with a severely failing LV may improve when LV dilatation decreases and STI increases through long-term LVAS support.

Key words: Long-term support — Left ventricular assist system — Profound heart failure — Echocardiography — Recovery of the heart

Introduction

The left ventricular assist system (LVAS) has been applied to selected patients with profound heart failure for maintenance of the systemic circulation and for promotion of recovery of the severely failing ventricles. However, it is unclear how long-term support of LVAS affects the severely failing left ventricle. In this study, we would like to clarify the effect of long-term LVAS support on the severely failing left ventricle from our recent clinical experience.

Patients and Methods

Patients

Since 1994, we have applied the Toyobo-NCVC LVAS (Toyobo, Osaka, Japan) to seven patients with profound heart failure. Of those, one patient died within 3 weeks because of severe infection. The other six patients were supported for more than three weeks. These six patients were enrolled in this study (Table 1). These patients were all males and were 17 to 53 years old. Their diagnoses were: valvular heart disease (VHD) in one, ischemic heart disease (IHD) in two, dilated phase hypertrophic cardiomyopathy (DHCM) in one, and dilated cardiomyopathy (DCM) in two. In all patients, myocardial damage was severe and we suspected that short-term support could not salvage their damage. In one patient, biventricular assist was performed because of coexisting severe right heart failure.

System

The Toyobo-NCVC ventricular assist system (VAS) consists of an air-driven, diaphragm-type blood pump and an automatic level control drive unit [1]. The pump is made of segmented polyether polyurethane. The adult-sized pump has a stroke volume of 70 ml, and a maximum output of 7 L/min. The left VAS (LVAS) was installed between the right-sided left atrium (LA) and the ascending aorta (Ao) and the right VAS (RVAS) was installed between the right atrium and the main pulmonary artery. The pump was positioned paracorporeally.

Hemodynamic Control

In the initial stage of LVAS pumping, total flow (bypass flow + natural heart output) was kept around $3 \, L \cdot min^{-1} \cdot m^{-2}$ to stabilize the general condition includ-

National Cardiovascular Center Research Institute, 5-7-1 Fujishiro-dai, Suita, Osaka 565, Japan

Table 1. Overall results: patients supported with ventricular assist devices

Patient number	Age	Gender	Diagnosis	Duration of severe heart failure[a]	Assist	Duration of assistance	Outcome
1	42	Male	VHD (Post-operative LOS)	About 1 month	BVAS	26 dyas	Discharge
2	53	Male	LOS due to IHD	Acute onset	LVAS	28 days	Weaned/died[b]
3	52	Male	LOS due to IHD	Acute onset	LVAS	95 days	Weaned/died[c]
4	17	Male	DCM	About 4 months	LVAS	89 days	Discharge
5	32	Male	DCM	About 2 months	LVAS	276 days	Not weaned/died[c]
6	45	Male	DHCM	About 5 months	LVAS	319 days	Not weaned/died[c]

VHD, valvular heart disease; IHD, ischemic heart disease; DCM, dilated cardiomyopathy; DHCM, dilated phase hypertrophic cardiomyopathy; LOS, low cardiac output syndrome; LVAS, left ventricular assist device; BVAS, biventricular assist device.
[a] Duration of hospitalization due to heart failure.
[b] Patient died of recurrence of heart failure.
[c] Patient died of multiple organ failure.

ing major organ functions [2]. After stabilization of hemodynamics, extubation and oral feeding were initiated and enlargement of activity of daily living was tried. Natural heart function was evaluated periodically by using echocardiography [3]. When the general condition became stable, exercise, including bicycle, was started to improve the generaly condition. During the exercise, the control parameters of the LVAS were fixed and the natural heart was induced to generate the excess output for accomplishing the exercise. When the natural heart could tolerate this load without deterioration of general condition, weaning from LVAS was conducted. In the weaning process, bypass flow was decreased gradually. If the natural heart showed good function under decreased bypass flow, the LVAS would be removed. When the natural heart function was insufficient for weaning, LVAS support was continued.

The ECG-triggered pumping mode was selected during the early stage of LVAS pumping to decrease the afterload to the natural heart. When the patient's general condition was stabilized and the weaning process was started, a fixed rate pumping mode was selected.

Echocardiographic Examination

Evaluation of the natural heart function was performed by echocardiography. One of the parameters for evaluation was natural heart size, indicated by the left ventricular diastolic dimension (LVDd). Systolic heart function was evaluated by the systolic time interval (STI) under LVAS pumping. This STI was calculated from the equation: ejection time (ET) divided by pre-ejection period (PEP) measured from the aortic valve movement. These parameters were measured under the ECG-triggered mode of LVAS pumping. Recovery of heart function could be monitored by this STI. We previously reported that the STI was useful

for estimation of the cardiac function of the LVAS patients [3].

Results

The overall results are shown in Table 1. In four patients, the natural hearts recovered and LVAS were removed after 1–3 months' support. Two of them (one DCM, one VHD) were discharged and are doing well now 2 years after removal. In one patient [low cardiac output syndrome (LOS) due to IHD], the heart functioned well after the removal of the LVAS. Unfortunately, he died of multiple organ failure due to thromboembolism. The other patient (LOS due to IHD) suffered from recurrent heart failure after the removal of the LVAS, and died. In the other two cases, recovery of the natural heart was insufficient and they could not be weaned from the LVAS.

In weaned cases, the heart size decreased after LVAS support. In contrast, the LVDd of unweaned cases showed unremarkable change. Changes in the LVDd in all cases are shown in Fig. 1. The LVDd of weaned cases decreased below 70mm within 4 weeks. In contrast, those of unweaned cases showed no marked decrease and stayed large.

In one representative weaned case, the aortic valve was not open at the beginning of LVAS support. On the 10th day, the ejection time increased markedly, but the pre-ejection period was long, which indicated electromechanical disturbance of the natural heart. On the 51st day, the aortic valve movement showed a long ejection time with a short pre-ejection period, which indicated recovery of the natural heart. Changes of the systolic time interval in all six patients are shown in Fig. 2. At the beginning of assistance, the STI was low (<0.7) in all cases. In the four weaned cases, the STI increased to >1.0 within 3 weeks. On the other hand, in the unweaned cases, the STI stayed at a relatively low value.

Fig. 1. Changes in left ventricular end-diastolic dimension

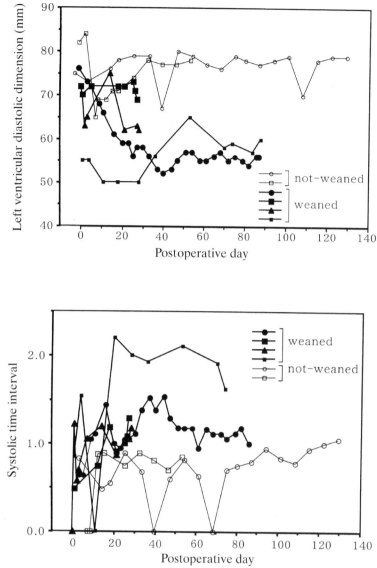

Fig. 2. Changes in the systolic time interval (STI, calculated by dividing the ejection time ET by the pre-ejection period PEP)

Pathologic findings in the myocardium from the right ventricle of one weaned case (no. 4, DCM case) were as follows. The myocardium at LVAS application showed prominent enlargement and vacuolar change of myocytes. At the time of removal, cell size had decreased to near normal, vacuolar change was reduced, and scatted interstitial fibrosis was seen in both the ventricles.

Discussion

A VAS can maintain the systemic circulation of a patient with profound heart failure and can buy time to allow the recovery of the damaged heart. Also, VASs have given good results in postcardiotomy cardiogenic shock cases [4–6]. However, the likelihood that the severely failing left ventricle will recover is unclear. Recently, bridges to heart transplantation have been performed successfully in many patients. The duration of support has become longer and longer because of the lack of donor hearts and the stability of patients' condition under LVAS support [7]. In a number of cases of prolonged support, reported by several groups, natural heart function recovered, and a few patients were weaned from LVAS successfully [8–13].

The influence of long-term LV support on the damaged myocardium is unclear. Our cases showed recovery of myocardium from damage after long-term support. Several researchers postulated, based on their experimental results, that long-term unloading of the LV by using an LVAS might have an adverse effect on the myocardium in normal hearts, such as atrophy [14,15]. Recently, several groups reported the possibility of recovery of the failing heart through long-term support. Frazier reported that long-term LV support by the TCI HeartMate may improve the cardiac function of DCM patients [11]. Also, the Berlin group reported that four patients were weaned from the Novacor LVAS after several months of support [12]. Further-more, the Cleveland Clinic group reported that chronic LV unloading with an implantable LVAS allows myocardial healing [13]. The possibility of recovery of damaged myocardium through long-term LV support should be researched precisely in further studies.

In our series, LV support was performed under LA-Ao bypass, in which complete reduction of the LV was difficult. When LV-Ao bypass is selected, the result after long-term support may be different from our results. More research is needed to clarify this point. Recently, the Berlin group pointed out that heart function recovered in the patients whose levels of anti-β_1-adrenoceptor autoantibodies decreased to zero [12]. Immunological reaction might have an impact on the myocardium in heart failure patients. Further studies are needed to clarify the pathogenesis of heart failure and pathophysiology of the failing heart under long-term mechanical support.

The accurate evaluation of LV function and the prediction of reversibility of LV function are difficult. Under LVAS pumping, the usual parameters of echocardiography such as fractional shortening are inadequate for the assessment of ventricular function, because the ventricular septum shows paradoxical movement. We used the STI as a practical parameter for the evaluation of whole LV function [3]. Although the STI is influenced by preload, afterload, and heart rate, patients with a high STI score could be weaned from the LVAS in acute profound heart failure, as we have reported. From this study, a decrease in LV size was one of the indicators of reversibility, and further, the STI indicated the reversibility of myocardial function. In one patient, recurrent heart failure occurred after the removal of the LVAS and finally he died. In this patient, weaning from an intra-aortic balloon pump (IABP) and catecholamine were performed; his heart tolerated the weaning process well and his general condition was satisfactorily maintained. Recurrence of heart failure might be induced by repeated heart attack due to ischemic heart disease, and the prediction of this kind of recurrence is difficult.

From these data, the cardiac function of the patient with a severely failing LV may improve when LV dilatation decreases and the STI increases due to long-

term LVAS (LA-Ao bypass) support. Long-term VAS support should be considered to promote the recovery of heart function in patients with profound heart failure.

References

1. Takano H, Nakatani T, Taenaka Y, Umezu M (1985) Development of the ventricular assist pump system: Experimental and clinical studies. In: Akutsu T (ed) Artificial heart 1. Springer, Tokyo, pp 141–151
2. Nakatani T, Sasako Y, Kumon K, Nagata S, Kosakai Y, Isobe F, Nakano K, Kobayashi J, Eishi K, Takano H, Kito Y, Kawashima Y (1995) Long-term circulatory support to promote recovery from profound heart failure. ASAIO J 41:M526–M530
3. Nakatani T, Takano H, Beppu S, Noda H, Taenaka Y, Kumon K, Kito Y, Fujita T, Kawashima Y (1991) Practical assessment of natural heart function using echocardiography in mechanically assisted patients. ASAIO Trans 37:M420–M421
4. Nakatani T, Takano H, Taenaka Y, Kumon K, Kito Y, Fujita T, Kawashima Y (1991) Clinical application of ventricular assist system (VAS) for post-cardiotomy profound heart failure: results and clinical consideration. Jpn J Artif Organs 20:342–348
5. Pae WE Jr. Miller CA, Matthews Y, Pierce WS (1992) Ventricular assist devices for postcardiotomy cardiogenic shock. J Thorac Cardiovasc Surg 104:541–553
6. Takano H, Nakatani T (1996) Ventricular assist system: Experience in Japan with Toyobo Pump and Zeon Pump. Ann Thorac Surg 61:317–322
7. Griffith BP, Kormos RL, Nastala CJ, Winowich S, Pristas JM (1996) Results of extended bridge to transplantation: Window into the future of permanent ventricular assist devices. Ann Thorac Surg 61:396–398
8. Holman WL, Bourge RC, Kirklin JK (1991) Circulatory support for seventy days with resolution of acute heart failure. J Thorac Cardiovasc Surg 102:932–934
9. Jacquet L, Zerbe T, Stein KL, Kormos RL, Griffith BP (1991) Evolution of human cardiac myocyte dimension during prolonged mechanical support. J Thorac Cardiovasc Surg 101:256–259
10. Scheinin SA, Capek P, Radovancevic B, Duncan JM, McAllister HA Jr, Frazier OH (1992) The effect of prolonged left ventricular support on myocardial histopathology in patients with end-stage cardiomyopathy. ASAIO J 38:M271–M274
11. Frazier OH (1994) First use of an untethered, vented electric left ventricular assist device for long-term support. Circulation 89:2908–2914
12. Theodoridis V, Muller J, Weng YG, Loebe M, Spiegelsberger S, Hennig E, Kaufmann F, Hetzer R (1996) Mechanical circulatory support (MCS) using implantable cardiac assist devices for more than 200 days. ASAIO J 42(2):33
13. Nakatani S, McCarthy PM, Kottke-Marchant K, Harasaki H, James KB, Savage RM, Thomas JD (1996) Left ventricular echocardiographic and histologic changes: Impact of chronic unloading by an

implantable ventricular assist device. J Am Coll Cardiol 27:894–901

14. Harasaki H, Zheng Z, Morimoto T, McMahon J (1985) Morphometric studies of chronic fibrillating heart. ASAIO Trans 31:73–78

15. Kinoshita M, Takano H, Taenaka Y, Mori H, Takaichi S, Noda H, Tatsumi E, Yagura A, Sekii H, Akutsu T (1988) Cardiac disuse atrophy during LVAD pumping. ASAIO Trans 34:208–212

Sympathetic Nerve Adjustment to Artificial Circulation

Tomoyuki Yambe[1], Shun-suke Nanka[1], Taro Sonobe[1], Shigeru Naganuma[1], Shin-ichi Kobayashi[1], Kazuhiko Shizuka[1], Makoto Watanabe[1], Akira Tanaka[2], Makoto Yoshizawa[2], Ken-ichi Abe[2], Makoto Miura[3], Kou-ichi Tabayashi[3], Hideki Takayasu[4], Kazutoshi Gouhara[5], Ken Naitoh[6], Hiroshi Takeda[7], and Shin-ichi Nitta[1]

Summary. To analyze the dynamical behavior of the autonomic nervous system while being driven by an artificial heart, sympathetic nerve discharges were analyzed by the use of nonlinear mathematics, including chaos and fractal theory. For the comparison of the natural and artificial circulation, a biventricular bypass type, total artificial circulation model was adopted under ventricular fibrillation in short-term animal experiments on four healthy mongrel dogs. After the implantation of a biventricular assist pneumatic pump, bipolar stainless steel bipolar electrodes were attached to the left renal sympathetic nerve via a retroperitoneal approach, to record the sympathetic nerve discharges. After amplifying the nerve activity with a preamplifier, the sympathetic discharges were further amplified with a main amplifier and integrated with a resistance–capacitance (R–C) integrator (time constant 0.1 s). After control natural-circulation data were recorded without biventricular assistance, ventricular fibrillation was induced electrically, and the biventricular bypass pneumatic pump was started, constituting the total artificial circulation model. Driving parameters for the bypass pumps were manually controlled to maintain the hemodynamic parameters within the normal range. Time-series data of the hemodynamics and sympathetic nerve discharges were recorded in the data recorder and calculated in a personal computer system (PC9801RA) through an analog–digital (A–D) converter. Even during artificial heart circulation, the reconstructed attractor of the sympathetic discharges in the phase space appeared to be a strange attractor, which is a feature of deterministic chaos. However, the Kolomosov–Sinai (KS) entropy of the reconstructed attractor decreased during artificial circulation, suggesting changes in the nonlinear dynamics in the autonomic nervous system. Various values of the KS entropy were observed according to the various drive rates of the artificial heart. Our results suggest that there is chaotic itineracy in the autonomic nervous system according to variations in the natural and artificial circulation, and artificial heart drive rate. These results suggest sympathetic nerve adjustments of the circulatory regulatory system in response to the artificial heart. It becomes possible to analyze the information-processing mechanism of the central nervous system by such an open loop experiment using an artificial organ. This mechanism is a focus of attention in the scientific community. We expect that this paper will contribute to understanding this field.

Key words: Chaotic itineracy — Chaos — Fractal — Kolomosov–Sinai (KS) entropy — Sympathetic nerve activity

Introduction

Some institutions have succeeded in supporting animals with total artificial hearts for more than one year [1,2]. As an aim of future research, it is important to design a more effective artificial heart. To that end, the influence of an artificial heart on the body needs to be made clear.

The body of a person implanted with an artificial heart shows dynamical behavior different from the normal body [3]. Until now, we have focused on the influence of an artificial heart on the body [4]. In the present study, we turned our attention to the autonomic nervous system, and measured sympathetic nerve activity during artificial heart circulation.

Recently, nonlinear dynamics in the cerebral nervous system have attracted attention [5]. In particular, a positive role is being investigated for deterministic chaos in the cerebral nerve mechanism. Because chaos shows that complicated behavior can arise in a simple system [6,7], it is thought that it is applicable to the analysis of the nerve mechanism. In this study, short-term experiments were performed on healthy mongrel dogs using artificial heart circulation, and time-series curves of sympathetic nerve activity were recorded. An artificial heart of the biventricular bypass type was selected, to compare the circulation of the artificial heart with the circulation of the natural heart. In addition, we changed the driving rate of the artificial heart,

[1] Department of Medical Engineering and Cardiology, Institute of Development, Aging and Cancer, Tohoku University, 4-1 Seiryo-machi, Aoba-ku, Sendai, Miyagi 980-77, Japan
[2] Graduate School of Engineering and [4] Information Sciences, Tohoku University, Aramaki, Aoba-ku, Sendai, Miyagi 980-77, Japan
[3] Department of Thoracic and Cardiovascular Surgery, Tohoku University School of Medicine, 1-1 Seiryo-machi, Aoba-ku, Sendai, Miyagi 980-77, Japan
[5] Department of Applied Physiology, Faculty of Engineering, Hokkaido University, Kita 13-jou, Nishi 8 choume, Kita-ku, Sapporo, Hokkaido 060, Japan
[6] Nissan Motor Company, Tokyo, Japan
[7] Faculty of Engineering, Tohoku-gakuin University, Sendai, Miyagi 983, Japan

and studied the non-linear dynamics of the autonomic nerve activity.

The results of nonlinear mathematical analysis of the autonomic nerve action potential were considered, together with our past research results, in terms of nonlinear mathematical theory, and nonlinear neural network theory. Information obtained about neural information-processing in biological systems is also reported.

Materials and Methods

After anesthesia was induced with thiopental sodium (2.5 mg/kg) and ketamine sodium (5.0 mg/kg) in four mongrel dogs weighing 15–35 kg, the left pleural cavity was opened through the fifth intercostal space, under mechanical ventilation. Electrodes were put in place for electrocardiography (ECG), and arterial blood pressure (BP) and left atrial pressure (LAP) were monitored continuously using catheters inserted into the artery and left atrium through the left femoral artery and left atrial appendage, respectively.

For left heart implantation, a polyvinyl chloride (PVC) cannula was inserted into the left atrium and descending aorta, and fixed by ligation. PVC cannulae were also inserted into the right atrium and the pulmonary artery, and they were fixed by ligature for right heart implantation. The left renal artery was exposed using a left retroperitoneal approach. The sympathetic nerve on the renal artery was exposed to light. A bipolar stainless steel electrode was attached to the renal sympathetic nerve, after the membrane of the nerve was removed.

Firstly, the nerve activity was amplified with a preamplifier, and recorded in a magnetic-tape data recorder through a main amplifer. The renal sympathetic nerve activity was integrated using a resistance–capacitance (R–C) integrator with a time constant 0.1 s. The integration waveform was also recorded on magnetic tape. The data provided was input into a personal computer through an analog–digital (A–D) converter. Integration, quantitative analysis, and nonlinear analysis were done. Nonlinear mathematical theory was used, and the time-series curve of sympathetic nerve activity was embedded into the phase space [3] using the procedure of Takens [7]. The embedding attactor of the sympathetic nerve discharges was used, and the fractal dimension and the Lyapunov exponent were calculated. The mathematical calculation methodologies were reported in [3–12].

After preparation, control time-series data were recorded with the artificial heart off, then the biventricular assist device was started, and ventricular fibrillation was induced electrically. After the stabilization of all the hemodynamic parameters, time-series data for the artificial heart were recorded. The artificial heart was manually controlled to maintain the hemodynamic parameters within the normal range, and maintained in a fixed-drive condition during the recording.

Results

With the artificial heart, all hemodynamic parameters were almost normal, and pump output was sufficient. The time-series data on hemodynamics and sympathetic nerve action potential were recorded satisfactorily. During artificial heart circulation, the heart was electrically fibrillated. Sympathetic nerve activity during artificial heart circulation was synchronized with the beat of the artificial heart. This synchronization of the sympathetic discharges was observed in all the experimental animals.

The attractor of the integration waveform of sympathetic nerve activity, reconstituted into the three-dimensional phase space, is shown in Fig. 1. The attractor is of opened form, and the dynamical system is described well. Fractal structure is observed in the disjunction of the trajectory. Similar structure was observed when one part of the reconstructed attractors was enlarged.

The disjunction of this trajectory was measured with the methodology of the Lyapunov exponents. Chaotic systems characteristically exhibit sensitive dependence on initial conditions. The Lyapunov exponent is a quantitative measure of this rate of separation. The largest Lyapunov exponents obtained with the various

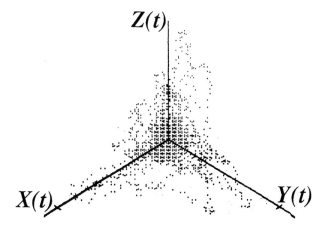

Fig. 1. Reconstructed attractor of the sympathetic nerve discharges embedded into three-dimensional phase space. The nerve action was recorded from the sympathetic nerve of the kidney. According to the methodology of Takens [7], the attractor was reconstructed. Time-series data of the nerve activity were embedded into three-dimensional phase space. An attractor of opened-up form was expressed. t, time

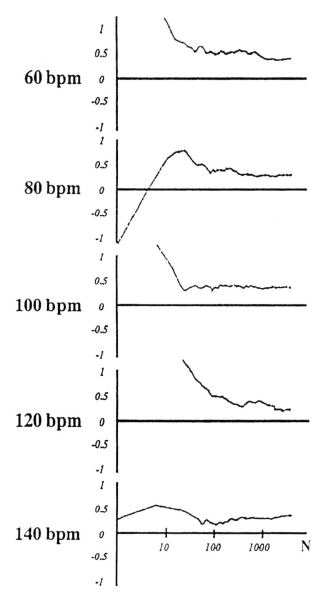

Fig. 2. Maximum Lyapunov exponents calculated from the sympathetic nerve discharges during total artificial circulation at various driving rates. The sum of the positive Lyapunov exponents indicates the Kolomosov-Sinai (KS) entropy of the reconstructed attractor in the phase space, suggesting information generation in the separated time series. bpm, beats per minute (driving rate)

driving rates of the artificial heart are shown in Fig. 2. Under all drive conditions, positive values for the maximum Lyapunov exponents were observed. Even if the driving rate of the artificial heart is changed, the chaotic dynamics of the sympathetic nerve is maintained. As shown in Fig. 2, a difference in driving rate influences the values of the Lyapunov exponents of the sympathetic nerve discharges. These data showed that driving conditions of the artificial heart influence

the nonlinear chaotic dynamics of the sympathetic nervous system.

Discussion

One of the major findings of this study is that the sympathetic nerve activity maintained chaotic dynamics, even during artificial heart circulation. The existence of chaos was confirmed by the following characteristics. First, it was possible to obtain a strange attractor. The reconstructed attractor was of open form, and the dynamical system appeared to be described well. Fractal structure was observed in the disjunction of the trajectory. Similar structure was observed when one part of the reconstructed attractors was enlarged. Fractal configuration is recognized by the occurrence of a strange attractor, which is a well-known characteristic of deterministic chaos. Second, the Lyapunov exponents were measured. The Lyapunov exponent is a quantitative measure of this rate of separation. If at least one Lyapunov exponent is positive, it strongly suggests chaotic dynamics. At every pump rate, the largest Lyapunov exponents were always positive. Even if the driving rate of an artificial heart is changed, the chaotic dynamics of the sympathetic nerve discharges is maintained. Variation in the driving rate influences the values of the Lyapunov exponents of the sympathetic nerve discharges. This shows that the driving rate of the artificial heart influences the nonlinear dynamics of the sympathetic nervous system.

Deterministic chaos is characterized by deterministic behavior, where irregular patterns obey mathematical equations and are critically dependent upon initial conditions [9–14]. The nonlinear dynamics of sympathetic nerves wander about the attractors, for which various values of the Lyapunov exponents were shown, according to the driving rate of the artificial heart. All these attractors are strange attractors which are characteristic of chaotic dynamics. In other words, the central nervous system, which mediates sympathetic nerve activity, wanders about various nonlinear attractors while maintaining chaotic dynamics.

Tsuda proposed the concept of "chaotic itineracy" as a mathematical model of the nonlinear dynamics of the central nervous system as part of his work on neural networks [9]. In phase space, a conditional function of the series wanders about the attractor of low entropy, as shown in Fig. 3. Such a highly advanced cerebral nerve mechanism as memory is likely to be expressed by this conception. If this algorithm explains the mechanism of nerve function, this concept is expected to apply universally in the central nervous system. Circulation drive controlled through the nervous system may also be relevant to this concept.

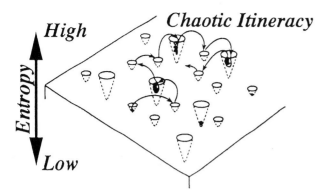

Fig. 3. Schematic diagram of "chaotic itineracy," a concept in nonlinear neural network science. This wanders about various attractors while maintaining the chaotic dynamics. As for the attractor, its KS entropy is lower than the transition course. To some extent, in the conditions with lower entropy, it becomes stable. Alteration of the artificial heart driving condition which answered the automatic control system brings transition of the attractor of the sympathetic nerve discharges

The dynamics of the sympathetic nerve controlling circulation wanders about various nonlinear chaotic attractors according to the drive rate of the artificial heart. However, catastrophe does not result from maintaining chaotic dynamics [13]. Upwards in the concept diagram (Fig. 3) represents increasing entropy, and downwards, lower entropy. For example, considering the case of a natural heart, an upward movement increases randomness, i.e., may be toward ventricular fibrillation. Conversely, cardiac arrest occurs at the lowest entropy. In a sense, the chaotic average condition in between these extremes becomes stable. Chaos is originally recognized by the time series running by oneself. Originally, the meaning of the notion of chaotic itineracy was that attractors in the phase space wandered by themselves without external stimuli. This concept may also be applied to the mechanical heart inside a biological system.

The notion of the edge of chaos is well-known in nonlinear dynamics. Chaos appears from one point by letting a parameter of the equation change. Such a phenomenon has been discovered in various fields. For example, in the genetic algorithms, the probability of survival rises with an increase in gene duplication rate, but survival probability suddenly drops if a certain point is reached [14]. When one tries to increase the probability of survival, development of chaotic dynamics is recognized, but when, furthermore, probability of survival is given, the system moves toward oscillation, and the probability of survival makes a sudden drop in the next generation. At the edge of chaos, there is oscillation, which is a low entropy con-

dition, more as recognized in this example, and a dynamic series tending toward catastrophe comes to mind next. In these conditions, chaotic dynamics maintains homeostasis and complexity.

Our results suggest that sympathetic nerve activity in the circulation of the artificial heart also produces chaotic itineracy according to the driving rate. By this mechanism, the characteristic of prediction impossibility is arrived at with stability. If the system had the characteristic of prediction impossibility, prospective behavior could not be predicted, because the system would be too complicated. If the system had the character of stability, we could easily predict the future. Therefore, these are mutually contradictory characteristics, generally. However, if the concept of chaotic itineracy is used, it can be explained logically. Chaotic dynamics are characterized by sensitive dependence on initial conditions; thus, we cannot predict future behavior, though the dynamics may fit a simple equation. Also, the chaotic dynamics has an attractor in the phase space; this indicates a measure of stability.

These phenomena indicate adaptation to the artificial heart of the central nervous system. It becomes possible to analyze the information-processing mechanism of the central nervous system by such an open loop experiment using an artificial organ. This mechanism is of interest to the advanced scientific community. We expect that our results will contribute to the evolution of this area of science.

In conclusion, sympathetic nerve activity shows chaotic dynamics with circulation driven by an artificial heart. This dynamics suggested chaotic itineracy according to changes in the driving rate of the artificial heart. It is thought that this mechanism accommodates both stability and prediction impossibility.

Acknowledgments. The mathematical methodology of this paper was discussed in the workshop "Various approaches to the complex systems" held at the International Institute for Advanced Studies. The authors thank Mr. Kimio Kikuchi for cooperation with experiments, and Miss Rie Sakurai and Mrs. Hisako Iijima for their excellent assistance and cooperation. This work was partly supported by a Grant-in-aid for Developmental Scientific Research (06558118, 07557309) and a Grant-in-aid for Scientific Research on Priority Areas (08234201), Research Grant for Cardiovascular Diseases from the Ministry of Heatlth and Welfare and Mochida Memorial Foundation.

References

1. Snyder AJ, Rosenberg G, Reibson J, Donachy JH, Prophet GA, Arenas J, Daily B, McGary S, Kawaguchi O, Quinn R, Pierce WS (1992) An electrically powered total artificial heart: over 1 year survival in the calf. ASAIO J 38:M707–M712

2. Abe Y, Chinzei T, Isoyama T, Mabuchi K, Matsuura H, Baba K, Kouno A, Ono T, Mochizuki S, Sun YP, Imanishi K, Yoshizawa M, Tanaka A, Uchiyama K, Fujimasa I, Atsumi K, Imachi K (1997) Long-term hemodynamics and pathophysiology in a total artificial heart goat survived for 532 days with 1/R control. Jpn J Artif Organs 26:21–26

3. Yambe T, Nitta S, Sonobe T, Naganuma S, Kakinuma Y, Izutsu K, Akiho H, Kobayashi S, Ohsawa N, Nanka S, Tanaka M, Fukuju T, Miura M, Uchida N, Sato N, Tabayashi K, Koide S, Abe K, Takeda H, Yoshizawa M (1995) Deterministic chaos in the hemodynamics of an artificial heart. ASAIO J 41:84–88

4. Yambe T, Nitta S, Sonobe T, Tanaka M, Miura M, Satoh N, Mohri H, Yoshizawa M, Takeda H (1990) Effect of left ventricular assistance on sympathetic tone. Int J Artif Organs 13:681–686

5. West BJ (1990) Fractal physiology and chaos in medicine. World Scientific, Singapore

6. Crutchfield JP, Farmer JD, Packard NH, Shaw RS (1986) Chaos. Sci Am 255:46–57

7. Goldberger AL, Rignery DR, West BJ (1990) Chaos and fractals in human physiology. Sci Am 259:35–41

8. Takens F (1981) Detecting strange attractors in turbulence. In: Rand DA, Young LS (eds) Lecture notes in mathematics. Springer, Berlin, pp 366–381

9. Tsuda I, Tahara T, Iwanaga H (1992) Chaotic pulsation in human capillary vessels and its dependence on mental and physical conditions. Int J Bifurc Chaos 2:313–324

10. Denton TA, Diamond GA, Helfant RH, Khan S, Karaguenzian H (1990) Fascinating rhythm — a primer to chaos theory and its application on cardiology. Am Heart J 20:1419–1440

11. Tsuda I (1990) Chaotic brain observation (in Japanese). Science, Tokyo

12. Pinsker HM, Bell J (1981) Phase plane description of endogenous neuroral oscillators in aphysia. Biol Cybern 39:211–221

13. Yambe T, Nitta S, Sonobe T, Naganuma S, Kakinuma Y, Kobayashi S, Tanaka M, Fukuju T, Miura M, Sato N, Mohri H, Koide S, Takeda H, Yoshizawa M, Kasai T, Hashimoto H (1994) Chaotic hemodynamics during oscillated blood flow. Artif Organs 18:633–637

14. Naitoh K (1995) Four group equation of genetic algorithm. JSME Int J Series-C 38:240–248

Pathological Study of a Goat That Survived for 532 Days with a Total Artificial Heart Using the 1/R Control Method

Kunihiko Mabuchi[1], Yusuke Abe[2], Sei-ichiro Shimizu[3], Kou Imachi[2], Tsuneo Chinzei[2], Hiroyuki Matsuura[1], Takashi Isoyama[1], Kazunori Baba[2], Kaoru Imanishi[2], Syuichi Mochizuki[2], Yen-Ping Sung[2], Tomotaro Tago[1], Akimasa Kono[2], Toshiya Ono[2], and Iwao Fujimasa[1]

Summary. A goat survived for 532 days with a pneumatically driven total artificial heart (TAH) that was controlled by the 1/R (reciprocal of peripheral resistance) method. Pathological observations were compared with those of long-surviving goats which had been fitted with TAHs that were operated with fixed driving parameters. The most striking pathological differences were observed in the liver. In the goat under study, congestion of the liver was not as severe as in the past cases in which the central venous pressure (CVP) was high, although fibrosis was prominent around the hepatic veins in many areas of the liver. In both kidneys, severe infarctions were prominent (as in the past cases), but a characteristic of this case was the existence of marked hemosiderosis at proximal tubules; however, this was not prominent in the spleen and liver. This suggested that the hemosiderosis was due to hemolysis in the blood pump rather than due to an increased destruction of erythrocytes in the spleen and liver. The pathological improvements in the liver are believed to have been due to a comparatively low CVP (approximately 5–10 mmHg) which was achieved by the use of the 1/R control method, even though the existence of pathological abnormalities in the kidneys and liver suggested that such long-term driving of the TAH may still cause hemolysis and some damage to the liver. This point requires further investigation.

Key words: Total artificial heart — 1/R control method — Pathological change — Central venous pressure — Centrilobular necrosis — Hemosiderosis

Introduction

A goat with a pneumatically driven total artificial heart that was controlled by the 1/R method [1] survived for a full 532 days. Because the goat survived for this long period, and because of the "high quality of life" of the goat during the postoperative survival period, it is believed that the 1/R control method has led

to important improvements. Before this 1/R control method was employed, the TAH system had been driven using a method in which the driving parameters of the right and left heart blood pumps were determined so that (1) the right heart blood pump could maintain a certain range of output (90–100 ml · min⁻¹·kg⁻¹), and (2) the left heart blood pump could push out all the venous return in accordance with the so-called Starling's law; in this method, once the driving parameters are thus determined, they basically remain unaltered [2]. The most serious problem in this latter control method has been the impossibility of controlling the central venous pressure (CVP) at a physiologically acceptable value, with the value usually rising to 15–30 mmHg [3]; in contrast, the 1/R control method made it possible to decrease the CVP to a comparatively low value (5–10 mmHg).

In this study, therefore, the pathological observations of the goat that survived for 532 days with a total artificial heart controlled by the 1/R method were compared with observations of long-surviving goats with a total artificial heart driven with fixed driving parameters [4] in order to clarify exactly what had been improved by the 1/R control method, and what still remains to be improved with regard to the control of the artificial heart system.

Materials and Methods

A comparison of pathological findings was performed between the goat that survived for 532 days using the 1/R method (#9403) and the longest surviving goat in the group with a total artificial heart operated with fixed driving parameters that survived for 344 days (goat #8304) [4,5]. The profiles of these two goats are given in Table 1. The artificial heart systems employed in the two experiments were basically the same, with the main difference being the control method for driving the artificial heart system. The 1/R control method basically involves altering the pump output in accordance with the change in peripheral resistance and aortic pressure. The pump output is determined by:

---

[1] Research Center for Advanced Science and Technology (RCAST), The University of Tokyo, 4-6-1 Komaba, Meguro-ku, Tokyo 153, Japan
[2] Institute of Medical Electronics, Faculty of Medicine, The University of Tokyo, 7-3-1 Hongo, Bunkyo-ku, Tokyo 113, Japan
[3] Department of Anatomy, Faculty of Medicine, The University of Tokyo

Table 1. Profiles of goats with total artificial hearts controlled by the 1/R method (goat no. 9403) or by fixed driving parameters (goat no. 8304)

	Experimental animal	
	#9403	#8304
Animal	Goat (female)	Goat (female)
Survival period	532 days	344 days
Artificial heart system		
Blood pump	Sac type (60 ml) (PVC-KIII)	Sac type (100 ml) (PVC-Cardiothane)
Valve	Jellyfish valve	Björk-Shiley valve
Driving system	Pneumatic driving system CORART 103[a]	As for #9403
Control method	1/R control method	Fixed driving parameters
CVP	5–10 mmHg	15–30 mmHg
Ascites	0 ml	13 700 ml
Pleural effusion	300 ml	600 ml
Cause of death	Pulmonary edema (due to acute left heart pump failure)	Chronic circulatory insufficiency

PVC, polyvinyl chloride.
[a] Aishin Cosmos.

$$CO(n+1) = \left(AoP.set(n+1) - RAP.set\right) \cdot \left(1/TPR\right)$$
$$+ CP \cdot \left(AoP - AoP.set(n)\right)$$

Here, CO(n + 1) = desired value of pump output
AoP = aortic pressure
AoP.set = set point of the aortic pressure
RAP.set = set point of the right atrial pressure
TPR = total peripheral resistance
CP = gain value of the compensation term

The value of Aop.set (n) is determined further by the following equation:

$$AoP.set(n) = p \cdot AoP.set(n-1) + (1-p) \cdot (AoP)$$

Here, $p = \exp(-t/\tau)$
t = sampling interval of the aortic pressure (2 s)
τ = time constant (12 h)

The driving parameters (the positive pressure, vacuum pressure, and the pumping rate) of both the right and left pumps are altered so that the total artificial heart system can maintain the set point of the stroke volume and preserve a balance between the right and left atrial pressures [1].

In the goat with fixed driving parameters, the outputs of the right and left heart blood pumps were respectively maintained at approximately 90–100 and 100–110 ml·min^{-1}·kg, and the CVP was elevated to 15–30 mmHg. In the goat controlled by the 1/R method, the outputs of the right and left heart blood pumps were altered after each beat in accordance with the values of the peripheral resistance and aortic pressure. The range of pump output altered much more widely than in the case of the goat with a total artificial heart that was operated with fixed driving parameters. The difference in the average value of pump output over the whole survival period was not significant, but a comparison of the pump outputs of the two goats at a similar resting state revealed a tendency for the pump output in the goat controlled by the 1/R method to be approximately 20%–30% higher than in the other goat; this meant that the CVP could be maintained at between 5 and 10 mmHg.

Comparison of the Pathological Findings

Liver

The most striking pathological difference was observed in the liver. Figure 1a shows the macroscopic and microscopic findings in the two cases. Macroscopically, the congestion and pathological changes were much less severe in the 1/R control case than in the goat with fixed driving parameters; the former appeared macroscopically almost normal. Under microscopic observation, however, basically the same pathological findings were observed in both cases, although the changes were much more prominent in the goat with fixed driving parameters than in the goat using the 1/R control method. In both cases, necrosis of the hepatic cells and fibrotic degeneration were prominent in many areas of the liver. However, these changes were patchy and were almost unobservable in some areas.

Kidney and Spleen

Significant differences in the pathological findings were also observed in the kidney and spleen. Although severe infarctions in both kidneys were prominent in both cases, a characteristic of the 1/R control case was the existence of marked hemosiderosis at proximal tubules without prominent hemosiderosis in the spleen. In contrast, in the goat with the system using fixed driving parameters, there was no marked hemosiderosis in the proximal tubules of the kidney, whereas it was very prominent in the spleen (Fig. 1b).

Bone Marrow

While the bone marrow was normal or rather hyperplastic in the 1/R control case, it was markedly

Fig. 1. Comparison of the microscopic pathological findings between the total artificial heart (TAH) goat that survived for 532 days using the 1/R method (#9403) and the longest surviving goat with a TAH operated with fixed driving parameters, which survived for 344 days (goat #8304): **a** patchy necrosis of the hepatic cells and fibrotic degeneration were prominent in many areas of the liver in both cases, although the changes were much more prominent in case #8304 than in case #9403; **b** there was marked hemosiderosis in goat #9403 at proximal tubules without prominent hemosiderosis in the spleen; in contrast, in goat #8304, there was no marked hemosiderosis in the proximal tubules of the kidney, but this was very prominent in the spleen; **c** the bone marrow was hypoplastic in goat #8304, but normal or rather hyperplastic in goat #9403

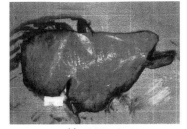
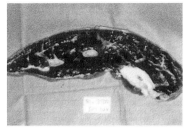

Liver (macro)   **Liver** (macro)

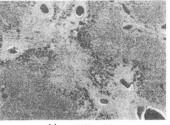
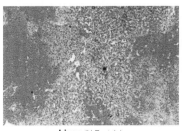

Liver (H.E. stain)   **Liver** (H.E. stain)

#9403　532 days
1/R control method

#8304　344 days
Fixed driving parameters   **a**

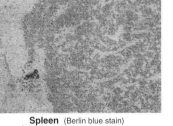
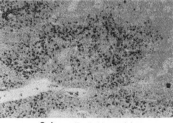

Spleen (Berlin blue stain)   **Spleen** (Berlin blue stain)

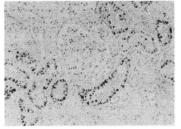
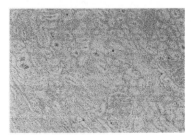

Kidney (Berlin blue stain)   **Kidney** (Berlin blue stain)

#9403　532 days
1/R control method

#8304　344 days
Fixed driving parameters   **b**

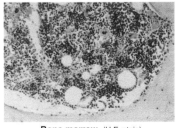
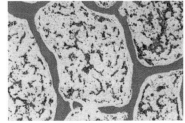

Bone marrow (H.E. stain)   **Bone marrow** (H.E. stain)

#9403　532 days
1/R control method

#8304　344 days
Fixed driving parameters   **c**

hypoplastic in the goat with fixed driving parameters (Fig. 1c).

Lung

In goat #9403, severe pulmonary edema (which was the cause of death) was prominent in the lung. A characteristic of both cases was that in several places hyalinization and calcification were observed in the arterioles which follow the terminal bronchiole near the alveoli.

Other Organs

No noteworthy abnormalities were found in any other organs in either goat.

Discussion

The following pathophysiological abnormalities have been observed in goats with TAH systems which were controlled using fixed driving parameters [6,7]: (1) elevation of CVP; (2) marked ascites; (3) congestive changes in the liver (focal necrosis and fibrotic degeneration of hepatic cells around the central veins); (4) pleural effusion; (5) decrease in the blood triiodothyronine (T_3) and thyroxine (T_4) levels; (6) anemia; (7) infarctions of organs due to thromboembolism; (8) infection. Of these, abnormalities (2) and (3) are believed to be due to the increase in the CVP, even though it has not yet been clarified why the CVP becomes so high in the animals with a TAH system controlled using fixed driving parameters. The improvements in the severity of the pathological liver abnormalities in the 1/R goat are believed to have been due to the comparatively low CVP which was achieved by the use of the 1/R control method. However, the fact that abnormalities still exist even in this case suggests that the CVP level (5–10mmHg) was still not satisfactory, and needs further improvement.

The hypoplasticity in the bone marrow and the marked hemosiderosis in the spleen in the goat with fixed driving parameters suggest that the main causes of the anemia in that goat were the decrease in the production of erythrocytes in the bone marrow and the increased destruction of erythrocytes in the reticuloendothelial system [8,9]. The causes of these abnormalities need further investigation, but the lack of these findings in the 1/R case suggests the involvement of high CVP [10].

Since no marked hemosiderosis could be observed in the spleen or liver, the hemosiderosis of the tubules in the 1/R case was probably due to increased hemolysis in the blood pump [11,12] rather than an increased destruction of erythrocytes in the reticuloendothelial system. It is not certain why hemolysis increased in this 1/R control case, although it may have been due to either (a) the greatly extended driving of the total artificial heart, or (b) the increased driving pressure and pulse rate (dP/dt).

Since calcification was evident at various locations in the blood pumps in both cases [4,13], the hyalinization and calcification in the arterioles of the lungs in both cases are believed to have been due to an embolism caused by calcified particles which were formed on and then came off the blood pump. However, this problem should be attributed not to the control of the TAH system but to the characteristics of the biomaterials which were used for the blood pumps.

The T_3 and T_4 levels in the blood of the longest surviving goat with a TAH using fixed driving parameters decreased without any abnormal findings being observed in the thyroid gland, a phenomenon which is observed in many patients with severe cardiac insufficiency. Although it is still unclear why the T_3 and T_4 levels in the blood in those cases, two possibilities can be considered: one possibility is that the release of T_3 and T_4 from the thyroid gland was suppressed due to either abnormal hemodynamics, such as increased CVP, or some humoral abnormality; and the other is that the blood level of the binding protein of T_3 and T_4 (which is produced in the liver) decreased significantly due to liver dysfunction following the cardiac insufficiency.

This study compared the pathological findings of only the two TAH goats which were, respectively, the longest survivors in their groups (i.e., controlled by either the 1/R method or with fixed driving parameters). Although virtually identical tendencies were observed in almost all long-term surviving goats in both control groups, the number of the experimental animals was rather small and further study is necessary before a definite conclusion can be reached.

Conclusion

It is believed that most of the pathological improvements in the TAH goat which was controlled by the 1/R method were due to the decrease in the CVP which was achieved by adoption of that method. However, the focal necrosis and fibrotic degeneration of hepatic cells around the central veins which still existed in the 1/R case suggests that the CVP level needs further improvement. The existence of prominent hemosiderosis in the proximal tubules suggests that it is also necessary to investigate further the optimum driving conditions in order to avoid hemolysis in the blood pump as well as to lower the CVP.

References

1. Abe Y, Chinzei T, Imachi K, Mabuchi K, Imanishi K, Isoyama T, Matsuura H, Senih G, Nozawa H, Kouno A, Ono T, Atsumi K, Fujimasa I (1994) Can total artificial heart animals control their TAH by themselves? One year survival of a TAH goat using a new automatic control method (1/R control). ASAIO J 40(3):M506–M509

2. Atsumi K, Sakurai Y, Fujimasa I, Imachi K, Nishizaka T, Mano I, Ohmichi H, Mori J, Iwai N, Kouno A (1975) Hemodynamic analysis on prolonged survival cases (30 days and 20 days) of total artificial heart replacement. ASAIO Trans 21:545–554

3. Imachi K, Fujimasa I, Nakajima M, Mabuchi K, Tsukagoshi S, Motomura K, Miyamoto A, Takido N, Inou N, Kouno A, Ono T, Atsumi K (1984) Overall analysis of the causes of pathophysiological problems in total artificial heart in analysis by cardiac receptor hypothesis. ASAIO Trans 30:591–596

4. Fujimasa I, Imachi K, Nakajima M, Mabuchi K, Tsukagoshi S, Kouno A, Ono T, Takido N, Motomura K, Chinzei T, Abe Y, Atsumi K (1986) Pathophysiological study of a total artificial heart in a goat that survived for 344 days. In: Nosé Y, Kjellstrand C, Ivanovich P (eds) Progress in artificial organs — 1985. ISAO Press, Cleveland, pp 345–353

5. Vasku J, Cerny J, Urbanek P, Dostal M, Dolezel S, Guba P, Vasku J, Smutny M, Sladek T, Filkuka J, Pavlicek V, Trubsek V, Bednarik B (1986) Central venous pressure in calves surviving several months with a total artificial heart. In: Nosé Y, Kjellstrand C, Ivanovich P (eds) Progress in artificial organs — 1985. ISAO Press, Cleveland, pp 386–392

6. Atsumi K, Fujimasa I, Imachi K, Nakajima M, Tsukagishi S, Mabuchi K, Motomura K, Kouno A, Ono T, Miyamoto A, Takido N, Inou N (1985) Long-term heart substitution with an artificial heart in goats. ASAIO J 8(3):155–165

7. Wanless IR (1994) Vascular disorders. In: MacSween RNM, Anthony PP, Scheuer PJ, Burt AD, Portmann BC (eds) Pathology of the liver (3rd edn). Churchill Livingstone, New York, pp 535–562

8. Vasku J (1984) Brno–experiments in long term survival with total artificial heart. J.E. Purkyne University, Medical Faculty, Brno

9. Kilbridge TM, Heller P (1969) Determinants of erythrocyte size in chronic liver disease. Blood 34:739

10. Kimber CL, Deller DJ, Lander H (1965) Megaloblastic and transitional megaloblastic anemia associated with chronic liver disease. Am J Med 38:767

11. Eichner ER (1992) Hemolytic anemia due to red blood cell fragmentation. In: Hurst JW (ed) Medicine for the practicing physician. Butterworth-Heinemann, Boston, pp 873–874

12. Wintrobe MM (1981) The red cell fragmentation syndromes. In: Wintrobe MM, Lee GR, Boggs DR, Bitbell TC, Foerster J, Athens JW, Lukens JN (eds) Lea and Febiger, Philadelphia, p 958

13. Imachi K, Chinzei T, Abe Y, Mabuchi K, Isoyama T, Baba K, Matsuura H, Imanishi K, Mochizuki S, Son Y, Kouno A, Ono T, Atsumi K, Fujimasa I (1996) A new hypothesis of the calcification mechanism on a blood contacting polymer membrane surface in the artificial heart. ASAIO J 42(2):16

The Role of Pulsatility in End-Organ Microcirculation After Cardiogenic Shock

Kin-ichi Nakata, Motomi Shiono, Yukihiko Orime, Mitumasa Hata, Akira Sezai, Hideaki Yamada, Satoshi Kashiwazaki, Mitsuru Iida, Mitsuhiro Nemoto, and Yukiyasu Sezai

Summary. To estimate microcirculation in end-organs in pulsatile- and nonpulsatile-assisted circulation, a comparison study was done using a swine model. Cardiogenic shock was brought on by ligation of left coronary artery branches. After cardiogenic shock, animals were divided into two groups: group P ($n = 7$), assisted by a pulsatile pump; and group NP ($n = 7$), assisted by a nonpulsatile pump. Stomach, epicardium, endocardium, liver, renal cortex, and renal medulla tissue blood flows, lactate, pyruvate, and the arterial blood ketone body ratio (AKBR) were measured. Epicardial and endocardial tissue blood flows recovered after assist in both groups. There were no significant differences between the groups. However, with the assist device, liver, renal cortex, renal medulla, and stomach mucous tissue blood flows in group P were significantly higher than those of group NP. In addition, AKBR recovered better in group P than in group NP. These results suggested that, with the uneven blood flow distribution in end-organs after cardiogenic shock, pulsatility was beneficial for recovering and maintaining function and microcirculation in end-organs in order to prevent multiple system organ failure.

Key words: Pulsatile flow — Nonpulsatile flow — Multiple system organ failure — Microcirculation — Cardiogenic shock

Introduction

Various types of nonpulsatile pumps have been developed and widely used in the clinical field not only as the main pump for cardiopulmonary bypass [1], but also as a postcardiotomy cardiac assist [2,3], because of their low cost and ease and simplicity of control. However, a few patients have died because of multiple organ failure [4,5] in spite of left ventricular assist device (LVAD) support. Therefore, appropriate device selection is one of the most important factors in obtaining better clinical results. To ascertain whether nonpulsatile assist is sufficient to recover and maintain end-organ function and microcirculation, or whether pulsatile assist is necessary, this experimental study was undertaken.

Second Department of Surgery, Nihon University School of Medicine, 30-1 Oyaguchi Kami-machi, Itabashi-ku, Tokyo 173, Japan

Material and Methods

The study was performed in 14 pigs (38–43 kg). Each animal was anesthetized with intravenous sodium pentobarbital (20 mg/kg) and ketamine chloride 1 mg/h). After tracheostomy and intubation, controlled mechanical ventilation was established under a tidal volume of 10–15 ml/kg. After median sternotomy, an inflow cannula of an LVAD was inserted into the left atrium through the left appendage, and an outflow cannula was inserted into the ascending aorta (Fig. 1). The animals were divided into two groups: group P ($n = 7$), assisted by a LVAD with a nonpulsatile pump (BP-80, BioMedicus, Minneapolis, MN, USA) for 3 h; and group NP ($n = 7$), assisted by an LVAD with a pulsatile pump (Zeon Medical, Tokyo, Japan) for 3 h. In both groups, a mean aortic pressure (AoP) of 110–120 mmHg was maintained.

An electromagnetic flow probe (FB type, Nihon Kohden, Tokyo, Japan) was placed into the ascending aorta, to measure native cardiac output (Fig. 1). To measure organ microcirculation, a laser regional flow meter was inserted into the epicardium, endocardium, liver, stomach mucous layer, renal cortex, renal medulla, and skin. In addition, the metabolic and chemical parameters lactate, pyruvate, and arterial ketone body ratio (AKBR) were evaluated. After the baseline recordings, the branches of the left anterior descending artery were ligated. A reduction of 60% in AoP compared with control was considered to constitute cardiogenic shock. Experimental results were expressed as mean ± SD. For statistical analysis, a paired t-test was used to analyze the diachronic shift in each group. The Scheffe method was used to analyze the relationship. A P value of less than 0.05 was judged to be statistically significant.

Results

Hemodynamic Changes

The mean AoP decreased significantly in cardiogenic shock, and it increased after assist in both groups. There were no significant differences between the two groups. Pulse pressure was 16.5 ± 9.0 mmHg in group NP, and 34.3 ± 3.7 mmHg in group P. These values were significantly different ($P < 0.05$) (Table 1). The assisted ratio [pump flow/(ascending aortic flow + pump flow)] of group NP was 49.0% ± 9.0%, and that of group P was 46.0% ± 5.0%. There was no statistical difference between the two groups.

Change of Microcirculation in Cardiogenic Shock

With cardiogenic shock, endocardial tissue blood flow decreased to 63% of the control value, epicardium to 62%, liver to 45%, stomach mucous tissue to 39%, renal cortex to 20%, renal medulla to 70%, and skin to 16% (Fig. 2).

Change of Microcirculation During Assisted Circulation

Tissue blood flows in endocardium and epicardium recovered to the preshock levels during assisted circulation, in both groups. There were no significant differences between the groups (Fig. 3). Tissue blood flows in the stomach mucous tissue and the liver recovered almost to control levels in group P. However, those of group NP did not recover to control levels; there was a statistically significant difference ($P < 0.05$) between the two groups (Fig. 4).

Tissue blood flows in the renal cortex in both groups were significantly decreased due to cardiogenic shock, and never recovered to the control level in either group. However, renal cortical blood flow was signifi-

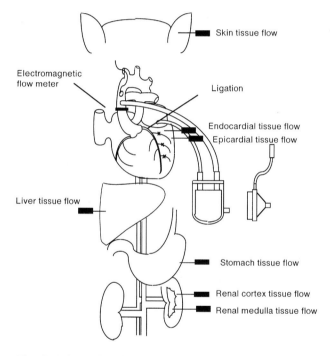

Fig. 1. Schematic drawing of experimental model *Rectangles*, tissue blood-flow meters

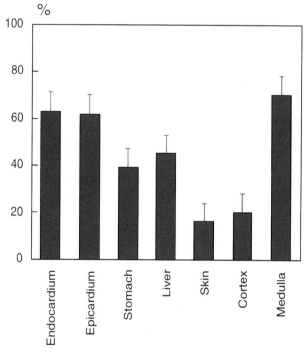

Fig. 2. Regional tissue blood flow distribution after cardiogenic shock

Table 1. Changes in aortic pressure and pulse pressure with cardiogenic shock and with nonpulsatile or pulsatile assist device

	Assist device	Control pressure (mmHg)	Shock (mmHg)	Assist (3h) (mmHg)
Aortic pressure	Pulsatile	126.3 ± 10.4	79.3 ± 1.8	105.6 ± 4.9
	Nonpulsatile	128.3 ± 9.4	80.1 ± 8.8	106.5 ± 3.3
Pulse pressure	Pulsatile	32.0 ± 7.8	22.6 ± 25.8	36.6 ± 4.6
	Nonpulsatile	30.5 ± 9.1	30.8 ± 6.4	14.3 ± 1.5

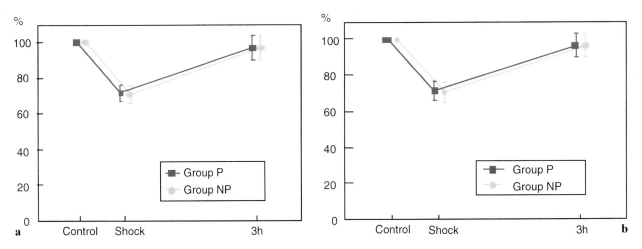

Fig. 3. Changes in epicardial (**a**) and endocardial (**b**) tissue blood flows with cardiogenic shock followed by pulsatile (*squares*) or nonpulsatile (*circles*) assistance for 3 h

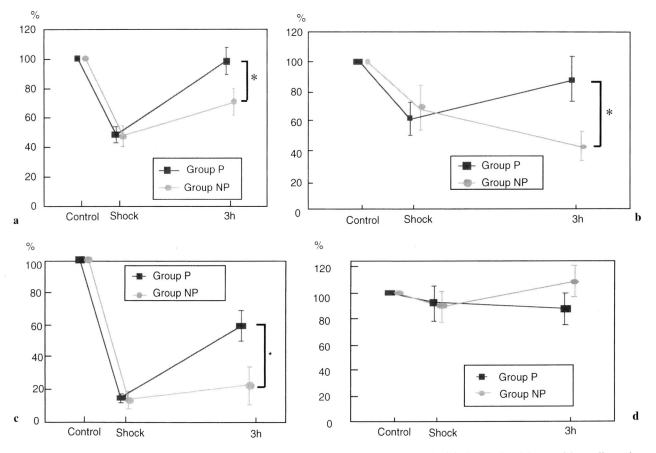

Fig. 4. Changes of stomach mucous (**a**), liver (**b**), renal cortex (**c**), and renal medulla (**d**) tissue blood flows with cardiogenic shock followed by 3 hours' pulsatile (*squares*) or nonpulsatile (*circles*) assistance. *, $P < 0.05$

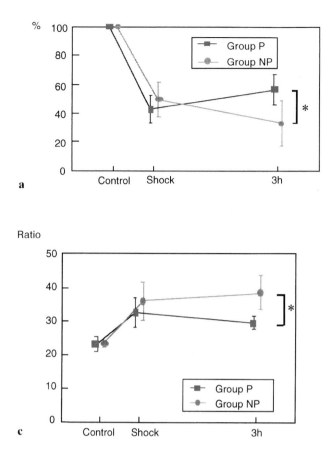

a

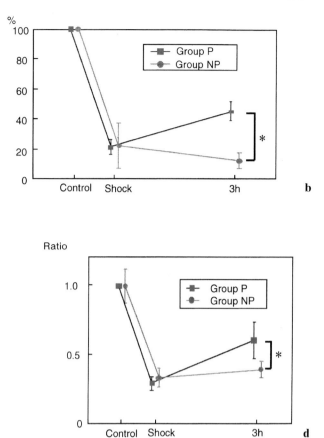

b

c

d

Fig. 5. a Changes in renal cartical blood flow as a percentage of total renal blood flow (cartex + medulla). **b** Changes in skin blood flow. **c** Changes in lactate: pyruvate ratio (L/P). **d** Changes in arterial blood ketone body ratio (AKBR).

Changes in **a–d** were brought on by cardiogenic shock, followed by assistance for 3 h with a pulsatile (*squares*) or nonpulsatile (*circles*) device. *$P < 0.05$

cantly higher in group P than in group NP after 3 hours' assist. Renal medullary blood flow decreased due to cardiogenic shock and recovered to control level after assist, and there was no difference between group P and group NP (Fig. 4). The distribution of tissue blood flow inside the kidney was reversed by cardiogenic shock because of the significant decrease in cortical blood flow. With the assist device, this uneven distribution significantly recovered in group P, while it showed no change in group NP (Fig. 5a). The tissue blood flow in skin decreased significantly in both groups due to cardiogenic shock. That of group P increased after assist; however, that of group P deteriorated (Fig. 5b).

Metabolic Change

The lactate: pyruvate ratio (L/P) increased due to cardiogenic shock and it did not recover to the control level in either group; however, the L/P in group P slightly decreased, whereas that of group NP in-

creased, during assist (Fig. 5c). The arterial blood ketone body ratio (AKBR) decreased in cardiogenic shock. The pulsatile assist device group had a tendency to improve more than the nonpulsatile group (Fig. 5d).

Discussion and Conclusion

No difference in regional endocardial or epicardial tissue blood flow was found between the pulsatile and nonpulsatile groups during the left heart bypass. In this study, the assist rate [pump flow/(ascending aortic flow + pump flow)] was around 50% in both groups. Due to this high assist rate, the left ventricular pressure was sufficiently decompressed in both groups, and this phenomenon caused a decrease in the intramyocardial pressure. Thus, this decreasing vascular resistance confers a significant advantage for overcoming ischemic coronary circulation. This seems to be the reason there were no significant differences between the two groups in heart tissue blood flow. In term of metabolic results, L/P reflects the oxygen supply to systemic tissue; the elevated L/P canused by cardiogenic shock decreased with pulsatile assistance, indicating an improvement in oxygen supply. The AKBR reflects the oxidation-reduction in liver mitochondria, and is widely used as a parameter of liver metabolism. With the assist, group P significantly recovered as compared with group NP. These data suggested that the pulsatile assist may improve splanchnic organ metabolic function, especially that of the liver. According to the measurements of kidney, stomach mucous, and liver tissue blood flows, the pulsatile assist gave significantly better flows than the nonpulsatile assist. These results suggest that the pulsatile assist was more effective for achieving the recovery of splanchnic organ microcirculation.

References

1. Noon GP, Sekela ME, Glueck J, Coleman CL, Fellowman L (1990) Comparison of Delphin and pumps. ASAIO Trans 36:M616–619
2. Noon GP, Ball JW, Short HD (1996) Bio-Medicus centrifugal ventricular support for postcardiotomy cardiac failure: A review of 129 cases. Ann Thorac Surg 61:291–295
3. Golding LAR (1992) Biomedicus centrifugal pump for mechanical cardiac support. In: Sezai Y (ed) Artifical heart: the development of biomation in the 21st Century. Saunders, Tokyo, pp 248–252
4. Orime Y, Hasegawa T, Kitamura S, Ohira M, Shino M, Hata H, Harada Y, Sezai Y (1990) Clinical application of left ventricular assist device: Retrospective evaluation of multiple organ failure. Artif Organs 14(Suppl 1):115–118
5. Noon GP (1991) Bio-Medicus ventricular assistance. Ann Thorac Surg 52:180–181

A New Index for Characterizing Pulsatility: Recovery of Renal Function

Hiroaki Konishi[1], Yoshio Misawa[1], James F. Antaki[2], Robert L. Kormos[2], and Katsuo Fuse[1]

Summary. The advantages of hemodynamic pulsatility are still controversial based on the evaluation of normal organ function under varying perfusion conditions. The development of the permanent nonpulsatile blood pump as a left ventricular assist device (LVAD) demands that the efficacy of pulseless perfusion in the recovery of end-organ function is verified. This study examined hemodynamic power as an index of mechanical forces applied to the blood, and also the recovery of renal function following a 30-min period of normothermic ischemia. Pigs were randomized into four groups. In all groups, acute renal ischemia was induced by clamping both renal arteries for 30 min. Reperfusion for 120 min was performed using either pulsatile perfusion, or pulseless perfusion at 65 ± 1.6 mmHg (groups I and II respectively) or 40 ± 1.1 mmHg (groups III and IV respectively). After reperfusion, renal blood flow (RBF) and hemodynamic power (HP $= \int P(t) \cdot Q(t) \, dt$, where P is renal artery pressure and Q is renal artery flow) in groups I, II, and III were significantly higher than in Group IV ($P < 0.01$ by analysis of variance). In terms of renal functional recovery, there was a significant positive correlation between hemodynamic power and renal oxygen consumption (VO_2) ($r = 0.96$, $P < 0.01$). It was concluded that high HP is important for promoting peripheral circulation. Under hypotensive conditions, pulsatile perfusion is more effective in delivering HP to the organ compared with pulseless perfusion.

Key words: Hemodynamic power — Pulsatile perfusion — Rotary blood pump — Left ventricular assist device

Introduction

Many studies have been performed to examine pulseless perfusion during the development of cardiopulmonary bypass (CPB) over the past 30 years. However, there is, as yet, no definitive conclusion regarding the consequences of pulsatile versus pulseless perfusion [1]. Currently, several rotary blood pumps, which are essentially nonpulsatile, are under development for use as a permanent left ventricular assist device (LVAD) [2]. This forces the debate to be re-solved. In this study we analyzed the difference between pulsatile and pulseless perfusion in terms of the effect on hemodynamic power (HP) [3]. We hypothesized that the benefit observed with pulsatile perfusion is related to a higher delivery of mechanical energy applied to the blood, and that HP can be used as an index of this energy delivery.

Materials and Methods

Surgical Preparation

A total of 20 pigs weighing 20–25 kg (40 kidneys) were used (Fig. 1). Following tracheal intubation, mechanical ventilation was initiated and general anesthesia was maintained with isofluorane in oxygen. Body temperature was kept at 38°C–39°C on a warming blanket. A central venous line was introduced via the right external jugular vein. Catheters to draw renal venous blood samples were introduced via the right and left femoral veins. A fluid-filled arterial catheter was placed via the right common carotid artery to measure the blood pressure in the upper body. Median laparotomy was made and an ultrasound flow probe (Transonics Systems, Ithaca, NY, USA) was applied to the right and left renal artery. The right femoral artery was cannulated to monitor the renal perfusion pressure using a microtip transducer (Millar Instruments, Houston, TX, USA) placed in the aorta at the level of the renal arteries. A blood reservoir was pressurized to maintain arterial blood pressure in the upper body after cross-clamping the aorta.

The extracorporeal circulation consisted of the following components: a centrifugal blood pump Bio-Pump, Medtronic Bio-Medicus, Medtronic, Eden Prairie, MN, USA), a collapsible reservoir, and a controller circuit to induce pulsatile or pulseless perfusion. A 12-Fr inflow cannula was inserted to the abdominal aorta and a 12-Fr outflow cannula was inserted to the left common iliac artery. Following a 30-min period of ischemia induced by clamping both renal arteries, reperfusion was initiated after clamping the thoracoabdominal aorta proximal to the renal arteries.

[1] Jichi Medical School, Department of Thoracic and Cardiovascular Surgery, 3311-1 Yakushiji, Minamikawachi-machi, Kawachi-gun, Tochigi 329-04, Japan
[2] University of Pittsburgh, Pittsburgh, PA, USA

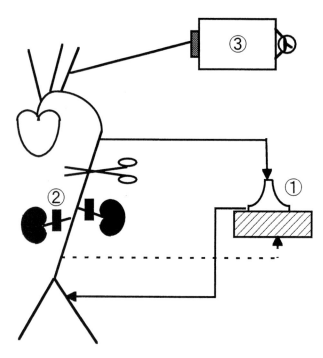

Fig. 1. Experimental procedure: *1*, centrifugal pump with controller; *2*, ultrasonic flow probes at renal arteries; *3*, pressurized reservoir bag

Hemodynamic Studies

Eight kidneys were studied in each group. During reperfusion, the systemic arterial pressure was kept constant at approximately 60 mmHg in all of the groups by a pressurized blood reservoir to avoid baroreceptor effects. Renal arterial pressure was regulated by the controller of the centrifugal pump at a mean pressure of 60 mmHg (group I pulsatile, group II pulseless) or 40 mmHg (group III pulsatile, group IV pulseless). Renal artery pressure and flow data were directly acquired into a PC-type computer. HP was calculated before ischemia and at 60, 90, and 120 min after reperfusion.

Renal Function Studies

Renal arterial and venous blood samples for blood gas analysis (Radiometer, Copenhagen, Denmark) were obtained before ischemia and at 0, 30, 60, 90, and 120 min after declamping the renal arteries and starting the pump. Renal oxygen consumption was determined by calculating concentration differences in arterial and venous blood samples.

Data Analysis

HP was calculated by the following equation, where P is renal artery pressure and Q is renal artery flow:

$$HP = \int P(t) \cdot Q(t) dt$$

All data were shown as means ± standard error of the mean ($n = 8$ in each of groups I, II, III, and IV). Comparisons between the different groups were performed by two-way repeated measures analysis of variance (ANOVA) and the Bonferroni corrected *t*-test (StatView version 4.5, Abacus Concepts, Berkeley, CA, USA).

Results

Preoperatively, the animals weighed 24 ± 2.2 kg. There was no difference among the groups.

Hemodynamic Analysis

Systemic arterial pressure from the right carotid artery was kept at 60 ± 5.5 mmHg among the four study groups. Renal artery pressure was regulated at 65 ± 1.5 mmHg (groups I and II) and 40 ± 1.1 mmHg (groups III and IV), respectively, by the controller attached to the centrifugal pump.

Renal blood flow (RBF) in group IV did not recover to the same extent as in groups I, II, and III ($P < 0.01$; ANOVA, Fig. 2). In the high-pressure groups, I and II, there was no difference in RBF between pulsatile and pulseless perfusion, but in the low-pressure groups, III and IV, pulsatile perfusion (group III) was superior to pulseless perfusion (group IV) for recovery of RBF. HP was reduced in group IV compared with group III ($P < 0.05$, Fig. 2).

Renal Function Analysis

Renal oxygen consumption was calculated from renal arterial and venous blood samples. During the recovery period, VO_2 remained low in all groups. However, VO_2 was highly correlated with HP ($P < 0.01$, $r = 0.96$, Fig. 3). This suggests that HP may be the first hemodynamic measure to indicate a decline in tissue perfusion.

Discussion

Currently, the effectiveness of pulseless or diminished pulse perfusion has gained renewed interest because of the development of implantable rotary blood pumps for permanent use as LVADs. There have been several studies describing the effects of a pulseless flow on end-organ function after ischemia and under hypotensive conditions [4]. Despite the efforts of these studies, the benefits of pulsatile perfusion remain controversial because it is not yet clear which

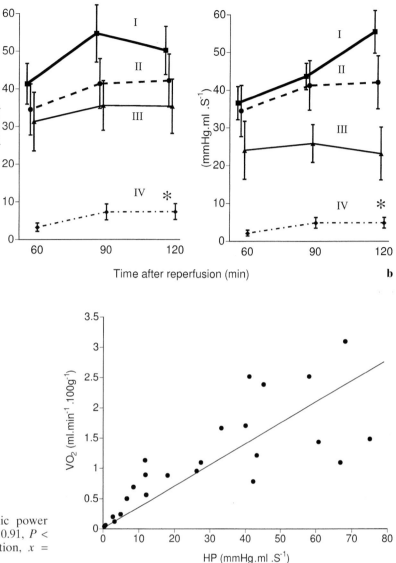

Fig. 2. a Recovery of renal artery flow (*P < 0.01). **b** Recovery of hemodynamic power (*P < 0.05). *I–IV,* groups I–IV (4 pigs in each)

Fig. 3. Relationship between hemodynamic power (*HP*) and oxygen consumption (*VO₂*) (r = 0.91, P < 0.01) y = 0.034 x (y = oxygen consumption, x = hemodynamic power)

hemodynamic characteristic is essential to maintain adequate peripheral circulation: flow, pressure, or pulsatility. Wright [3] pointed out the problems inherent in this kind of study in comparing pulsatile flow with pulseless flow. The most important point is the lack of understanding of the basic mechanical properties of the left ventricle and major arteries, and of the interactions between them which optimize the transmission of mechanical energy from the heart to the tissues. He proposed to make use of the concepts of hemodynamic power and vascular impedance.

In this study we hypothesize that the essential difference between pulsatile and nonpulsatile perfusion is the energy delivered to the peripheral circulation. This study indicates that, if a high mean arterial blood pressure can be maintained during the recovery phase, the effect of pulsatility may be minimal with respect to renal function. We postulate this because the force applied to the blood under these conditions is high enough to maintain adequate peripheral circulation. However, at a low perfusion pressure, pulsatile perfusion may be necessary to recover normal renal blood flow and promote normal function within a shorter period of time than pulseless perfusion. Under conditions of critical organ perfusion, HP with pulsatile perfusion is higher than with pulseless perfusion for the same mean pressure. The higher HP in pulsatile perfusion is in turn associated with improved end-organ function under hypotensive conditions.

In conclusion, HP may prove to be a comprehensive and sensitive determinant of adequate end-organ perfusion, because HP is dependent on pressure, flow, and pulsatility.

References

1. Hickey PR, Buckley MJ, Philbin DM (1983) Pulsatile and nonpulsatile cardiopulmonary bypass: review of a counterproductive controversy. Ann Thorac Surg 36:720–737
2. Butler KC, Maher TR, Borovetz HS, Kormos RL, Antaki JF, Kameneva M, Griffith BP, Zerbe T, Schaffer FD (1992) Development of an axial flow blood pump LVAS. ASAIO J 38:M296–M300
3. Wright G (1994) Hemodynamic analysis could resolve the pulsatile blood flow controversy. Ann Thorac Surg 58:1199–1204
4. Nakata K (1996) Effect of pulsatile and nonpulsatile assist for microcirculation in major organs after cardiogenic shock. Jpn J Cardiovasc Surg 25:158–164

Discussion

Dr. Vasku:
Dr. Yambe shows that he is doing exact analysis of the sympathetic signals. It shows that it seems that the sympathetic drive increases after total artificial heart. We have had the same experience and similar experience is shown also in the paper by Dr. Mabuchi. It's very important that central venous pressure and the general sympathetic drive by this 1/R system of driving in his laboratory practically normalizes the whole vascular periphery. We have done similar with stimulation of right atrium and with pharmacological treatment. This is very important because then you can prolong the survival which was very well shown. I much appreciate these two papers which are dealing with the pulsatile problem because they confirm that the pulsatile hemodynamics during the heart assist is very important. The pulsatile system is much more effective. I appreciate this very much.

Dr. Yambe:
We've been analyzing the central nervous system discharge during artificial circulation. In this paper, we want to describe the nerve information processing system in the central nervous system by the use of the artificial heart. So, for the next meeting we will do another experiment and present the paper.

Dr. Müller:
Perhaps I didn't get the point of your talk, but perhaps you can explain, with an example, how you can use the pathologic nervous drive for controlling an artificial heart?

Dr. Yambe:
As we showed in our slide, during chaotic dynamics it shows the stability and the complicated forecast impossibility. The robust characteristics were maintained by chaotic dynamics, but if it disappeared to the upper side or lower side at the very high entropy or very low entropy, and, if you, for example, choose the heart with higher KS-entropy, the very upper state is ventricular fibrillation. And if you use the chaotic dynamics you make the circulation healthy, and we use these chaotic dynamics in the central nervous system by the use of the artificial heart.

Dr. Nosé:
Based upon our experience and initial 2 weeks after implantation of a total artificial heart we have high venous pressure. However, after 2 weeks, that becomes normal. The only way we can control the venous pressure is a pumping capacity of the pump set lower than the body weight of the animal. I am sure your animal body weight is the same, so it means your pump performance is down. That is the only thing I can think about. There is nothing to do mysterious chaotic nervous control or whatever, because just pump cannot provide enough flow. That is the way I assume. What is your opinion? What is a chaotic thing?

Dr. Yambe:
If the state of the circulation is changed, the attractor in the phase space has changed as we have shown in this paper, but this is only acute experiments. I cannot mention the chronic experiments, but if your animal changes state, these attractors showing chaotic dynamics are changed. Our point is explaining the change of the state of your hyperacute phase, or acute phase or chronic states. It may be explained by the nonlinear mathematical methodology, I think.

Dr. Nosé:
With artificial heart pumping, the animal will not change. OK and it means something is wrong. You are generating microclots or your pump is doing something wrong. If you have a good pump, it will not cause any change to the recipient. I would like to ask a question to Dr. Nakata. I wrote a textbook 20 years ago and if the blood flow is going down, first blood flow to the skin and the muscles goes down, and second the flow to the splanchnic areas decreases, so this is exactly what we have been saying for the last 15 years. For nonpulsatile perfusion, you have to get at least 20% more blood flow then, the other physiology becomes the same. I believe Dr. Yada is in the audience and I am sure he agrees with me.

Dr. Yada:
I read your paper. In my experimental study, the total output was the same for the pulsatile group and

nonpulsatile group. For the same cardiac output, this is the experimental condition, pulsation is effective for microcirculation.

Dr. Müller:
I think there is another important point. Insertion of a nonpulsatile pump in a human leads always to a modulation of the nonpulsatile flow by the pulsatile flow of the native heart. That means you will never have a pure constant flow. You will get a modulated pulsatile flow.

Dr. Nosé:
Well, I think if we implant a steady flow pump to the pumping ventricle, the patient will have a very difficult time to get steady flow; they're getting pulsatile flow. And I think one of the most important things Dr. Konishi mentioned today is hemodynamic power. I'm very glad you mentioned this particular parameter.

Dr. Yambe:
Only one comment: I would say that we don't think we reach the steady state during artificial circulation. Dr Nosé wanted to question to me about this. Every day the central nervous system changes. And sympathetic nerve discharge was mediated by central nervous system so I think it changes every day, it changes all the time. So these parameters were showing these dynamics.

Part VII
Engineering

Further Development of the Moving-Actuator Type Total Artificial Heart

Byoung Goo Min[1], Jae Mok Ahn[1], Chan Young Park[2], Yung Ho Jo[1], Won Woo Choi[2], Hyun Jung Kim[4], Seong Keun Park[1], Jong Jin Lee[2], Jae Soon Choi[2], Kyong Sik Om[2], Jongwon Kim[4], Jun Keun Chang[2], Hee Chan Kim[1], Won Gon Kim[3], Joon Ryang Roh[3], and Yong Soon Won[5]

Summary. The electromechanical total artificial heart (TAH) developed at Seoul National University Hospital was verified as acceptable for human implantation through several successful animal experiments. In the last two years (1994–1996), the TAH was redesigned to be small (600–650 ml, total volume) and lightweight (approximately 950 g), and also improved to overcome three practical problems encountered in the animal experiments. First, we implemented modifications to the blood-pump housing to resolve the anatomical problem made apparent through the construction of a three-dimensional model of the TAH, the human thoracic cavity, and the large vessels, from magnetic resonance images and Angiogram-Computer tomography. Second, the intraventricular surface of the blood sacs was modified with fibrinolytic and anti-infective surface treatments. Third, the mechanism of regulation of cardiac output (CO) was improved by analyzing the measured pressure in the interventricular volume space (IVP). It proved beneficial to achieve the regulation of CO in response to the physiological demand, and to prevent atrial collapse due to the suction. The IVP, which accurately reflected the hemodynamic parameters, was used to predict the preload condition. These three improvements will assist in the application of the newly developed implantable electromechanical artificial heart for long-term implantation.

Key words: Total artificial heart — Pressure of interventricular volume — Cardiac output

Introduction

The moving-actuator total artificial heart (TAH) has unique characteristics: first, the moving-actuator type electromechanical pump, consisting of a high-energy-efficiency brushless d.c. motor inside the actuator, and two polyurethane blood sacs; and second, the usage of the interventricular air-volume space as an internal compliance chamber for balancing and active filling.

The entire TAH system consists of the internal control unit based on a microcontroller (Intel, 87C196KD, CA, USA), a tether-free electrical energy source (transcutaneous energy transmission [TET]), and a tether-free communication system (transcutaneous information transmission [TIT]).

In this paper, our research group has focused on improving the pump system for better fit and blood compatibility, and refining the control algorithms. At a preclinical stage, these are very important factors. The performance and reliability of the newly developed TAH was evaluated through a series of mock circulation tests and animal experiments, with very encouraging results.

Materials and Methods

Pump System

The moving-actuator type blood pump consists of three major parts: the actuator, the right ventricle, and the left ventricle, as shown in Fig. 1. The energy convertor is a small, high-efficiency brushless d.c. motor (S/M594-05, Sierracin/Magnedyne, CA, USA) located inside the actuator. This actuator moves back and forth during a full stroke, together with the motor.

The pump dimensions and materials selected for all mechanical components were designed to achieve a 5-year operational life. The motor housing was made from an aluminum alloy (duralumin) to reduce the total weight of the pump, and steel (S45C) was used for the rack.

Each ventricle is a smooth, seamless, segmented polyurethane (SUP; Pellethane, Dow Chemical, MI, USA) blood sac with an elliptical shape. The pump is a semi-rigid mesh-reinforced polyurethane. When the actuator moves to the left and contracts the left ventricular sac, the right sac inflates by way of the inflowing venous return with moderate active filling, and vice versa.

[1]Department of Biomedical Engineering, College of Medicine, [2]Department of Biomedical Engineering, College of Engineering, [3]Department of Thoracic Surgery, College of Medicine, and [4]Department of Biomedical Engineering, Institute of Biomedical Engineering, Seoul National University, 28 Yungun-Dong, Chongno-Ku, Seoul 110-744, Korea
[5]Department of Thoracic Surgery, College of Medicine, Ehwa Women's University, 11-1 Daehyun-Dong, Seodaemun-Ku, Seoul 120-750, Korea

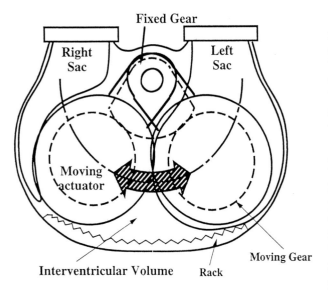

Fig. 1. The moving-actuator type blood pump

Instead of an external compliance chamber, the bottom part (anterior part) of the pump housing was made flexible using a compliance window to allow expansion and compression of the internal air in the interventricular volume space. This flexible window compensates for the change in the pressure of the interventricular space (IVP) to prevent atrial collapse.

Model of the Human Thoracic Cavity and the TAH

Accurate and detailed three-dimensional measurements of the human thoracic cavity were necessary to optimize the design of the new model of the TAH. Magnetic resonance imaging (MRI) and Angiogram-Computer tomography images were obtained from healthy volunteers at 3-mm intervals from the peak of the aortic arch to the diaphragm. The average ages of 3 men and 6 women were 62 and 47, respectively. The images acquired were used to reconstruct a three-dimensional thoracic cavity using ISG Allegro (ISG Technologies, Toronto, Canada). The contours of target organs, such as the aortic arch, pulmonary trunk, left ventricle, right ventricle, left atrium, right atrium, superior vena cava, and inferior vena cava, were defined using the different gray levels of the MRI images. The resulting contour lines in each slice of the image were reconstructed into a three-dimensional model using a volume-reconstruction algorithm implemented in ISG Allegro. In particular, the pulmonary trunk and the aortic arch were reconstructed carfully within the thoracic cavity to measure the relative direction and position of the respective remnants for TAH implantation.

Based on the anatomical fitting constraints of the reconstructed three-dimensional model of the thoracic cavity and remnants, a solid model of the Korean TAH, comprising the energy converter, outer case, two blood sacs, and chamber [1,2], was realized using a Unigraphics (LG-EDS, Seoul, Korea) computer-aided design (CAD) system installed on an HP 715–100 workstation.

Enhancement of Biocompatibility

Surface modification techniques were used for improving the blood compatibility of the blood-contacting surfaces of the implanted TAH. In order to improve the thromboresistance of the polyurethane, we introduced, in collaboration with Dr. Matsuda's group at the National Cardiovascular Center, Osaka, Japan, a new method for immobilization of Lumbrokinase (LK) extracted from earthwarm on substrate. It is based on the photochemical conversion of the phenylazido group to the highly reactive phenylnitrene upon ultraviolet (UV) light irradiation [3]. The procedures are as follows. First, an aminated polymer, partially derivatized with a photoreactive phenlyazido group in its side chains, was coated onto a polyurenthane surface. Subsequently, the surface was exposed to the UV light. Second, to induce the carboxyl group on the UV light treated surface, maleic acid ether copolymer (MAcMEC) was added. After the reaction, LK was immobilized on the resulting coated polyurethane surface with 1-ethyl-3-(3-dimethylaminopropyl) carbodiimide (EDC) in aqueous solvent. Electron spectroscopy for chemical analysis (ESCA) and water contact angle measurement before and after sequential surface reactions, revealed that LK was immobilized successfully.

Cardiac Output Regulation Algorithm

To regulate the cardiac output of the totally implantable TAH, a control algorithm was developed to maintain left–right output balance, as well as to control the cardiac output according to physiological demand. The new control algorithm is based on the analysis of the measured pressure of the interventricular volume space (IVP). During one heart cycle, the volume of the interventricular space is changed dynamically by the difference between the ejection volume of one ventricle and the inflow volume of the other. Cardiac output is regulated by five control variables to control: the actuator's speed and moving angle; right systolic speed and right end–systolic brake time; left systolic speed and left end-systolic brake time; and left asymmetry. The new algorithm uses a combination of these five control variables, determined at each stroke termination, to regulate the nagative peak of the IVP. From many analytical studies and the mock circulation tests, we confirmed that the changes in the IVP directly reflected the atrial pressures according to the volume difference between the inflow and outflow, as shown in Fig. 2.

Based on the measured IVP, cardiac output is regulated by five control variables to control: the actuator's speed and moving angle; right systolic speed and right end-systolic brake time; left systolic speed and left end-systolic brake time; and left asymmetry [4]. An adequate combination of these five control variables is determined at each stroke termination through the Proportional-Integral derivative (PID) controller, to regulate the negative peak of the IVP at the predetermined level (rIVP).

The predetermined level, rIVP, at each diastolic phase, was initialized to maintain the right and left atrial pressures at around −3 mmHg and 10 mmHg, respectively. To maintain a well-balanced pump output, the automatic control adjusts an asymmetric amount of the moving-actuator stroke angle, which provides a different net output from the two ventricles.

Modification of Filling Conditions Using the IVP

With the flexible window attached to the anterior wall of the semirigid housing of the TAH, the filling conditions fall into one of the following two categories according to the volume occupied by air in the interventricular space: (1) If the interspace between the two ventricles is vented to the atmosphere, the inflow volume is determined by the atrial pressure and inflow resistance including the valves (passive filling); (2) In the case of complete ventricle sealing after total removal of the air, the inflow volume of one ventricle depends on the other sac's outflow volume (active filling).

Therefore, for the maximal cardiac output delivery without atrial collapse, a compromise between the passive and active filling conditions can be obtained by changing the amount of air. There is approximately 100–110 ml air for the compensation of right and left cardiac output, including approximately 15 ml of air corresponding to the flexible window; in addition, there is about 80 ml of lubricant oil for lubrication of the moving actuator and heat dispersion in the interventricular space.

The flexible window functions to compensate the volume difference of approximately 15 ml by moving itself inward and outward passively according to the IVP, and thereby reduces the negative peak pressure, IVP. For example, a high left-atrial pressure means increased venous return to the left ventricle, resulting in increased IVP; whereas a low atrial pressure represents decreased venous return to the corresponding

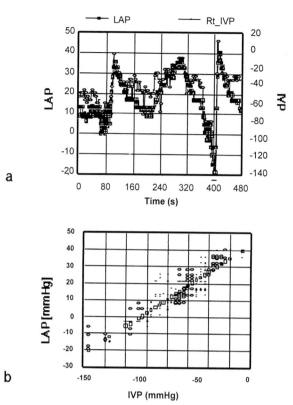

Fig. 2. Relationship between left atrial pressure (*LAP*) and the pressure of the interventricular colume (*IVP*): **a** with time; *upper trace*, LAP, *lower trace*, IVP; **b** LAP vs IVP ($y = 0.55 + 51.6$; $r = 0.88$; SD = 5.2)

ventricle, and the peak IVP decreases to a negative value within the range −35–−70 mmHg. At the same time, the peak IVP is less negative because of the window's expansion and compression. The IVP waveform was measured using an absolute pressure sensor (Mpx7200AP, Motorola, AZ, USA) with temperature compensation.

Results

Pump System and Model of the TAH and Human Thoracic Cavity

A three-dimensional model of the thoracic cavity was acquired by the volume reconstruction of target organs from 15–20 frames of MRI images. To solve the anatomic fitting problems, the pulmonary artery and aortic arch were reconstructed inside a chest cavity model. With this reconstruction of great vessels, accu-

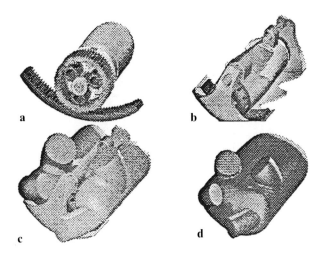

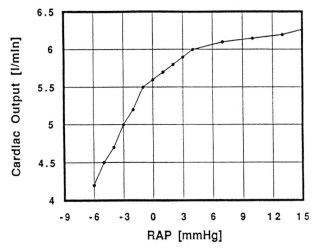

Fig. 3. a Solid model of energy convertor and rack gear of Korean total artificial heart (TAH); **b** outer case assembled to (**a**); **c** two blood sacs for left ventricle and right ventricle assembled in the correct positions, and **d** solid model of assembled Korean TAH

Fig. 4. Starling's cardiac output response to a preload change from −6 mmHg to 15 mmHg. *RAP*, right atrial pressure

rate three-dimensional information on their position and orientation for connection to the TAH was derived.

Figure 3 shows the newly developed TAH moving-actuator: the energy convertor, outer case, blood sacs, and the outer chamber. The solid model of the TAH, constructed by CAD, made it possible to verify the anatomical fit by comparing the three-dimensional constraints with the reconstructed thoracic cavity model. The TAH was designed and refined based upon these findings, which describe the geometrical dimensions of the pericardial space and the great vessel geometry for orthotopic cardiac replacement devices.

Enhancement of Biocompatibility

A polyurethane surface containing immobilized Lumbokinase (LK) was prepared by sequential surface reactions: photochemical fixation of poly (allyamine hydrochloride), then surface graft of MAcMEC, and finally LK immobilization. The blood compatibility of the LK-immobilized surface was demonstrated by in vitro and ex vivo studies. Less fibrinogen was adsorbed from whole blood on the LK-immobilized surface than onto the polyurethane control surface, possibly due to the fibrinolytic activity of the immobilized LK. The LK-immobilized surface showed less platelet adhesion than the MAcMEC-grafted surface without LK. The suppression of platelet adhesion, together with the low fibrinogen adsorption from the whole blood, indicates in vitro thromboresistance and thrombolysis by the immobilized LK.

Cardiac Output Regulation Algorithm

The performance of the automatic control algorithm was assessed through a series of in vitro experiments. The atrial pressures were measured using a pressure gauge at the position before each valve, and recorded by a polygraphy system (CG-5591; Fukuda Denshi, Tokyo, Japan).

With the proposed PID control method using the IVP, a plot of the in vitro cardiac output response to changing preload is shown in Fig. 4. The cardiac output increases in response to an increase in the right atrial pressure (RAP) from −3 to 6 mmHg, and the resultant response is similar to Starling's curve. Since the lowest value of the RAP, −3 mmHg, is experimentally due to the fluctuation pressure generated at the moment of valve opening or closing, it is not significant for regulation of the physiological demand. The preload sensitivity depends upon the aortic pressure and could be enhanced or reduced by adjustment of the reference IVP level.

Modification of Filling Conditions Using the IVP

Detection of the occurrence of atrial collapse was performed for the left and right ventricular diastolic phase through analysis of the IVP. The regulation of cardiac output based upon the maximum filling rate, as estimated by the IVP, provided an optimal cardiac output for a given venous return.

The preload-sensitive response was achieved by analyzing the measured IVP waveforms. Figure 3 in the paper by Jo, this volume, shows that the IVP waveforms directly reflect the filling condition of both the left and right sacs. These results show that out TAH has the unique characteristic of having no separate compliance chamber. This is one of the most important features in terms of the system's reliability as well as its simplicity.

Fitting Trials

The feasibility of implantation of the TAH into small animals was verified in preliminary in vivo animal experiments. Five sheep weighing about 60 kg each were successfully implanted with a TAH for 1–3 days, with a reasonably acceptable fit. There was not thrombus formation inside grafts, cuffs, right or left ventricles, or polymer valves.

Conclusions

The development of a total artificial heart (TAH) suitable for humans has been brought closer to reality with the help of the three-dimensional reconstruction of the structure of soft tissues inside the human thoracic cavity, together with a CAD system for TAH design. For the control of cardiac output of a totally implantable electromechanical TAH, an adaptive automatic control algorithm, using the interventricular pressure, was developed and tested in vitro and in vivo. Cardiac output was increased from 4.2 to 6.3 l/min with 80–120 mmHg of aortic pressure according to

an increase of preload. The left atrial pressure was maintained under 15 mmHg, and the right atrial pressure, 0–5 mmHg.

In the animal experiments, the resultant cardiac output and preload-sensitive response to the physiologic variations were satisfactory. Our moving-actuator type pump demonstrated the feasibility of engineering a TAH for implantation into small animals. Before commencing long-term survival experiments, we need to undertake further extensive studies for the improvement of the pump's function and raliability.

References

1. Cheon GJ, Kim HC, Min BG, Han DC (1990) A new type of the motor-driven blood pump for artificial heart. Artif Organs 112:473–475
2. Min BC, Kim HC, Lee SH, Chang JK, Choi JW, Kim JW, Seo KP, Rho JR, Ahn H, Kim SW, Olsen DB (1991) Design of moving-actuator total artificial heart (Korean Heart). Artif Heart 3:229–234
3. Sugawara T, Matsuda T (1994) Novel Surface graft copolymerization method with microorder regional precision. Macromolecules 27:7809–7814
4. Kim HC, Lee SH, Kim IY, Min BG, Kim JW, Choi JW, Kim JT, Jung DY (1990) Optimal and physiological control for the new moving-actuator type electromechanical total artificial heart. Artif Organs 14: 103–105

Discussion

Dr. Nosé:

In the history of the total artificial heart development, any device which incorporates the so-called suction pump principle failed, and the only surviving devices are passive-fill devices, and I can see you went through all kinds of difficulties. Why not use a simple compliance chamber and then eliminate all of your headaches? I know you started that direction with window; make a bigger window and put the compliance chamber.

Dr. Min:

We want to have a very small pump, and with a small pump, to get higher cardiac output, the only way is to have a very high heart rate, normally like 100, or above 140. In that case, I think even with commercially available valves, we cannot have sufficient filling with such a very short period, so, we need a certain amount of active filling in a case of low atrial pressure. But, as I described various times, this suction, as long as we know that there is suction or not, we can control the velocity of the actuator and we can control the suction.

Dr. Nosé:

With commercially available tissue valves, you can get sufficient fill with pulses of 150 to 160 beats per minute, and if that can be achieved, why do you have to go through such a difficult process? And your pump is not so small.

Dr. Min:

It's now in the range of 550 to 600 ml, and not only small, but the important thing is its A-P dimension, like 5.5 cm. I have seen many actual laboratory tests of various artificial hearts, and they say that even with commercially available valves it's very difficult to achieve complete filling at low filling pressure and within a short time. As an example, if the right atrial pressure is 5 mmHg and the valve pressure drop is about 5 mmHg, then there is pressure difference of zero. So, we need some sort of small degree of active filling in this case.

Dr. Nosé:

My colleague presented yesterday, if you have 5 mm of preload and the time required to fill the 50 cc chamber is only 180 ms to 220 ms, that will give you an adequate pulse rate.

Dr. Umezu:

Ok, I think he'd like to reconsider and to discuss it with you later on.

Dr. Nawrat:

What kind of valves do you use in your artificial heart?

Dr. Min:

I think it is going to be published in *The European Journal of Artificial Organs* soon. It's a floating type and flapping. It's triangular, but the membrane moves back and forth. It's similar to a jellyfish valve but there is no attached point, so it's moving and flapping.

Dr Umezu:

I guess it was presented in the last symposium. Please check the book *Artificial Heart 5*.

The "Cool Seal" Concept: A Low-Temperature Mechanical Seal with Recirculating Purge System for Rotary Blood Pumps

Kenji Yamazaki[1], Toshio Mori[2], Jun Tomioka[3], James F. Antaki[1], Philip Litwak[1], Osamu Tagusari[1], Bartley P. Griffith[1], Hitoshi Koyanagi[4], and Robert L. Kormos[1]

Summary. A critical issue facing the development of an implantable, rotary blood pump is the maintenance of an effective seal at the rotating shaft. Mechanical seals are the most versatile type of seal in wide industrial applications. However, in a rotary blood pump, the typical seal life is much shorter than required for chronic support. Seal failure is related to adhesion and aggregation of heat-denatured blood proteins which diffuse into the lubricating film between seal faces. Among the blood proteins, fibrinogen plays an important role due to its strong propensity of adhesion and low transition temperature (Td), around 50°C. Once exposed to temperatures exceeding 50°C, fibrinogen molecules fuse together by multiattachment between heat-denatured D-domains. This quasipolymerized fibrin increases the frictional heat which proliferates the process into seal failure. If seal-face temperature is maintained well below 50°C, a mechanical seal would not fail in blood. Based on this "cool seal" concept, we developed a miniature mechanical seal made of high thermally conductive material (SiC), combined with a recirculating purge system. Although purge consumption is less than 10 ml/day, a large supply of purge fluid is recirculated behind the seal face to augment convective heat transfer. An ultrafiltration filter integrated in the recirculated purge system continuously purifies and sterilizes the purge fluid. The seal system was subsequently incorporated into our intraventricular axial flow blood pump (IVAP). Ongoing in vivo evaluation of this system has demonstrated good seal capability over 150 days. The "cool seal" system can be applied to any type of rotary blood pump (axial, diagonal, centrifugal, etc.), and offers a practical solution to the shaft-seal problem, and to heat-related complications, which currently limit the use of implantable rotary blood pumps.

Key words: Low-temperature mechanical seal — Rotary blood pump — Implantable assist device

[1] Artificial Heart/Lung Research, University of Pittsburgh Medical Center, 300 Technology Drive, Pittsburgh, PA 15219, USA
[2] Sun Medical Technology Research Corporation, 1-3-11 Suwa, Nagano 392, Japan
[3] Waseda University, 3-4-1 Okubo, Shinjuku-ku, Tokyo 169, Japan
[4] Tokyo Women's Medical College, 8-1 Kawada-cho, Shinjuku-ku, Tokyo 162, Japan

Introduction

A critical issue facing the development of an implantable, rotary blood pump is the maintenance of an effective seal at the rotating shaft. Mechanical seals are usually the most versatile type of seal for industrial applications (Fig. 1). However, in a rotary blood pump, the typical seal life is much shorter than required for chronic circulatory support. The unique properties of blood which lead to seal failure are related to adhesion and aggregation of heat-denatured blood proteins which diffuse into the lubricating film between seal faces. To solve the problem related to heat denaturation of blood proteins, we recently developed a "cool-seal" system; a low-temperature mechanical seal combined with a recirculating purge system to augment convective heat transfer. The seal system is currently incorporated in our intraventricular axial flow pump (IVAP prototype no. 9). The IVAP was implanted in a calf and an in vivo seal durability test was performed.

Material and Methods

A miniature mechanical seal was constructed which comprised a SiC seat ring and carbon graphite seal ring. The outer diameter is 8 mm, and the inner diameter is 5 mm. The inside of the seal faces are designed to be flushed by recirculating purge fluid. The seal system was incorporated into our intraventricular axial flow blood pump (IVAP prototype no. 9, Fig. 2). Purge fluid (sterile water) is introduced into the motor case through a purge inflow port. This serves to cool the motor coil, lubricate and cool the journal bearings, and directly flush the inside of the mechanical seal faces. The fluid then returns to the purge outflow port (Fig. 3). The purge fluid is recirculated between the blood pump and a paracorporeal purge reservoir, through flexible inflow and outflow purge tubing. The recirculating purge system is shown in Figs. 4 and 5. It consists of a purge reservoir (0.8l), a purge fluid pump (MasterFlex L/S; IL, USA), and an ultrafiltration filter (Nikkiso, FLX-12WG, Tokyo, Japan). The total circulating purge fluid volume was 1l. The purpose of

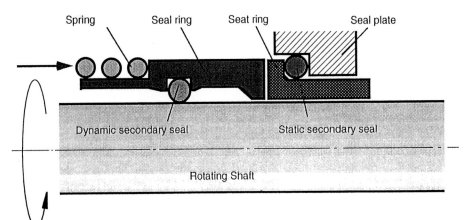

Fig. 1. Configuration of typical mechanical seal

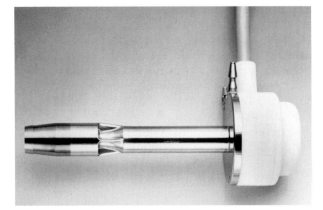

Fig. 2. Intraventricular axial flow pump (IVAP) prototype no. 9

the ultrafiltration filter is to continuously sterilize and purify the purge fluid by removal of bacteria, viruses, pyrogens, and any possible contamination by blood proteins. The intraventricular axial flow pump was implanted in a calf, and an in vivo seal system durability test was performed. After pump implantation, the purge flow rate to the blood pump was maintained at approximately 50–70 ml/min by a flow regulation valve within the bypass circuit. The purge pressure was maintained at about 100–150 mmHg. Purge fluid consumption was measured by periodically checking the fluid level at the purge reservoir. Paired samples of purge fluid (base control, and after 100 h) were taken for analysis to detect contamination by blood elements. The difference of chloride ion concentration of the samples was measured by ion chromatography

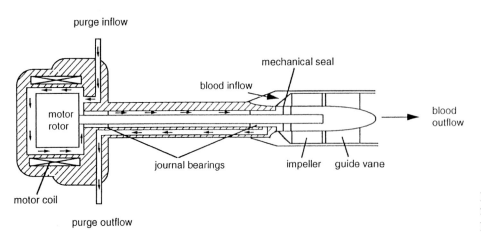

Fig. 3. A schema of purge fluid circulation inside the pump

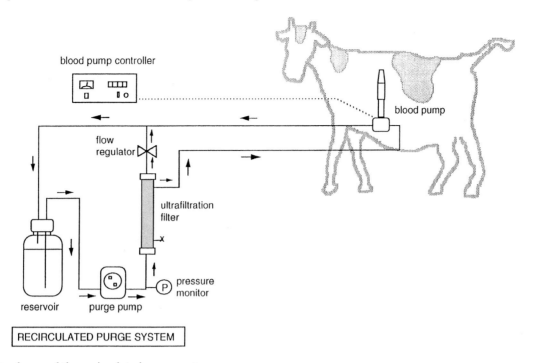

Fig. 4. A schema of the recirculated purge system

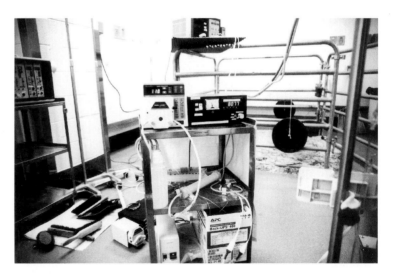

Fig. 5. A photograph of the recirculated purge system

(ICA-3030; Toa, Tokyo, Japan). The chloride ion concentration of the blood serum was measured simultaneously. The serum contamination into the purge fluid was calculated from these data. The electric power consumption of the blood pump was monitored during the experiment to assess indirectly the viscous friction in the seal system. Plasma free hemoglobin was measured periodically for evaluation of hemolysis.

Results

The chloride concentration above control of the purge fluid sample taken at 100 h was 0.2 mg/l. The concentration of chloride ion of the blood serum was 120 mEq (4200 mg/l). The blood serum contamination into the purge fluid at 100 h was 0.048 ml (about 0.01 ml/day). The temperature of the purge fluid in the reservoir was maintained below 30°C without any additional cooling methods. The average purge fluid consumption was 10 ml/day.

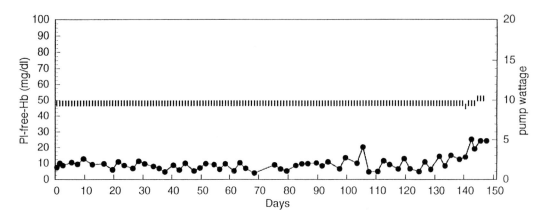

Fig. 6. Pump wattage (*striped trace*) and plasma free hemoglobin (*Pl-free-Hb, circles*) during the in vivo experiment

The motor power consumption of the blood pump was quite stable (approximate 9.6 W) during 150 days of operation (Fig. 6).

Plasma free hemoglobin remained in an acceptable range (mean plasma free hemoglobin was 9.9 mg/dl).

Discussion

Mechanical seals are the most versatile type of seals for rotating shafts in industrial applications. Mechanical seals, in principle, consist of two plane faces arranged perpendicular to the axis of a rotating shaft (Fig. 1). To keep leakage to an acceptable level in the current application, it is necessary that the two faces mate with a very small clearance, less than 1 μm. To maintain proper seal function and to keep frictional heat generation and wear within acceptable limits, an appropriate lubricating liquid film must be maintained between the two seal faces. However, in a rotary blood pump, the typical seal life is much shorter than that required for chronic support. Seal failure is related to adhesion and aggregation of heat-denatured blood proteins which diffuse into the lubricating film between the seal faces. Blood proteins denature in a temperature range from 50°C to 100°C. Among the blood proteins, fibrinogen plays an important role due to its strong propensity of adhesion and low transition temperature (Td), around 50°C. Once exposed to temperatures exceeding 50°C, fibrinogen molecules fuse together by multiattachment between heat-denatured D-domains. This quasi-polymerized fibrin increases the frictional heat and impairs optimal lubrication, which exacerbates the process, resulting in seal failure. Heat-denatured blood proteins eventually build up inside the seal faces, then invade into the bearing gap and clog it. Eventually the pump will cease to work.

The "Cool Seal" Concept

We hypothesize that if seal-face temperature is maintained well below 50°C to prevent the heat denaturation of blood proteins, a mechanical seal would not fail in blood. To achieve this "cool seal" system, a heat balance must be established between the heat generated at the seal faces and heat dissipated from them (Fig. 7).

The heat generation at the faces (Q_g) is approximated by

$$Q_g = \mu \, D_m \, n \left(F_s + \Delta p \times A_f \times B \right)$$

where

μ = friction coefficient
D_m = effective mean diameter of sealing interface
n = rotational speed
F_s = spring force
Δp = differential pressure across seal
A_f = area of sealing interface
B = balance ratio of mechanical seal

The heat dissipation from the seal $[Q_d \, (= Q_g)]$ is given by

$$Q_d = m \, k \, A \tanh \left(m \, l \right) \times \Delta T$$

where
$m = \sqrt{hc/kA}$
k = thermal conductivity of seal
A = cross-sectional area perpendicular to heat flow
h = heat transfer coefficient
l = axial length of seal ring heat transfer surface
c = circumference of heat transfer
ΔT = temperature rise at seal face (T_f) over surrounding fluid (T_b)

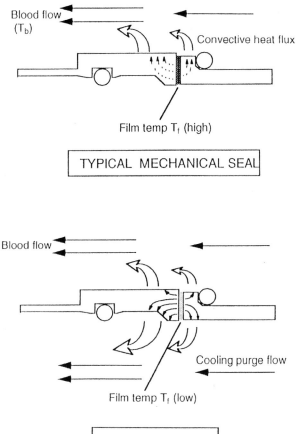

Fig. 7. Heat balance consideration of mechanical seal

over 150 days. However, several questions remain: did the seal work well as a result of the "cool seal" system? The mechanism is not fully understood since we do not have data specifically on the seal surface temperature (this would be extremely difficult to obtain experimentally). The "flushing" of transport proteins out of the seal annulus might be very important in the cooling within the seal system. Rather than state definitively that this is a thermal phenomenon, we have stated a new hypothesis based on our successful results — the combined transport of heat and proteins out of the seal annulus.

In summary, the "cool seal" system, comprising a mechanical seal with a recirculating purge system, has the following advantages:

1. It prevents heat denaturation of blood proteins and heat-induced hemolysis.

2. It cools the motor coil and bearings, thus reducing the dependence upon heat dissipation into the blood stream and surrounding tissue.

3. It helps sweep away any possible contamination of blood elements from the seal annulus. The ultrafiltration filter integrated in the recirculated purge system continuously purifies and sterilizes the purge fluid.

4. The recirculating feature of the system provides a high purge flow rate, yet results in minimal purge fluid consumption (<10 ml/day). This also enables easy maintenance (purge reservoir change is required once per month).

5. The recirculated purge system can be used as a monitoring system of seal function. Seal failure can be detected at an early stage by analyzing blood contamination into the purge fluid. It provides advance warning for corrective action to be taken to avert catastrophic blood pump failure.

6. If sufficient vacuum pressure is applied to the purge return tubing, purge consumption into the blood side can be virtually eliminated. In this situation, the purge circuit will behave as a complete closed loop. Periodical disinfectant procedure can then be performed to sterilize the whole purge circuit by irrigation (e.g., with sodium hypochlorite solution).

7. It can be applied to any type of rotary blood pump (axial, diagonal, centrifugal, etc.).

The disadvantage of the recirculated purge system is its complexity: it requires a purge fluid reservoir, a purge fluid pump, and inflow and outflow purge fluid tubing. Seal life and reliability are the most important issue for the seal system. Though these elements require periodic maintenance, the complexity of the recirculating purge system does not impair the total system reliability. If the purge recirculation is stopped for some reason, the mechanical seal can well maintain its seal capability for a couple of days of more. This provides sufficient time for

To maintain the seal face temperature at a low level, it is important to increase heat dissipation from the seal faces, while minimizing heat generation within them. To minimize heat generation, it is advisable to select a seal ring pair with a low friction coefficient, to minimize seal dimensions and rotational speed, and to optimize seal face loading. To increase the heat dissipation efficiency, it is important to select high thermally conductive material for the seal rings, and to maximize convective heat transfer by eliminating blood stagnation around the seal area. To maintain the seal face temperature at around 45°C (allowing a safety margin of about 5°C below 50°C), the temperature rise above the surrounding blood should be less than 8°C. This minimal allowable differential temperature might make it difficult to maintain an optimal heat balance at the seal faces without additional cooling methods.

The most efficient method to control the seal face temperature is to introduce a large supply of purge fluid behind the seal faces to improve convective heat transfer. The seal system functioned well in blood for

corrective action on the paracorporeal purge system to be taken.

Extended seal life can be obtained by proper design (appropriate seal configuration, materials, environmental controls, etc.); proper fabrication (precise, accurate, stiff, and balanced construction of shaft, bearings, etc.); and proper operation (optimal pressure–velocity factor, appropriate lubricating conditions, etc.) The operating conditions for blood sealing (pressure 100 mmHg, seal face velocity 1.2–5.0 m/s) are much less rigorous than the conditions in typical industrial applications, where pressures can exceed several thousand mmHg, and velocities can be well above 10 m/s. In spite of these severe operating conditions, it is encouraging that some recently introduced mechanical seals have demonstrated an average seal life of more than 5 years.

If the problem of heat denaturation of blood proteins at seal faces is completely solved, blood sealing would become an easy task. The "cool seal" system described here offers a practical solution to the shaft-seal problem, and to heat-related complications, which currently limit the use of implantable rotary blood pumps.

Discussion

Dr. Reul:
If you are going to follow this concept you will never have a totally implantable system without skin perforation for the purge fluid.

Dr. Yamazaki:
That's correct. A skin perforation is prerequisite for our system. We are developing a sink button made of carbon material as an ideal skin interface. Although a TETS (transcutaneous energy transmission) system can eliminate skin perforation, it would require additional components (secondary coil, telemetry system, internal battery, internal controller) to be implanted. I believe that reduces the advantage of the compactness of a rotary blood pump, and affects the reliability of the total pump system. I think a percutaneous system with a reliable skin button might be a better method to realize a totally implantable LVAD.

Dr. Sipin:
I guess you will have an external purge reservoir. If you recirculate the purge fluid it takes heat from the pump and from the body, so you will have to have a heat exchanger. You will have to cool the purge fluid. The best you can do is to get it warmer than the atmospheric air unless you put in a refrigerator.

Dr. Yamazaki:
The power consumption of the pump was less than 10 W. So optimal heat balance can be easily maintained without a heat exchanger. The purge reservoir was placed paracorporeally at room temperature, and the heat-dissipating efficiency was good enough to maintain the purge fluid temperature between 25° and 30°C.

Dr. Sipin:
But then you will need a large reservoir. The smaller the temperature difference, the larger the reservoir would have to be to bring your temperature down.

Dr. Yamazaki:
I used an 800-ml water reservoir, and the temperature of the purge reservoir was well maintained below 30°C throughout the experiment. The reservoir can be made small enough to be incorporated into a compact console.

Remote Energy Transmission for Powering Artificial Hearts and Assist Devices

Tofy Mussivand, Albert Hum, and Kevin S. Holmes

Summary. A high-capacity transcutaneous energy transfer (TET) system has been developed for implantable devices including artificial hearts and ventricular assist devices. The TET system provides more accurate self-tuning capabilities, increased power delivery, improved reliability, and a reduced size, in comparison with previous designs. The design of the TET was optimized with: (1) microprocessor-controlled tuning; (2) a current-sensing transformer; and (3) a reduced component count (4 versus 11 integrated circuits and 15 versus 51 discrete components). Based on these optimisations, the system efficiency has been increased through a 20% reduction in the power required to operate the circuit. The reduced component count has also provided a 40% reduction in the overall footprint of the circuitry. Circuit reliability has been improved by the reduction in complexity and component count. In vitro evaluation of the system has demonstrated its capability to deliver 44–120 watts at a d.c. input of 12–17 volts with coil spacings (in air) from 4 to 14 mm. In the spirit of cooperation, the developed system is also being made available to other research groups, for use with their respective devices. In conclusion, the developed TET delivers increased power (up to 120 watts), with a reliable design, that is efficient, and compact. Further in vitro and in vivo evaluations are ongoing.

Key words: Transcutaneous energy transfer — Artificial heart — Ventricular assist — Reliability — Efficiency

Introduction

The ability to power implanted medical devices such as artificial hearts and assist devices poses a difficult challenge. Early devices used pneumatic actuation systems which were connected to the implanted device via drivelines which passed through the patient's skin and tissue to the implanted device. This approach, unfortunately, left patients tethered to a bulky pneumatic console, thus confining them to the hospital. As the need for portable systems that would allow patients to leave the hospital became apparent, electric systems were developed. While electric systems offer portability, these systems need to be powered via a wire through the skin, since a suitable implantable power source capable of supplying the long-term power requirements of these systems has not yet been developed. Unfortunately, the use of a wire through the skin and tissue to power an implanted device faces one of the major obstacles encountered and never adequately solved with the pneumatic drivelines, namely infection. Infection and related difficulties remain one of the major complications with the use of artificial hearts and assist devices, and some investigators have suggested that with the use of chronic externalized lines, infection becomes inevitable [1]. One manner in which to overcome this problem is through the use of transcutaneous energy transfer.

Transcutaneous energy transfer (TET) is a concept pioneered in the 1960s by Schuder and colleagues [2]. Basically, the concept involves electromagnetic induction between two wire coils separated by a skin and tissue layer. The Cardiovascular Devices Division (CVD) of the University of Ottawa Heart Institute has concentrated on developing a system for use with artificial hearts, ventricular assist devices, and other implantable medical devices. The resulting TET system has been evaluated (in vitro, in vivo, and in cadavers) by CVD and other centres (including the University of Utah, Abiomed, Cleveland Clinic/Nimbus, Milwaukee Heart Project, and the Helmholtz Institute for Biomedical Engineering), as previously reported [3–5].

The developed system is designed primarily to overcome previously identified limitations to the use of TET systems, including: (1) extreme susceptibility to metal objects coming into contact or near the external coil, resulting in complete or partial shutdown of energy transfer [6]; (2) low power-transfer efficiency, resulting in unacceptable levels of heat generation by the electronics that would be implanted in the patient; and (3) high sensitivity to small variations in coil coupling that occur during normal breathing and body motion [7]. The developed system overcame the issue of the impact of metal objects, by utilising a unique external coil configuration which provides a continuous magnetic field, thereby blocking the effects of metal objects on the power transfer process. The external coil configuration utilises a three-dimensional spiral

Cardiovascular Devices Division, University of Ottawa Heart Institute, 1053 Carling Avenue, Room H560B, Ottawa, Ontario, K1Y 4E9, Canada

construction (truncated cone shape) for the wire turns of the coil, as opposed to a planar toroidal construction. This shape prevents a metal object which provides a path of least resistance from shorting out all of the wire turns simultaneously, as is possible with a planar toroidal construction. More recently, the design has undergone major optimisations to provide a more efficient, responsive, and reliable system, all within a smaller physical size.

Materials and Methods

The developed system utilises an internal and an external wire coil to form a transcutaneous air-core transformer, operated by an internal and an external electronic module. The external coil is driven by a power source (power supply or external battery pack) which drives an oscillator circuit located on the external electronic module. Energy is electromagnetically coupled through the skin and tissue to the implanted internal coil. The resulting alternating current (a.c.) at the internal coil is then converted to a direct current (d.c.) by the internal electronic module for power delivery to the implanted device. The design optimisation process concentrated on implementing a microcontroller-based tuning system, to allow for faster and more accurate tuning of the system, thus improving the overall efficiency of the power-transfer process during dynamic loading conditions.

Microcontroller Tuning. The microcontroller tuning circuit is essentially used to determine the optimal amount of energy to be supplied to the external coil at any given time. The tuning circuitry utilises two inputs, the input voltage to the oscillator and the load current derived from a current-sensing transformer at the output of the oscillator. Based on these inputs, the on-time and subsequently the frequency of the oscillator is determined on an ongoing basis, to provide optimum power-transfer efficiency at all times. This determination is implemented using preset minimum and maximum values, as well as a lookup table stored on the microcontroller. Each individual system has the lookup table generated experimentally to take into account any variations due to component tolerances, which could have a significant impact on achieving optimal tuning characteristics.

Current-Sensing Transformer. The current-sensing transformer is used to determine the reflected load current which enables the timing of the oscillator to be optimised. The use of a current-sensing transformer offers immunity to switching noise from the field effect transistor (FET) which drives the external coil. The current-sensing transformer also provides important electrical isolation between the drive circuitry and the sensing circuitry.

In Vitro Testing. The system was tested with the totally implantable ventricular assist device being developed in this laboratory [8]. The microcontroller tuning circuit was assessed to determine overall function, power transfer capability, and system response to load variation.

Power Transfer Capability. The power transfer capability was assessed using a test fixture which allowed the coils to have calibrated coil separations (in air) for a series of measurements under various loading conditions. Measurements were taken for coil separations of 4, 10, and 14mm and input voltages of 12 and 17V. Measurements were taken at delivered powers of 10, 20, 40, 60, 80, 90, 100, and 120W.

Response to Load Variation. Since the developed system is primarily intended for use with systems that have cyclical loading characteristics, the response time of the tuning circuitry was measured. To measure response time, the system was connected to a programmable load generator (PLZ303W; Kikusui Electronics, Yokohama, Japan). The load generator was programmed for a two-stage cyclical load of 1A for 50ms followed by a 3A load for 5ms. Response time and the accuracy of the tuning circuit was measured.

Results

The high-capacity TET system has been designed, developed, fabricated, evaluated, and patented in the United Kingdom, the United States, and Canada. The design is capable of transcutaneously providing power to devices such as artificial hearts and ventricular assist devices, with increased reliability, responsiveness, and efficiency.

The overall footprint of the circuit design has been reduced by 40%, through a reduction in the number of components from 11 integrated circuits (ICs) and 51 discrete components to 4 ICs and 11 discrete components. The reduced component count has provided improved efficiency over previous designs, by reducing the operating power requirements of the electronic circuitry by 20%. A significant improvement is also expected in the overall reliability of the electronic circuitry, due to the reduction in both complexity and component count of the circuitry.

Results from the evaluation of power-transfer capability are shown in Fig. 1. The implementation of the microcontroller tuning allowed increased power-delivery capabilities by providing faster and more precise tuning control. The microcontroller tuning circuit

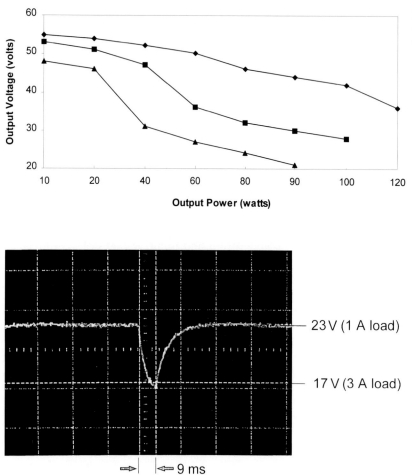

Fig. 1. Power delivery versus output voltage for various coil spacings: *diamonds* 4mm; *squares* 10mm; *triangles* 14mm

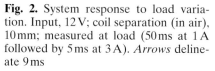

Fig. 2. System response to load variation. Input, 12 V; coil separation (in air), 10mm; measured at load (50ms at 1 A followed by 5ms at 3 A). *Arrows* delineate 9ms

improved the overall efficiency and power-transfer capability in comparison with a fixed tuning system, by shifting the power transfer curve (efficiency versus delivered power) such that at a given efficiency, the power delivery was increased. For example, at a coil spacing of 5mm, the delivered power for the microcontroller-tuned system was approximately 5W greater along the entire efficiency curve than that of the fixed tuning system. More importantly, the microcontroller-tuned system allows optimal power transfer efficiency over an entire range of loading conditions, whereas fixed tuning operates at optimal efficiency only within a narrow band of loading conditions, outside of which the power-transfer efficiency is severely degraded. The developed system can provide up to 120W of delivered power (at 17V d.c. input with 4mm coil spacing). The system response time to load variation was measured to be approximately 9ms, while utilising a pulsatile load of 50ms at 1 A followed by 5ms at 3 A (Fig. 2). Further design

optimisation is ongoing in preparation for in vivo evaluation and subsequent clinical utilisation.

Discussion

The development of totally implantable artificial hearts and ventricular assist devices is currently viewed as an important step in the evolution of mechanical circulatory support. This type of device will offer an improved quality of life for the patient, and provide clinicians the ability to release patients from the hospital, after device implantation and recovery. This aspect in especially important in the era of cost consciousness in the health care field. Transcutaneous energy transfer systems will play a vital role in the development of these totally implantable devices by eliminating the need for percutaneous connections to power these devices and the inherent risk of infectious complications. As a gesture of goodwill and collaboration, the investigators have made, and continue to make, this system available to other investigators for use with their respective devices.

References

1. Pennington DG (1996) Extended support with permanent systems: Percutaneous versus totally implantable. Ann Thorac Surg 61:403–406
2. Schuder JC, Stephenson HE, Townsend JF (1961) High-level electromagnetic energy transfer through a closed chest wall. In: 1961 IRE International Conv. Rec (part 9). vol 9, pp 119–126
3. Mussivand T, Holmes KS, Hum A, Keon WJ (1996) Transcutaneous energy transfer with voltage regulation for rotary blood pumps. Artif Organs 20:621–624
4. Mussivand T, Hum A, Diguer M, Holmes KS, Vecchio G, Masters RG, Hendry PJ, Keon WJ (1995) A transcutaneous energy and information transfer system for implanted medical devices. ASAIO J 41:M253–M258
5. Mussivand T, Miller JA, Santerre JP, Belanger G, Rajagopalan KC, Hendry PJ, Masters RG, Holmes KS, Robichaud R, Keaney M, Virginia VM, Keon WJ (1993) Transcutaneous energy transfer system performance evaluation. Artif Organs 17:940–947
6. Geselowitz DB, Hoang QTN, Gaumond RP (1992) The effects of metals on a transcutaneous energy transmission system. IEEE Trans Biomed Eng 39:928–934
7. Miller JA, Belanger G, Mussivand T (1993) Development of an autotuned transcutaneous energy transfer system. ASAIO J 39:M706–M710
8. Mussivand T, Masters RG, Hendry PJ, Keon WJ (1996) Totally implantable intrathoracic ventricular assist device. Ann Thorac Surg 61:444–447

New Insight into the Fracture and Wear Problems of a Mechanical Heart Valve — In Vitro Microstrain, Creep Rupture, and Wear Studies

S.H. Teoh

Summary. Reports on strut fracture of mechanical heart valves with the tilting disk design and wear marks on the occluder have prompted a detailed study of the forces and strains that are associated with the closing and opening of the valves. Using the finite element method (FEM), the site of stress concentration and the relative magnitudes of the stresses and strains on the upper strut of a St. Vincent's mechanical heart valve were located. With microstrain gauges and appropriate instrumentation, the actual forces on the struts were evaluated in vitro using a pulse simulator. The maximum stress at the site of stress concentration of the titanium valve housing was 51 MPa. This is well below the fatigue endurance limit of titanium. The imposed stress on the occluder by the upper strut was less than 2 MPa. Using computational creep rupture analysis, it was found that this is below the lower stress limit of polyacetal, which is the material used for the occluder. This work gives new insight into why no fracture of the plastic disk occluder has been reported for in vivo cases of similar design where the valve has been operating in the heart for more than 20 years. From in vitro wear studies and ex vivo examination of an explanted valve (17 years 5 months; Björk-Shiley valve), the wear debris size of polyacetal was in the range of 30 μm, which was believed to be of a range tolerable in the cardiovascular system.

Key words: Mechanical heart valve — Fracture and wear — In vitro strains — Creep rupture of polyacetal — Wear debris — Björk-Shiley tilting disc prosthesis — Finite element method

Introduction

In recent years there have been some reports on strut failure [1] of mechanical heart valves with a tilting disk design. These have been traced to the poor quality of welding at the root of the metallic struts. Disk fractures, though low in incidence, have also been reported. For example, fracture of disks made from pyrolytic carbon has been reported for the Björk-

Shiley tilting disk [2] and also for the Edwards-Duromedics bileaflet valves [3]. However, the excellent wear resistance and biocompatibility of pyrolytic carbon have made this implant material very popular over the last decade. Plastic occluder materials such as polyacetal have been used since as early as 1969 [4]. Unlike the brittle ceramic pyrolytic carbon material, the plastic occluder is ductile. No reports of mechanical failure of any sort for the Björk-Shiley polyacetal tilting disk heart valves have been found in the literature [5]. More than a hundred Björk-Shiley polyacetal disk prostheses have been examined by Montero et al. [6]. Their report recorded that, apart from the low thromboembolic rate of the plastic occluder, no patients had to undergo reoperation because of fracture or dislodgment of the disk occluder or severe hemolysis. However, wear marks, in particular those caused by accelerated in vitro life tests on the plastic occluder, have caused some concerns [7,8]. Nevertheless, the question remains as to why the older-design Björk-Shiley polyacetal disk prostheses have survived for so long (exceeding 17 years of in vivo experience). Figure 1 shows an explanted valve (17 years 5 months) of this type taken from a patient who died of a disease not related to the heart.

There are still concerns about (a) the imposed stresses on the struts and on the occluder (b) the durability of the polyacetal disk of mechanical heart valves, and (c) the design stress limits of the implant materials. These have prompted a detailed study of the forces associated with the closing and opening in a St Vincent's mechanical heart valve of similar design to the Björk-Shiley polyacetal tilting disk prosthesis, except that it is machined from a block of pure titanium without welding of the struts, and the contact areas between the struts and the occluder have been increased to reduce contact stresses [8]. With the availability of microstrain gauges and the finite element method (FEM) to locate the areas of maximum stress, it is now possible to conduct in vivo and in vitro experiments on prosthetic heart valves [9,10]. Creep rupture data and computational analysis have enabled the prediction of design stresses for the plastic occluder [11,12]. This, together with the wear assessment of materials used in mechanical heart valves [13], has provided new insight

Centre for Biomedical Materials Applications and Technology (BIOMAT), Institute of Materials Research and Engineering, Mechanical and Production Engineering Department, National University of Singapore, 10 Kent Ridge Crescent 119260, Singapore

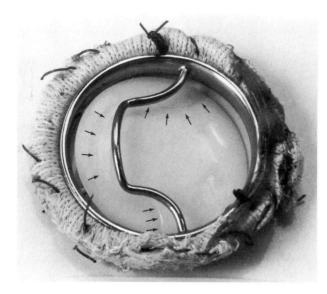

Fig. 1. Explanted Björk-Shiley Delrin tilting disk prosthesis, 17 years 5 months. The *arrows* indicate the wear groove made by the upper strut

into the fracture and wear problems of the mechanical heart valves.

Materials and Methods

In Vitro Microstrain/FEM

A 29-mm St. Vincent's mechanical heart valve with a polyacetal occluder was used. The in vitro experiment using a pulse simulator (MHL 6891, Vivtro Systems, Canada) has been described previously [10]. Two microstrain gauges (EA-05-015DJ-120, Micro-Measurements, USA) of gauge length 3.2 mm were attached to the upper strut, 4.5 mm away from the root of the titanium housing. FEM was carried out on the Intergraph Randmicas Package. Young's modulus for titanium was taken to be 107 GPa and Poisson's ratio, 0.34.

Creep Rupture and Computational Modelling

Details of the creep rupture studies and computational modelling have been published [12]. Dead weights were used and the stress applied varied from 20 to 80 MPa. The polyacetal (Delrin 500; Du Pont) used is the same as that of the plastic occluder of the St. Vincent's mechanical heart valve. A range of temperatures from 20°C to 80°C were used as a means to predict the long-term durability of the polyacetal. In addition, a set of specimens were also tested in saline solution (0.9% NaCl) at 37°C to study the effect of NaCl solution on the creep fracture behaviour. Design

stress predictions were based on a three-element mechanical model in conjunction with an energy failure criterion. This results in a nonlinear equation between time to failure (t_f) and applied stress (σ_{ap}):

$$\ln t_f = \ln\left\{1/(C\,B)\ln\left[\tan h\left(B\sigma_{ap}/2\right)/\tan h\left(B\,H/2\right)\right]\right\}$$

where C = constant related to activation energy, B = constant related to the activation volume, and $H = \sigma_{ap} - [2E_a(R - \sigma_{ap}/E_e)]^{1/2}$, where E_a = anelastic modulus, E_e = elastic modulus, and R = resilience of the material (defined as the maximum elastic stored energy before fracture). It can be seen that when the applied stress equals ($E_e\,R$), immediate fracture occurs (SX), but when it equals $[R/(1/E_e + \frac{1}{2}E_a)]^{1/2}$, the material sustains the load indefinitely (SN). The significance of the first equation is that one can obtain SX and SN from just creep rupture data.

Wear Assessment

The explanted polyacetal occluder was examined under scanning electron microscopy (SEM) (Joel LSM-T330A). Prior to SEM examination, the specimen was sputter gold coated in a vacuum evaporator (Joel JEF-4X).

Results and Discussion

Figure 2 shows a typical oscilloscope trace of the strain recorded on the arms of the titanium strut. On valve closure, a sharp peak (75–150 $\mu\varepsilon$) was initially seen, which subsided quickly to a plateau (31–42 $\mu\varepsilon$). This was due to the sudden surge in the left ventricular pressure (217–240 mmHg) on valve closure for about 0.26 s. When the valve opened, small multiple peaks (20–63 $\mu\varepsilon$), indicative of vibrations, were noted on the left side of the valve. This observation gives valuable information on the transient forces that may be related to slight flow disturbances on the left side of the valve during the opening period, caused, perhaps, by the sliding action of the occluder. When the valve was closed, the occluder exerted a pressure that was transmitted to the base of the upper strut as well as to the lips of the valve housing. In the worst possible case, all the load can be considered to have been transmitted to the bottom face of the upper strut as a point load acting at the midspan of the upper strut. The FEM results indicate that the maximum stress occurs at the root of the junction between the valve housing and the upper strut (indicated by X in Fig. 3). The maximum peak stress ranges from 25–51 MPa and the steady stress range is 10–14 MPa. This is well below the fatigue endurance limit of pure titanium (345 MPa). The stress on the occluder on valve closure can be calculated by assuming that the upper strut supports the

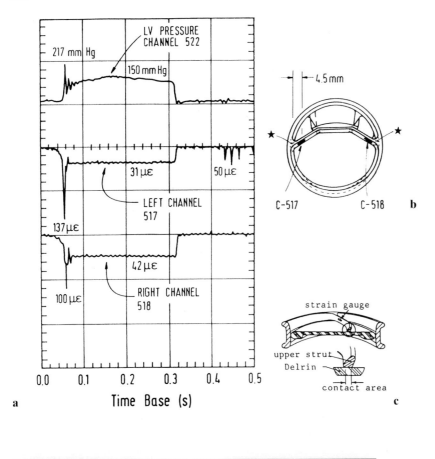

Fig. 2. a Typical oscilloscope trace during in vitro microstrain measurements of a 29-mm St. Vincent's mechanical heart valve in a pulse simulator: *top trace*, left ventricular pressure; *middle trace*, strain, left channel; *bottom trace*, strain, right channel. **b** Diagram of the heart valve housing. *Stars*, locations of maximum stress concentration. **c** Cross sections shwoing locations of strain gauge and contact area

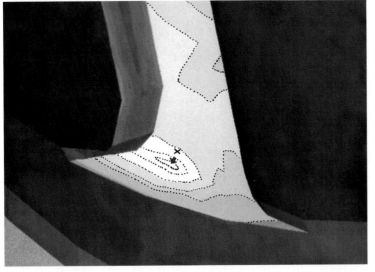

Fig. 3. Finite Element Method (FEM) analysis of the upper strut. Position X indicates location of maximum stress concentration

entire load. The peak left ventricular pressure of 240 mmHg over an orifice diameter of 26.1 mm will generate a force of 17.1 N on the surface of the occluder. The imposed stress on the occluder is calculated to be about 2 MPa (17.1/8.73, where the denominator is the contact area between the upper strut and the occluder). This value is an overestimate as the lip area of the valve housing also supports the force on

closure. It is now left to see whether this stress level (<2 MPa) is below the endurance stress limit of polyacetal.

Figure 4 shows the creep rupture time versus applied stress for various temperatures ranging from 20°C to 80°C. It can be seen that saline solution has the significant effect of reducing the lower stress limit (SN) from 20 MPa (at 37°C in air) to about 5 MPa (at

Fracture and Wear in Mechanical Heart Valve   351

Fig. 4. Modelling the creep rupture behaviour of polyacetal. In air unless otherwise stated: *open circles*, 20°C; *triangles*, 37°C in air; *slashed closed circles*, 37°C in saline solution; *squares*, 60°C; *closed circles*, 80°C

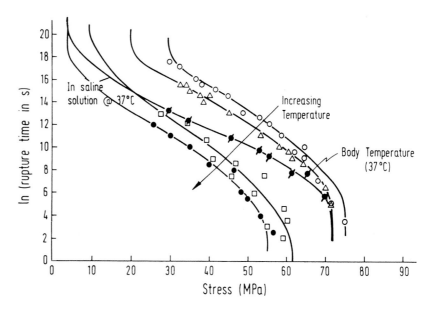

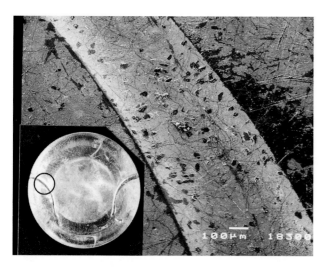

Fig. 5. Scanning electron micrograph of the explanted valve showing wear debris in the groove structure. *Bar*, 100 μm

37°C in saline solution). This value can be predicted if the polyacetal is subjected to a high temperature, 80°C. These results indicate that if the imposed stress is less than 5 MPa, the material will not fail prematurely by creep fracture and will sustain the applied stress indefinitely under saline conditions. Therefore, it can be seen that the imposed stress on the plastic occluder is far below the lower stress limit of Delrin. This probably explains why there has not been any report of disk fracture using this plastic material as the occluder for the last two decades. However, this is on the assumption that sodium chloride is the dominant stress-reducing factor as compared to the other chemi-

cals in the human blood. A more complete picture would be gained by conducting the creep fracture experiments in a blood environment, a topic for future work.

Figure 5 shows the SEM picture of the explanted valve. A deep groove of about 1.2 mm can be seen. This represents the impression worn out by the upper strut of the Björk-Shiley prosthesis on the occluder. Its is remarkable that having suffered such a deep groove the plastic occluder did not fracture. A ceramic occluder would have fractured. However, it is not hard to understand since the fracture toughness of polyacetal is about 4 MPa·m$^{-1/2}$ and that of pyrolytic carbon is only about 1 MPa·m$^{-1/2}$. This means that the plastic occluder is about four times more resistant to crack propagation than pyrolytic carbon. The size of the wear debris, about 30 μm, is of a magnitude measured during in vitro testing of Delrin [13]. This size appear to be of a range tolerable in the cardiovascular system, since the valve has been in operation for more than 17 years.

References

1. Lindblom D, Björk VO, Semb KH (1986) Mechanical failure of the Björk-Shiley valve. J Thorac Cardiovasc Surg 92:894–907
2. Novenberg DD, Evans RW, Gundersen AE, Abellera RM (1977) Fracture and embolization of a Björk-Shiley disc. J Thorac Cardiovasc Surg 74:925–927
3. Klepetko W, Moritz A, Mlczoch J, Schurawitzki H, Comanig E, Wolner E (1989) Leaflet fracture in Edwards-Duromedics bileaflet valve. J Thorac Cardiovasc Surg 97:90–94

4. Björk VO (1972) Delrin as an implant material for valve occluders. Scan J Thorac Cardiovasc Surg 6:103–107

5. Lindblom D (1988) Long-term clinical results after aortic valve replacement with the Björk-Shiley prosthesis. J Thorac Cardiovasc Surg 95:658–667

6. Montero CG, Rufilanchas JJ, Juffe A, Burgos R, Ugarte J, Figuera D (1984) Long-term results of cardiac valve replacement with the Delrin disc model of the Björk-Shiley valve prosthesis. Ann Thorac Surg 37:328–336

7. Clark RE, Swanson WM, Kardos JL, Hagen RW, Beauchamp RA (1987) Durability of prosthetic heart valves. Ann Thorac Surg 26:323–335

8. Teoh SH, Martin RL, Lim SC, Lee KH, Mok CK, Kwok WC (1990) Delrin as an occluder material. ASAIO Trans 36:M417–M421

9. Riner WG, Christopher RA, Golter LB, Sadler TR Jr, Serkes KD (1975) In vivo strain measurements of a prosthetic aortic valve. J Thorac Cardiovasc Surg 70: 732–734

10. Teoh SH, Lee KH, Nugent AH, Goh KS (1993) In vitro measurement of a mechanical heart valve in a pulse simulator. ASAIO J 39:929–932

11. Teoh SH (1994) Predicting the life and design stresses of medical plastics under creep conditions. In: Kambic HE, Yokobori AT Jr (eds) Biomaterials mechanical properties. ASTM STP 1173, American Society for Testing and Materials, Philadelphia, pp 77–86

12. Teoh SH (1993) Effect of saline solution on the creep fracture of Delrin. Biomaterials 14:132–136

13. Teoh SH, Lim SC, Yoon ET, Goh KS (1994) A new method for in vitro wear assessment of materials used in mechanical heart valves. In: Kambic HE, Yokobori AT Jr (eds) Biomaterials mechanical properties. ASTM STP 1173, American Society for Testing and Materials, Philadelphia, pp 43–52

Basic Study Towards the Establishment of a Fabrication Technology for a Vacuum-Formed Blood Pump

Mitsuo Umezu[1], Manoja Ranawake[2], Tadasuke Nakayama[1], Tomoyuki Ohnuma[1], Kazushige Iinuma[1], Yoshitaka Ueda[1], Makoto Arita[1], Takayuki Kido[3], Toshihiko Kijima[3], Chisato Nojiri[3], and John Woodard[2]

Summary. An adult-sized pump has been developed based on our experience with the development of a pediatric-type ventricular assist pump using the vacuum-forming process. During the scale-up process, large oscillations of pressure and flow were observed, which resulted from the substitution of a trileaflet valve for a bileaflet valve in the inflow position. At the pump inlet, an in vitro study using a high-speed video camera indicated that the oscillation was induced by expansion of the flexible sinus of Valsalva during early systole. As the valve leaflets subsequently opened, a large pressure spike was induced and the oscillation commenced. This phenomenon could be reduced by using a thicker wall section for the sinus of Valsalva, or using a bileaflet valve in the inlet position.

Key words: Ventricular assist device — Vacuum forming method — Trileaflet valve — Bileaflet valve — Polyurethane valve

Introduction

The vacuum-forming method has well-known advantages in reducing manufacturing time as well as simplifying a manufacturing process. We started the development of our first vacuum-formed ventricular assist pump in 1992, by reference to the results achieved by Dr. Kolff's group [1], and our pediatric-type blood pump was completed in 1993 [2,3]. Based on experience, we have scaled up the pump to adult size as shown in Fig. 1. Throughout this scale-up porcess, we have experienced considerable difficulty, especially in the development of a suitable polyurethane (PU) inlet valve. This paper deals with the design of a vacuum-formed valve at the pump inlet.

Materials and Methods

The two different-sized pumps used in this investigation had dome-shaped diaphragms with different diameters (ϕ; 51 mm and 70 mm). The stroke volumes were 20 ml and 65 ml, respectively. The outlet valve design was the same for both pumps except that the valve diameter for the pediatric-type was 13.6 mm, while that for the adult type was 19 mm. In our present procedure, PU sheets (E380, Miractran, Tokyo, Japan) with a thickness ranging from 0.2 to 6 mm were chosen. Heat was applied to the PU sheet at a temperature of 410°C before applying a vacuum pressure of −70 mmHg. For the fabrication of valve leaflets and the conduit with Valsalva sinuses, 0.3-mm and 4-mm PU sheets were used, respectively. The duration of the heating depended on the sheet thickness, as listed in Table 1. In the adult-type pump, identical trileaflet valves were mounted at both inlet and outlet positions, whereas a bileaflet valve was employed in the inlet position of the pediatric type. Further fabrication methods were described elsewhere [4].

Results and Discussion

Mechanism of Oscillation of the Inlet PU Valve

The adult-type pump produced an extraordinarily high oscillation of the inlet flow and pressure during the pump-systolic phase, as shown in Fig. 2d and f. The flow and pressure waveforms measured at the inlet of the pediatric type appear in Fig. 2c and e for comparison. A high-speed video camera (Fastcam-ultima01, Photoron, Tokyo, Japan) was set up beside the mock circulatory system to measure the oscillation phenomenon at 500 frames per second. It was seen that the first pressure spike (arrow **A** in Fig. 2f) and the second (arrow **B**) were generated from different causes. The first spike was produced by an initial elevation of the pump inner pressure. At the time, the leaflets did not close completely as filling had not finished. At this critical moment diastolic and systolic phases overlapped. This phenomenon has been observed in other pulsatile pumps. In the pediatric-type pump, this was

[1] Department of Mechanical Engineering, Waseda University, 3-4-1 Ohkubo, Shinjuku-ku, Tokyo 169, Japan
[2] CHAD Research Laboratories Pty Ltd, PO Box 264, Surry Hills, Sydney, NSW 2010, Australia
[3] Research and Development, Terumo Corporation, Kanagawa 259-01, Japan

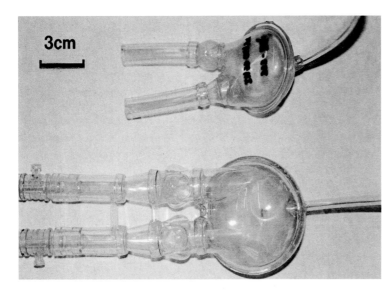

Fig. 1. Two sizes of vacuum-formed ventricular assist devices (*upper*, pediatric-type; *lower*, adult-type)

Table 1. Manufacturing condition for each element during vacuum forming process

Element		Pediatric type	Adult type
Diaphragm	Thickness[a]	0.5	0.5
	Duration[b]	30	30
Housing	Thickness	3	4
	Duration	100	170
Inlet valve leaflet	Thickness	N/A	0.2 0.5 0.7
	Duration	(Bileaflet valve)	15 30 50
Inlet valve conduit	Thickness	3	2 3 4 6
	Duration	100	85 100 170 220
Outlet valve leaflet	Thickness	0.3	0.5
	Duration	20	30
Outlet valve conduit	Thickness	3	4
	Duration	100	170

[a] Thickness (mm), thickness of the polyurethane sheet before vacuum forming process.
[b] Duration (s), duration of the heating (410°C).

also observed, as indicated by arrow **X** in Fig. 2. The first pressure spike was caused as the inlet valve closed by reversed flow.

The video film revealed that the oscillation phenomenon was induced from the second pressure spike (arrow **B**). Speculation as to the mechanisms is as follows:

1. The pump housing as well as the junction between the housing and valve conduit were deformed by the systolic drive pressure.
2. Subsequently, the sinuses in the inflow valve conduit were expanded.
3. As the valve leaflets and sinuses of Valsalva were composed as one body, the leaflets were forced to open.
4. High pressure generated by the systolic drive pressure passed through the leaflets toward an inlet cannula.
5. This pressure was tranferred in the inlet cannula and a reflected wave returned toward the pump. The oscillation was thus started.

A separate in vitro test using a bileaflet valve indicated that there was no oscillation phenomenon, even if the conduit with Valsalva sinuses was employed. In the bileaflet valve, the leaflets were not forced to open, because two leaflets and the conduit were isolated by the way the pump was constructed. Therefore, the large oscillation did not occur.

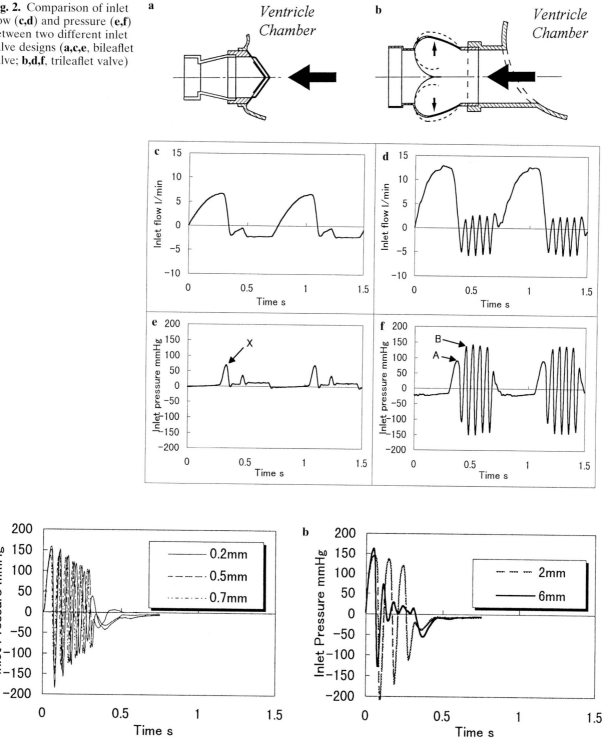

Fig. 2. Comparison of inlet flow (**c,d**) and pressure (**e,f**) between two different inlet valve designs (**a,c,e**, bileaflet valve; **b,d,f**, trileaflet valve)

Fig. 3. Effects of leaflet and Valsalva-conduit thickness on inlet pressure change. **a** The thickness of the polyurethane (PU) Sheet for the fabrication of the leaflet was changed: *solid line*, 0.2 mm; *dashed line*, 0.5 mm; *dotted line*, 0.7 mm. **b** The thickness of the Valsalva conduit was changed: *dashed line*, 2 mm; *solid line*, 6 mm

Trials to Reduce the Oscillation Phenomenon

To reduce the oscillation phenomenon, we developed identical PU valves with different leaflet and conduit-wall thicknesses. Figure 3a shows the effects of leaflet thickness on inlet pressure. Although the PU sheet thickness before vacuum forming was changed from 0.2 to 0.7 mm, there was no distinct difference among the valves and oscillation could not be restrained. On the other hand, as shown in Fig. 3b, the second pressure spike could be reduced using a thick (6-mm) PU sheet. This result appears to support the postulated oscillation mechanism.

Conclusions

When trileaflet PU valves are designed using flexible materials, deformation of the components should be taken into consideration, otherwise unexpected flow dynamics may be induced. To reduce the oscllation of the inlet pressure we could explore solutions such as a thick conduit, or a valve design other than a trileaflet type. These options will need further investigation.

References

1. Yu LS, Klinkman J, Robinson P, Bishop D, Kolff J, Versteeg F, Burns G, Yuan B, Kolff WJ (1989) Soft artifical ventricles (abstract). Artif Organs 13:393
2. Ranawake M, Umezu M, Nojiri C, Kijima T, Majima S, Horiuchi K, Shimazaki Y, Ohnuma T, Moribe T, Akutsu T (1994) An inexpensive vacuum-formed ventricular assist device. In: Goh JCH, Nather A (eds) Proceedings of 8th International Conference on Biomedical Engineering. National University of Singapore, pp 219–221
3. Ranawake M, Nojiri C, Kijima T, Kido T, Majima S, Horiuchi K, Hagiwara K, Shimazaki Y, Ohnuma T, Moribe T, Umezu M, Kolff WJ, Akutsu T (1996) Investigation of a ventricular assist device for serial production. In: Akutsu T, Koyanagi H (eds) Heart replacement: artifical heart 5, Springer, Tokyo, pp 341–344
4. Umezu M, Ranawake M, Nakayama T, Kobayashi K, Kido T, Nojiri C, Kijima T, Fujimoto T, Akutsu T (1996) Improvement of fabrication process of vacuum formed valves for ventricular assist device. Jpn J Artif Organs 25(1):43–47

Discussion

Dr. Nosé:

I would like to ask a question to Dr. Umezu. As you know, Dr. Kolf has been working with vacuum-forming devices for many years. Dr. Kolf is my teacher, and he asked my help to find a company to make a vacuum-formed pump device. I contacted many companies, but they always refused because quality assurance of the vacuum pump parts is nightmarish and they said they could not make reproducible parts with the method. How have you dealt with this problem of quality assurance?

Dr. Umezu:

We are at the initial stage of our trial, and, as I mentioned in my transparency, the quality control seems good as compared with our conventional solution casting method. But a deviation still remains there, so we are discussing the problem, as you pointed out, of how to decrease the deviation of the characteristics. One of the problems is that we have to glue several components and I think this part has more difficulties as compared with the vacuum-forming process. Therefore, I would like to find a way to eliminate the gluing process. Maybe we will show you some more results in the near future. Thank you.

Dr. Reul:

Yuki, I also strongly disagree with your statement. If you control your initial sheet material thickness well and if you control your process parameters correctly, then the quality control of thermoforming is much easier than dipping.

Dr. Nosé:

No, what I said is not my opinion, it's the manufacturing company's opinion.

Dr. Reul:

Yes, development takes a long time, but it can be done. And I have an additional question to Dr. Umezu. Are you really talking about a 6 mm wall thickness of your conduit? This is enormous.

Dr. Umezu:

Yes, before this trial, I couldn't believe it either, and I think it is too thick. Therefore I would like to change and discard the concept of the trileaflet valve with the sinus of Valsalva at outlet position.

Dr. Reul:

I have a question to Dr. Teoh. I congratulate you on your very nice paper but it was very short and I missed, actually, your final suggestions. Are you suggesting that we go back to plastic materials for heart valves due to your recent findings? Or what can we learn from your talk?

Dr. Teoh:

The basis of my talk was to try to find what could be the possible reasons for such a long in vivo experience of the first few designs of the Bjork-Shiley tilting disk valve. I didn't have a chance to present my conclusions, but what I wanted to show was the fact that it is true, and if you look at the statistics, Delrin has got very good cardiovascular experience as a mechanical heart valve, although I realize in the literature Delrin polyacetal has been a disaster in hip joint replacement. That is because of the imposed stresses which no one has really done too much work on. So I am proposing the fact that if the imposed stresses are low, below, in my estimate 5 MPa, it should last for a long time.

Dr. Rosenbaum:

You were talking about the stresses. Are you talking about the steady state stresses or Herzian stress, the impulse stress?

Dr. Teoh:

This is a very first approximation. I am taking the peak load from the in vitro FEM analysis, so the peak load is a dynamic load. As you look at the dynamic load and the steady state load, it is roughly about four times that of the steady state load. So I am taking the worst case.

Dr. Rosenbaum:

So you really are taking the Herzian stress application?

Dr. Teoh:

Yes.

Part VIII
New Approaches

A Review and Assessment of Investigative Methods for Mechanically Induced Blood Trauma: Special Aspects in Rotary Blood Pumps

Heinrich Schima[1,2], Georg Wieselthaler[2], Ilse Schwendenwein[1], Udo Losert[1], and Ernst Wolner[2]

Summary. In the last decade, enormous progress in the development and clinical use of cardiac assist devices has been made. Membrane pumps are already used routinely in clinical practice for implantation times of over a year, and some rotary pumps have attained reasonable quality for medium-term application. However, blood compatibility and thrombogenicity are still crucial problems, and thrombotic events in patients are still being reported. In rotary pumps with fast-spinning rotors and high-velocity gradients, thrombi can obtain characteristics different to those observed with membrane pumps. With unsatisfactory design or improper working conditions, small thrombi frequently may be released to the blood stream. This paper discusses the currently available models to assess mechanical blood trauma, and suggests design strategies to avoid thrombus formation. Finally, it considers in vitro and in vivo approaches to the evaluation of the performance and the safety of these pumps.

Key words: Biocompatibility — Hemolysis — Thrombogenesis — Numerical model — In vitro test — Microembolus

Introduction

In recent years the development of blood pumps has made enormous progress. Membrane pumps have been successfully used for long-term clinical purposes. Advanced rotary pumps in various designs have been developed, and some of them have already been applied in animal trials lasting up to several months [1–3].

Certainly, important topics remain to be solved. Percutaneous leads and vent tubes bear increased risks of infection, and also the management of the power cable sometimes leads to considerable problems. Further, the adaptation of pumping activity to physiological demand has to be further improved. The size and complexity of the currently available clinical systems is another limiting factor, which is being addressed by intensive research on rotary pumps.

Without a doubt, blood compatibility, thrombus formation, and release of emboli remain the most crucial problems with most devices, although they are less frequently observed than several years ago [4,5]. The valves, conduits, and connectors are the most critical locations for material accumulation in membrane pumps, as seen after explantation. In rotary pumps, the locally elevated velocity gradients and smooth surfaces create an enhanced risk for releasing undetected microemboli. Even if the pump itself and the conduits are free from major depositions at explantation, considerable numbers of thrombi may have already been released to the patient [6]. In particular, the bearing/sealing areas and stagnation points at vane-connecting structures are locations of major risk for platelet aggregation and thrombus formation.

During pump development and evaluation of various products, the authors observed a high potential for microembolus generation with some of the designs, and concluded that widely used methods such as hemolysis tests, pump inspection, and macroscopic autopsy may not offer sufficient sensitivity to detect small aggregates, which may lead to complications in the human neurocerebral system.

Therefore, a revised view on the currently available models and theories of mechanically induced blood trauma is given, including the limitations of their application for pump development. Currently available design strategies for bearing systems, and the specific danger of microembolus generation in high-speed rotary pumps are discussed and illustrated with a case from the authors' experience. Finally, some strategies to evaluate microthrombogenicity in vitro and in vivo are considered.

Theories of Mechanically Induced Blood Trauma

Blood compatibility is influenced both by biochemical factors associated with the pump surface materials and the physical properties of the flow-field — shear gradients and thermal effects. Lack of adequate physical properties can lead to mechanical damage to the blood, which is usually discussed in respect of

[1]Center of Biomedical Research and [2]Department of Cardio-Thoracic Surgery, General Hospital of the University of Vienna, Waehringer Guertel 18, A-1090 Vienna, Austria

hemolysis (destruction of erythrocytes) and of platelet activation and deposition.

Hemolysis and its implications for pump design have been intensively investigated in the past three decades, resulting in a number of theories and models, and derived guidelines for design. Although these theories are partially inconsistent and even contradictory, they have helped to improve the hemolytic properties of these pumps.

For platelet activation and thrombus deposition, however, far less data suitable for device engineering are available. This may be due to the enhanced complexity of thrombus formation owing to fluid-mechanical and biochemical pathways [7,8]. Quite often, low hemolysis levels were taken as a guarantee of low platelet activation. Usually, for the pragmatic design of pumps, stagnation areas and gaps are avoided and very smooth surfaces are used; alternatively, very rough surfaces have been recommended to obtain stable, adhering layers of proteins, with excellent clinical results [9].

Models of Mechanically Induced Hemolysis

For engineering approaches to pump design and optimization, a mathematical equation for blood trauma would be highly desirable. With such a formula, computer programs could be used to optimize the design of cardiovascular devices in a straightforward fashion [10,11]. Of course, the characteristics of such a formula (such as thresholds at short exposures, weighting of

stress amount, and time span, recirculation, and recovery effects) is crucial for the reliability of the whole optimization process. Wrong grading of these effects would lead to very different implications for optimization of design and working points.

Yet, within the available data and models, considerable contradictions are observed. Intensive engineering work on the mechanical stability of erythrocytes was performed in the 1960s [12–18], especially by Blackshear and co-workers. They designed a number of kinds of apparatus to expose blood to different types of shear stress and surface contact, and worked out a model of blood trauma, which allowed them to construct an impeller pump with excellent hemodynamic properties, the former Medtronic impeller pump (Minneapolis, MN, USA) [19]. Additional important work was done by Leverett, Hellums, and colleagues [7,8,20]. In their theories, erythrocyte destruction depended on exposure time, shear value, and laminar/turbulent characteristics, but with a considerable level of tolerable stress for short exposures (Fig. 1). Following these data, actual hemolysis would be less influenced by shear exposure in regular flow areas but would rather be caused by destruction of blood cells in particular localizations, called "hot spots." Following this theory, the geometrical design of vane shape may have less influence on hemolysis than singular imperfections at a seal or in a high-flow area.

Later, Wurzinger and co-workers did some experiments using a cylindrical shear-flow apparatus, in which they could expose blood in single passages to

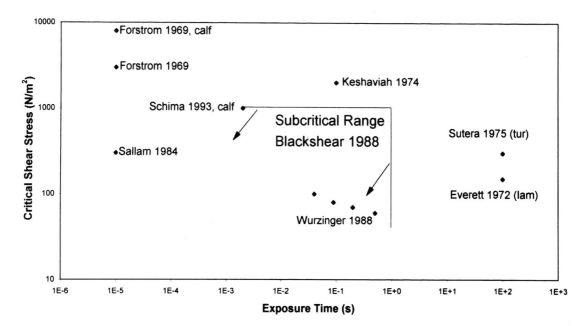

Fig. 1. Critical levels of shear-stress/exposure-time for hemolysis, as found in literature ([18,21], see text for restrictions). *lam*, laminar; *tur*, turbulent

shear stress at variable short exposure times [21,22]. These data were used to derive a formula for hemolysis and applied to heart valves [23] and to initial, rather simple calculations on blood pumps [10,24]. However, as shown by the authors, this formula leads to an excessive overestimation of hemolysis. This was demonstrated by applying it to simple structures such as throttles in in vitro test circuits [25]. The shortcomings in the formula may be caused by artifacts due to the sealing in the original test device of Wurzinger, which was not considered to be of high importance at that time [21]. Figure 1 shows a synopsis of hemolysis thresholds at various shear values and exposure times for singular exposures. Huge differences can be observed, which can only partially be explained by differences in flow-field settings and chosen species.

All of these tests suffered from difficulties in exposing blood under well-defined conditions to reiterated short duration exposure. Therefore, mostly experiments with single passages at high hemolyzing levels were performed, to provide measurable levels of hemolysis, with subsequent extrapolation to lower shear and shorter time periods. Oscillating flow-fields, repeated passage, and also the distribution of erythrocytes in terms of age and fragility would have to be taken into account when calculating an index of hemolysis for a single geometry or a whole device [26]. Such approaches were recently taken by Yeleswarapu, Akamatsu, and Umezu and their colleagues [27–29]. It remains to be seen whether these theories lead to formulas applicable to device optimization.

In conclusion, numerical approaches to calculate the hemolytic potential of devices have to be taken with great caution. For practical development and evaluation of pumps, in vitro tests are now routinely performed, under standardized conditions [30,31].

Models of Mechanically Induced Thrombus Formation

Compared to hemolysis theories, less data and fewer models are available for platelet activation and thrombus deposition. The reasons seem to be: first, the far more complex mechanisms and chemical interactions of thrombus formation; second, greater difficulties in designing experiments without artifacts caused by chemical surface reactions; and third, the fact that platelet activation and the deposition of material usually take place at different locations. Additionally, surface quality and geometry change with material deposition.

Intensive studies on mechanical platelet injury were performed by Hellums, Forstrom, and their colleagues in the seventies [7,8,32,33]. Numerical data on shear-time dependencies of released substances were reported also by Wurzinger and co-workers [21,22]. For

the concept of thrombus growth, a two-stage model was established, in which the platelets were damaged and activated in areas of high shear with subsequent deposition in zones of limited washout [34,35]. Mass transport and mixing effects came into consideration, obviously stimulated by the intensive work done in arteriosclerosis research [e.g., 36]. Affeld et al. established a numerical model of platelet adhesion at stagnation points [37]. Recently, Rappitsch and Perktold constructed an extensive finite-element model with implementation of kinetics of mass transfer, which allows the study of the interaction between geometry, flow mechanics, mixing effects, and the local concentrations of physiological and pharmacological components [38]. However, up to now, these approaches have not been applied to complex structures, and their experimental validation will be an even more difficult task than that of hemolysis models. If such validation is carried out in animal models, the differences in platelet aggregation [39] and fibrinolysis mechanisms [40] in different species must be taken into account.

Thrombogenicity of Pump Bearing and Seals and Current Strategies to Avoid Thrombus Formation

The bearing and seals are the most critical locations for thrombus formation. Depending on the design, several factors promoting platelet activation and thrombus formation may coincide:

Because of the small distance involved, the transition between the stationary and the rotating part of the pump leads to large velocity gradients and exaggerated levels of shear stress.

Friction between the bearing/seal elements and the lubricating fluid causes local spots of high temperature, which can even lead to degradation of proteins.

Especially in centrifugal pumps, the bearing/seal is usually placed in the center of the pump, where flow stagnation and enormous residence times for recirculating blood elements occur.

If material degradation occurs (e.g., fraying of rubber, cracks), these imperfections become sources of material deposition.

Variable and pulsatile loads on the bearing/seals may lead to large variability in thrombogenicity.

In the worst case, platelets are captured for extended time periods within areas of high shear at elevated temperatures.

A number of strategies have been applied to pumps with mechanical bearings to circumvent these difficulties. An overview is given in Table 1:

Table 1. Strategies to minimize thrombus formation in the bearing/seal area of rotary blood pumps

Minimization of bearing and seal gaps
Frequent liftoff of the bearing
Flushing of seals with purging/cooling fluid
Highly polished surfaces, especially of the parts near the gaps
High flow velocities
Reduction of velocity differences (=radius of the shaft)
Reduction of heat generation
Controlled growth of an adherent, stable thrombus

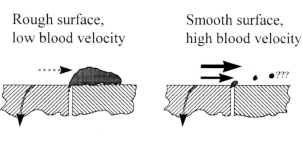

Fig. 2. Factors influencing thrombus size and number: gap width, surface roughness, and local velocity gradients

The seal gaps may be minimized by providing a very precise fitting between the parts. The remaining gap width should be at least smaller than the diameter of the blood cells.

The diameter of the bearing is kept small to minimize the local velocities and velocity gradients.

In an opposite strategy, several pump designs have very loose fittings, providing a liftoff of deposited material nearly every heartbeat. Potential depositions may be washed off before gaining a critical size.

In nonpermanent pumps, the seal may be flushed by purging fluids, which keep blood from entering the seal gap. Seals with impressively low demand for purging fluid could be designed. Such fluid can also be used to cool the bearing, which, however, requires considerable purging flow.

In axial pumps, bearings are positioned in regions of large flow velocities. In combination with careful surface smoothing, depositions would be washed into the bloodstream, when still at a small size.

Finally, controlled thrombus growth and stabilization of persistent depositions may be included into the pump design. At the moment, however, it remains unknown whether the final size and surface quality of such a deposition can be predicted with acceptable reliability.

The question remains, whether these strategies really do decrease the amount of thrombus to acceptable magnitudes, or whether they only shift the problem to the dissemination of numerous mini- and microthrombi (Fig. 2). Certainly, such small thrombi may cause less-serious embolization, and may be dissolved to some extent by the fibrinolysis system. Nevertheless, they may well lead to transitory ischemic attacks (TIAs), as known from patients with carotid stenosis and devices already in clinical use [4,6], and also to more generalized prolonged, reversible neurological deficits (PRINDs). Further, such emboli may not lead to symptoms in animal experiments (except for the very peculiar histology), but nevertheless be a potential danger to patients.

Only in pumps with a completely magnetically suspended rotor, currently being developed by several groups [41–43], can a narrow transition between stationary and moving parts be avoided; but even in these designs, sudden impacts may cause touching, and furthermore, gradual deposition can influence the flowfield and trigger progressing thrombus growth.

In Vivo and In Vitro Thrombus Evaluation

Until now, animal experiments have been the most reliable and widely used tool to evaluate the thrombotic potential of pumps. Usually, this potential is evaluated by monitoring proper organ function during the experiment, by inspection of the pump after the end of the experiment, and by macroscopic autopsy findings and spot-check histological investigations. However, these methods are obviously not sensitive enough to find microscopic emboli, which do not cause conspicuous behavior in animals and remain undetected in intensive care patients, but may well cause at least minor problems in conscious humans with their enhanced cerebral functions [6,44].

Several years ago, the group of Mohammad developed a procedure to simulate thrombus growth in vitro, based on an absolutely atraumatic uptake of bovine blood and controlled heparinization [45]. This technique was adopted for the evaluation of rotary pumps by the authors [46]. It allows us to mimic at least the deposition growth, which takes place within the first few days of device application, usually within 2 h of pumping. Even an enhanced protocol using hypercritical settings can be used, yet with limitations in quantitative standardization. The depositions grow in the setup at the same locations as they do in vivo, with similar shape and microstructure. However, it remains to be validated that the mechanisms of deposition are comparable in all aspects to those in vivo. Therefore, with this test, it is possible to evaluate hemolysis and basic thrombogenic behavior.

Experience with a Sliding Bearing

Here, the pitfalls of microthrombogenicity and its evaluation in vivo and in vitro are illustrated using an example from our development work. Because of reports of low hemolysis in such designs [47], a pump head with an axle-less rotor was developed, in which the pump rotor was coupled by permanent magnets to the motor unit, and stabilized with three sliding elements (Fig. 3). In in vitro tests, the favorable hemolytic properties of the system could be proven [48], and the pump remained free of thrombi in our in vitro setup. In two subsequent animal experiments, the pump was used for 2 and 3 days, respectively. Both animals did wake after the operation, but exhibited hyperuremia and did not really recover. In the autopsy and the standard histology, no relevant thrombi were observed.

A modification of our in vitro test, however, demonstrated the disastrous thrombogenic behavior of this pump. We introduced blood bags with an integrated filter net (from Medos, [Aachen, Germany]; filter size 10×15cm, mesh width 100μm) into the test circuit (Fig. 4). Running the tests using our thrombogenicity test protocol [46], we found large numbers of small thrombi within this net, with a still-thrombus-free pump head. Obviously, the sliding elements did create small plaques, which could not stay in place because of the smooth surface and the large velocity gradients. It should once again be emphasized that this behavior

was observed together with a low hemolysis (index of hemolysis IH = 0.0046 g/100l).

Figure 5 gives an example of such thrombi. In this case they were generated by a commercially available pump (test time 2h), probably because of reuse, even though it had undergone intensive cleansing. Gross inspection of the pump showed only tiny layers at the seal and fluid behind the seal within two hours in the test circuit.

Possible Strategies to Improve the Assessment of Mechanically Induced Thrombogenicity

Based on these experiments and also on clinical experience with currently available long-term and short-term assist devices, the following strategies for assessing mechanically induced thrombogenicity and the eventual microthrombotic risk with blood pumps may help to improve the understanding of these problems, and by this, the performance of the devices:

— Approaches to improved hydrodynamical and mathematical models of platelet activation and deposition, including the statistical and random aspects of such procedures [38,49]. Such efforts are certainly extremely challenging; however, the practical outcomes within an acceptable time may remain limited.
— Use of full magnetic bearings to avoid points with excessive shear.
— Better understanding of the biochemical pathways of platelet activation, including modern techniques of platelet aggregometry and specific receptor investigation [50–52].
— Standardization of in vitro test protocols on thrombogenicity, and adaptation of test circuits for embolus detection [46]. Such standardization may

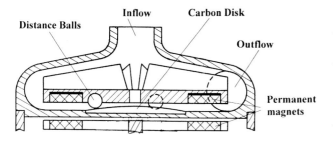

Fig. 3. Axle-less rotor with sliding bearings

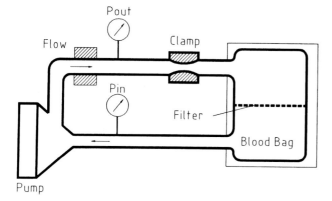

Fig. 4. Schematic drawing of a mock-loop for microthrombus evaluation, including a filter

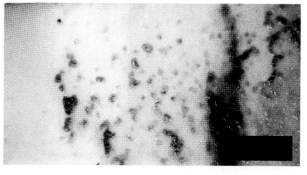

Fig. 5. Emboli found in the filter of the blood bag after an in vitro evaluation of a rotary blood pump (mesh width 100μm)

be aggravated by the statistical character of thrombus trigger events.

— Inclusion of various working points and pulsatile and nonpulsatile bearing loads into the test protocols.

— Refinement of autopsy protocols and histological investigations, which currently may often not be specific enough to give complete insight into the problems [6,44].

— Extended use of detection apparatus for microemboli in experimental and clinical situations. For ex vivo tests, optical test methods have been developed [53]. Devices based on the spectral analysis of Doppler ultrasound are already available for diagnoses in the transcranial position and for carotid and vertebral arteries, with further refinements under development [54–56].

By the use of such methods specifically aiming at the potential thrombogenicity of these devices, better understanding of the performance and the relevant parameters of hemodynamics in blood pumps should become possible, leading to further improvement of these already highly developed devices.

Acknowledgments. This work was sponsored by the Ludwig-Boltzmann Institute of Cardiosurgical Research. We want to thank cordially the many people who established and performed blood tests in our laboratory, and especially Dr. J. Antaki, Dr. P. Blackshear, Dr. K. Butler, Dr. R. Jarvik, Dr. S. Mohammad, Dr. M.M. Müller, and Dr. Y. Nosé for their stimulating discussions.

References

 1. Taenaka Y, Wakisaka Y, Masuzawa T, Tatsumi E, Toda K, Miyazaki K, Eya K, Baba Y, Nakatani T, Ohno T, Nishimura T, Takano H (1996) Development of a centrifugal pump with improved antithrombogenicity and hemolytic property for chronic circulatory support. Artif Organs 20:491–496

 2. Jarvik RK (1995) System considerations favoring rotary artificial hearts with blood-immersed bearings. Artif Organs 19:565–570

 3. Kaplon RJ, Oz MC, Kwiatkowski PA, Levin HR, Shah AS, Jarvik RK, Rose EA (1996) Miniature axial flow pump for ventricular assistance in children and small adults. J Thorac Cardiovasc Surg 111(1):13–18

 4. Körfer R, el Banayosy A, Posival H, Minami K, Korner MM, Arusoglu L, Breymann T, Kizner L, Seifert D, Kortke H (1995) Mechanical circulatory support: The Bad-Oeynhausen experience. Ann Thorac Surg 59(2 Suppl):s56–62

 5. Wagner WR, Johnson PC, Kormos RL, Griffith BP (1993) Evaluation of bioprosthetic valve-associated thrombus in ventricular assist device patients. Circulation 88(5):2023–2029

 6. Curtis JJ, Walls JT, Boley TM, Schmaltz RA, Demmy TL (1992) Autopsy findings in patients on post-

 7. Hellums JD, Hardwick RA (1981) Response of platelets to shear stress — a review. In: Hwang NHC, Gross DR (eds) Hemovascular rheology: the physics of blood and vascular tissue. Sijthoff and Noorhoff, Amsterdam, pp 160–183

 8. Hellums JD, Peterson DM, Stathopoulos NA, Moake JL, Giorgio TD (1987) Studies on the mechanisms of shear-induced platelet activation. In: Hartmann A, Kuschinsky W (eds) Cerebral ischemia and hemorheology. Springer, Berlin, pp 80–89

 9. Dasse KA, Chipman SD, Sherman CN, Levine AH, Frazier OH (1987) Clinical experience with textured blood-contacting surfaces in ventricular assist devices. ASAIO Trans 10(3):418–425

10. Bludszuweit C (1995) Three-dimensional numerical prediction of stress loading of blood particles in a centrifugal pump. Artif Organs 19:590–596

11. Antaki JF, Ghattas O, Burgreen GW, Beichang H (1995) Computational flow optimization of rotary blood pump components. Artif Organs 19:608–615

12. Rand RP (1964) Mechanical properties of the red cell membrane: II. Viscoelastic breakdown of the membrane. Biophys J 4:303–316

13. Williams AR (1973) Viscoelasticity of the human erythrocyte membrane. Biorheology 10:313–319

14. Forstrom RJ (1969) A new measure of erythrocyte membrane strength: The jet fragility test. PhD thesis, University of Minnesota, Minneapolis St. Paul

15. Sallam AM, Hwang NHC (1984) Human red blood cell hemolysis in a turbulent shear flow: contribution of Reynolds shear stresses. Biorheology 21:783–797

16. Blackshear P (1966) Contribution to the meeting. In: Mechanical devices to assist the failing heart. National Academy of Science, New York, pp 113–120

17. Dorman F, Bernstein EF, Blackshear PL, Sovilje R, Scott DR (1969) Progress in the design of a centrifugal cardiac assist pump with transcutaneous energy transmission by magnetic coupling. ASAIO Trans 15:441–448

18. Blackshear PL, Blackshear GL (1987) Mechanical hemolysis. In: Skalak R, Chien S (eds) Handbook of bioengineering. McGraw-Hill, New York, pp 14.1–14.17

19. Bernstein EF (1978) A centrifugal pump for circulatory assist. In: Unger F (ed) Assisted circulation. Springer, Berlin, pp 231–242

20. Leverett LD, Hellums JD, Alfrey CP, Lynch EC (1972) Red blood cell damage by shear stress. Biophys J 12:157–173

21. Wurzinger L, Opitz R, Eckstein H (1986) Mechanical blood trauma. In: Affeld K, Schichl K, Yoganathan A (eds) Nonpulsatile blood pumps — Summary of the ESAO Workshop. Hermann-Foettinger Institut der Technischen Universitaet Berlin, Berlin, pp 30–44

22. Wurzinger LJ (1986) Die Bedeutung der fluid-mechanisch induzierten viskösen Metamorphose der Blutplättchen für die Abscheidungsthrombose. Inaugural dissertation, Technical University of Aachen

23. Giersiepen M, Wurzinger LJ, Opitz R, Reul H (1990) Estimation of shear-stress-related blood damage in heart valve prostheses — in vitro comparison of 25 aortic valvs. Int J Artif Organs 13(5):300–306

24. Papantonis D (1991) Numerical prediction of the shear stresses and of the mean stay time for radial flow

cardiotomy centrifugal ventricular assist. ASAIO J 38:M688–690

impellers. In: Schima H, Thoma H, Wieselthaler G, Wolner E (eds) Proceedings of the international workshop on rotary blood pumps, Vienna, Sept 9–11, 1991, pp 63–69

25. Schima H, Müller MR, Tsangaris S, Geihseder G, Schlusche C, Losert U, Thoma H, Wolner E (1993) In-vitro testing of blood pumps: comparison of tubing and throttle as flow-resistors in regard to blood trauma. Artif Organs 17(3):164–170

26. Hashimoto S (1989) Erythrocyte destruction under periodically fluctuating shear rate: comparative study with constant shear rate. Artif Organs 13(5):458–463

27. Yeleswarapu KK, Antaki JF, Kameneva MV, Rajagopal KR (1995) A mathematical model for shear induced hemolysis. Artif Organs 19:576–582

28. Umezu M, Yamada T, Fujimasu H, Fuhimoto T, Ranawake M, Nagawa A, Kijima T (1969) Effects of surface roughness on mechanical hemolysis. Artif Organs 20:575–578

29. Tamagawa M, Akamatsu T, Saitoh K (1996) Prediction of hemolysis in turbulent shear orifice flow. Artif Organs 20:553–559

30. Müller MR, Schima H, Engelhardt H, Salat A, Olsen DB, Losert U, Wolner E (1993) In vitro hematological testing of rotary blood pumps: Remarks on standardization and data interpretation. Artif Organs 17(2):103–110

31. Takami Y, Nosé Y (1996) Recommended practice for assessment of hemolysis in continuous flow blood pumps. Draft for ASTM Guideline F04-40-101, Baylor College, Houston (in process of certification)

32. Forstrom RJ, Voss GO, Blackshear PL (1974) Fluid dynamics of particle (platelet) deposition for filtering walls: Relationship to atherosclerosis. J Fluids Eng, June 1974:168–172

33. Blackshear P, Kenneth J, Bartley W, Forstrom RJ (1993) Fluid dynamic factors affecting particle capture and retention. Ann N Y Acad Sci 270–281

34. Schmid-Schönbein H, Wurzinger LJ (1988) Über die Schultern von Eberth und Schimmelbusch auf Blutgerinnung und gestörte Strömung gesehen. Haemostaseologie 8:146–148

35. Wurzinger LJ, Schmid-Schönbein H (1987) Surface abnormalities and conduit characteristics as a case of blood trauma in artificial internal organs. In: Leonard EF, Tiritto VT, Vroman L (eds) Blood contact with natural and artificial surfaces. New York Academy of Sciences, New York, pp 316–333

36. McIntire LV, Tay RTS (1989) Concentration of materials released from mural platelet aggregates: Flow effects. In: Yang WJ, Lee CJ (eds) Biomedical engineering. Hemisphere, New York, pp 229–245

37. Affeld K, Reininger AJ, Gadischke J, Grunert K, Schmidt S, Thiele F (1995) Fluid mechanics of the stagnation point flow chamber and its platelet deposition. Artif Organs 19:597–602

38. Rappitsch G, Perktold K (1995) Computer simulation of convective diffusion processes in large arteries. J Biomech 29:207–215

39. Jain NC (1993) Essentials of veterinary hematology. Lea and Febinger, Philadelphia

40. Dodds WJ (1989) Hemostasis. In: Kaneko JJ (ed) Clinical biochemistry of domestic animals, 4th edn, Academic, San Diego, pp 274–315

41. Allaire PE, Kim HC, Maslen EH, Olsen DB, Bearnson GB (1996) Prototype continuous flow ventricular assist device supported on magnetic bearings. Artif Organs 20(6):582–590

42. Hart RM, Filipenco VG, Kung RTV (1996) A magnetically suspended hydrostatically stabilized centrifugal blood pump. Artif Organs 20(6):591–596

43. Akamatsu T, Tsukiya T, Nishimura K, Park CH, Nakazeki T (1995) Recent studies of the centrifugal blood pump with a magnetically suspended impeller. Artif Organs 19(7):631–634

44. Vasku J (1996) Brain and spinal cord lesions in the long-term TAH pumping (abstract). 6th International symposium on artificial heart and assist devices. Tokyo

45. Swier P, Bos WJ, Mohammad SF, Olsen DB, Kolff WJ (1990) An in vitro model to study the performance and thrombogenicity of cardiovascular devices. ASAIO Trans 35:683–687

46. Schima H, Siegl H, Mohammad SF, Huber L, Müller MR, Losert U, Thoma H, Wolner E (1993) In vitro investigation of thrombogenesis in rotary blood pumps. Artif Organs 17(7):605–608

47. Ohara Y, Nosé Y (1994) The next generation Baylor C-Gyro pump: Antithrombogenic "free impeller" design for long-term centrifugal VAD. Artif Organs 18(3):238–243

48. Schima H, Schmallegger H, Huber L, Birgmann I, Reindl C, Schmidt C, Roschal K, Wieselthaler G, Trubel W, Losert UM, Wolner E (1995) An implantable seal-less centrifugal pump with integrated double-disk motor. Artif Organs 19:639–643

49. Hoover WG, Pierce TG, Hoover CG, Shugart JO, Stein CM, Edwards AL (1994) Molecular dynamics, smoothed-particle applied mechanics and irreversibility. Comput Math Appl Vol 28, Nr 10:155–174

50. Müller MM, Salat A, Pulaki S, Schreiner W, Huber G, Stangl P, Losert E, Wolner E (1995) Influence of hematocrit and platelet count on impedance and reactivity of whole blood for electrical aggregometry. J Pharmacol Meth 34:17–22

51. Konstantopoulos K, Grotta JC, Sills C, Wu KK, Hellums JD (1995) Shear induced platelet aggregation in normal subjects and stroke patients. Thromb Haemost 74(5):1329–1334

52. Goto S, Salomon DR, Ikeda Y, Ruggeri ZM (1995) Characterization of the unique mechanism mediating the shear dependent binding of soluble van Willebrand factor of platelets. J Biol Chem 270(40):23353–23361

53. Solen KA, Mohammad SF, Pijl AJ, Swier P, Monson RD, Olsen DB (1990) Detection of microemboli by constant-pressure filtration during in vitro circulation of bovine and human blood. Artif Organs 14(6):446–470

54. Moehring MA, Ritcey A (1996) Sizing emboli in blood using pulse Doppler ultrasound — I: Verification of the EBR model. IEEE Trans Biomed Eng 43:572–580

55. Markus HS, Tegeler CH (1995) Experimental aspects of high intensity transient signals in the detection of emboli. J Clin Ultrasound 23:81–87

56. Jansen C, Ramos LM, van Heesewijk JP, Moll FL, van Gijn J, Ackerstaff RG (1994) Impact of microembolism and hemodynamic changes in the brain during carotid endarterectomy. Stroke 25:992–997

Discussion

Dr. Nitta:
At first, could you briefly tell us about the ultrasound microthrombus diagnostic method you mentioned?

Dr. Schima:
There are devices available which are based on statistics, and I know from a study, I think it was in Pittsburgh, they were using such equipment. It was a device you can use with clinical ultrasound equipment to detect microthombi by statistical means. It's a very complex system but it is available.

Dr. Nitta:
Are you talking about some microscopic apparatus to detect the microthombi?

Dr. Schima:
No. It's a standard ultrasound.

Dr. Nitta:
Standard ultrasound? About 3 or 4MHz?

Dr. Schima:
Yes. There was an article in June's *IEEE Journal* on the basic function of these devices.

Dr. Morsi:
Forgive me for asking you a rather primitive question because I am new to this area. Are you suggesting that we cannot get rid of thrombus formation at all, regardless of what we do?

Dr. Schima:
Well, I think there are devices which perform suitably well, at least in animals, otherwise it would be impossible to have such rotary pumps devices running for over half a year.

Dr. Morsi:
Does this mean we can live with some level of thrombus formation?

Dr. Schima:
It's an interesting point to discuss with physicians what level of microthrombi is acceptable! I think there must be numbers available from artificial heart valves, where these ultrasound detection systems were already used.

Dr. Morsi:
But you personally don't know the level of it?

Dr. Schima:
No, I don't know. But we have experienced patients with TIAs and this is a rather disturbing experience.

Dr. Nitta:
In my opinion, if you use a commercially available ultrasound apparatus using around 3MHz to 5MHz, I don't think the resolution is high enough to detect the microthrombi.

Dr. Schima:
These systems have a special evaluation unit. They different absorption levels at two different ultrasound frequencies and compare that, so it's a completely different technology.

Dr. Reul:
Are you talking about the so-called HITS, high-intensity transcranial signals, to identify these microthrombi?

Dr. Schima:
Well, that's one approach. I saw in an exhibition 3 or 4 years ago such a device which at that time was combined with neural networks and learning curves and it was a very expensive and complex thing. At the moment, new techniques are underway.

Dr. Reul:
And another question is, are you able to quantify the amount of microthrombi found in these filters?

Dr. Schima:
We did count them so we could estimate how often a microthrombus is generated. But it certainly is a question of getting these data reproducible, also the devices in reproducible quality.

Dr. Reul:
So you need more statistics, probably.

Dr. Schima:
There need to be a lot of statistics included, and I think that even the production of some of these industrially available pumps varies from time to time.

Dr. Reul:
And have you been able to correlate specific design features of a certain pump to the amount of thrombus formation? Like the seating configuration or gap width.

Dr. Schima:
The data I presented here about the in vitro tests are rather preliminary. They give information on geometric and material imperfections. And they show that low hemolysis results say nothing or practically nothing about the risk of thrombus formation.

Remote Monitoring and Control of Artificial Hearts and Assist Devices

Tofy Mussivand, Albert Hum, Kevin S. Holmes, Paul J. Hendry, Roy G. Masters, and Wilbert J. Keon

Summary. A system to control and monitor implanted devices, such as artificial hearts and assist devices, from remote sites using telephone lines and other public communications networks has been developed. The developed system was successfully demonstrated during the G7 Ministerial Conference on the Information Society in Brussels. The system allowed specialists at the Berlin Heart Institute to remotely monitor the operating parameters of a prototype ventricular assist device which was located in Ottawa, Canada. The personnel on both sides of the Atlantic were able to see changes in the performance of the device and consult on its operating characteristics. This demonstration, which utilised an ATM (asynchronous transfer mode) communication network, represented the first transatlantic communication for this type of medical device information. Additional demonstrations of the technology have been conducted from Ottawa (Canada) to Geneva (Switzerland) and Whitehorse (Canada). The developed system was recently enhanced to allow for similar control and monitoring using standard telephone lines and cellular telephone networks. In conclusion, by utilizing the developed technologies it may now be possible to provide future artificial heart patients with increased freedom and improved quality of life, as opposed to the strict travel zone and residence limitations that are currently imposed in out-of-the-hospital studies. The technology could also have a positive impact on health costs during the utilisation of implantable medical devices.

Key words: Remote monitoring — Artificial heart — Ventricular assist — Communications — Control methods

Introduction

Rapid progress in the development of mechanical circulatory support systems such as artificial hearts and ventricular assist devices has occurred during the last decade. These technologies have advanced from experimental use to the point where some insurance carriers and third-party payers consider use of certain devices as an acceptable and a reimbursable treatment. Some patients are now even able to be discharged and return home with certain portable ventricular assist devices. As advances continue in this field, further efforts are needed towards developing systems that allow future recipients of these devices the ability to return to relatively normal lifestyles, no matter where they reside. One manner in which this goal can be achieved is by utilising advances in other fields such as the telecommunications area.

The Cardiovascular Devices Division of the University of Ottawa Heart Institute has developed a system for remotely monitoring and controlling implanted medical devices. The developed system is currently being tested for application with devices such as artificial hearts and ventricular assist devices. The system can provide health-care professionals the ability to monitor and/or control the function of an implanted device, without the need to bring the patient into the hospital. This type of system can also have an important impact on the patients' quality of life, by allowing patients to return to their homes, no matter where they live, without the concern that their location will hinder their ability to remain in close contact with medical personnel knowledgeable in these types of systems.

Materials and Methods

The system consists of two distinct communication systems: (1) the first system (local system) allows data communication through the skin and tissue from the implanted device to the outside of the body; and (2) the second system (remote system) allows communication from the area immediately outside of the body to remote locations such as a hospital or research centre. A description of each of these systems follows:

Local System

Data communications between an implanted device and the outside of the body represent a complex challenge. While the simplest approach would be to run a cable from the implanted device through the skin and tissue to the outside of the body, this approach is unacceptable for several reasons. First, infection associated with this type of percutaneous connection has been identified as a serious complication, leading to morbid-

Cardiovascular Devices Division, University of Ottawa Heart Institute, 1053 Carling Avenue, Room H560B, Ottawa, Ontario, K1Y 4E9, Canada

ity and in some cases even mortality [1]. Some investigators suggest that infection is inevitable with the use of such chronically externalised connections [2]. Second, this approach is aesthetically unacceptable and creates an unneeded burden on patients who would be required to maintain care of the exit site after they have been discharged from the hospital. Third, this approach would create unnecessary limitations on the patients' activities. Finally, percutaneous lines will require ongoing care, repeat hospital visits, and utilisation of healthcare professionals' time, and thus can be extremely costly.

To overcome these issues, several alternative approaches were assessed. Data communications to and from the inside of the body, without the need for percutaneous connections, can be achieved by utilising modulated energy forms such as light, electromagnetic waves, and ultrasound [3]. The light method (optical) was applied for the developed system, by utilising an infrared wavelength. Infrared (IR) data communications through the skin and tissue offers the significant benefit of a high level of immunity to electrical noise, which is a major consideration considering the life-critical nature of implantable devices such as artificial hearts and assist devices.

The developed local system consists of two small (2.6-cm diameter) transmitter/receiver modules, one connected to the implanted device and located subcutaneously, and the other directly over the top of the implanted module at the outside of the body. Each module consists of multiple infrared receiver and transmitter components. The configuration of multiple components is designed in such a way that the impact of misalignment and/or off-axis rotation of the two modules is greatly reduced. In addition, the use of multiple components provides system redundancy, ensuring that the communications link remains functional should one of the transmitter or receiver components fail. The IR components on each of the modules are encapsulated in an optically clear, saline-resistant epoxy resin which provides optimal optical transmission properties and gives the implanted module vital protection from biodegradation.

Data communications between the two modules is accomplished by using a frequency shift keying (FSK) data communications protocol. The developed system functions as follows: a digital data stream of 0–5-V transistor–transistor logic (TTL) signals is fed into a frequency shift keying generator which converts each digital bit (1 or 0) to a specific sinusoidal frequency. This sinusoidal data stream is sent to the IR transmitters which convert the electrical signal into a modulating IR signal (890-nm wavelength), which is then directed to the IR receivers on the other side of the skin and tissue barrier. After passing through the skin and tissue, the IR signal is picked up by the IR receiv-

ers and converted back into an electrical sinusoidal data stream. A frequency shift keying demodulator then converts the sinusoidal data stream back into the original digital data stream. Simultaneous bidirectional communications at rates up to 9600 Baud is achieved by utilising two separate operating frequencies: (1) outside to inside, and (2) inside to outside.

Remote System

The remote system consists of a wearable external controller which can be worn on a belt, similar to a pager. This device is connected via a wire cable to the external transmitter/receiver module and serves two purposes. First, this device contains a liquid crystal display (LCD) unit which allows data from the implanted device to be directly displayed, thus providing important information on the patient to healthcare professionals and other care givers. This component also provides warning messages and/or alarms for the patient to take specific actions after he/she has been discharged from the hospital. Second, the device provides an interface to connect the unit to public communications systems (phone lines, asynchronous transfer mode systems, satellites, etc.) to allow monitoring and control of the device from distant locations.

The current configuration of the wearable external controller was developed specifically for the totally implantable ventricular assist device (VAD) being developed in this laboratory; however, this unit could easily be configured to meet the requirements of a wide range of implanted medical devices. The unit provides a visual display of text, numerical data, and graphics (i.e., waveforms) obtained from the implanted device. In the current configuration designed for the VAD, the following data are displayed on the LCD: beat rate, systolic fraction, operating voltages (systole and diastole), and various warning messages, as well as error-checking information on the IR data transfer including the number of data packets received, number of error-free data packets received, and the overall data transfer error rate. Additionally, a waveform representing the motion of the blood-pumping diaphragm within the VAD is displayed, to allow healthcare personnel to monitor and optimise operation of the device by overriding default operating settings if necessary.

The current wearable external controller also has an RS-232C port which allows the unit to be directly connected to a personal computer to allow advanced control and monitoring functions via custom-developed, device-specific software. This feature has been utilised to monitor data from the VAD, during ongoing in vitro and in vivo experiments with the device.

Results

A system for remotely monitoring and controlling implanted medical devices such as artificial hearts and ventricular assist devices has been designed, fabricated, and evaluated. The system provides the capability to access an implanted device from a remote location via public communication networks, for monitoring and control purposes. The system includes the ability to: remotely obtain operating status from an implanted device, download operating commands, implement the downloaded commands, and obtain confirmation of the command implementation.

The local system used for IR data communications between the implanted device and the outside of the body has been evaluated both in vitro and in vivo. Initial studies to assess IR performance in cadavers were also conducted [4]. IR data transmission through human skin and tissue (thickness up to ~25 mm) has been achieved with error rates of less than 10^{-5}. Studies of IR data transmission were also conducted in porcine and bovine tissue to ensure adequate operation in the animal models used for evaluation of the various components of the VAD. While human tissue provided a considerably better medium for IR transmission than either porcine or bovine tissue, acceptable transmission performance was obtained in each of the animal models. The system has been utilized for a series of bovine implants of the totally implantable ventricular assist device being developed by this laboratory, and it provided the ability to both control and

monitor the implanted device successfully [5]. The system has also been assessed and utilized by a number of research groups [6] for use with their respective artificial heart devices.

The capability of the remote system, which allows the local system to be connected to public communications systems for control and monitoring of the implanted device from distant locations, has also been demonstrated. During the G7 Ministerial Conference on the Information Society in Brussels (February 24, 1995), the system was utilised to allow specialists at the Berlin Heart Institute to remotely monitor the operating parameters of a prototype ventricular assist device located at our laboratories in Ottawa, Canada. The personnel on both sides of the Atlantic were able to see changes in the performance of the device and consult on its operating characteristics, utilising an asynchronous transfer mode (ATM) communication network. Similar demonstrations of the technology have been conducted from Ottawa (Canada) to Whitehorse (Canada) (July 6, 1995) and Geneva (Switzerland) (October 4, 1995).

Recently, the ability to control and monitor the device over standard phone lines has been implemented and utilised in our laboratories. On July 5, 1996, a demonstration of this capability was presented to 11 delegates from the Medical Research Council of Canada (MRC), the Natural Sciences and Engineering Council of Canada (NSERC), and Industry Canada. This successful demonstration highlighted the ability of the system to remotely monitor and control a VAD

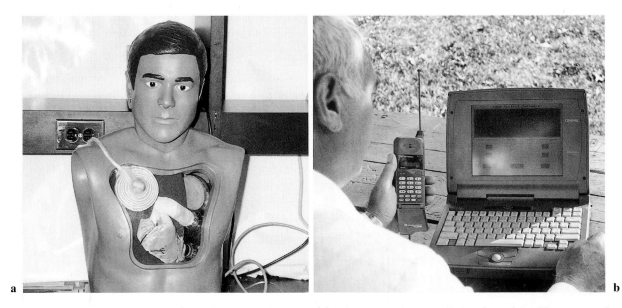

Fig. 1. A prototype ventricular assist device in the laboratory (**a**) being remotely controlled and monitored by a researcher located in a park over 1 mile from the laboratory (**b**). Interconnection was established by utilising a cellular telephone and a portable computer

located in the laboratory from another room, using a standard telephone line. During the demonstration, changes (increase and decrease) to the beat rate of the VAD were downloaded over the telephone line, implemented in the VAD and successfully reported back to the remote location. Further refinements to utilise cellular telephone networks have also been implemented and are currently being assessed. Figure 1 shows the prototype ventricular assist device in the laboratory (on the left) being monitored and controlled via a cellular telephone network, by a researcher located in a park over a mile away from the laboratory.

Discussion

As the use of medical devices such as artificial hearts, ventricular assist devices, and other implantable medical systems (pacemakers, defibrillators, neuromuscular stimulators, drug delivery systems, etc.), becomes more widespread, it is becoming necessary to be able to monitor and control these devices non-invasively. Currently, in North America, out-of-the-hospital patients with implantable ventricular devices have strict travel zone and residence limitations that limit their ability to truly return to society with a normal lifestyle. By utilising technologies such as the developed system, patients with such devices would not need to return to hospital repeatedly to have the status of their implanted system status assessed; this could instead be accomplished by patients simply connecting their external wearable controller to a phone jack (or other public communications system), and authorised healthcare personnel would be able to monitor and control the implanted device remotely. By allowing these patients a more normal lifestyle, which is less dependent on repeated visits to the hospital, the recipients of these devices would obtain an improved quality of life. Additionally, cost savings to the healthcare system could certainly be envisioned by reducing the number of hospital visits simply to assess the function of these systems.

Conclusions

The use of IR data communications provides an acceptable means to control and monitor implanted devices from the outside of the body, without the need for percutaneous connections. The developed system highlighted the capability of such a system to operate at required data rates (up to 9600 Baud), through a typical skin thickness with acceptable data reliability (error rates $<10^{-5}$). Since an IR system requires minimal operating power, is not affected by electrical interference, and provides satisfactory performance under typical operating conditions, this methodology provides an excellent solution for the control and monitoring of implanted medical devices.

Control and monitoring of implanted medical devices from distant locations utilising public communications systems (ATM, phone lines, cellular networks) has been demonstrated to be feasible with the developed system. This capability could offer substantial opportunities for future implantable devices that require detailed post-discharge monitoring by eliminating the need for patients to visit the hospital repeatedly. This aspect can also help to reduce the burden on patients from rural areas and those who travel by ensuring that advanced medical assessment is possible over great distances using existing public communications networks.

In conclusion, the use of various technologies and public communications networks provides the ability to control and monitor implantable medical devices readily, both locally and over great distances, as demonstrated by the developed system. Ultimately, the widespread utilisation and success of these capabilities will greatly depend on identifying specific applications which provide improved patient outcome, cost savings to the healthcare system, improved convenience and quality of life to the patient, and/or optimised delivery of healthcare service. In the case of artificial hearts and assist devices, it is believed that some, if not all, of these criteria will be met through utilisation of technologies such as the developed system.

References

1. Holman WL, Murrah CP, Ferguson ER, Bourge RC, McGiffin DC, Kirklin JK (1996) Infections during extended circulatory support: University of Alabama at Birmingham experience 1989 to 1994. Ann Thorac Surg 61:366–371
2. Pennington DG (1996) Extended support with permanent systems: Percutaneous versus totally implantable. Ann Thorac Surg 61:403–406
3. Jeutter DC (1982) Biomedical telemetry techniques. Crit Rev Biomed Eng 7:121–174
4. Miller J, Mussivand T, Belanger G, Hendry P, Masters RG, Keaney M, Walley V, Keon WJ (1992) Performance evaluation of a transcutaneous infrared telemetry system. ASAIO Abstr 21:39
5. Mussivand T, Masters RG, Hendry PJ, Keon WJ (1996) Totally implantable intrathoracic ventricular assist device. Ann Thorac Surg 61:444–447
6. Mussivand T, Hum A, Diguer M, Holmes KS, Vecchio G, Masters RG, Hendry PJ, Keon WJ (1995) A transcutaneous energy and information transfer system for implanted medical devices. ASAIO J 41:M253–M258

Fractal Dimension Analysis of Heart Rate Variability with Left Ventricular Assist Device

Shunsuke Nanka[1], Tomoyuki Yambe[1], Taro Sonobe[1], Shigeru Naganuma[1], Shin-ichi Kobayashi[1], Kou-ichi Tabayashi[2], Makoto Miura[2], Makoto Yoshizawa[3], Hideki Takayasu[4], and Shin-ichi Nitta[1]

Summary. We analyzed heart rate variability by nonlinear mathematics, including fractal theory, to evaluate the hemodynamic stability of left ventricular assistance. A left ventricular assist device (LVAD) was implanted from the left atrium to the descending aorta in four long-term experiments using healthy adult goats. After the implantation procedure, these goats were placed in a cage, and then extubated after the anesthesia was terminated. All time-series data were recorded with the animals awake. The LVAD was driven in internal mode (INT) at a rate of 50–60 bpm, counterpulsation mode (CP), and copulsation mode (CoP). Electrocardiograms were recorded. To assess the heart rate variability with the LVAD, we calculated the fractal dimension by the box-counting method. During left ventricular assistance, fractal dimensions were decreased. This result suggests that the hemodynamics during LVAD use have decreased fractal characteristics. A system which has fractal structures is said to have the characteristics of stability when stimuli are fed from outside. During LVAD use, we must carefully control the hemodynamic parameters to compensate for any unexpected stimuli received from outside.

Key words: Left ventricular assist device (LVAD) — Heart rate variability — Fractal dimension

Introduction

Mandelbrot proposed the concept of "fractal" in 1975 [1,2] to describe the complexity of various natural phenomena and shapes. We can also describe the complexity of physical and biological phenomena as a whole, not as decomposed parts, by the use of fractal and chaos theory. This concept is expected to be useful for understanding the complexity of natural structures.

There are many reports [3–6] which show that nonlinear mathematics, including fractal theory, is essential for the understanding of complex systems (like physical and biological systems) as a whole. In order to evaluate the stability of hemodynamics under left ventricular assistance, we analyzed heart rate variability by nonlinear mathematics, including fractal theory.

Materials and Methods

Animal Experiments

Four goats weighing 60–70 kg were used in the experiments. They were fasted for 2 days before the experiments. The animals were anesthetized in normal fashion with tracheotomy and halothane inhalation on a respirator. Electrocardiogram (ECG) electrodes were attached to the legs. The left pleural cavity was opened by a left fifth rib resection. Arterial blood pressure was monitored continuously with a catheter inserted into the left internal thoracic artery. Central venous pressure was monitored with a catheter through the internal thoracic vein. For left artificial heart implantation, the intercostal arteries were separated to free the descending aorta.

The outflow cannula was sutured to the descending aorta and the inflow cannula was inserted into the left atrium through the left atrial appendage. Both cannulae were connected to a pneumatically driven, sac-type blood pump. Pump output was measured by an electromagnetic flowmeter attached to the outflow cannula. Heparin (5000 IU) was injected into the vein and infusion was continued at approximately 1000 IU/h.

After attachment, the left ventricular assist device (LVAD) was operated in an internal mode at a rate of 50–60 beats per minute. The chest was then closed and the LVAD positioned on the chest wall. The goats were then placed in a cage and extubated after awakening. Data recording was done while awake, 0.5–1.0 day after the operation, to eliminate the influence of anesthesia. ECG and other hemodynamic parameters were recorded with thermal recorders and magnetic tape.

[1] Department of Medical Engineering and Cardiology, Division of Organ Pathophysiology, Institute of Development, Aging, and Cancer, Tohoku University, 4-1 Seiryo-machi, Aoba-ku, Sendai, Miyagi 980, Japan
[2] Department of Thoracic and Cardiovascular Surgery, Tohoku University School of Medicine, Sendai, Miyagi 980-77, Japan
[3] Department of Electrical Engineering, Graduate School of Engineering, Tohoku University, Sendai, Miyagi 980-77, Japan
[4] Graduate School of Information Sciences, Tohoku University, Sendai, Miyagi 980, Japan

Initially, left ventricular assistance was carried out in internal mode, and then it was switched to a counterpulsation mode or copulsation mode. The ECG was recorded after the ECG and other hemodynamic parameters were stabilized. The pump flow rate was manually operated to maintain blood flow within the normal range. Other hemodynamic parameters were also kept in the normal range during data recording.

Analysis Method

Fractal dimension analysis was used in this study to evaluate the characteristics of fractals associated with the heart rate [7]. Fractal dimensions were calculated by various analytical methods [8]:

1. Changing the coarse graining level
2. Using the fractal measure relations
3. Using the correlation function
4. Using the distribution function
5. Using the power spectrum

In this study, we calculated the fractal dimension by the changing the coarse graining level, using a technique called the box-counting method. Before calculating the fractal dimension, the time-series data of the ECG were reconstructed in a phase plane. By the use of a return map on a beat-to-beat basis, the heart rate was embedded into a two-dimensional phase plane. At first, we quantified the time-series data on a beat-to-beat basis. As shown in Fig. 1(1), the value of one beat is plotted on the x-axis and that of the next beat is plotted on the y-axis. Then, the phase plane is divided

into several squares with side length r. The number of squares that contain at least one point is denoted as the number $N(r)$. If r and $N(r)$ are known,

$$r^{-D} \propto N(r)$$

where D represents the dimension of this structure of the return map. For a fractal structure, the D value would be a fraction.

Results

ECG and other hemodynamic parameters were recorded while the animals were awake, and the values obtained were considered to fall within the normal range. Positive pressure, negative pressure, and systolic duration were controlled with the driving console to keep these parameters of the pneumatically driven, sac-type blood pump within the normal range. All these parameters were easily controlled within the normal range during data recording. Exceptions, in which the ECG was not clearly recorded by electromyelography, were removed from the analysis.

The fractal dimension analysis of the heart rate was calculated with a personal computer by the use of the box-counting method. With the LVAD, the fractal dimension (about 0.8) was significantly lower than that with natural circulation, and this lower value was found with all three driving modes: internal, counterpulsation, and copulsation. In the other situations, natural heart rate variability shows 1.0–2.0 dimension (Fig. 2).

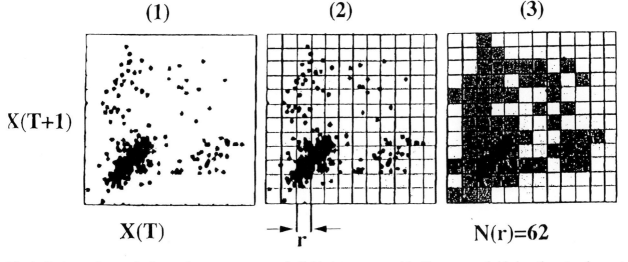

Fig. 1. Box counting method: step *1*, return map; step *2*, divide into square grid with squares of side length *r*; step *3*, count the number of squares which contain at least one point, and denote this number $N(r)$

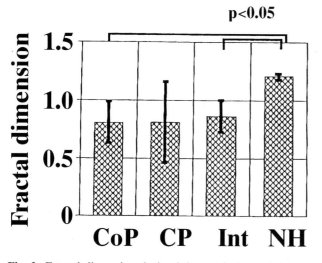

p<0.05

Fig. 2. Fractal dimension during left ventricular assistance. *CoP*, copulsation mode; *CP*, counterpulsation mode; *Int*, internal mode; *NH*, natural heart

During LVAD operation, we must carefully control the hemodynamic parameters to compensate for unexpected stimuli fed from outside.

Conclusion

We found that, compared with normal circulation, the heart rate showed a reduction in fractal dimension in all LVAD driving modes. Therefore, during LVAD operation, we must carefully control the hemodynamic parameters to compensate for unexpected stimuli fed from outside.

Acknowledgments. This paper was presented, in part, at the Artificial Organs Japan meeting, 1995. The authors thank Mr. Kimio Kikuchi for cooperation with experiments, and Mrs. Hisako Iijima and Miss Rie Sakurai for their excellent assistance and cooperation.

Discussion

A return map shows the relation of one cycle to the next cycle [8]. In this study, we showed how one beat R-R interval influences the next beat R-R interval under left ventricular assistance. A high fractal dimension suggests that one beat R-R interval would relate less to the next R-R interval, and the R-R interval would come to be random. A low fractal dimension indicates a higher degree of regularity, and less variability. Systems with low fractal dimensions would show less stability in response to unexpected stimuli fed from the outside [9]. It is desirable to have an intermediate fractal dimension for the circulation, under which the environment could accommodate unexpected stimuli fed from the outside.

In this study, we found that the heart rate showed a decrease of fractal dimension in all LVAD driving modes compared with that under normal circulation. This result suggests that one beat R-R interval has an increased influence on the following beat and that the heart period is more cyclic, under left ventricular assistance. This indicates that the hemodynamics during LVAD operation have decreased fractal characteristics. A fractal dimension indicates the number of nonlinear dynamic parameters contribution to the time-series data [8]. Recent reports from our group showed that rhythmic fluctuations of the hemodynamics were significantly changed during artificial circulation compared with the natural circulation [9–12]. A system that has fractal structures is said to have stability when stimuli are fed from the outside.

References

1. Mandelbrot BB (1975) Les objects fractals; forme, hasard et dimension. Flammarion, Paris
2. Mandelbrot BB (1982) The fractal geometry of nature. Freeman, New York
3. Goldberger AL, Rigney DR, West BJ (1990) Chaos and fractals in human physiology. Sci Am 259:35–41
4. Tsuda I, Tahara T, Iwanaga H (1992) Chaotic pulsation in human capillary vessels and its dependence on mental and physical conditions. Int J Bifurc Chaos 2:313–324
5. Denton TA, Diamond GA, Helfant RH, Khan S, Karageunzian H (1990) Fascinating rhythm — A primer chaos theory and its application to cardiology. Am Heart J 20:1419–1440
6. Crutchfield JP, Farmer JD, Packard NH, Shaw RS (1986) Chaos. Sci Am 255:46–57
7. Yambe T, Nanka S, Naganuma S, Kobayashi S, Akiho H, Kakinuma Y, Ohsawa N, Nitta S, Fukuju T, Miura M, Uchida N, Tabayashi K, Tanaka A, Yoshizumi N, Abe K, Takayasu M, Takayasu H, Yoshizawa M, Takade H (1995) Can the artificial heart make the circulation become fractal? Int J Artif Organs 18(4):190–196
8. Takayasu H (1990) Fractals in the physical sciences. Wiley, Chichester, pp 1–26
9. Yambe T, Nitta S, Sonobe T, Naganuma S, Kakinuma Y, Kobayashi S, Tanaka M, Fukuju T, Miura M, Sato N, Mohri H, Koide S, Takeda H, Yoshizawa M (1994) New artificial control method from the neurophysiological point of view. In: Akutsu T, Koyanagi H (eds) Heart replacement — Arificial heart 4. Springer, Tokyo, pp 353–356
10. Yambe T, Kobayashi S, Nanka S, Naganuma S, Nitta S, Matsuki H, Abe K, Yoshizawa M, Fukuju T, Takeda H, Hashimoto H (1996) Fluctuations of the hemodynamic derivatives during left ventricular assistance using oscillated blood flow. Artif Organs 20(6):637–640

11. Yambe T, Nanka S, Sonobe T, Naganuma S, Kobayashi S, Akiho H, Kakinuma Y, Yukita K, Mitsuoka M, Chiba S, Ohsawa N, Haga Y, Idutsu K, Nitta S, Fukuju T, Miura M, Uchida N, Sato N, Tabayashi K, Tanaka A, Yoshizumi N, Abe K, Takeda H, Takayasu M, Yoshizawa M, Takayasu H (1996) Fractal dimension analysis of chaos in hemodynamics with artificial heart. Heart replacement — Artificial heart 5, Springer, Tokyo, pp 315–318

12. Yambe T, Nanka S, Sonobe T, Naganuma S, Kobayashi S, Akiho H, Kakinuma Y, Mitsuoka M, Chiba S, Ohsawa N, Haga Y, Idutsu K, Nitta S, Fukuju T, Miura M, Uchida N, Sato N, Tabayashi K, Tanaka A, Yoshizumi N, Abe K, Takayasu M, Takayasu H, Yoshizawa M (1995) Chaotic behavior of hemodynamics with ventricular assist system. Int J Artif Organs 18(1):17–21

Parameter Optimization Approach to Estimation of E_{max} Under Cardiac Assistance

Makoto Yoshizawa[1], Shozo Iemura[1], Akira Tanaka[1], Ken-ichi Abe[1], Hiroshi Takeda[2],
Yoshito Kakinuma[3], Hiroshi Akiho[3], Tomoyuki Yambe[3], and Shin-ichi Nitta[3]

Summary. A new method for less invasive and beat-by-beat estimation of the maximum ventricular elastance (E_{max}) is proposed. The method (*parameter optimization method*) needs only two measurements: aortic pressure and flow. In the estimation process, the least squares method was applied to an identity equation based on a simple electrical circuit model of the systemic circulation. In the model, the left ventricular elastance was approximated by a linear time function. In in vivo experiments using an adult goat, the error in estimation of aortic flow was usually less than about 2 l/min. The stability of estimation was also good at each beat, except where there was arrhythmia.

Key words: Ventricular elastance — E_{max} — Cardiac assistance — Parameter optimization method — Estimated maximum elastance

Introduction

The maximum elastance (E_{max}) is considered a good index for evaluation of the contractility of the ventricle. It may be possible to use E_{max} to determine the proper timing for weaning patients from the left ventricular assist device (LVAD). However, most traditional methods for obtaining E_{max} require invasive measurements of parameters such as left ventricular volume (LVV) and pressure (LVP). Yoshizawa et al. [1] proposed a method using only aortic pressure (AOP) and flow (AOF). This method does not require a sudden change in phase of the LVAD [2]. However, the method is not practical because its reliability depends strongly on the data obtained at only two instants.

In the present study, another method is proposed for the estimation of E_{max} without direct measurement of LVV and LVP in the patient under cardiac assist-

[1] Department of Electrical Engineering, Graduate School of Engineering, Tohoku University, Aoba, Aramaki, Aoba-ku, Sendai, Miyagi 980-77, Japan
[2] Department of Electrical Engineering, Tohoku Gakuin University, Tagajo, Miyagi 985, Japan
[3] Department of Medical Engineering and Cardiology, Institute of Development, Aging and Cancer, Tohoku University, Sendai, Miyagi 980-77, Japan

ance with the LVAD. This method is called the *parameter optimization method*, since a key point of the method is to optimize unknown parameters included in an identity equation derived from a model of the systemic circulation. The method also does not need a sudden change in phase of the LVAD. In vivo experiments have been carried out to examine the adequacy of the method.

Methods

Parameter Optimization Method

Assume that the systemic circulation can be modelled as shown in Fig. 1. The left ventricle is assumed to be represented by a time variant elastance [$E(t)$]. The system dynamics from LVP [$e(t)$] to AOP [$p(t)$] is assumed to be expressed by a series combination of a resistance (r) and an inductance (L).

Let V_0 denote the volume-axis-intercept of the line expressing the end-systolic pressure and volume relation (ESPVR). The quantity $v(t)$ shown in the figure (unbiased left ventricular volume) denotes a subtraction of V_0 from LVV:

$$v(t) = \text{LVV} - V_0 \qquad (1)$$

Moreover, assume that in the ejecting phase, the left ventricular elastance $E(t)$ can be approximated by a linear time function

$$E(t) = at + b \qquad (2)$$

From the definition of elastance, the unbiased ventricular volume $v(t)$ can be represented by

$$v(t) = \frac{p(t) + i(t)r + i(t)L}{E(t)} \qquad (3)$$

From Eq. 2 and differentiation of Eq. 3 with respect to t, AOF [$i(t)$] is given by

$$i(t) = \Big[\big\{ p(t) + i(t)r + i(t)L \big\} a \\ - \big\{ \dot{p}(t) + \dot{i}(t)r + \ddot{i}(t)L \big\}(at + b) \Big](at + b)^{-2} \qquad (4)$$

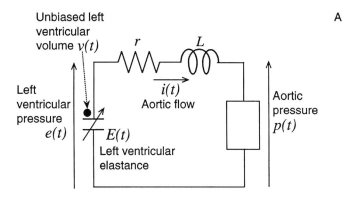

Fig. 1. Electrical circuit model of the systemic circulation

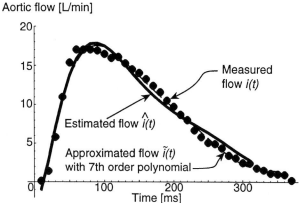

Fig. 2. Estimation of aortic flow $i(t)$ in an adult goat with the ventricular assist device off. Aortic flow: measured, $i(t)$ (*dot*); estimated by parameter optimization method, $\hat{i}(t)$ (*solid line*); approximated using 7th order polynomial function, $\tilde{i}(t)$ (*broken line*)

To the extent that the initial assumptions are exactly correct, Eq. 4 is an identity equation including four unknown parameters — a, b, r, and L — which holds for any time t. If the estimates $\hat{a}$, $\hat{b}$, $\hat{r}$, and $\hat{L}$ are respectively used instead of true values a, b, r, and L in the right hand side of Eq. 4, this side can be regarded as an estimate $[\hat{i}(t)]$ of $i(t)$ as follows:

$$\hat{i}(t) = \left[\left\{ p(t) + i(t)\hat{r} + i(t)\hat{L} \right\}\hat{a} \right.$$
$$\left. - \left\{ \dot{p}(t) + i(t)\hat{r} + \ddot{i}(t)\hat{L} \right\}\left(\hat{a}t + \hat{b}\right) \right]\left(\hat{a}t + \hat{b}\right)^{-2} \quad (5)$$

Optimal values of the estimates $\hat{a}$, $\hat{b}$, $\hat{r}$, and $\hat{L}$ can be obtained to minimize the flow estimation error (δ). The error δ is defined as the root mean square value of the difference between the measured $i(t)$ and its estimate $\hat{i}(t)$ within the ejecting phase, and is given by

$$\delta = \sqrt{\frac{1}{N_2 - N_1 + 1} \sum_{k=N_1}^{N_2} \left\{ i(t_k) - \hat{i}(t_k) \right\}^2} \quad (6)$$

where $t_k = k\Delta t$, $\Delta t = 10\,ms$ (a sampling period), and N_1 and N_2 are the numbers corresponding to the start and the end of estimation, respectively. The time origin ($t = t_k = 0$ or $k = 0$) is set to the beginning of ejection.

Once two parameters, $\hat{a}$ and $\hat{b}$, out of four are obtained, E_{max} can be estimated as

$$E_{max} \simeq \hat{a}t_{es} + \hat{b} \quad (7)$$

where t_{es} is the end-systolic time (the end of ejection).

In our calculations, the mathematical processing language *Mathematica* (Wolfram Research, Champaign, IL, USA) was employed. In particular, its least squares function *FindMinimum* was used to find the optimal parameters. Its curve-fitting function *Fit* with the order of 5 to 7 was also used to eliminate measurement noises included in $p(t)$ and $i(t)$, and to yield their approximates $\tilde{p}(t)$ and $\tilde{i}(t)$. To calculate the values of Eqs. 4–6, $\tilde{p}(t)$ and $\tilde{i}(t)$ were applied instead of $p(t)$ and $i(t)$.

Experiments

In vivo experiments using an adult goat weighing 50 kg were carried out with the chest open. The LVAD was placed between the left atrium and the descending aorta and driven by a pneumatic driver in synchronization with the electrocardiogram. The drive conditions used in the experiments were the counterpulsation (CP) mode with a systolic delay of 40% of the cardiac cycle, and the copulsation (CoP) mode with a systolic delay of 10 ms. AOP and LVP were measured by a catheter-tip type pressure sensor at the ascending aorta. AOF was measured by an electromagnetic flow meter at the same position. The data acquisition rate was 100 Hz.

The left anterior descending coronary artery was occluded for 1 min to evaluate the effect of the LVAD on the estimated E_{max}.

Results

Estimation of Flow Rate

Figure 2 shows an example of estimations of AOF. In the present study, the lower and upper limits of the estimation range, N_1 and N_2, were respectively set to time 0 and the time corresponding to 85% of the duration of ejection. The reason for choosing 85% will be mentioned later.

Figure 2 demonstrates that the approximated AOF, $\tilde{i}(t)$, obtained from the 7th order polynomial function, almost coincided with the measured AOF, $i(t)$, except in the neighborhood of the peak. The estimated AOF, $\hat{i}(t)$, obtained from the parameter optimization method, was quite similar to the measured $i(t)$. The flow estimation error δ given by Eq. 6 was 0.88 l/min in this example.

Estimation of E_{max}

Figure 3 shows the change in E_{max} estimated by the parameter optimization method (upper trace) and the error δ (lower trace), with heartbeat, when the LVAD was shutting down (Fig. 3a) and when the LVAD was running (Fig. 3b). The rectangle depicted by broken lines indicates the duration of the coronary arterial occlusion, 1 min. In Fig. 3b, the drive mode was copulsation (CoP) in the intervals corresponding to the rectangles depicted with solid lines. Arrhythmia occurred during the interval between the 135th beat and 167th beat with the LVAD running. This caused the failure of the estimation of E_{max} for that period and

generated a large δ. Hence, the data were not plotted during this interval.

Discussion

Estimation of Flow Rate

The flow rate error δ can be regarded as a quantitative index to evaluate the adequacy of estimation of E_{max}, as long as the proposed assumptions are absolutely correct. As shown in Fig. 3 as well as Fig. 2, δ was less than 2 l/min at almost all times. This value is small in comparison with the average peak value (about 17 l/min) of AOF.

However, when the end limit of estimation N_2 was set closer to the time corresponding to the exact end of ejection instead of 85% of ejection, δ suddenly became

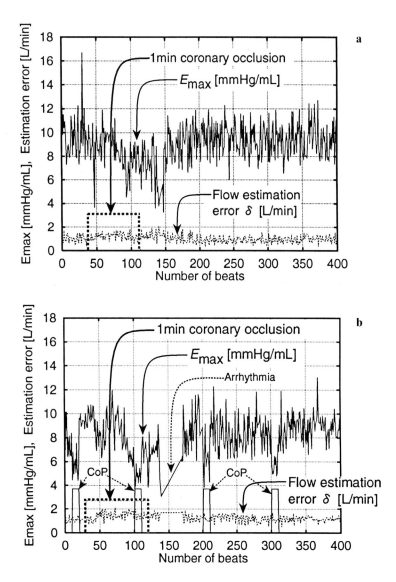

Fig. 3. Effect of an 1-min coronary occlusion (*broken lines*), **a** with the left ventricular assist device off, and **b**, on. The *upper traces* in **a** and **b** are the maximum elastance E_{max} (mmHg/ml), as estimated by the parameter optimization method. The *lower traces* are the flow estimation error δ (l/min). In **b**, the *solid lines* delineate periods in which the drive mode was copulsation (*CoP*)

larger. This implies that the ventricular elastance $E(t)$ may become far from linear as the time t approaches end-systole. If $E(t)$ is not linear and has a peak before end-systole, E_{max} obtained from Eq. 7 will be an overestimate. However, this overestimation will be able to be modified if the position of the peak can be estimated. In a future study, it would be worth estimating the peak position at the time when δ becomes abruptly larger as N_2 is increased.

Effect of Coronary Arterial Occlusion

In Fig. 3a it can be seen that the value of E_{max} estimated by the parameter optimization method has a large degree of scatter. Nevertheless, the values of E_{max} tended to decrease from the 80th beat (about 45 beats after the start of occlusion) and returned to the previous level at the 150th beat (about 40 beats after the end of occlusion). On the other hand, the phenomenon of a decrease in E_{max} is less apparent with the LVAD on (Fig. 3b) than with it off (Fig. 3a). This could imply that the effect of cardiac assistance with the LVAD prevented E_{max} from decreasing, if the period of arrhythmia is ignored.

Four periods of obvious decrease in E_{max}, corresponding to the CoP mode, can be found in Fig. 3b. However, these values are erroneous since the estimation is impossible in principle due to interference by the outflow of the LVAD on AOP.

In the same way as the previous method [1], the present method can execute the beat-by-beat estimation of E_{max} without direct measurement of either LVV or LVP, and without any change in afterload. The improvement over the previous method is that the estimation accuracy could be evaluated quantitatively as the error δ, and its value had a tendency to be small.

Conclusion

The important point of the parameter optimization method is that $E(t)$ is assumed to be a linear time function (Eq. 2). In further studies, this point must be verified. Moreover, the value of E_{max} estimated by the proposed method must be compared with that estimated by another method using LVV and/or LVP.

References

1. Yoshizawa M, Abe K, Sato D, Takeda H, Yambe T, Nitta S (1994) Less invasive E_{max} estimation under cardiac assistance based on angular frequency method. Proceedings of 16th Annual International Conference of the IEEE Engineering in Medicine and Biology Society, pp 107–108, Nov. 3–6, 1994, Baltimore, MD, USA
2. Nitta S, Yoshizawa M, Yambe T, Tanaka M, Hiroshi T (1995) A less invasive E_{max} estimation method for weaning from cardiac assistance. IEEE Trans Biomed Eng 42(12):1165–1173

Development and Clinical Application of Silicon-Coated, Leak-Free Oxygenator with a Built-in Hemoconcentration Function

Hiroshi Nishida[1], Masahiro Endo[1], Hitoshi Koyanagi[1], Katsuyuki Kuwana[2], and Hikaru Nakanishi[2]

Summary. We have developed a new membrane oxygenator with a hemofiltration (HF) function and applied it clinically in open heart surgery. The hollow fiber units for gas exchange (effective surface area $2.23\,m^2$) and HF ($0.61\,m^2$) were combined in concentric circles in a cylindrical housing (outer diameter 95 mm, length 40 mm). The total priming volume was only 190 ml. This oxygenator was completely resistant to serum leakage even after hydrophilic treatment, because we adopted an ultrathin ($0.2\,\mu m$) silicon-coated polypropylene hollow fiber membrane, which has been used in the intravascular oxygenator (IVOX) for gas exchange. Both units possess a blood-outside perfusion system. All blood flows in a radial direction from around the central core to the surrounding hollow fiber units, first to the HF section and then to the gas exchange area. Filtered fluid was easily collected through a stopcock mechanism. We confirmed excellent in vitro performance (O_2 transfer rate 312 ml/min at a blood flow rate of 6 l/min; HF rate 3.5 l/h at a blood flow rate of 4 l/min with 25% hematocrit and 200 mmHg transmembrane pressure; pressure drop 62 mmHg at a blood flow rate of 4 l/min), and lasting effectiveness of HF due to continuous wash-out by the total blood flow, with no adverse effects, in an in vivo study in a mongrel dog. The system was then used, with informed consent, on a 44-year-old male patient, who underwent cardiopulmonary bypass (CPB) for coronary artery bypass grafting. This new membrane oxygenator was used safely without any significant problems. The CPB circuit was simplified and handling of CPB and collection of filtered fluid were markedly facilitated. In conclusion, this durable, combined system was able to achieve excellent and simplified HF together with gas exchange of blood. It was useful not only in CPB during open heart surgery, but also in cases of extracorporeal membrane oxygenation (ECMO) and venoarterial bypass, because most patients who need such assistance have impaired renal function and fluid overload.

Key words: Hollow fiber — Oxygenator — Hemoconcentrator — Blood-outside flow mode — Silicon coating

Introduction

Hemoconcentrators using hemofiltration have been widely used to raise the hematocrit of blood diluted with priming solution and crystalloid cardioplegic solution. This is done to avoid homologous blood transfusion during open heart surgery. Since both the membrane oxygenator and hemoconcentrator are devices made of hollow fibers, we decided to develop a combined device, an oxygenator with a hemofiltration function. We have finished the developmental stage through trial manufacture of prototypes 1 to 4. The basic concepts in design and principal goal have been reported previously [1]. We recently applied this new membrane oxygenator clinically after confirming satisfactory in vitro and in vivo performance of prototype 4 [2]. This report describes the clinical version of this combined device and the results of its clinical application, together with its theoretical advantages in handling and performance.

Advantages

Advantages in Handling

Simple Circuit

The additional parallel circuit for the hemoconcentrator required in the conventional system (Fig. 1a) is unnecessary.

One Less Pump

The roller pump for the hemoconcentration circuit can be eliminated because the main roller pump for systemic circulation also perfuses the oxygenator and hemoconcentrator at the same time (Fig. 1b).

Reduced Priming Volume

The total priming volume of the combined system is only 190 ml (Fig. 1b), approximately 200 ml less than the overall total priming volume of a conventional oxygenator, hemoconcentrator, and extra circuit for hemofiltration (Fig. 1a).

[1] Department of Cardiovascular Surgery and Cardiopulmonary Bypass, The Heart Institute of Japan, Tokyo Women's Medical College, 8-1 Kawada-cho, Shinjuku-ku, Tokyo 162, Japan
[2] Senko Medical Instruments Manufacturing, 3-23-13 Hongo, Bunkyo-Ku, Tokyo 113, Japan

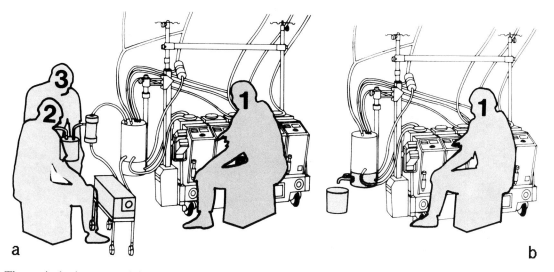

Fig. 1. Theoretical advantage of the system: **a** complex conventional system; **b** oxygenator with built-in hemoconcentrator

Easy Collection of Filtered Fluid

Filtered fluid can be easily collected by simply opening the stopcock. By closing and opening the stopcock, hemofiltration can be easily stopped and started whenever desired (Fig. 1b).

Fewer Personnel to
Handle Cardiopulmonary Bypass

The perfusionist can concentrate on the oxygenator and the blood level in the reservoir without worrying about an extra circuit for hemofiltration (Fig. 1b).

Theoretical Advantages in Performance

Because the blood flow rate through the hemoconcentrator portion is the same as the systemic blood flow rate, the flow, 4–6 l/min, is significantly larger than that obtained with a conventional blood-inside, perfusion-type hemoconcentrator, 200–500 ml/min. This significantly higher blood flow rate assures improvement in the performance of the hemoconcentrator.

Theoretical Advantages in Durability

Durability of Oxygenator

Serum leakage cannot occur even with long-term usage or after hydrophilic treatment of the device, because silicon-coated (0.2-μm thickness) polypropylene microporous hollow fibers, which have been used in the intravascular oxygenator (IVOX) [3,4], were adopted in the oxygenator part of this device.

Durability of Hemoconcentrator

Because a larger amount of blood always washes out the blood-contacting surface of the hollow fibers for hemofiltration, clogging or sealing by protein accumulation in the micropores in the hollow fibers, which leads to a drop in hemofiltration performance, is significantly less with the combined system than with the blood-inside perfusion mode.

In Vitro Performance of Prototype 4

We have developed four prototypes, and their in vitro performance was evaluated in a mock circulation using bovine blood. The performance of prototype 4 (Fig. 2), the final prototype, was as follows.

The oxygen transfer rate (Fig. 3) was 312 ml/min at a blood flow rate of 6 l/min with a hematocrit of 35%. The ultrafiltration rate (Fig. 4) was 3.5 l/h at a blood flow rate of 4 l/min with 25% hematocrit and 200 mmHg transmembrane pressure; and 2.0 l/h with 100 mmHg transmembrane pressure. A linear relation between the ultrafiltration rate and transmembrane pressure was maintained even under high transmembrane pressure in prototype 4. We consider that this phenomenon was the result of the radial flow direction in prototype 4. This characteristic may be beneficial when considering the situations under which this combined device will be used. In this combined device, transmembrane pressure will reach much higher levels because of the significantly greater blood flow higher levels because of the significantly greater blood flow through the device.

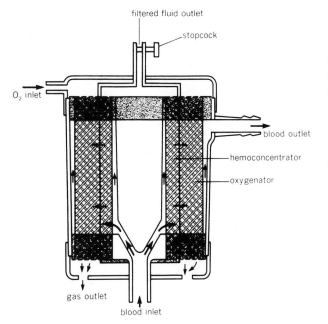

Fig. 2. Diagram of prototype 4

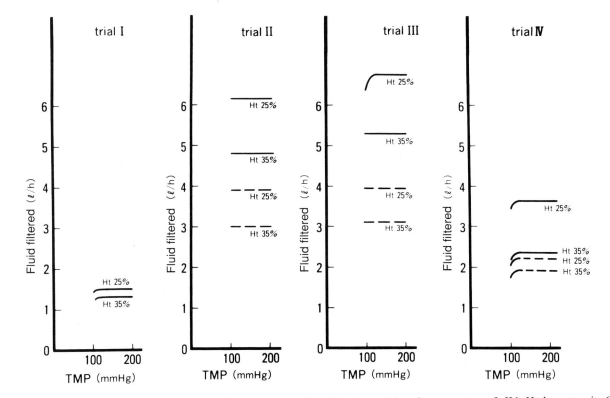

Fig. 3. Oxygen transfer rate at various blood flow rates. Q_B, blood flow rate. Bovine blood; oxygen saturation of blood on the venous side 65%; hemoglobin 12 g/dl; temperature 37°C. Trials I–IV correspond to prototypes I-IV. *Areas* are the effective membrane surface area

Fig. 4. Ultrafiltration rate against transmembrane pressure (*TMP*) in four trials using prototypes I–IV. *Ht*, hematocrit; Q_B, blood flow rate: *solid lines*, 4 l/min; *dashed lines*, 2 l/min; bovine blood, 37°C. *Trial I*, 0.49 m² cross-wind fibers; *Trial II*, 0.46 m², straight; *Trial III*, 0.45 m², straight-loop; *Trial IV*, 0.50 m², cross-wind fibers

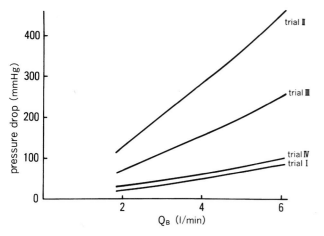

Fig. 5. Pressure drop at various blood flow rates in four trials. Conditions as in Fig. 3

The pressure drop (Fig. 5) was 62 mmHg at a blood flow rate of 4 l/min and 99 mmHg at a blood flow rate of 6 l/min. This value was nearly the same as that with prototype 1 and significantly lower than those observed with prototypes 2 and 3. We consider this degree of pressure drop is acceptable for clinical application.

Clinical Version

We considered the performance of prototype 4 satisfactory for clinical application. Therefore, we have developed a clinical version with a heat exchanger (Figs. 6, 7) based on the design of prototype 4. All blood flows first longitudinally in the small gap between the central core and the surrounding hollow fiber bundle, and then in a radial direction toward the surrounding hollow fiber units, first to the hemofiltration section and then to the gas exchange area. This blood path enabled the coexistence of excellent performance and a small pressure drop.

Clinical Application

A 44-year-old male patient, with informed consent, underwent cardiopulmonary bypass for double coronary artery bypass grafting using this new membrane oxygenator with the built-in hemoconcentrator. We incorporated a back-up oxygenator and hemoconcentrator in a parallel fashion. The operation was completed safely, and the performance of the oxygenator, heat exchanger, and handling were satisfactory. The performance of hemofiltration was lower than expected from the results of the in vitro study, probably due to incomplete hydrophilization of the hollow fibers of the hemoconcentrator under sterile conditions. We believe this problem can be easily solved.

Discussion

There is a great demand to decrease or abolish homologous blood transfusion in open heart surgery to avoid various blood-borne infections and to avoid homologous blood transfusion-related complications such as graft-versus-host disease and anaphylactic response. A hemoconcentrator with a hemofiltration function has been widely employed as the most simple and useful device to remove excessive fluid from blood diluted with priming solution and crystalloid cardioplegic solution. The hemoconcentrator is structurally very similar to a membrane oxygenator in terms of artificial organs incorporating a hollow fiber unit, except for its hydrophilic characteristics. The conventional hemoconcentrator is separate from the membrane oxygenator which has hydrophobic characteristics. The blood flow mode also differs. The oxygenator utilizes a blood-outside perfusion mode, while the hemoconcentrator employs a blood-inside perfusion mode. This makes the whole system and handling unnecessarily complex, and collection of filtered fluid cumbersome. With this background, we arrived at the concept of combining these two hollow fiber units into a single housing using silicon-coated hollow fibers. The adoption of this silicon-coated hollow fiber unit makes this development possible because the hollow fibers for the oxygenator have to be completely resistant to serum leakage, even after treatment to make the hollow fibers for hemofiltration hydrophilic.

The circuit and its setup were significantly simplified. Starting and stopping hemofiltration and the collection of filtered fluid are extremely easy because of the stopcock mechanism and continuous flow around the hollow fibers for hemofiltration. The combined device is highly durable, with respect to not only the oxygenator but also the hemoconcentrator, because of the continuous wash-out by the significant amounts of fluid in the total bypass flow. Therefore, this simple combined device is useful for assisted circulation requiring long-term oxygenation such as venoarterial bypass and extracorporeal membrane oxygenation (ECMO), because the patients who require those methods of assistance need management of circulating blood volume due to associated impaired renal function.

As a next step, we have started the development of a detachable, blood-outside, perfusion-mode

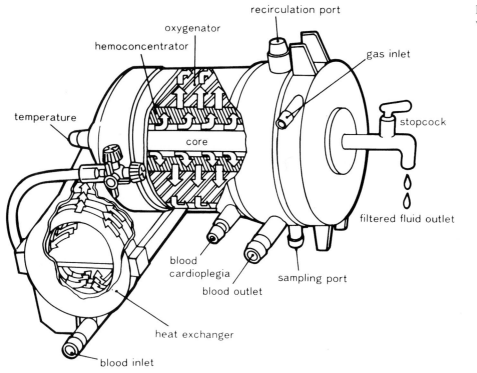

Fig. 6. Diagram of clinical version

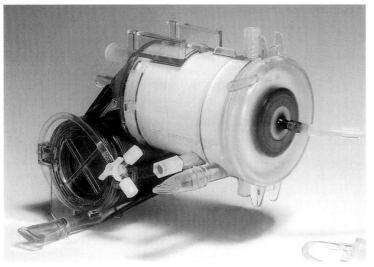

Fig. 7. Photo of clinical version

hemoconcentrator, as shown in Fig. 8, to make the most of its excellent performance and characteristics. We can easily connect and disconnect this hemoconcentrator to and from the oxygenator according to the preference or need of the physician and perfusionist.

Conclusion

This durable, combined system was able to achieve excellent and simplified hemoconcentration, together with gas exchange with blood. It is useful not only in cardiopulmonary bypass during open heart surgery,

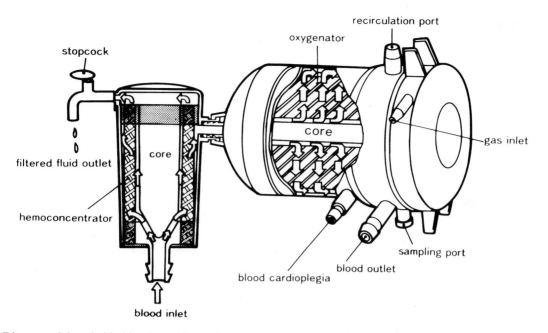

Fig. 8. Diagram of detachable blood-outside, perfusion-mode hemoconcentrator connected to the oxygenator

but also in extracorporeal membrane oxygenation and venoarterial bypass. Most patients in this category who need these types of assisted circulation have impaired renal function and fluid overload.

References

1. Nishida H, Endo M, Koyanagi H, Suzuki S, Kuwana K, Nakanishi H (1995) Oxygenator with built-in hemoconcentrator: a new concept. Artif Organs 19:365–368

2. Nishida H, Endo M, Koyanagi H, Suzuki S, Nakanishi H, Kuwana K (1995) Development of an oxygenator with built-in hemoconcentrator. Jpn J Artif Organs 24:620–623

3. Conrad SA, Zwischenberger JB, Eggerstedt JM, Bidani A (1994) In vivo gas transfer performance of the intravascular oxygenator in acute respiratory failure. Artif Organs 18:840–845

4. Tao W, Biandi A, Cardenas VJ, Niranjan SC, Zwischenberger JB (1995) Strategies to reduce surface area requirements for carbon dioxide removal for an intravenacaval gas exchange device. ASAIO 41:M567–M572

Discussion

Mr. Mullaly:
A question to Dr. Nishida. A very interesting concept. I'm interested in the pressure drop across the device. The pressure measured at the outled versus the pressure at the inlet.

Dr. Nishida:
In prototype four about 90 mmHg at the flow rate of 6 liters per minute.

Mr. Mullaly:
And what is the rate of hemofiltration that you were able to achieve in the test procedure and in the clinical application?

Dr. Nishida:
In vivo study, the performance of hemofiltration is 6 liters per hour. So 1 liter per 10 minutes.

Mr. Mullaly:
Quite adequate.

Dr. Nishida:
Yes.

Dr. Schima:
I have a question for Dr. Yoshizawa: Have you made an estimation about the accuracy of your E_{max} determination?

Dr. Yoshizawa:
I think the accuracy depends on the assumption of the wave form of the elastance. We can evaluate the accuracy, not directly, but indirectly with the level of flow rate error between the estimated flow and the true flow.

Dr. Sipin:
That was very interesting, but couldn't you get the same result with a commercial hemofilter and oxygenator, and why do you have a combined unit?

Dr. Nishida:
You mean the detachable type?

Dr. Sipin:
The commercial hemofilter is available for the use of patients with kidney problems, like dialyzers. The idea is to get the fluid out of the blood, so you have a hemoconcentration if you remove the plasma.

Dr. Nishida:
You mean the purpose of this kind of development?

Dr. Sipin:
Yes.

Dr. Nishida:
As I mentioned in my presentation, the handling is improved and performances is improved, so that's why we developed such an instrument.

Part IX
From Pulsatile to
Nonpulsatile

Magnetically Suspended Centrifugal Pump as an Implantable Ventricular Assist System

Kazunobu Nishimura[1], Tomoyuki Yamada[1], Satoshi Kono[1], Sadatoshi Yuasa[1], Tomonori Tsukiya[2], Teruaki Akamatsu[2], Tsugito Nakazeki[3], Takayoshi Ozaki[3], and Toshihiko Ban[1]

Summary. We have been developing a magnetically suspended centrifugal pump (MSCP) for long-term use. The pump eliminates the need for a shaft seal. The shaft seal limits the life of conventional centrifugal pumps due to blood leakage and thrombus formation around the shaft. An in vitro hemolysis test revealed that the MSCP was less harmful than the Biopump with respect to destruction of blood components. In an ongoing series of animal experiments, pumps have been placed extracorporeally in sheep for extended times. So far, seven sheep have under gone implantation of the MSCP, for up to 46 days. The pump flow rate was 2.5–5.0 l/min under a pressure head of 100–140 mmHg. In parallel with the animal experiments, we have started to develop an implantable version for long-term use. The size and weight was markedly reduced (82 mm in total diameter, 50.5 mm in width, and 420 g in weight). A sensorless system which eliminates the flow meter and/or pressure sensors has also been investigated and showed good correlation to direct measurement in vivo. The power required was 15 W (9 W for magnetic suspension and control system, 6 W for driving motor), and this will be reduced to 12.5 W in the future. The implantable version of the MSCP is a promising device for long-term clinical use.

Key words: Magnetically suspended centrifugal pump (MSCP) — Ventricular assist system (VAS) — Implantable assist device — Sensorless system

Introduction

Centrifugal pumps have been used as a ventricular assist in patients with profound heart failure, even those awaiting heart transplantation. The advantages of centrifugal pumps over pulsatile assist devices are simplicity and low cost. Centrifugal pumps currently available have a shaft and seal, which causes blood leakage and thrombus formation around the shaft, and therefore pump heads need to be replaced every 48 to 72 h.

To overcome the problems around the shaft, we have been developing a magnetically suspended centrifugal pump (MSCP), the impeller of which is suspended within the casing with magnetic forces produced by permanent magnets and electromagnets [1–3]. Eliminating the shaft would increase the life expectancy of the pump in theory. So far, we have reported on the in vitro pump performance of the MSCP [2–3], hemolysis tests [4], and ex vivo animal experiments [5]. The hemolysis test showed that the MSCP was less harmful than the Biomedicus pump (Medtronic Bio-Medicus, Minneapolis, MN, USA) with respect to destruction of blood components. In an ongoing series of animal experiments to test the long-term use of the MSCP, pumps have been extracorporeally placed in sheep. To date, seven sheep have undergone implantation of MSCPs, and the longest survival was 46 days. The pump flow rates during these experiments were 2.5–5.0 l/min under a pressure head of 100–140 mmHg.

Since the assist device should be placed inside the body for long-term use, we have stared to develop an implantable type of MSCP, with reduced size, weight, and requirement for electrical power. This paper describes a new version of the MSCP in combination with technical innovations essential for an implantable system.

Pump Structure

The basic structure of the implantable type of MSCP has not changed greatly compared with an old version (extracorporeal type). Figure 1 shows the implantable type of MSCP. The mechanism of magnetic suspension of the impeller is the same as in the old version. The pump is composed of three parts: a motor unit, a pump housing, and a magnetic bearing. The pump housing has an impeller inside that pumps blood in and out. The magnetic bearing contains three electromagnets and gap sensors, which contributes to the reduction in size, as the old version contained four electromagnets. The rotor of the motor and

[1] Department of Cardiovascular Surgery, Kyoto University Faculty of Medicine, 54 Kawahara-cho Shogoin, Sakyo-ku, Kyoto 606, Japan
[2] Department of Mechanical Engineering, Kyoto University Faculty of Engineering, Yoshida-honmachi, Sakyo-ku, Kyoto 606, Japan
[3] NTN Corporation, 1578 Higashi-kaizuka, Iwata, Shizuoka 438, Japan

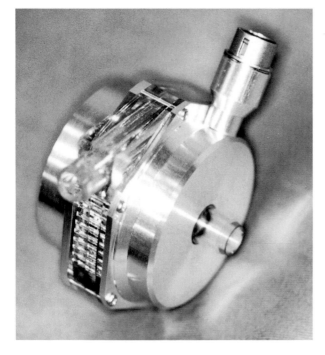

Fig. 1. Implantable version of magnetically suspended centrifugal pump (MSCP). The inlet and outlet of the pump are both 10 mm in inner diameter. A cable connector emerges from the top of the pump (*upper right*)

Table 1. Specifications of extracorporeal and implantable versions of magnetically suspended centrifugal pump

	Extracorporeal version	Implantable version
Total size (diameter × width)	86 × 80 mm	82 × 50.5 mm
Size of impeller (diameter × width)	50 × 10 mm	unchanged
Weight	700 g	420 g
Power required (total)	32 W	15 W
Motor	8 W	6 W*
Magnetic suspension	10 W	5 W
Control	14 W	4 W

* Pumping conditions: pump flow, 5 l/min; pressure head, 100 mmHg.

corresponding side of the impeller have 24 pairs of permanent magnetic that produce magnetic attraction. On the opposite side of the impeller, electromagnets produce contrary magnetic force against the permanent magnets so as to float the impeller inside the casing. Three sensors detect the gap between the impeller and the pump casing so that the gap and instability of the impeller can be actively controlled. Previous studies showed that a gap of 0.15–0.2 mm is optimal to minimize hemolysis [5]. The motor unit

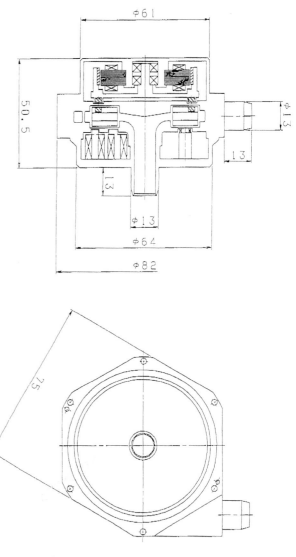

Fig. 2. Blueprint of implantable type of MSCP. Numbers are in mm; φ, diameter

contains a d.c. brushless motor and a rotor. The specifications of the extracorporeal type and the implantable type are listed and compared in Table 1. Figure 2 illustrates a blueprint of the implantable type. Another point of redesign is that the implantable type has only one cable connector from the pump to a driver, while in the extracorporeal type two connectors were used: from the motor and from the magnetic bearing.

Sensorless System and In Vivo Results

It is mandatory to establish a system that measures pump flow rate and pressures for controlling the operation of the pump. Furthermore, minimizing the number of the sensors required for a circulatory assist system could reduce the incidence of infection and thrombus formation. We have devised a method for measuring flow rate and pressure difference in the MSCP by utilizing motor current and motor speed [6].

When the loss of energy through mechanical friction in a pump is negligible, the relationship of the pump flow rate and the motor current at a given motor speed should be linear. The MSCP is suitable for applying this principle because it has no rotating shaft or seal. In addition, the pressure difference through the pump could be calculated from a characteristic curve of the pump as a function of flow rate and motor speed. Thus, at a given motor speed, the flow rate and pressure difference in the pump can be measured. However, the relationship of the pump flow rate and the motor current varies depending on fluid viscosity, because the

gap between the impeller and the casing is extremely narrow (0.2 mm), which should influence the loss of energy due to friction in fluid. Nonetheless, we attempted to establish a calibration system of flow measurement by simple clamping of an outflow tube of the pump. The credibility of the sensorless system was investigated in vitro and in vivo. Figure 3 shows the simultaneous measurement of the pump flow rate derived from both direct measurement using an electromagnetic flow probe and estimation using the sensorless system. The estimate of the pump flow obtained by calculation correlated well with that of the actual measurement. In an animal experiment in which the pump flow rate was continuously measured by the two methods for over a month, the sensorless system was reliable throughout. The calibration was required once a day, as fluid viscosity did not fluctuate much.

Discussion

Other groups have been developing different types of centrifugal pumps for long-term use, and have reported durations of implantation from 1 to 6 months [7–8]. Characteristics of our MSCP include complete suspension of the impeller by magnet coupling and active control of the impeller position in the pump casing. These features enabled the MSCP to survive for an extended period and allowed the development of an accurate, sensorless system of measuring the pump flow rate because the MSCP has no rotating shaft or seals, and thus, loss to mechanical friction inside the pump is negligible [6].

The results of animal experiments using the extracorporeal version are to be reported elsewhere. Table 2 summarizes the results of chronic animal experiments. To date, seven sheep have undergone implantation of MSCPs and the longest survival was 46 days. Plasma free hemoglobin was within an acceptable range. The main cause of termination was embolism,

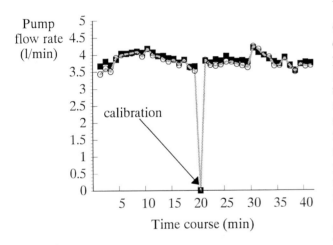

Fig. 3. Simultaneous measurement of the pump flow rate by electromagnetic flow probe (*squares*) and the sensorless calculation system (*circles*) in sheep experiment. Measurements were carried out throughout the period of 40 min, 20 min before and 20 min after calibration

Table 2. Results of long-term use of magnetically suspended centrifugal pump in animals

Animal number	Duration (days)	Maximum free Hb (mg/dl)	PT (s)	Cause of termination
1	14	18	19.3–20.5	Infection
2	15	15	19.5	Embolism
3	27	16	18.7–21.0	Intestinal impairment
4	46	16	16.0–17.9	Embolism
5	14	11	13.7	Embolism
6	15	9	17.3	Respiratory failure
7	37	11	14.7–22.8	Embolism

Hb, hemoglobin; PT, prothrombin time.

although thrombus formation inside the pump was observed in only one sheep at the termination. We have now changed the coating of the pump surface from silicon to heparin and are expecting better results thereafter.

There are several obstacles to overcome in placing the pump inside the body. One of the most important factors is reduction in size and weight to fit the body. We have achieved this chiefly by making the magnet bearing thinner than that of the old version. We also decreased the diameters of the inlet and the outlet of the pump from 12 mm to 10 mm in this version. The width of the pump is now 50.5 mm, which allowed it to be positioned on or in the abdominal wall. Next, the requirement for electrical power has to be minimized. With the new version, the total power required was decreased to about 15 W. In the future, the power required should be further reduced by changing the amplifier controlling the magnet bearing from a linear type to a switching type with lower loss of electrical power. In addition, as we have previously stated, the integrated use of permanent and electromagnets in the magnet bearing (the so-called null-power system) could reduce the power required to suspend the impeller [2].

It was demonstrated that the sensorless system developed to estimate the pump flow rate and the pressure difference was useful and accurate enough for clinical settings. All we need for measurement are the motor current and the pump speed, both of which are currently monitored all the time during the experiment. Thus, we are able to eliminate the need for a flow probe. At present, the calibration method for the system is not suitable for an implantable device, because the clamping of the outflow tube is necessary. However, we are investigating the possibility of measuring the fluid viscosity, which is crucial for calibration, by fluctuating the impeller for a short time. If successful, this will allow the complete establishment of a viable implantable system in the near future.

In conclusion, the implantable version of the MSCP is a promising device for long-term clinical use.

Acknowledgments. The authors thank Mr M. Watanabe of Takeda Hospital, and T. Ohnishi and Y. Wada in the Department of Engineering, Kyoto University, for their support during the animal experiment. Secretarial help by Miss E. Hatanaka is also acknowledged.

References

1. Akamatsu T, Nakazeki T, Ito H (1992) Centrifugal blood pump with a magnetically suspended impeller. Artif Organs 16:305–308
2. Akamatsu T, Nakazeki T (1993) Recent development of a centrifugal blood pump with a magnetically suspended impeller. In: Akutsu T, Koyanagi H (eds) Heart replacement, artificial heart 4. Springer, Tokyo, pp 305–308
3. Akamatsu T, Tsukiya T, Nishimura K, Park CH, Nakazeki T (1995) Recent studies of centrifugal blood pump with a magnetically suspended impeller. Artif Organs 19:631–634
4. Nishimura K, Park CH, Akamatsu T, Yamada T, Ban T (1996) Development of a magnetically suspended centrifugal pump as a cardiac assist device for long-term application. ASAIO J 42:68–71
5. Park CH, Nishimura K, Yamada T, Mizuhara H, Akamatsu T, Tsukiya T, Matsuda K, Ban T (1995) Development of a magnetically suspended centrifugal pump — in vitro and in vivo assessment ASAIO J 41:M345–350
6. Tsukiya T, Akamatsu T, Nishimura K, Park CH (1996) Indirect measurement of flow rate and pressure difference and operation mode of the centrifugal blood pump with magnetically suspended impeller. Jpn J Artif Organs 25:249–254
7. Taenaka Y, Wakisaka Y, Masuzawa T, Tatsumi E, Toda K, Miyazaki K, Eya K, Baba Y, Nakatani T, Ohno T, Nishimura T, Takano H (1995) Development of a centrifugal pump with improved antithrombogenicity and hemolytic property for chronic circulatory support. Artif Organs 20:491–496
8. Nakazawa T, Makinouchi K, Ohara Y, Ohtsubo S, Kawahito K, Tasai K, Shimono T, Benkowski R, Damm G, Takami Y, Glueck J, Noon GP, Nosé Y (1996) Development of a pivot bearing supported sealless centrifugal pump for ventricular assist. Artif Organs 20:485–490

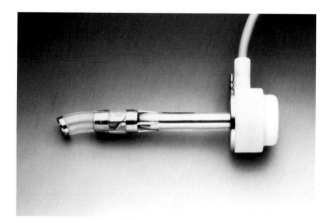

Fig. 1. A photograph of the intraventricular axial flow blood pump (IVAP) prototype no. 8

recirculated between the blood pump and extracorporeal purge fluid reservoir (800 ml) through inflow and outflow purge tubing. The priming volume of the purge system is 1 l. Purge fluid consumption is less than 10 ml/day. The blood-contacting surface of the pump was carbon-coated to enhance antithrombogenicity.

Animal Experiments

IVAP prototype no. 8 pumps were implanted in two calves weighing 90 kg (no. 8 #1), and 59 kg (no. 8 #2). IVAP prototype no. 9 was implanted in a calf weighing 78 kg (no. 9). Anesthesia was maintained with 2% isoflurane. The chest was entered via the left fifth intercostal space. The pericardial sac was widely opened, Xylocaine (100 mg) was injected intravenously, and two, 2-0 braided Dacron, pledgetted, valve-type sutures were placed around the circumference of the LV apex as purse-string sutures. After a bolus of heparin (3 mg/kg), the LV apex was incised and cored with a puncher. The pump was inserted into the left ventricular cavity and the purse-string sutures were tied. There was no difficulty inserting the outlet cannula past the aortic valve. The pump was started at 5000 rpm and the pump speed was gradually increased up to 9000 rpm. Arterial pressure, left atrial pressure, and left ventricular pressure were monitored during the surgical implantation of the pump. The motor was placed into the space at the phrenicocostal angle. Only minimal ventricular arrhythmias (PVC) were observed during this procedure; normal sinus rhythm was maintained easily. The electrical drive cable and purge lines were tunneled subcutaneously to the dorsolateral abdominal wall. Extubation was carried out approximately 1.5 h after the operation. The calves were able to stand up, eat, and drink soon after the surgery. The chest drainage tube was removed on the first postoperative day. The activated clotting time was kept 50% higher than the preoperative level by heparin drip infusion for a couple of days; following that, coumarin was orally administered. In the chronic stage, treadmill exercise (20 min walking) was performed twice per week, and we investigated possible arrhythmia during exercise.

Results

In all three calves, the pump systems were very stable throughout the experiments. We lost one calf (prototype no. 8 #1) due to pneumonia on day 26. A second calf (prototype no. 8 #2) was electively sacrificed on day 30 to analyze the pump and evaluate possible end-organ damage. The other calf (prototype no. 9) is still surviving at 150 days.

Hemodynamic Results

Arterial pressure, left atrial pressure, and left ventricular pressure, monitored during surgical implantation of the pump, are shown in Fig. 2. When the outlet cannula passed the aortic valve and the pump was turned off, the aortic pressure waveform resembled that of aortic insufficiency, due to a regurgitant flow through the pump. The pump was started at a low speed, around 5000 rpm, and the pressure waveform returned to the normal pattern. The pulse pressure became smaller as the rotational speed increased. At 9000 rpm, the pressure waveform became an almost nonpulsatile pattern. The pump rotational speed was kept at 8000–9000 rpm during the experimental period.

Hematological Data

Hematological data from three experiments are shown in Fig. 3. The plasma free hemoglobin (Hb) remained at normal levels (mean plasma free hemoglobin, prototype no. 8 #1: 8.9 mg/dl; prototype no. 8 #2: 6.0 mg/dl; prototype no. 9: 9.9 mg/dl). The lactate dehydrogenase (LDH) enzyme levels also remained in an acceptable range (mean LDH, prototype no. 8 #1: 976 IU/l; prototype no. 8 #2: 1018 IU/l; prototype no. 9: 1121 IU/l).

Other Laboratory Findings

During experiments (even during treadmill exercise), arrhythmia was hardly detected in any of the three calves. There was no hepatic or renal dysfunction, as measured by bilirubin, blood urea nitrogen, and creatinine levels. Appropriate coagulation control was maintained by coumarin at a dose of 5–10 mg/day.

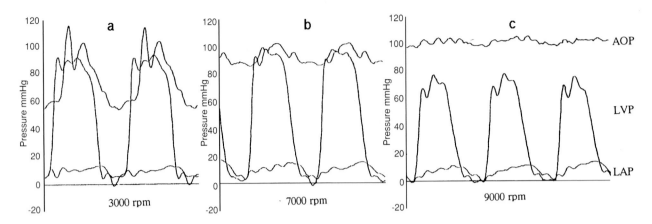

Fig. 2. Hemodynamic data at different pump rotational speeds: **a** 3000 rpm: the aortic pressure (*AoP*) wave form (*upper trace*) resembles an aortic regurgitation pattern: **b** 7000 rpm: the pulsation of aortic pressure decreased; **c** 9000 rpm: the aortic pressure wave form became almost a nonpulsatile pattern. *Middle traces*, left ventricular pressure (*LVP*); *lower traces*, left atrial pressure

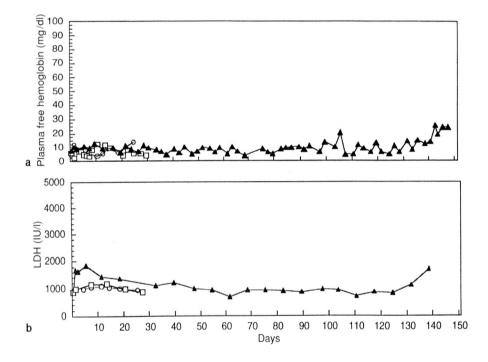

Fig. 3. Hematological data from in vivo experiments in calves with implanted IVAP: prototype no. 8 (*circles*, calf #1; *squares*, calf #2) or prototype no. 9 (*triangles*). **a** plasma free hemoglobin data; **b** lactate dehydrogenase (*LDH*) data

Pump System

In all three experiments, there was no pump failure and the pump operation was very stable throughout the experiments. Pump wattage changes were minimum. Purge fluid consumption was 24 ml/h in prototype no. 8 (purged-lip seal system), and less than 10 ml/day in prototype no. 9 (mechanical seal with recirculating purge system).

Postmortem Examination

The pump (motor part) was placed in the costophrenic angle at the 5th–6th costal level. In both no. 8 #1 and #2, the outlet cannula was smoothly passed through the aortic valve, and there was no interference between the pump and the mitral apparatus (Fig. 4). The pump was held in the correct position at two points of support. One was the pump base which was fixed at

Fig. 4. A photograph of the heart at postmortem examination after 30 days of support (no. 8 #2)

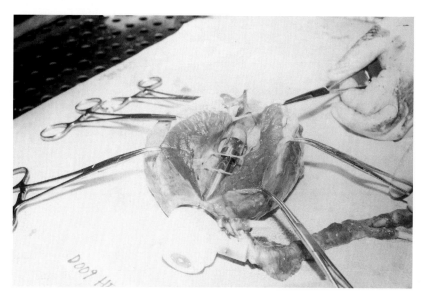

the LV apex, and the other was the outflow cannula which was supported by the fibrous annulus of the aortic valve. In no. 8 #1, though a small whitish thrombus (3 × 4mm) was found at the inflow guide-vane, a part which had not been coated with heparin, there was no other thrombus, even at the LV apex. In no. 8 #2, both the LV cavity and the pump were entirely free from thrombus formation. There was no major thromboembolism in vital organs in either no. 8 #1 or #2.

Discussion

The IVAP was designed as an implantable LVAD for use as a bridge to heart transplantation. The IVAP can be implanted with a minimally invasive, rapid procedure, which will be valuable especially in emergent cases. At the time of heart transplantation, there would be less adhesion around the heart because it does not have either an inflow or an outflow conduit outside of the heart. For clinical application, dilated cardiomyopathy is considered to be a good indication for use of this pump.

Mechanically induced hemolysis and shaft seal reliability are two major issues in developing an axial flow blood pump. The IVAP demonstrated a low hemolysis rate (in vitro, normalized index of hemolysis 0.005g/100l [6]; in vivo, plasma free Hb < 10mg/dl). In prototype no. 8, a purged-lip seal was used [6]. A lip seal requires continuous purging at a flow rate of more than 10ml/h for safe operation. This higher purge fluid consumption requires frequent maintenance during support. In addition, the estimated seal life is limited to several months. To solve these problems of the

purged-lip seal system, we developed a new mechanical seal with a recirculating purge system. This system demonstrated good seal performance for over 150 days. It is based on the "cool seal" concept; it keeps the temperature of the seal faces cool to prevent heat denaturation of blood proteins and maintains appropriate seal performance (details are described by K. Yamazaki et al. in this volume). In this system, purge fluid consumption can be minimized (<10ml/day), which enables easy maintenance (purge reservoir change is required less than once per month). Furthermore, this seal system has the potential to extend the seal life for years.

References

1. Yamazaki K, Kitamura M, Eishi K, Kawai A, Kobayashi S, Endo M, Koyanagi H (1990) A new left ventricular assist device — a miniature intraventricular axial flow blood pump (in Japanese). J Clin Exp Med 154:133–134
2. Yamazaki K, Kitamura M, Shiikawa A, Eishi K, Kawai A, Nojiri C, Endo M, Koyanagi H (1991) A new left ventricular assist device — a miniature intraventricular axial flow blood pump (in Japanese). Jpn J Artif Organs 20:705–710
3. Yamazaki K, Umezu M, Koyanagi H, Kitamura M, Eishi K, Kawai A, Tasugari O, Niinami H, Akimoto T, Nojiri C, Tsuchiya K, Mori T, Iiyama H, Endo M (1992) A miniature intraventricular axial flow blood pump that is introduced through the left ventricular apex. ASAIO Trans 38:679–683
4. Yamazaki K, Umezu M, Koyanagi H, Fujimoto T, Kitamura M, Nojiri C, Murayama Y, Ohtake Y, Shiozaki H, Mori T, Iiyama H, Hashimoto A, Endo M (1993) Development of a miniature intraventricular axial flow blood pump as a fully implantable LVAD for bridge use.

In: Akutsu T, Koyanagi H (eds) Heart replacement. Artificial heart 4. Springer, Tokyo, pp 273–278

5. Yamazaki K, Umezu M, Koyanagi H, Outa E, Ogino S, Otake Y, Shiozaki H, Fujimoto T, Tasugari O, Kitamura M, Hachida M, Nishida H, Nojiri C, Kawai A, Niinami H, Sakata K, Nakajima K, Hashimoto A, Endo M, Iiyama H, Mori T, Tsuchiya K (1993) Development of a miniature intraventricular axial flow blood pump. ASAIO Trans 39:224–230

6. Yamazaki K, Kormos R, Mori T (1995) An intraventricular axial flow blood pump integrated with bearing purge system. ASAIO Trans 41:327–332

Improvements in the Design of the Monopivot Magnetic-Suspension Blood Pump

Takashi Yamane[1], Masahiro Nishida[1], Toyoki Orita[1], Toshihiko Kijima[2], and Jun Maekawa[2]

Summary. A monopivot magnetic-suspension blood pump with an impeller suspended by permanent magnets instead of ball-bearings or seals has been developed. The magnetic coupling has been strengthened to prevent impeller lift-off and motor decoupling, and the extent of magnetic suspension has been reduced without losing stability. The impeller shape has been replaced by a closed-type hollow impeller to remove any thrombogenic flow obstruction at the inlet. The vane discharge angle has been increased to reduce hemolysis, based on the results of flow visualization of the gap flow profile. Recently, the magnetic coupling was replaced by a direct-drive mechanism, which reduces the total pump size to half the previous size. Finally, hemolysis testing of the latest model, DD1, revealed that DD1 causes only a slightly higher level of hemolysis than a regular extracorporeal centrifugal pump.

Key words: Centrifugal blood pump — Magnetic suspension — Direct drive — Totally implantable artificial heart — Closed impeller

Introduction

Currently available extracorporeal centrifugal blood pumps can be used only for a few days, mainly due to heat generation and subsequent hemolysis or thrombus formation around the shaft. The authors have been developing a monopivot magnetic-suspension blood pump with an impeller suspended by permanent magnets instead of ball-bearings or seals. The impeller cannot be maintained in a given position in three-dimensional space by permanent magnets alone; it also requires a mechanical contact (Fig. 1). The motor driving torque is transmitted to the impeller through the magnetic coupling. To maintain the gap clearance between the impeller and the housing, a ceramic pivot is provided at the bottom center of the impeller. To maintain the positioning of the impeller shaft, magnetic suspension is provided at the pump inlet. The magnetic suspension is achieved using rare-earth magnets and is magnetized axially.

Prototype Models

For the initial model, to verify the principle of magnetic suspension, a multidisk impeller similar to the BioPump (Medtronic Bio-Medicus, Minneapolis, MN, USA) was used (Fig. 2a). Though the extent of magnetic suspension was reasonably large, it was able to generate a pressure similar to that with the BioPump-80 at a given rotational speed (Fig. 2b).

The prototype series used a semi-open impeller of 50 mm in diameter; that is, one side of the impeller was covered by a disk or an impeller shroud. For the first prototype model, the magnetic force was designed to be small to minimize the pivot wear. During pump performance testing, the impeller lifted off at a pressure of approximately 80 mmHg, since the fluid dynamic lifting force became larger than the axial

[1] Mechanical Engineering Laboratory, Namiki 1-2, Tsukuba, Ibaraki 305, Japan
[2] Terumo Corporation, 1500 Inokuchi, Nakai-machi, Kanagawa 259-01, Japan

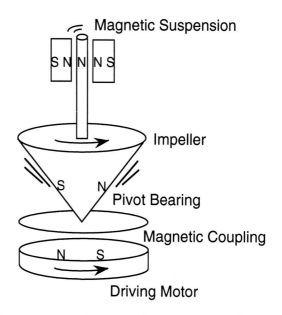

Fig. 1. Concept of monopivot magnetic-suspension pump. *N*, north pole; *S*, south pole

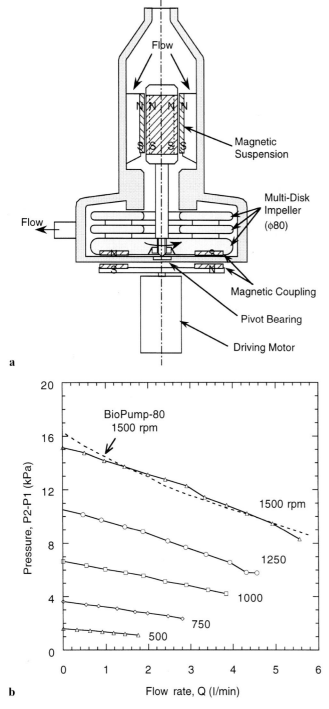

Fig. 2a,b. Initial model (φ80 × L105 multi-disk impeller, 26 × 26 × 47 d.c. motor). **a** Schematic drawing; **b** Pressure–flow curve (water) at various pump speeds

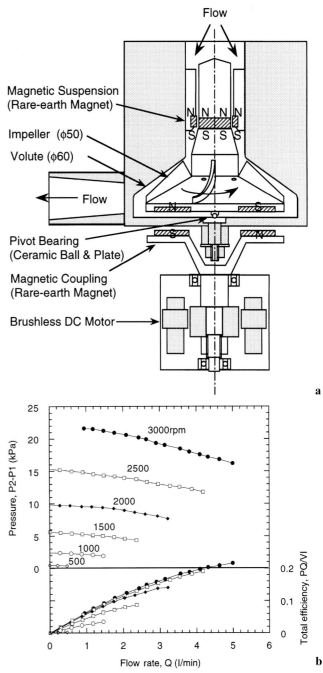

Fig. 3a,b. Prototype model (φ50 × L57 semi-open impeller, φ38 × L22 brushless d.c. motor). **a** Schematic drawing, **b** Pressure–flow curve (45 wt% glycerol, 37°C) at various pump speeds. The *lower panel* shows the total pump efficiency. *Q*, flow rate; *P1, P2*, pressures at inlet and outlet; *VI*, electric power input

magnetic force of 6.3 N. Washout holes were not effective in preventing the lift-off phenomenon. With further improvement, the axial pivot force of the magnetic coupling was increased to 10.0 N [1].

Finally, the length of the suspension magnet was reduced from 20 mm to 5 mm (Fig. 3a). The radial stiffness or radial stability, evaluated from the natural frequency, was not affected much by the magnet

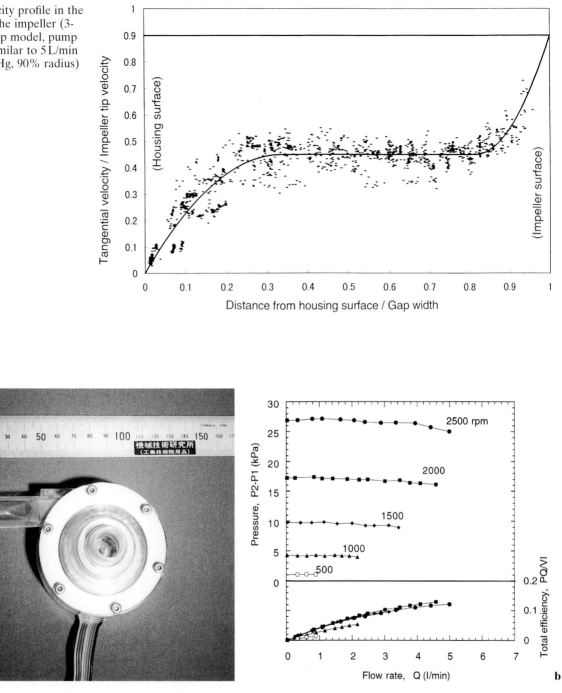

Fig. 4. Velocity profile in the gap behind the impeller (3-times scale-up model, pump condition: similar to 5 L/min and 100 mmHg, 90% radius)

Fig. 5a,b. Direct-drive model DD1 (impeller size, ϕ50 × L32; 4 vanes; housing size including motor, ϕ74 × L44; weight 435 g; volume 163 ml; inlet and outlet diameters, 15 mm) **a** Top view, **b** Pressure–flow curve (45% (w/w) glycerol, 37°C) at various pump speeds. The *lower panel* shows the total pump efficiency

length. The necessary pressure and flow (100 mmHg and 5 l/min) was attained in a steady state at a rotational speed of 2700 rpm. The total efficiency reached 22% for a 45 wt% glycerol solution having the same viscosity as blood (Fig. 3b).

Quantitative Flow Visualization

These models were only for engineering purposes. They did not have antithrombogenic structures, especially at the inlet, and the magnets were directly

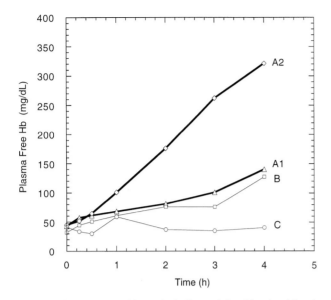

Fig. 6. Time course of hemolysis (heparinized bovine blood, 37°C; Pump settings: 5 l/min, 100 mmHg). A1: DD1, 4-vane model, well adjusted; A2: DD1, 8-vane model, not well adjusted; B: BioPump-80; C: control. *Hb*, hemoglobin

exposed to blood and stained easily. To assess hemocompatibility, flow visualization analysis was conducted. A special fluid, NaI, whose refractive index matches with the acrylic resin, was the working fluid for the 3-times scale-up pump model, and SiO_2 beads were added as tracer particles. The particles were illuminated by a 5-W laser light, and images recorded using a high-speed video camera. Particle-tracking velocimetry algorithms were applied to evaluate the flow vectors. With the intention of assessing hemolysis, the velocity profile was measured in the gap between the moving impeller surface and the stationary housing wall. Results revealed that the gap flow has a core region of low shear in the gap center and that high shear exists only near the walls (Fig. 4; [2]). Thus, the shear is determined not by the gap clearance, but by the impeller speed. Therefore, it was decided that the impeller speed should be reduced in subsequent models.

Recent Improvements and Hemolysis Testing

Model DD1 (Fig. 5a) uses a closed-type hollow impeller [3] to reduce thrombogenic flow obstruction at the inlet. A closed-type impeller has the fluid-dynamic effect of suppressing impeller lift-off compared with the semi-open impeller. In the light

of the expected shear in the gap, the discharge angle of the vane was increased from 22.5° to 72.7°. As a result, the necessary pressure and flow (100 mmHg, 5 l/min) could be attained at a rotational speed of 1900 rpm, 30% lower than that in the prototype (Fig. 5b).

Moreover, model DD1 is combined with a direct-drive mechanism, reducing the pump size by replacing the motor and coupling magnets with stator coils. The impeller is driven directly by the rotating magnetic field generated by the thin stator coils. The heat generation and pivot wear were comparatively small [4].

Hemolysis testing was conducted over 4 h with two DD1 models and a regular extracorporeal centrifugal pump, the BioPump-80. The first DD1 had four vanes and was well adjusted regarding the center of rotation and gap clearances. Since the gap clearance between the impeller and the housing was only 0.4–0.6 mm, a slight inclination of the impeller or manufacturing errors could cause rotational friction. The second DD1, with eight vanes, was adjusted only roughly and had a small amount of rotational friction. The blood was bovine venous blood which was filtered, heparinized, and maintained at a temperature of 37°C. It seems that despite the different number of vanes, when well adjusted, the DD1 generated a level of hemolysis almost as low as the BioPump-80 did, though when not so well adjusted, three times more hemolysis was generated (Fig. 6).

Conclusion

A monopivot magnetic-suspension blood pump with an impeller suspended by permanent magnets instead of ball-bearings or seals has been developed. The strength of the magnetic coupling and the extent of magnetic suspension have been improved. The impeller shape has been changed to a closed type and the vane discharge angle has been increased to reduce hemolysis, based on the results of flow visualization of the gap flow profile. Recently, the magnetic coupling was replaced by a direct-drive mechanism, which reduces the total pump size to half the previous size. Finally, hemolysis testing of the latest model, DD1, revealed that the DD1 causes only a slightly higher level of hemolysis than a regular extracorporeal centrifugal pump.

Acknowledgments. The authors express their thanks to Kanetec Co., Ltd. for manufacturing prototype models and to Chiba Precision Corporation, Ltd. for manufacturing direct-drive models.

References

1. Yamane T, Ikeda T, Orita T, Tsuitsui T, Jikuya T (1995) Design of a centrifugal blood pump with magnetic suspension. Artif Organs 19:625–630
2. Yamane T, Clarke H, Nishida M, Orita T, Asztalos B, Kobayashi T (1996) Flow visualization study for the design of rotary blood pumps — velocity profile in the gap between the impeller and housing. In: Proceedings, Waseda International Congress of Modeling and Simulation Technology for Artificial Organs, Waseda, Tokyo, pp 42–43
3. Tanaka S, Yamakoshi K, Kamiya A, Tajima H, Yokoyama Y, Kusakabe M (1985) A new seal-less centrifugal blood pump. Jpn J Artif Organs 14:1126–1129
4. Yamane T, Nishida M, Kijima T, Maekawa J (1997) New mechanism to reduce the size of the mono-pivot magnetic-suspension blood pump: Direct drive mechanism. Artif Organs 21:620–624

Discussion

Dr. Nosé:

In 1971, I made a so-called totally biolized pump with glutaraldehyde cross-linked natural tissues and the implant the pump passively, in the serial way, not the bypass way, and one of the calves survived for five and a half years. So I think your system should work for long periods of time without any thrombus formation.

Dr. Wolner:

When I visited you at that time in Cleveland, I saw such a calf, so that was a big mistake not to mention your previous work.

Dr. Nosé:

No, it's OK. And also I'm very happy that he is using a nerve cuff electrode. For a long time many groups tried to stimulate the muscle, and that is not an efficient method.

Dr. Wolner:

If you allow me a comment on this, you are right that it is much better to stimulate the nerve; however, it is also much more difficult to stimulate the nerve. It looks so easy but it must be done by microsurgery techniques, and it is much easier to take a wire through the muscle than to fix four electrodes on the nerve. Sometimes if you are not so experienced, you can also have some nerve damage. And we know from the patients of Dr. Thoma, with stimulation of the femoral nerve and the sciatic nerve, when the patient then moves too much they had problems with these electrodes. So, that's a very difficult problem. But carousel stimulation is superior to simple bipolar stimulation.

Dr. Nosé:

In 1962, I used monopolar biphasic nerve trunk stimulation, and it did work. The most important issue was not to mobilize the nerve; the cuff electrode should be implanted loosely around the nerve and its nutritional tissues together. It was very simple. Maybe, going back to that kind of simple method might work better than what you have achieved.

The DeBakey/NASA Axial Flow Ventricular Assist Device

Michael E. DeBakey[1] and Robert Benkowski[2]

Summary. An implantable, nonpulsatile, axial flow ventricular assist device (VAD) is currently under development as a joint project between the Baylor College of Medicine and the NASA/Johnson Space Center. The project was initiated after a NASA engineer underwent a heart transplant in 1984. In 1989 a memorandum of understanding was signed, and 1993 was the first year of funding for this project. Since then, more than 50 configurations have been designed, fabricated, and tested. To date, the pump has been optimized in terms of hydraulic efficiency, hemolysis, and thrombosis. The pump requires less than 10 W to deliver 5 l/min against 100 mmHg. A normalized Index of Hemolysis of less than 0.003 mg/dl has been achieved and several configurations have been thrombus-free after 2 weeks' ex vivo implantation. Following the success of the ex vivo experiments, a series of in vivo experiments has been initiated with the goal of 6 months', thrombus-free implantation.

Key words: Axial flow ventricular assist device — DeBakey/NASA

Introduction

For more than three decades the development of a mechanical pump to assist or replace heart function, as a means of restoring and maintaining circulation in patients with irreversible cardiac failure, has constituted an important objective of our research endeavors. As early as 1963, before Congress at Senator Lester Hill's Committee, Michael E. DeBakey first proposed the need of the National Institutes of Health's (NIH) support for this type of research endeavor:

"Experimentally, it is possible to completely replace the heart with an artificial heart, and animals have been known to survive as long as 36 hours. This idea, I am sure, could be reached to full fruition if we had more funds to support more work, particularly in the bioengineering area." [1]

Congress fortunately responded enthusiastically to this proposal, but the leadership at NIH, was less than enthusiastic but accepted the mandate from Congress and proposed sponsoring feasibility studies. This is reflected by the warning to researchers and lobbyists that "if too much money was authorized, we wouldn't spend it" [2]. This is further reflected by the fact that Congress, in 1967, increased the appropriations for this purpose by $10 million following the recommendation made in the Report on the President's Commission on Heart Disease, Cancer, and Stroke [3], which Michael E. DeBakey had the privilege of chairing. Also, Dr. DeBakey appeared before the Subcommittee of the Committee on Appropriations, chaired by Senator Lister Hill [4]; the leadership of the NIH circumvented these efforts by renaming the program "The Artificial Heart—Myocardial Infarction Program." By this means about half the funding was diverted to other heart research. From time to time during the next few decades, the program was reassessed and reevaluated with varying degrees of support. Nonetheless, it has been sustained, and researchers in the field have made considerable progress.

Our initial research efforts were directed toward both cardiac replacement and ventricular assist devices (VAD). It soon became apparent that the development of a mechanical pump for total cardiac replacement was associated with a large number of problems that would require a broad range of long-term investigations [3–5]. Accordingly, this group directed its efforts primarily toward the development of a pump for support of the failing left ventricle [6–9].

This conviction was reinforced by impressive results after clinical application of a left ventricular device, the first of which took place in 1963 [8]. It was in a patient requiring aortic valve replacement who had cardiac arrest the next day and was resuscitated but then had left ventricular failure with severe pulmonary edema. A left ventricular assist device, consisting of a double lumen tube with a blood chamber and a compressible bladder with ball valves at each end to provide unidirectional flow, was implanted by attachment of the inlet tube to the left atrium and the outlet tube to the descending thoracic aorta. During the next few

[1] Chancellor Emeritus, Olga Keith Wiess Professor of Surgery, Distinguished Professor of Surgery and Director of the DeBakey Heart Center and [2] Department of Surgery, Baylor College of Medicine, One Baylor Plaza, Houston, TX 77030, USA

days, the pulmonary edema cleared impressively although the patient died on the fourth postoperative day, probably from brain damage occurring during the cardiac arrest [8].

The second and more highly gratifying experience occurred in a 37-year-old woman suffering from heart failure caused by severe aortic insufficiency and mitral stenosis requiring both aortic and mitral valve replacement on August 8, 1966. Because the patient could not be weaned from the heart-lung machine, a left ventricular assist device was installed. This gas-energized, synchronized pump is of hemispherical design with a Dacron-reinforced Silastic-molded diaphragm separating the gas chamber from the blood chamber, and it had been demonstrated experimentally to be safe and effective [10,11]. The inlet cannula for the pump was attached to the left atrium, and the outflow was attached to the right axillary artery. With a pump flow rate of 1200 ml/min, it became possible to wean the patient off the heart-lung machine. During the next 9 days, the patient continued to improve, and on the tenth day, after reduction in flow to 350 ml/min and finally terminating pump flow with no increase in left atrial pressure and stable blood pressure, the pump was removed. The patient was discharged in satisfactory condition and resumed normal activities as a hairdresser [12]. Unfortunately, she was killed in an automobile accident 6 years later.

The concept is now well established that left ventricular bypass assist devices, by reducing left atrial pressure and therefore left ventricular end-diastolic pressure, reduce left ventricular strain, relieve pulmonary congestion, and increase arterial oxygen tension. Improvement in cardiac output, with increase in coronary perfusion, thus enhances myocardial recuperation. Moreover, providing better systemic organ perfusion corrects metabolic disturbances.

The ventricular assist device has, however, an important additional conceptual value, and that is, it provides supplemental cardiac output in patients whose cardiac failure is not correctable by medical or surgical means. According to the American Heart Association, more than 60 million Americans have some form of cardiovascular disease and more than 2 million Americans are living with heart failure, with 500 000 new cases diagnosed each year. Heart transplantation, which is the most effective method of treating many of these patients, is restricted to less than 2500 annually by availability of donors. The number of patients in this category who could use a new heart or be helped by cardiac assistance is estimated to approach 60 000. A fully implantable ventricular assist device, including its drive mechanism and energy source, with no extracorporeal tethering, would meet this need. This is believed to be an objective attainable by means of the axial flow ventricular assist device to be described later.

In 1984, Michael E. DeBakey performed a heart transplant on a NASA engineer. The patient was fortunately able to resume his normal activities at the NASA Johnson Space Center and became interested in our experimental laboratory investigations on the artificial heart. This led to a collaborative effort with some NASA engineers, who at first worked voluntarily on their free time, but in 1988, a joint collaborative NASA/Baylor project was formalized. The design strategy of this combined effort was to develop a miniature blood pump that would meet all the physiologic and biocompatibility requirements for supplementing cardiac output.

This has led to the development of an axial flow pump that is 86 mm in length and 25 mm in diameter, and weighs 95 g (Figs. 1–3). A brushless dc motor stator surrounds the middle of the flow tube. The components from left to right (the direction of blood flow) are, first, the flow straightener, which is stationary and acts as the front-bearing support. The inducer-impeller is the only moving component of the pump. Downstream of the impeller is the diffuser, which is stationary and contains the rear bearing. The diffuser slows the high tangential velocity blood by redirecting it axially, and thus resulting in a pressure build of the fluid. The stator on the outside of the flow tube spins a magnetic field. The impeller contains rare earth magnets in the blades and acts as the rotor of this brushless motor. This results in a pump with *no* seals and *no* valves. To achieve 5 l/min flow against 100 mmHg pressure, the inducer/impeller spins at approximately 10 000 rpm while requiring less than 10 W of input power [13].

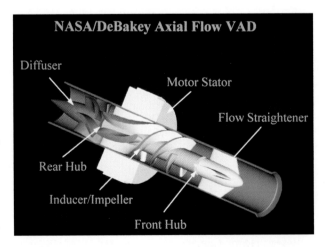

Fig. 1. Drawing showing configuration of the DeBakey/NASA axial flow pump

Fig. 2. Photograph showing disassembled components of the DeBakey/NASA axial flow pump. The diameter of the coin (*lower right*) is about 17 mm

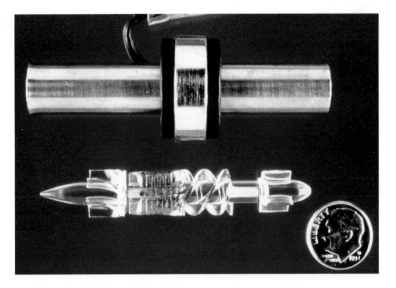

Fig. 3. Photograph of assembled DeBakey/ NASA axial flow pump with centimeter ruler to show its relatively small size

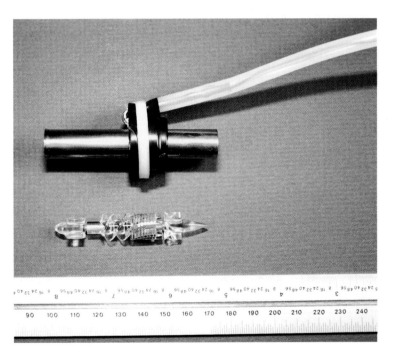

Materials and Methods

To optimize the hydraulic performance and hemolysis of the pump, our group performed extensive computational fluid dynamics analysis jointly with NASA — Ames Research Center [14]. The flow simulation requires about 24 h of computational time on a Cray supercomputer. Based on the Computational Fluid Dynamics (CFD) results, Ames suggested the addition of an inducer similar to that of the pumps on the Space Shuttle main engines. There is a strong similarity between pumping blood where the red blood cells rupture at low pressure and pumping liquid rocket fuels that vaporize easily and cause cavitation in the pumps. With the addition of the inducer section to the impeller, the pressure gradient along the tips of the blades was improved with a resulting increase in pump efficiency and reduction of the normalized Index of

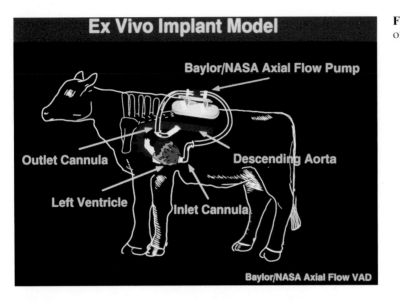

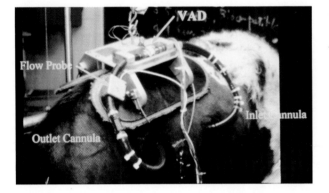

Fig. 5. Photograph showing paracorporeal implant of DeBakey/NASA axial flow pump located on a saddle on the back of a calf. *VAD*, ventricular assist device

Hemolysis by almost an order of magnitude. The hemolytic characteristics of the pump were further improved by independently optimizing blade inlet angles, outlet angles, number of blades, and clearances to produce a pump with a normalized Index of Hemolysis below 0.003g/100l, which is well within acceptable limits [15].

Besides hemolysis, the most challenging task in developing an axial flow pump is the elimination of thrombosis. To meet this challenge, Michael E. DeBakey's group implanted pumps in calves paracorporeally where they could be replaced easily and in a timely manner (Figs. 4, 5). The initial pumps were screened in 2-day tests in which the pumps were exchanged every 48h. Using this method, the authors quickly eliminated from the test matrix pumps that did not exhibit desirable antithrombogenic properties. Pumps passing the 2-day screening test were then subjected to the 2-week screening tests, which were also performed paracorporeally [15–17].

Results

A normalized Index of Hemolysis below 0.003g/100l was ascertained with the optimized inlet and outlet blade angles [15]. Seven pumps passed the 2-week screening test and showed no thrombus or only slight thrombus in the hub areas of a few pumps. All the pumps showed stable performance, with a flow averaging between 4 and 5l/min, requiring 7–8W. The calves were in excellent health, exercised regularly, and exhibited normal hepatic and renal function. Additionally, one pump passed the 30-day test without thrombus formation. Because of the long lengths of polyvinylchloride (PVC) cannulae in paracorporeal experiments, the duration of these tests is limited. For experiments with a scheduled duration of longer than 30 days, in vivo testing is preferred since long-term graft material can be used. In vivo testing with the DeBakey/NASA VAD has been initiated. Flow between 5 and 6l/min has been maintained, and this requires an input power between 6 and 7W. Experiments are scheduled for durations of 30 days, 90 days, and longer.

Discussion

The next phase of investigations will be directed toward intracorporeal implantation in animals for several specific purpose. The first purpose is to deter-

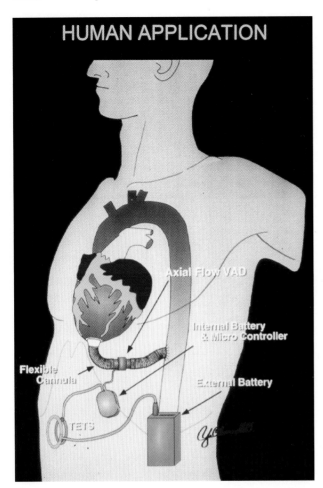

Fig. 6. Drawing showing a proposed surgical method of complete intracorporeal clinical application of the DeBakey/ NASA axial flow pump, rechargeable subcutaneously. *TETS*, Transcutaneous Energy Transfer System

mine if the evidence of short-term safety and efficacy in regard to pump flow and blood compatibility can be sustained for a much longer period of time — 6 months to 1 year. The second is to determine the adequacy and perhaps the most effective technologic surgical procedure of implantation among several alternative methods. The final purpose is to determine the most satisfactory materials for the various component parts of the pump and its connections for both biocompatibility and durability.

Conclusion

If these studies establish the long-term safety, efficiency, and durability of this axial flow pump, its clinical application will have more liberal indications than exist at the present time for ventricular assist devices. In addition, for example, for temporary use for transient but recoverable cardiac failure resulting from myocardial infarction, cardiac operations or other causes, and for bridging to transplantation, it can have more widespread use in the much greater proportion of patients with chronic irreversible heart failure, estimated to number more than 50000. Its application for these patients would be as a permanent left ventricular assist device (LVAD) with all components inside the body and a rechargeable battery placed subcutaneously (Fig. 6). Supplementing the defective cardiac output of these patients (with an ejection fraction of less than 15) with an additional 3000–4000 ml/min could restore the resting cardiac output to normal levels, and thus relieve the patient of manifestations of chronic heart failure and allow the resumption of reasonably normal activities. Because of the small size of the pump, which consequently causes little displacement of tissues in the thoracic cavity, it could also be easily used for both right and left ventricular assistance in patients requiring such support. Finally, it is extremely cost-effective since it can be manufactured, according to estimates that these authors have been given, for less than $25000.

References

1. Senate Subcommittee on the Committee on Appropriations for 1964 (1963) Hearings of Department of Health, Education, and Welfare Appropriations. Government Printing Office, Washington, DC, p 1402
2. Strauss MJ (1984) The political history of the artificial heart. N Engl J Med 310(5):332–336
3. The President's Commission on Heart Disease, Cancer, and Stroke (1964) Vol I, Superintendent of Documents, U.S. Government Printing Office, Washington, DC, December 1964, p 7
4. Hearing before the Subcommittee on Appropriations (1964) United States Senate, U.S. Government Printing Office, Washington, DC
5. DeBakey ME, Hall CW (1964) Toward the artificial heart. New Scientist 22:538–541
6. Hall CW, Liotta D, DeBakey ME (1967) Artificial heart — present and future. In: Research in the service of man: biomedical knowledge, development, and use. U.S. Government Printing Office, Washington, DC, pp 201–216
7. Kennedy JH, DeBakey ME, Akers WW, Ross JN Jr, O'Bannon W, Beker LE, Lewis CW, Adachi M, Alfrey CP, Spargo WJ, Fergun JJM (1973) Progress toward an orthotopic cardiac prosthesis. Biomater Med Dev Artif Organs 1(1):3–56
8. DeBakey ME, Liotta D, Hall CW (1966) Prospects for and implications of the artificial heart and assist devices. J Rehabil 32:106
9. DeBakey ME, Dietrich EB (1969) Cardiac assistors. In: Cooper P (ed) Surgery annual. Appleton Century-Crofts, New York, pp 433–449

10. DeBakey ME, Liotta D, Hall CW (1966) Left-heart by-pass using an implantable blood pump mechanical device to replace the failing heart. Chapter 18, National Research Council, Washington, DC
11. DeBakey ME (1971) The artificial heart: total replacement. Transplant Proc 3:1445
12. Hall CW, Liotta D, DeBakey ME (1967) Bioengineering efforts in developing artificial hearts and assistors. Am J Surg 114:24–30
13. Hall CW, Liotta D, DeBakey ME (1968) Review of cardiac booster pumps. In: Levine SN (ed) Advances in biomedical engineering and medical physics, vol I. Interscience, New York, pp 61–75
14. DeBakey ME (1971) Left ventricular bypass pump for cardiac assistance. Am J Cardiol 27:3–11
15. Kawahito K, Damm G, Benkowski R, Tasai K, Shimono T, Takatani S, Nosé Y, Noon GP, DeBakey ME (1996) Ex vivo phase 1 evaluation of the DeBakey/NASA axial flow ventricular assist device. Artif Organs 20(1):47–51
16. Nosé Y, Shiono M, Ohtsubo S, Ohara Y, Tasai K, Kawahito K, Nakazawa T, Benkowski R, Damm G, Glueck J, Takatani S, Noon G, DeBakey ME (1995) Recent trends in the development of non-pulsatile cardiac prostheses. In: Sezai Y (ed) Progress in the artificial heart. Axel Springer, Tokyo, pp 67–102
17. Mizuguchi K, Damm G, Benkowski R, Aber G, Svjkovsky P, Glueck J, Takatani S, Nosé Y, DeBakey ME (1995) Development of an axial flow ventricular assist device: in vitro and in vivo evaluation. Artif Organs 19(7):653–659

Discussion

Dr. Olsen:

Dr. DeBakey, based upon 60 years of work in this field, and your chosen field of cardiac surgery where you have had frequent need for these sorts of devices, would you perhaps look into your crystal ball and tell us what do we need in the future? Where should we spend some of our efforts in the immediate future?

Dr. DeBakey:

I don't think these scientists need any advice. I must tell you, I've been tremendously impressed with the scientific work that was presented here during the past two days. They are doing a great job. Perhaps I am biased, but I sincerely believe that a great deal of additional research on the total artificial heart is not needed. The experimental work that has been done was very useful because it gave us the basis for actually developing a mechanical device for assisted circulation.

As you know, it has already been expressed at this meeting that with the use of these very small devices, if they ultimately develop as we hope they will (and there is every good indication to believe that they will), there will be less and less need for removing the heart. These devices can be easily used for both right ventricular bypass and left ventricular bypass. And we have already heard about examples of how, with the use of the left ventricular assist device, it has actually been possible to remove the device and have the patients with cardiomyopathy lead reasonably normal lives. This is most impressive. I am more and more convinced that this will lead to widespread use of this device. The estimates of the number of people in chronic heart failure who could use some kind of help, beyond the relatively ineffective treatment of the medical specialists, are considerable because if you take away lasix, they have very little left. I could conceive in the future that from 50 000 to 100 000 patients in the United States alone would be able to use a left ventricular assist device. You will be able to convert a large number of these patients who now cannot do anything, but can survive with general medical therapy for perhaps a year or two at a cost of a great deal of money. And if you can convert them with this device to be independent, you will not only save a lot of money, but you will also increase the quality of their lives. These are people in their sixties and seventies, and they are growing in number, not only in our country, but in Japan and Europe, so there is a large proportion of patients who will be able to use this type of device. I really believe that the time will come when we will be able to apply it to a large proportion of the patients who need this type of support.

Dr. Watson:

Dr. DeBakey, I wonder whether you would share with us, your interest, of course, is in mechanical systems but also in fundamental science, and I wonder if you would share the reason that you were given the Lasker Award and the principle that has led to so many advances in surgery.

Dr. DeBakey:

I think that the important consideration in the advancement of any clinical development is the basic science knowledge that is being developed. And those of us who are in the clinical field and are eager to improve our clinical ability to deal with clinical problems must be in a position to translate this knowledge as best we can. This simply means that as clinicians we should keep up with the basic science work that is taking place because it is going to be our responsibility to use that knowledge and to put it into proper perspective and, of course, proper application. That means we will need to maintain our scientific capabilities. I am very gratified to see what has been taking place here over the last two days. The work that Dr. Wolner just showed us is a good example of how scientific work is moving ahead the knowledge to be used in clinical application. This is the way that we progress. And it is very gratifying for me to see how many of the scientists who made presentations at this meeting are reflecting that capability.

Part X
Posters

The Design of a Linear Oscillatory Actuator for an Artificial Heart

Tomoyuki Honda[1], Mayumi Hashimoto[1], Masaya Watada[1], Koh Imachi[2], and Daiki Ebihara[1]

Summary. For an implantable total artificial heart (TAH), it is desirable to reduce the rated capacity, and therefore size, of the power supply. Use of a linear oscillatory actuator (LOA) driven by constant current should decrease the capacity needed for the power supply. Therefore, the authors calculated the thrust characteristics required for the LOA to drive a pusher-plate type total artificial heart (TAH), then simulated the aortic pressure and the flow rate to verify the calculation. In the simulation, the systolic/diastolic (S/D) ratio became constant at 0.25, and the S/D ratio and cardiac output were insensitive to alterations in the excitation time ratio (the ratio between the excitation time and the period of the excitation current). This insensitivity should permit the failsafe operation of the TAH system in case of a defect in the position sensors.

Key words: Design — Total artificial heart — Linear oscillatory actuator (LOA) — Thrust characteristics

Introduction

In a total artificial heart (TAH), the actuator and power supply must be made small to allow implantation of the whole system, which includes a battery and an energy converter. The size of the power supply is related to its capacity. One way to decrease the necessary rated capacity is to drive a linear oscillatory actuator (LOA) within the TAH using alternating current at a constant level. This paper reports (a) the method of calculation used to obtain the required thrust characteristics of the LOA, using a circuit to represent the systemic circulation, and (b) the verification of this method.

Basic Structure

Figure 1 shows the cutaway view of the LOA [1]. The mover consists of two magnets and three inductors. The stator surrounds the mover, which in turn con-

tains an excitation coil. As the excitation alternating current flows, the mover is driven forward and backward. Figure 2 shows the basic concept of the TAH. A pump is placed on each side of the LOA, one for systemic circulation and the other for pulmonary circulation. The pumps are pushed alternately by the pusher plates located on both ends of the mover, and they pump the blood to both circulatory systems. The design of this TAH system takes advantage of the ability of the LOA to generate linear reciprocating motion directly, without using conversion mechanisms.

Method

To allow implantation of the whole TAH, including the controller, it is necessary to decrease the rated capacity of the power supply. Equation 1 expresses the rated capacity of the power supply for driving the LOA, the circuit of which can be represented as the series connection of a resistor R and an inductor L:

$$P_{\text{PowerSupply}} = \max\left(Ri^2 + Li\frac{di}{dt} \right)[\text{VA}] \tag{1}$$

where i, R, and L are the excitation current, resistance, and inductance of the LOA, respectively. The excitation current determines the thrust force of the LOA [2]. Driving the LOA with a constant current is the method used to reduce the rated capacity of the power supply. To design the LOA for constant current drive, we need to determine the level of thrust force needed. This paper aims to establish the method for calculating the required thrust force of the LOA with constant current drive.

Systemic circulation can be represented by the simple equivalent circuit shown in Fig. 3. The circuit consists of a parallel circuit with a resistor and a capacitor. Resistance R represents the peripheral resistance, and capacitance C the compliance of blood vessels. The aortic pressure AoP can be calculated on the assumption that TAH-driven blood flow follows the waveform shown in Fig. 4. Therefore, the thrust force necessary for the LOA can be calculated. A stable

[1]Musashi Institute of Technology, 1-28-1 Tamazutsumi, Setagaya-ku, Tokyo 158, Japan
[2]The University of Tokyo, 7-3-1 Hongo, Bunkyo-ku, Tokyo 113, Japan

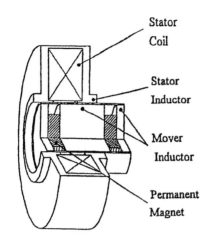

Fig. 1. Cutaway view of the linear oscillatory actuator (LOA)

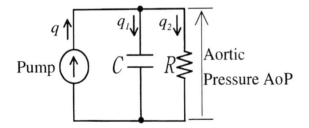

Fig. 2. Basic concept of total artificial heart incorporating LOA

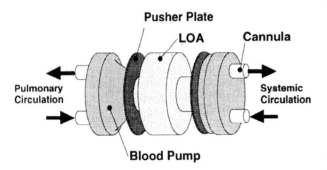

Fig. 3. Circuit representing the systemic circulation. C, capacitance representing compliance of blood vessels; R, resistance meaning peripheral resistance; q is flow rate

sinusoidal state is assumed for the aortic pressure. The flow rate, in ml/s, is

$$q = q_{max} \sin(\omega_1 t) = q_{max} \sin\left(\frac{\pi}{t_1} t\right) \quad (0 < t < t_1)$$

$$= 0 \qquad\qquad (t_1 < t < T) \quad (2)$$

where q_{max} is the maximum flow rate. The aortic pressure AoP is expressed as the summation of the prod-

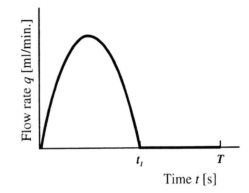

Fig. 4. Flow rate waveform. T, is the period of the flow rate

ucts of the Fourier-transformed flow rate and the total impedance of the equivalent circuit:

$$AoP = \sum_n q_n Z_n \exp\left\{ j\left(\omega t + \theta_{qn} + \theta_{Z_n}\right)\right\}[\text{mmHg}]$$

$$Z_n = \frac{R}{1 + jn\omega CR} = \frac{\sqrt{R^2 + \left(n\omega CR^2\right)^2}}{1 - \left(n\omega CR\right)^2} \exp\left(j\theta_{Z_n}\right)[\Omega]$$

$$\theta_{Z_n} = \tan^{-1}\left(-n\omega CR\right)[\text{rad}] \qquad (3)$$

where n is the order of harmonics, Z is the total impedance of the equivalent circuit, q is the flow rate, θ_q is the phase of the flow, and θ_z is the phase of the impedance. The required thrust force can be calculated from the resultant aortic pressure. Equation 4 shows the required thrust force F in Newtons, taking into consideration the loss at the outlet of the pumps and the inertia of the mover:

$$F = A \cdot \left(AoP + \gamma\zeta\frac{v^2}{2g}\right) + m\ddot{x}\,[\text{N}] \qquad (4)$$

where A is the area of the pusher-plates; γ is the specific weight of water; ζ is the coefficient of loss; v is the velocity at the outlet of the pump; g is gravitational acceleration; m is the mass of the mover; x is the displacement of the mover.

In real applications, the LOA will be controlled by the filling of the pulmonary artery, therefore the cardiac output and the systolic:diastolic (S/D) ratio were the parameters used in this calculation [3].

Results

Figure 5 shows the thrust force required for the LOA calculated using this method. Although the thrust force of LOA must increase in proportion to the cardiac output, the influence of both the loss at the pump

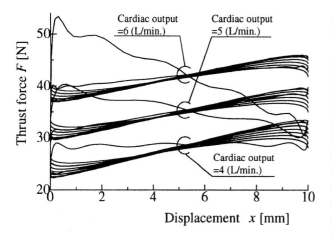

Fig. 5. Calculated thrust characteristics at set cardiac outputs: 6 l/min (*upper traces*), 5 l/min (*middle traces*), and 4 l/min (*lower traces*). The excitation ratio was in the range 0.1–0.9

outlet and the inertia of the mover becomes more marked as the S/D ratio decreases.

The results of the calculation of the thrust characteristics were verified using simulation of the LOA driving a pusher-plate type TAH. We selected the calculated thrust force characteristics obtained at a cardiac output of 5 l/min and an S/D ratio of 0.5 (see Fig. 5). Adopting these as the input, the aortic pressure and flow rate were obtained by simulation, using the equivalent circuit shown in Fig. 3. In this simulation, the excitation time ratio — that is, the ratio between the excitation time and the period of the excitation current — was varied between 0.3 and 0.7, and the cardiac output was maintained at a set level, 4, 5, or 6 l/min. Figures 6, 7, and 8 show the results with cardiac output set at 4, 5, and 6 l/min, respectively. Note that although the intended thrust characteristics, predicated on a cardiac output of 5 l/min and an S/D ratio of 0.5, were applied to the simulation, the results indicate a variable flow rate and aortic pressure.

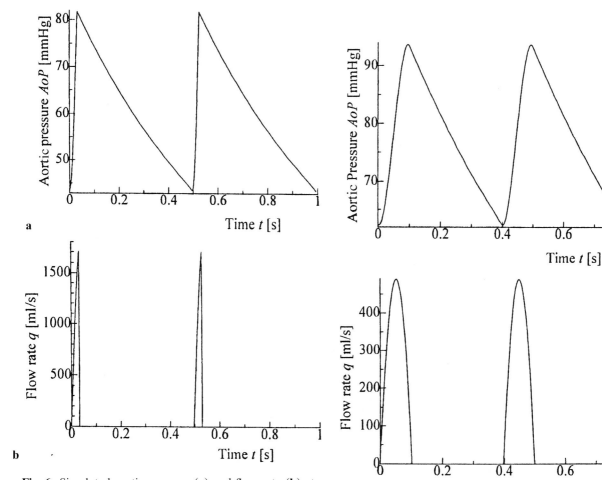

Fig. 6. Simulated aortic pressure (**a**) and flow rate (**b**) at a cardiac output of 4 l/min. The excitation time ratio (excitation time: duration of excitation current) of the LOA was 0.3–0.7

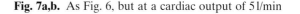

Fig. 7a,b. As Fig. 6, but at a cardiac output of 5 l/min

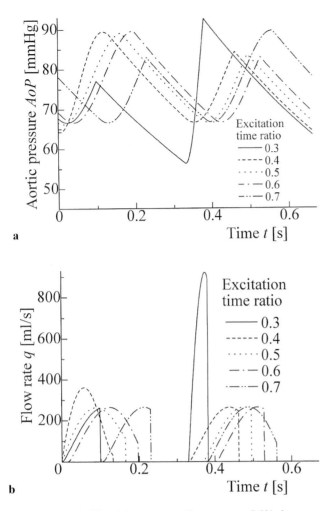

Fig. 8a,b. As Fig. 6, but at a cardiac output of 6 l/min

ance, thrust characteristics for constant current drive were calculated. The S/D ratio was held constant in each simulation, whereas the excitation time ratio (the ratio between the excitation time and the period of the excitation current) varied between 0.3 and 0.7. The reason for this difference is that the greatest acceleration of the mover occurs at the stroke end, because the simulated aortic pressure is stable despite the large variation. The difference arises because of the error generated by Fourier transformation on Eq. 3; fluctuations in the flow rate waveform and impedance of the equivalent circuit are magnified by a power of twenty is this calculation.

A notable fact of the results is that the excitation time ratio is independent from the S/D ratio of flow rate in this simulation with constant current drive. Therefore, the cardiac output is proportional to the heart rate, if the peripheral resistance varies. The stability of the S/D ratio and cardiac output, however, ensure the safety of the system against the failure of the position sensor or the controller. Once an error signal is detected, the input signal of the energy conversion system from the controller could be switched into the one from the basic oscillator, and the TAH would be able to maintain the required cardiac output and the aortic pressure of the patient.

Discussion

Constant-current drive for the LOA is a desirable design characteristic to incorporate into the totally implantable TAH. In the simulation of LOA perform-

References

1. Ebihara D, Watada M, Imachi K (1992) Development of a single-winding linear oscillatory actuator. IEEE Trans Magn 28:3030–3032
2. Watada M, Yanashima K, Oishi Y, Ebihara D, Dohmeki H (1993) Improvement on characteristics of linear oscillatory actuator for artificial hearts. IEEE Trans Magn 29:3361–3363
3. Snyder AJ, Rosenberg G, Pierce WS (1993) Noninvasive control of cardiac output for alternately ejecting dual-pusherplate pumps. Artif Organs 16:189–194

Reintroduction of the Jarvik/CardioWest Total Artificial Heart as a Bridge to Transplant

Ricardo J. Moreno-Cabral[1], Robert M. Adamson[1], Walter P. Dembitsky[1], Pat O. Daily[1], Francisco A. Arabía[2], and Jack G. Copeland III[2]

Introduction

The first clinical application of the Jarvik total artificial heart (TAH) as a bridge to transplant was reported by Copeland et al. in 1985 [1].

Our cardiac transplantation program was initiated in 1985. Two years later we used the Jarvik 7/70 TAH for the first time at our institution. We implanted the device in two additional patients before its clinical use was temporarily suspended in the United States by the Food and Drug Administration (FDA).

In 1994 we reintroduced the Jarvik 7/70 TAH to our program when the FDA authorized a few centers to continue clinical research under the CardioWest Company from Tucson, Arizona.

Patients and Methods

CardioWest TAH

The CardioWest TAH is the Jarvik 7 pneumatic ventricle with Medtronic Hall valves, actuated by the Utah drive controller and monitored by the Cardiac Output Monitoring and Diagnostic Unit (COMDU), which are essentially the same systems extensively reported as the Symbion TAH [2–4]. We used the Symbion controllers in our first three patients and the CardioWest refurbished units since 1994.

Patients

The six patients were all men. Their ages ranged from 36 to 62 years with a mean age of 55. The diagnosis was acute allograft failure in three, refractory graft rejection in one, acute myocardial infarction with postinfarct ventricular septal defect in one, and extensive right ventricular infarct in the last patient (Table 1).

[1] Department of Cardiovascular Surgery, Sharp Memorial Hospital, 7901 Frost Street, San Diego, CA 92123, USA
[2] Arizona Health Science Center, 1501 North Campbell Avenue, Tucson, AZ 85712, USA

Surgical Technique

The TAH is implanted through a median sternotomy under full cardiopulmonary bypass. Our preference is to cannulate the venae cavae directly with Pacifico cannulae. The heart is excised; care is taken to leave the great arteries long by dividing them at the level of the valve commissures. The atria are divided at the atrioventricular (AV) junction leaving the annuli in situ and with some rim of ventricular muscle, which is tailored further once the heart is removed, to provide tissue with maximal strength. The technique is otherwise fairly similar to that reported by Jarvik et al. [5]; we cut the atrial cuffs straight in the areas of the interatrial septum to facilitate a hemostatic suture line. Teflon felt is used to reinforce the suture lines.

Anticoagulation

Low-molecular-weight Dextran is started at the end of the operation and continued at a rate of 25 cc per hour, usually during the initial 6–12 h. If bleeding is not a problem, we then start heparin, with a target activated partial thromboplastin time (aPTT) of no greater than 40 s. Warfarin is initiated, usually within 24 h after starting the heparin so that the time of heparin is minimized. The heparin drip is continued until the International Normalized Ratio (INR) is at least 3–3.5. The target INR is between 4 and 5. Aspirin: 325 mg of enteric coated aspirin is given per 150 000 platelets. Ticlopidine is substituted for patients intolerant to aspirin. Dipyridamole is given at 100 mg p.o. q. 6 h per 100 000 platelets. Pentoxifylline (Trental) is given at a dose of 400 mg p.o. q. 8 h unless the fibrinogen remains elevated, in which case the dose is increased to 800 mg po every 8 h.

The anticoagulation protocols are modified if there is excessive bleeding and the patient requires reexploration.

Results

Duration of Support

The TAH was used from 1 h to 29 days. The patient who was supported for 1 h developed endobronchial

Table 1. Jarvik/CardioWest total artificial heart (TAH) as a bridge to transplant

Patient (age, sex)	Diagnosis	Date of implant	Duration of support
1. 36 M	Acute graft failure	June 15, 1987	12 days
2. 57 M	Acute graft failure	December 29, 1987	5 days
3. 59 M	Acute graft rejection — on ECMO	January 31, 1988	16 hours
4. 60 M	Acute graft failure — on ECMO 36 hours	April 13, 1994	1 hour
5. 62 M	After repair of infarct/ ventricular septal defect with RV/LV failure	February 17, 1996	18 days
6. 54 M	Acute RV infarct status post coronary artery bypass graft	April 6, 1996	29 days

M, male; ECMO, extracorporeal membrane oxygenation; RV/LV, right/left ventricle.

Table 2. Results

Patient	Complications	Survival posttransplantation	Cause of death
1	Coagulopathy, tamponade	Alive for 1 year, 1 month	Noncompliance, rejection
2	Coagulopathy	Alive at 9 years	—
3	Coagulopathy, pulmonary hypertension	Not bridged	Pulmonary hypertension, multiple organ failure
4	Coagulopathy, pulmonary hypertension, hemorrhage, multiple organ failure	Not bridged	Pulmonary thrombosis Hemorrhage, multiple organ failure
5	None	Alive at 7 months	—
6	Coagulopathy, renal failure	Alive at 5 months	—

hemorrhage secondary to pulmonary hypertension and diffuse pulmonary thrombosis. The TAH was ineffective owing to persistent bleeding and high pulmonary pressures.

One patient who was supported for 16h also developed supra-systemic pulmonary pressures and a severe coagulopathy, making the TAH ineffective.

The remaining four patients, supported between 5 and 29 days, were bridged to transplant.

Complications

The most common complication was coagulopathy which occurred in all but one patient. Tamponade requiring decompression occurred in one patient and reversible acute renal failure in one. The two patients supported less than 1 day developed multiple organ failure (Table 2). There were no thromboembolic complications of clinical significance.

The cause of death was pulmonary hypertension and coagulopathy in the two patients who could not be bridged to transplant, and non-compliance with chronic cardiac rejection 13 months after transplant in one patient.

Survival

One patient is alive 9 years after he was bridged to transplant with the TAH. The last two patients bridged in 1996 are also alive and well.

Comment

A clear indication for the use of the TAH is acute cardiac allograft failure when no other donor heart is available. This was the indication for use in four of our six patients: three of them with graft failure immediately after orthotopic transplantation and one with refractory rejection 1 month after transplantation.

The two patients with acute myocardial infarctions had severe structural damage to the right ventricle, precluding isolated left ventricular support.

The main complication was postoperative bleeding and the results were unfavorable on two patients who had been on extracorporeal membrane oxygenation (ECMO) prior to TAH implant. Both had severe pulmonary hypertension, and at autopsy we found diffuse microvascular pulmonary thrombosis in the patient who had been on ECMO for 36 h [6].

This experience suggests caution with the application of this technology on ECMO patients, as we were unsuccessful in two of our cases. The favorable results with the rest of our patients have encouraged us to continue using the CardioWest TAH as a bridge to a second transplant for patients with acute graft failure, and for patients with left ventricular failure associated with severe right ventricular dysfunction. The survival was 100% for patients who could be bridged to transplant.

References

1. Copeland JG, Emery RW, Levenson MM, Copeland J, McAleer MT, Riley JE (1985) The role of mechanical support and transplantation in the treatment of patients with end-stage cardiomyopathy. Circulation 72 (Suppl II):7–12

2. Joyce LD, Johnson KE, Pierce WS, DeVries WC, Semb BK, Copeland JG, Griffith BP, Cooley DA, Frazier OH, Cabrol C (1986) Summary of the world experience with the clinical use of total artificial hearts as heart support devices. J Heart Transplant 5:229–235

3. Rabago G, Gandjbakhch J, Pavh A, Bors V, Corbi P, Leger P, Levasseur JP, Vaissier E, Szefner J, Cabrol C, Cabrol A (1993) Bridge to transplant with the Symbion total artificial heart. In: Hanley & Belfus (ed), Cardiac surgery: state of the art reviews, vol 7, no. 2. Hanley & Belfus, Philadelphia, pp 439–446

4. Pifarré R, Sullivan HJ, Montoya A, Blakeman B, Calandra DB, Costanzo-Nordin MA, Lonchyna V, Hinkamp T, Walenga JM (1993) Bridge to transplantation with the total artificial heart: the Loyola experience. In: Cardiac surgery: state of the art reviews, vol 7, no. 2. Hanley and Belfus, Philadelphia, pp 447–455

5. Jarvik RK, DeVries WC, Semb BK, Koul B, Copeland JG, Levinson MM, Griffith BP, Joyce LD, Cooley DA, Frazier OH (1986) Surgical positioning of Jarvik-7 artificial heart. J Heart Transplant 5:184–195

6. Adamson RM, Dembitsky WP, Daily PO, Moreno-Cabral RJ, Copeland JG (1996) Immediate cardiac allograft failure: ECMO versus total artificial heart support. ASAIO J 42:314–316

Application of Adaptive Pole Assignment Method to Vascular Resistance-Based Control for Total Artificial Heart

Akira Tanaka[1], Makoto Yoshizawa[1], Ken-ichi Abe[1], Tomoyuki Yambe[2], and Shin-ichi Nitta[2]

Summary. A new vascular resistance based adaptive controller has been developed. A primary function of this controller is automatic adaptation for changes in cardiovascular dynamics with time, or for variation among individuals. Experiments were executed in a mock circulatory system. These experiments revealed that the proposed control system was able to automatically adjust cardiac output to maintain aortic pressure in accordance with artificial changes in peripheral vascular resistance.

Key words: Total artificial heart — Vascular resistance-based control — Adaptive control — Adaptive pole assignment method — ARMA model

Introduction

One of the most difficult problems in controlling the total artificial heart (TAH) is how to decide the reference value of cardiac output. This problem may be solved by using peripheral vascular resistance (R) because R is directly controlled by the remaining cardiovascular center through the autonomic nervous information, even after replacing the natural heart with the TAH.

Abe et al. [1] have successfully implemented this approach by using the $1/R$ control method. In this method, cardiac output depends linearly on the reciprocal of R (that is, the peripheral vascular conductance). However, the method requires a searching process to establish the coefficient depending on individual differences and experimental conditions. This constraint prevents us from applying the method to clinical use because the process must be done in a trial and error manner [2].

To cope with this defect, in the authors' previous study [3], a new adaptive controller based on vascular resistance was developed. However, this controller could not always keep the resulting closed-loop system stable because the controller operates by using the inverse system of an identified plant model.

To guarantee the stability of the closed-loop system in the present study, a controller has been developed by using the adaptive pole assignment method.

Methods

Structure of Controller

In our controller, the stroke volume of the right heart is automatically changed so that the difference between the right and left arterial pressures is kept constant, to maintain the balance of cardiac outputs of both sides of the heart. In contrast, the stroke volume of the left heart is automatically controlled to be constant by adjusting the filling and ejecting drive pressures.

In this situation, the cardiovascular system driven by a TAH can be roughly regarded as a two-input and two-output system, as shown in Fig. 1 (C).

Assume that the dynamics of $(HR, R) \rightarrow AOP$ in Fig. 1 (C) at the k-th beat can be expressed by the ARMA (auto-regressive moving average) model given by

$$A\left(z^{-1}\right)AOP\left(k\right) = B\left(z^{-1}\right)HR\left(k\right) + C\left(z^{-1}\right)R\left(k\right) \quad (1)$$

where $A(z^{-1})$, $B(z^{-1})$ and $C(z^{-1})$ are polynomials with coefficients a_1, a_2, b_1, b_2, c_1 and c_2 as follows:

$$A\left(z^{-1}\right) = 1 - a_1 z^{-1} - a_2 z^{-2} \quad (2)$$

$$B\left(z^{-1}\right) = b_1 z^{-1} + b_2 z^{-2} \quad (3)$$

$$C\left(z^{-1}\right) = c_1 z^{-1} + c_2 z^{-2} \quad (4)$$

The controller of the TAH [Fig. 1 (A)] manipulates the drive rate (HR) so that the aortic pressure (AOP) may approach its artificially given reference value ($AOP**$), by eliminating the disturbance effect of R on AOP. The aim of control is to satisfy Eq. 5 by manipulating $HR(k)$:

$$D\left(z^{-1}\right)AOP\left(k\right) = K \cdot B\left(z^{-1}\right)AOP** \quad (5)$$

where

$$D\left(z^{-1}\right) = 1 + \sum_{i=1}^{n_D} d_i z^{-i}, \quad K = \frac{D\left(1\right)}{B\left(1\right)} \quad (6)$$

[1] Department of Electrical Engineering, Tohoku University, Sendai 980-77, Japan
[2] Department of Medical Engineering and Cardiology, Institute of Development, Aging, and Cancer, Tohoku University, Sendai 980-77, Japan

Fig. 1. Circulatory control system after replacement of the natural heart with a total artificial heart (*TAH*). *AOP*, aortic pressure; *CO*, cardiac output; *HR*, heart drive rate; *R*, peripheral vascular resistance

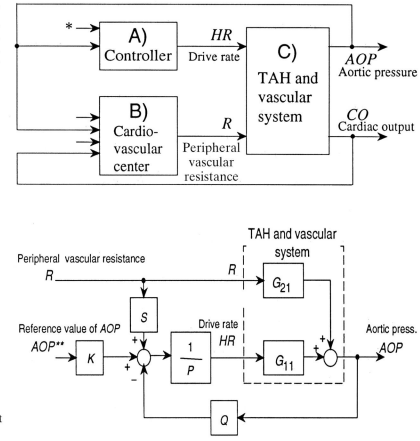

Fig. 2. Structure of the pole assignment controller

To guarantee the stability of the resulting closed-loop system, the coefficients d which are in the n_D-th order polynomial $D(z^{-1})$ should be chosen so that all poles of the closed-loop system are inside a unit disc. If the controller (A) is designed so that the manipulation of R directly affects the change in cardiac output (CO) with little change in AOP, it is possible that the cardiovascular center (B) can manipulate R to cause CO to approach its reference value CO^*, which we cannot know but the center can.

Identification Part

To adapt the controller of the TAH (A) to changes in cardiovascular dynamics such as time variation or individual differences, the controller estimates the coefficients included in Eqs. 2–4 by use of the least squares method given by

$$\hat{\theta}(k) = \hat{\theta}(k-1) - \frac{\Gamma(k-1)\xi(k)}{1+\xi^T(k)\Gamma(k-1)\xi(k)}e(k) \quad (7)$$

where $\hat{\theta}(k)$ is a coefficient vector of Eq. 1, $\Gamma(k)$ is a time-varying gain matrix, $\xi(k)$ is a data vector consisting of variables of Eq. 1, and $e(k)$ is an estimation error

of $AOP(k)$. $\Gamma(k)$ is changed so that its trace may be constant to avoid numerical overflow and underflow.

Pole Assignment Control Part

Figure 2 shows structure of the pole assignment controller. To guarantee stable closed-loop poles [4], the drive rate $HR(k)$ is determined in a real-time fashion to satisfy

$$P(z^{-1})HR(k) = K \cdot AOP^{**} - Q(z^{-1})AOP(k)$$
$$+ S(z^{-1})R(k) \quad (8)$$

where

$$P(z^{-1}) = 1 + \sum_{i=1}^{n_P} p_i z^{-i} \quad (9)$$

$$Q(z^{-1}) = \sum_{i=0}^{n_Q} q_i z^{-i} \quad (10)$$

$$S(z^{-1}) = \sum_{i=0}^{n_S} s_i z^{-i} \quad (11)$$

subject to

$$A(z^{-1})P(z^{-1}) + B(z^{-1})Q(z^{-1}) = D(z^{-1}) \quad (12)$$

$$B\left(z^{-1}\right)S\left(z^{-1}\right)+C\left(z^{-1}\right)P\left(z^{-1}\right)=0 \qquad (13)$$

To obtain a solution of Eqs. 12, 13 in a real-time fashion, in the present study, the order of Eq. 9 to Eq. 11 were set such that $n_p = 1$, $n_Q = 1$, $n_s = 1$. Hence, explicit expression of $HR(k)$ included in Eq. 8 is

$$HR\left(k\right)=\frac{1}{b_1+b_2}AOP^{**}-p_1HR\left(k-1\right)-q_0AOP\left(k\right)$$
$$-q_1AOP\left(k-1\right)+s_0R\left(k\right)+s_1R\left(k-1\right) \qquad (14)$$

Experiments

The proposed controller was implemented on a personal computer system (PC-9801RA; NEC, Tokyo, Japan). Experiments were executed in a mock circulatory system consisting of water tanks, tubes, and two (left and right) air-driven ventricular assist devices.

The maximum volume of each device was 60 ml. Each stroke volume was automatically regulated to approach the reference value by means of proportional/integral (PI)-control of air pressure.

To examine the vascular resistance-dependent behavior of the proposed controller, R was changed as a rectangular wave form by manually manipulating a tap placed on the corresponding tube. In nature, R is varied by the cardiovascular center.

Results

Figure 3 shows the variation of the cardiovascular parameters with the number of beats.

In itially, it took about 20 beats for the parameter vector $\hat{\theta}$ to converge to the steady state value from the zero vector. In Fig. 3, the transient state for the initial 100 beats is not depicted.

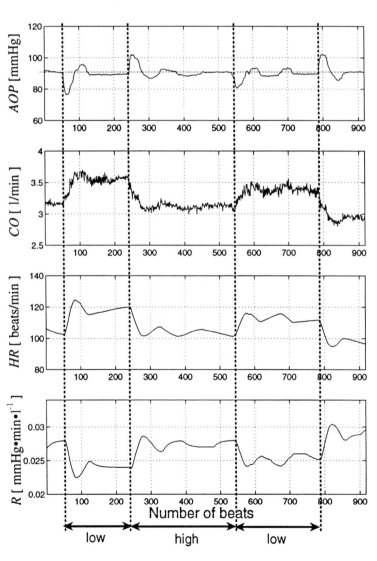

Fig. 3. Results of experiments in mock circulatory system

The vertical broken line indicates the time when the sudden change in R occurred. It can be seen that a decrease in R yielded an increase in CO, and vice versa, so as to maintain AOP at its reference value $AOP^{**} = 90\,mmHg$. This resulted in behavior similar to that with $1/R$ control.

Discussion

The $1/R$ control method needs to determine the value of the control parameter in a trial-and-error manner. As previously reported, the closed-loop system will easily diverge if the value of this parameter is not correct [2]. On the other hand, because of the adaptation mechanism, the method proposed here can avoid this trial-and-error searching process, with the exception that the value of AOP^{**} must be set for each individual. However, this process may not be difficult because it is easy to measure and analyze the recipient's AOP before implantation of the TAH.

The difference between the previous controller in [3] and the present one is that we have introduced the adaptive pole assignment method. In the previous controller, even if the coefficients represented by Eq. 1 of the plant can be successfully identified, the stability of the closed-loop system cannot be guaranteed because the inverse system of the plant is explicitly employed. On the other hand, the controller proposed here can make the closed-loop system always stable as long as the plant identification is completed.

Of course, if the identification is not sufficiently completed or not realized, the resulting control behavior will become inappropriate. This may occur in two situations. One is the case where the plant is in a transient state after an abrupt change in conditions. This case includes the initial state. The other situation is where the plant cannot be modelled by the linear model proposed here. If the actual cardiovascular dynamics are strongly nonlinear, the proposed adaptive controller will not be applicable.

To cope with such misidentification, the error $e(k)$ between AOP and its estimated value must be always monitored, and the feedback loop should be cut as soon as possible if the absolute value of $e(k)$ is beyond a given threshold. The value of the summation of b_1 and b_2 in Eq. 3 expresses the contribution of HR to AOP. Hence, the feedback loop should be also cut if the value becomes low.

The proposed method requires continuous measurements of flow and pressure. Because of low reliability of measuring these values inside the body in the long term, it would be difficult to apply our method to an implantable artificial heart at present. In the future, however, this defect will be improved because it is possible to extract hemodynamic parameters from more reliable signals such as the position of the pusher plate and the electrical voltage or current of the actuator, by using mathematical estimation methods [5,6].

Conclusion

In the present study, the adequacy of control behavior of the proposed adaptive control system could be roughly ascertained in a mock circulatory system. A number of animal experiments and further refinements, especially for nonlinearity of the plant model or the condition of persistent excitation [4], are needed before the system can be applied to clinical use.

References

1. Abe Y, Imachi K, Chinzei T, Mabuchi K, Imanishi K, Isoyama T, Yonezawa T, Kouno A, Ono T, Atsumi K, Fujimasa I (1993) Reciprocal of the peripheral vascular resistance (1/R) control method for the total artificial heart. In: Akutsu T, Koyanagi H (eds) Artificial heart 4. Springer, Tokyo, pp 349–351
2. Yoshizawa M, Hashiya H, Takeda H, Yambe T, Nitta S (1993) Simulation study on 1/R control strategy of the artificial heart. In: Sezai Y (ed) Artificial heart 1993. Harwood Academic, Chur, pp 123–127
3. Tanaka A, Yoshizawa M, Abe K, Yambe T, Nitta S, Takeda H, Chinzei T, Fujimasa I, Abe Y, Imachi K (1995) Design of adaptive control system for total artificial heart. Jpn J Artif Organs 24(5):976–981
4. Goodwin GC, Sin KS (1984) Adaptive filtering prediction and control. Prentice-Hall, Englewood Cliffs
5. Holzer S, Scherer R, Schmidt C, Schwendenwein I, Wieselthaler G, Noisser R, Schima H (1995) A clinical monitoring system for centrifugal blood pumps. Artif Organs 19(7):708–712
6. Snyder AJ (1987) Automatic electronic control of an electric motor-driven total artificial heart. Dissertation, Pennsylvania State University

Relationship Between Atrial Pressures and the Interventricular Pressure in the Moving Actuator Type Total Artificial Heart

Y.H. Jo[1], W.W. Choi[2], J.M. Ahn[1], S.K. Park[1], J.J. Lee[2], K.S. Om[2], J.S. Choi[2], W.K. Kim[3], Y.S. Won[4], H.C. Kim[1], and B.G. Min[1]

Summary. The right and left atrial pressures are important parameters in the automatic control of a total artificial heart (TAH) within normal physiological ranges. Our TAH is composed of a moving actuator, right and left ventricles, and the interventricular space (IVS) enclosed by a semirigid housing. During operation of the TAH, the IVS volume is changed dynamically by the difference between the ejection volume of one ventricle and the inflow volume of the other. Therefore, the change in pressure of the IVS is related to both right and left atrial pressures. We measured the interventricular pressure (IVP) waveform using a pressure sensor and attempted to estimate indirectly the changes in atrial pressures. This method has the advantage that the sensor does not contact the blood directly. Furthermore, the IVP waveform has a zero baseline in each pump cycle, thus the pressure measurements are free from transducer drift problems because the peak pressure can be measured from these baseline values. From in vitro experiments, we found that the IVP waveform contained several useful parameters such as negative peak IVP value, dP/dt on the initial break, and the area enclosed by the profile for each stroke, each of which are associated with the left and right atrial pressures and the filling conditions of the ventricles. The measured atrial pressures were linearly related to the negative peak value of the interventricular pressure.

Key words: Total artificial heart — Interventricular pressure — Atrial pressure — Moving actuator

Introduction

The left atrial pressure (LAP) is about 8 mmHg (2–12 mmHg) [1] in the healthy human, and dyspnea occurs when the LAP is over 20 mmHg. Moreover, pulmonary edema occurs when the LAP is over 30 mmHg. On the other hand, atrial collapse, normally prevented by ventricular inflow, occurs when the right atrial pressure drops below atmospheric pressure (0 mmHg). Under normal circumstances, the human heart maintains atrial pressures precisely within the physiological range using spontaneous regulation of the heart itself, neuronal regulation through the sympathetic and parasympathetic nervous systems, and humoral regulation by factors such as hormones [2].

For automatic control of the total artificial heart (TAH), one important objective is to obtain precise information on the atrial pressures, and regulate those pressures within the desired range. In this paper, we estimated in vitro and in vivo the right and left atrial pressures from the pressure waveform obtained using a pressure sensor located in the interventricular space (IVS).

Materials and Methods

Materials

Our TAH is composed of a moving actuator, right and left ventricles, and an IVS enclosed by a semirigid polyurethane housing. There is a flexible window (7 cm × 5 cm) attached to the anterior surface of the TAH in order to prevent excessive negative pressure generation in the IVS. The window has a role of damping the pressure changes by moving itself inward and outward passively about 5 mm according to the interventricular pressure (IVP). Therefore, the window has an effective volume-compensation capacity of about 15 mℓ of IVS (Fig. 1).

The TAH contains about 100 ml air as a compliance chamber for the compensation of the right and left cardiac output balance, and 80 ml lubricant oil for lubrication of the moving actuator and heat dispersion from the actuator to the TAH wall. We used water instead of blood as a circulating fluid. A polygraph (MCS — 5000, Fukuda Denshi, Tokyo, Japan) was used to display various signals. A flow meter (T 201 2-channel ultrasonic bloodflow meter, Transonic Systems, NY, USA) was used to measure the inflow and the outflow.

[1] Department of Biomedical Engineering, College of Medicine, [2] Interdisciplinary program, Biomedical Engineering, and [3] Department of Thoracic Surgery, College of Medicine, Seoul National University, 28 Youngun-Dong, Chongno-Ku, Seoul 110-744, Korea
[4] Department of Thoracic Surgery, College of Medicine, Ehwa Women's University, 11-1 Daehyun-Dong, Seodaemun-ku, Seoul 120-750, Korea

Fig. 1. The flexible window (7 cm × 5 cm) (*arrows*) attached to the anterior surface of the total artificial heart. The interventricular space contains about 100 ml air (*broken arrow*) and 80 ml lubricating oil, and the volume-compensation capacity of the window is 15 ml

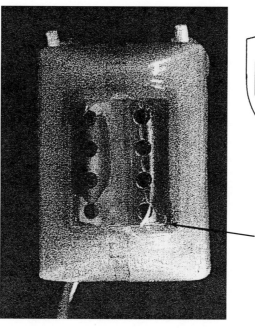

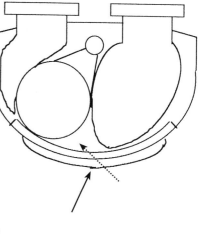

Methods

To analyze the characteristics of the IVP waveform, we settled on a mock circulation system with synchronization of pressures (IVP, aortic pressure, and right and left atrial pressures), a flows (aortic outflow, pulmonary outflow, and right and left atrial inflows), and the motor direction signal; a break signal indicated the actuator position. The direction signal shows high state in right stroke period and the break signal shows high state during the motor stopping period.

Results and Discussion

Principle of the IVP Waveform Generation

During operation of the TAH, the IVS volume is changed dynamically by the difference between the ejection volume of one ventricle and the inflow volume of the other, because the volume of the moving actuator is constant [3]. For example, during left systole, the ejection volume of the left ventricle is larger than the inflow volume into the right ventricle in the initial phase. The volume difference is partly compensated by passive inward movement of the window, and the remaining volume difference is reflected in an increase in IVS volume. Therefore, the interventricular volume pressure (IVP) is decreased in the initial phase (Fig. 2).

The IVP negative peak is observed when the inflow volume is the same as the ejection volume. Because the dynamic volume of both ejecting and filling ventricles is not changed. The IVP increases again in the

final phase because the inflow volume is larger than the ejection volume.

Relationship Between Atrial Pressures and the IVP

We already mentioned that the IVP waveform reflects the diastole filling status at that moment. Because the atrial pressure influences the filling condition of the blood sac, we can estimate the atrial pressures from the IVP waveform at both pump strokes. During left systole, the IVP waveform reflects the volume of blood filling the right sac and the right atrial pressure, and vice versa during right systole.

Figure 3 shows the IVP waveform at various right atrial pressures (RAP) but constant left atrial pressure (LAP), and also shows both rates of outflow over the same period. The IVP negative peak values at left systole decrease linearly (i.e., become more negative) with the decrease in RAP from 10 mmHg to −5 mmHg.

Figure 4 shows the relationship between LAP and IVP with time, and Fig. 5 is a linear regression graph of LAP against IVP. The correlation was marked ($r = 0.88$). We performed an experiment with a male sheep weighing 55 kg to confirm the in vitro tests. Figure 6 shows the time course of LAP (lower trace), the IVP at the right stroke (upper trace, circles joined by broken line) and the aortic pressure (middle trace).

As with the in vitro results, the in vivo finding indicates that we can use the IVP negative peak value as a useful parameter to satisfy the goal of maintaining control of atrial pressures within the desired range. This is an important consideration, given that the pa-

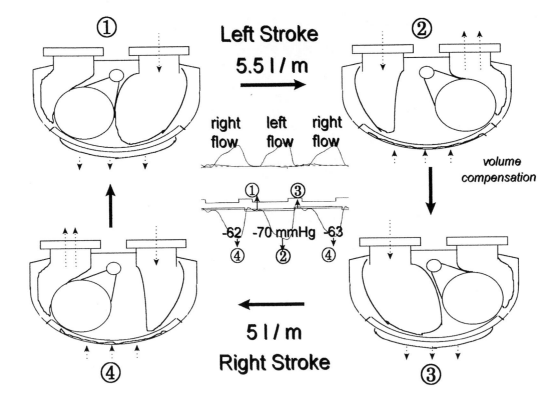

Fig. 2. The principle of the interventricular pressure (IVP) waveform generation. The *circled numbers* on the IVP waveform (*lower trace*) correspond to the respective part of the pump cycle

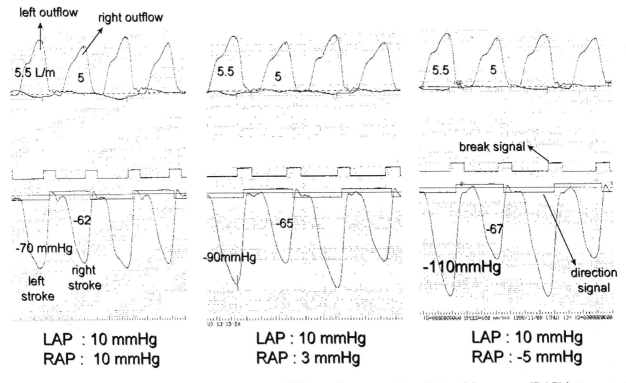

Fig. 3. In vitro tests. Interventricular volume pressure (IVP) waveforms at various right atrial pressures (RAP) but constant left atrial pressure (LAP). Rates of outflow over the same period are also shown

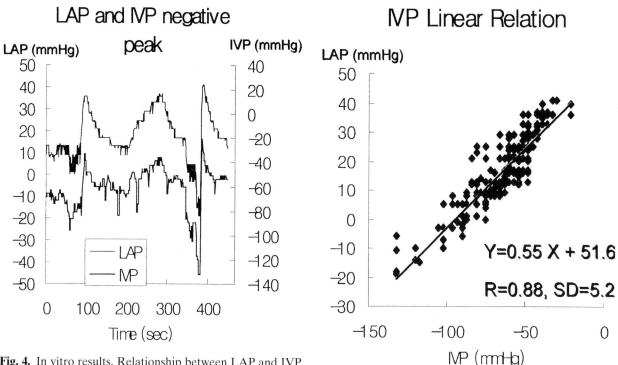

Fig. 4. In vitro results. Relationship between LAP and IVP with time

Fig. 5. In vitro results. Linear regression of LAP against IVP

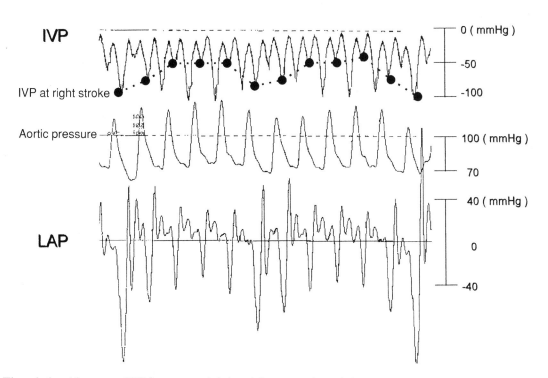

Fig. 6. The relationship among IVP (*upper trace*), left atrial pressure (*LAP*) (*lower trace*), and aortic pressure (*middle trace*). The IVP at the right pump stroke is indicated by *circles* linked by *dotted line*

tient needing TAH implantation has a high LAP and an active filling device such as our TAH has a suction problem.

This method has the advantages of avoiding thrombogenesis and bacterial niche formation, and increasing the long-term reliability of the pressure sensor, because it does not contact blood directly.

Conclusion

We showed that the IVP waveform represented the volume difference between the right and left blood sacs, and especially the filling status of the diastolic blood sac. We also showed by both in vitro and in vivo

tests that the IVP negative peak value will be a good information source for the control of the TAH, because the IVP negative peak value has a strong correlation with both right and left atrial pressures.

References

1. Grossman W (1986) Cardiac catheterization and angiography, 3rd edn. Lea and Febiger, Philadelphia
2. Schmidt RF, Thews G (1989) Human physiology. Springer, New York
3. Chun G (1988) A study on the mechanical design of motor-driven artificial heart. Ph.D dissertation, Seoul National University, Seoul

Progress in Developing a Permanent Totally Implantable Pulsatile Impeller Total Artificial Heart

K.X. Qian and M. Zheng

Summary. For heart replacement or biventricular assist, the impeller total artificial heart (TAH) has many advantages as compared with the diaphragm TAH: it needs no valves and no diaphragms; its volume and weight can be reduced and minimized because its output can be enlarged by increasing the rotating speed; the volume equilibrium of both pumps can be achieved naturally, due to the self-modulation property of the impeller pumps; etc. Further improvements have recently been made to the authors' implantable pulsatile impeller TAH: (1) the driving brushless d.c. motor and the left and right pumps are now compacted into one unit; thus the system has only one moving part, which rotates without contact with the stator, by using magnetic suspension so as to eliminate mechanical wear; (2) the logarithmic spiral impeller vanes are now manufactured by computerized wire-cut according to their design analytical expressions, thus improving the accuracy and dynamic balance of the rotor; and (3) to reduce or eliminate the need for anticoagulation therapy, all the blood-contacting surfaces in the pumps and cannulae have been bonded with heparin. The impeller TAH is at present unique: it is driven by a single motor, both pumps eject blood simultaneously, and volume equilibrium can be achieved without the need for a separate control.

Key words: Impeller pump — Total artificial heart — Blood compatibility — Mechanical reliability — Magnetically suspended motor

Introduction

The impeller total artificial heart (TAH) was developed and reports published in the mid-1980s [1,2], but its in vivo evaluation began in the early 1990s, at first in pigs [3,4] and then in calves (Fig. 1), as a biventricular assist device. As compared with the traditional diaphragm TAH, the impeller TAH has many inherent advantages in simplicity, implantability, biocompatibility, reliability, and so forth. It promises to be a viable alternative to, and to have more applications than, the problematic diaphragm TAH. With the recently developed magnetically suspended motor, the

Institute of Biomedical Engineering and Artificial Heart Laboratory, Jiangsu University of Science and Technology, Jiangsu 212013, China

impeller TAH will be able to be used in long-term and permanent experiments.

Prototype of the Impeller TAH

Device Description

The impeller TAH is driven by a single motor with double output shafts, on which the left and right impellers are fixed. As a square-wave voltage is introduced into the motor coil, both impellers rotate at a periodically changed speed, and the left and right pumps produce a pulsatile blood flow. The systolic and diastolic pressures in the aorta and pulmonary main artery can be adjusted by controlling the voltage peak and valley values. The left and right pumps eject blood simultaneously without the need for compliance chambers. Since the left and the right pumps deliver the same blood volume, but against different pressures, the left and right impellers have different dimensions (Fig. 2). Volume equilibrium in both pumps is achieved naturally, due to the self-modulation property of the impeller pump; that is, the flow rate increases if the afterload decreases, and vice versa. The seals and the bearings in the prototye of the impeller TAH are similar to those used in the Biopump (Medtronic Bio-Medicus, Eden Prairie, MN, USA), with the exception that an improvement was made by substituting the ball bearing in the Biopump with a slide bearing.

Advantages of Impeller TAH

As compared with the traditional diaphragm TAH, the impeller TAH has many inherent advantages in:

1. *Simplicity*. The device has only one moving part. It needs no valves and no diaphragms.
2. *Implantability*. The volume and the weight of the impeller TAH can be reduced and minimized because its output can be enlarged by increasing the rotation speed.
3. *Biocompatibility*. Because of its simplicity and relative large ratio between flow rate and the blood

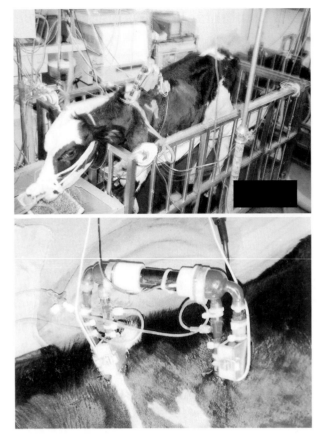

Fig. 1. The biventricular assist experiment in calves with an impeller total artificial heart (TAH)

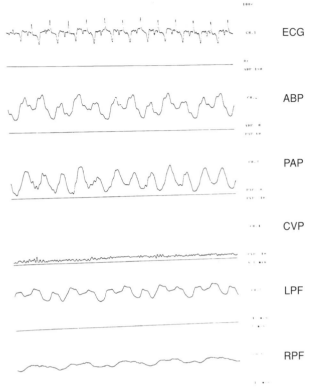

Fig. 3. Physiological measurements of biventricular assisted animals. From *top* to *bottom*: ECG, arterial blood pressure (ABP), pulmonary arterial pressure (PAP), central venous pressure (CVP), left pump flow (LPF), right pump flow (RPF)

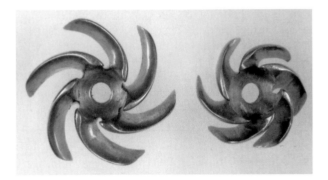

Fig. 2. The left impeller (*left*) and the right impeller (*right*)

chamber volume, the impeller TAH has better anti-thrombogenesis and resistance to hemolysis than the diaphragm TAH.

4. *Simultaneous ejection*. The impeller TAH is driven by a single motor, and the left and the right pump eject the blood simultaneously, without a need for compliance chambers.

5. *Volume equilibrium*. In the impeller TAH, there is no need for controlling the volume equilibrium of both pumps; because the impeller pump has the ability to self-modulate, its output flow changes according to its afterload.

6. *Hemodynamics*. The impeller TAH can produce a pulsatile flow, thus it can maintain a pulsatile perfusion, so as not to increase the resistance in the microcirculation, as nonpulsatile flow is acknowledged to do. Furthermore, the impeller TAH has no back-flow and can increase the diastolic pressure; this is beneficial for increasing the perfusion in the coronary artery, and for facilitating the recovery of the natural heart during biventricular assist.

7. *Reliability*. The impeller TAH has only one moving part, thus increasing its reliability. The sole problem, bearing wear, promises to be solved by the development of a magnetically suspended motor.

First Results of In Vivo Studies

In both 6-h acute experiments in five pigs and survival experiments in three calves lasting for up to 1 week, the biventricular assist impeller TAH demonstrated its excellent biocompatibility: no blood damage or organ dysfunction was detected in the animals. The physiological measurements during the experiments indicated the suitability of the device for the animals (Fig. 3). By autopsy, neither severe thrombus nor serious embolus formation was found, either in the pump or the vessels.

On the basis of previous results obtained with the authors' left ventricular assist impeller pump, which enabled experimental animals to survive for up to 2 months [5,6], the impeller TAH has been prepared for applications of a few months' duration.

Improved Type of the Impeller TAH

The initial goal of research and development toward a TAH is to assist or replace the natural heart for periods up to several years. In developing such a permanent impeller TAH, some new advances have been achieved recently.

To overcome the main obstacle of bearing wear, a magnetically suspended motor is now in investigation. On the opposite sides of a disc, which is connected to the rotor axis, two magnetic rings are embedded, one for driving and the other for suspending (Fig. 4). The disc is driven by a motor coil to rotate, and its axial position is maintained by suspending the coil to avoid any contact with the stator. Since both coils with iron cores attract the disc, no radial bearing is needed. The same principle for suspension has been successfully employed in the Kyoto University Centrifugal Pump

[7–9]. The magnetic suspension principle promises to overcome, finally, the obstacle of bearing wear.

To achieve stability of the suspended rotor, the accuracy and the dynamic balance of the rotor has been improved by manufacturing the impeller with computerized wire-cut, according to their analytical expressions.

Lastly, for further improvement of the blood compatibility of the device, particularly for reducing or eliminating anticoagulation therapy in experiments or clinical applications, all the blood-contacting surfaces in the pumps and cannulae have been bonded with heparin.

Discussion

It has been controversial whether nonpulsatile perfusion will detrimentally increase the resistance in the microcirculation. Thus, the question arises whether a rotary TAH is possible, because most experts consider the rotary pump nonpulsatile. However, it is not true that a rotary pump can only produce a nonpulsatile flow. Over the past 12 years, our group has published numerous papers about pulsatile impeller assist and total artificial hearts. Regretably, this work has so far largely been ignored and disregarded.

The impeller TAH is continuously being developed and improved. It meets with almost all the requirements of a TAH. With a magnetically suspended motor, the newly devised impeller TAH promises to have long-term and permanent application.

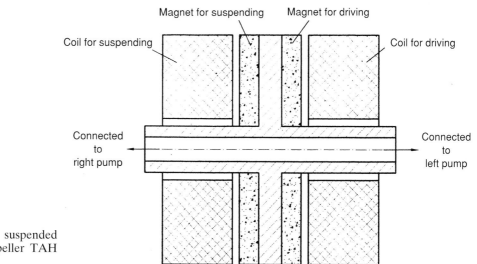

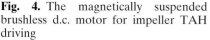
Fig. 4. The magnetically suspended brushless d.c. motor for impeller TAH driving

Acknowledgments. This work is supported by the Chinese National Foundation for Natural Sciences.

References

1. Qian KX, Pi KD, Wang YP (1982) Toward an implantable total impeller heart. ASAIO Trans 33(3):704–707
2. Qian KX (1990) A new total heart design via implantable impeller pumps. J Biomater Appl 4(4):405–418
3. Qian KX, Wang SS, Chu SH (1994) In vivo evaluations of pulsatile impeller total heart. ASAIO Trans 40(2):213–215
4. Qian KX, Wang SS, Chu SH (1996) Haematological variations in experimental pigs during biventricular assistance with impeller total heart. J Med Eng Phys 18(1):67–69
5. Qian KX, Zheng M (1997) Chronic left ventricular assist in calves with a pulsatile impeller pump. ASAIO J 43(1):89–91
6. Qian KX, Zheng M. Long-term survival of calves with a left ventricular assist impeller pump. J Med Eng Phys (in press)
7. Akamatsu T, Nakaxzedi T, Itoh H (1992) Centrifugal blood pump with a magnetically suspended impeller. Artif Organs 16(3):305–308
8. Akamatsu T, Tsukiya T, Nishimura K, Park CH, Nakazeki T (1995) Recent studies of the centrifugal blood pump with a magnetically suspended impeller. Artif Organs 19(7):631–634
9. Park CH, Nishimura K, Yamada T, Mizuhara H, Akamatsu T, Tsukiya T, Matsuda K, Ban T (1995) A magnetically suspended centrifugal pump. ASAIO J 41:M345–350

The Combined Use of Extra-Aortic Balloon Counterpulsation and a Ventricular Assist Cup for Acute Heart Failure in Dogs — Effects on Regional Blood Flow

Atsuhiro Mitsumaru[1], Ryohei Yozu[1], Shinichi Taguchi[1], Hiroshi Odaguchi[1], Ryuichi Takahashi[1], Tadashi Omoto[1], Hiroshi Yoshito[2], Katsuki Kanda[2], Yoko Tsutsui[2], Nobumasa Tsutsui[2], and Shiaki Kawada[1]

Summary. We evaluated the applicability and effectiveness of support with a combination of an extra-aortic balloon (EAB) and a ventricular assist cup (VAC), using an acute heart failure model. Under general anesthesia, ten adult dogs were used. Through median sternotomy, an EAB was placed around the ascending aorta and a VAC in the pericardial cavity. After heart failure was induced by the administration of propranolol, on–off tests of devices were performed as follows: EAB only; VAC only; and both devices in operation. Regional blood flows (RBFs) in both ventricles and in the liver, kidney, and brain were measured using a colored microsphere technique. Aortic flow and cardiac output were also measured. In the heart failure model, aortic flow and cardiac output decreased to 65% and 66% of the control value, respectively. With assistance by the EAB only, RBFs in both ventricle and brain increased significantly. With only the VAC on, RBFs in all but the left ventricle significantly increased. With both the EAB and the VAC on, all five RBFs significantly increased. These results suggest that the combination of EAB and VAC is applicable and effective, and would be a very promising implantable device for chronic heart failure.

Key words: Heart assist device — Counterpulsation — Acute heart failure model — Regional blood flow — Colored microsphere

Introduction

A circulatory assist device without any blood-contacting surfaces would be desirable. Recently, we developed the extra-aortic balloon (EAB), which improved both myocardial oxygen supply and demand balance with the endocardial viability ratio. However, the influence of the extra-aortic balloon counterpulsation (EABC) at the ascending aorta on regional blood flows (RBFs) in the other vital organs is still unknown. We also developed the ventricular assist cup (VAC) to assist circulation during the systolic phase. In this study, we assessed the effect of the VAC combined with the EAB from the viewpoint of RBFs, using the acute heart failure model in dogs.

Materials and Methods

The VAC consists of a urethane membrane, a stainless steel wire, and a urethane cup. The membrane is bonded to the edge of the cup and designed so that it fits to the inside of the cup when deflated. The wire prevents the membrane from pushing out the ventricles and divides the membrane into two parts. The VAC has the connecting port at the bottom and is connected to a pneumomatic ventricular assist device driving a console (VCT 20, TOYOBO, Osaka, Japan). The components of the EAB were described in detail in our previous report [1]. The EAB has a polyurethane balloon, fitted inside the balloon holder. Extra-aortic balloon counterpulsation (EABC) is generated by inflating and deflating the balloon in the holder, which grips the ascending aorta. The balloon catheter is connected to the pulsatile bypass pump (Avco, Cranberry, NJ, USA). The timing of balloon inflation and deflation is synchronized with the dicrotic notch of the aortic pressure and the end of diastole, respectively.

Ten adult mongrel dogs weighing 11.3–14.5 kg were used in this study. They were anesthetized with sodium pentobarbital (25 mg/kg i.v.), intubated, and mechanically ventilated with room air at tidal volume 15 ml/mg and a rate of 12 per minute. The anesthesia was continued by additional administration of sodium pentobarbital and pancuronium bromide. Median sternotomy was performed. Magnetic blood flow probes (Nihon Kohden, Tokyo, Japan) were placed around the innominate artery and the distal aorta. A Swan-Ganz catheter (93-631-5.5F, Baxter, Irvine, CA, USA) was inserted from the right femoral vein to the pulmonary artery. Cardiac output was measured by a cardiac output computer (SAT-2-100, Baxter). A fluid-filled catheter was inserted from the right upper pulmonary vein to the left atrium for administration of colored microspheres. Two epicardial leads were placed on the inflow and outflow portion of the right ventricle and connected to a polygraph (RPM-6008M,

[1] Department of Surgery, Keio University, 35 Shinanomachi, Shinjuku-ku, Tokyo 160, Japan
[2] Tokai Medical Incorporated, 1485 Sarayashiki, Taragacho, Kasugai, Aichi 486, Japan

Nihon Kohden). The signal from the epicardial lead was delivered to two driving consoles through the polygraph to synchronize the devices with the heart. A catheter was placed into the left femoral artery and connected to a syringe pump (CFV-3200, Nihon Kohden) for withdrawal of a reference blood sample. Another catheter was placed into the left femoral vein for administration of drugs and fluid. The EAB was placed around the ascending aorta. The VAC was placed in the pericardial cavity to cover both ventricles.

After the installation of the two devices, the control data were obtained. Then, acute heart failure was induced by administration of propranolol hydrochloride (Sigma, St. Louis, Mo, USA; 2 mg/kg i.v. and 50 µg/kg continuous i.v.). After hemodynamic parameters were stabilized, the hemodynamic parameters were measured with the device(s) off, and repeat measurements were obtained 20 min after the device(s) were turned on. In all ten dogs, these on–off tests were performed in three ways. In test 1, the EAB only was used. In test 2, the VAC only was used. In test 3, both the EAB and VAC were used. The aortic blood flow was calculated by the addition of the blood flow values obtained with two magnetic flow probes. Cardiac output was determined by the average of three to five measurements. During measurement, the respirator was temporarily turned off.

In this study, polystyrene microspheres of seven different colors (E-Z Trac, Los Angeles, CA, USA) with a diameter of 15 µm were used. Before each injection, five million colored microspheres were mixed with 10 ml of normal saline and agitated in a vortex mixer for 1 min. In each phase of an on–off test, colored microspheres were injected into the left atrial catheter for 10 s and the catheter was flushed with 10 ml of normal saline. Ten seconds before the injection, the reference blood sample was withdrawn from the catheter placed into the left femoral artery at a speed of 10 ml/min for 90 s. After the completion of measure-

ments, the dogs were killed with potassium chloride. After death, tissue samples were obtained from a free wall of the left ventricle, a free wall of the right ventricle, the liver, the kidney and the left hemisphere. RBFs were also calculated using the colored microsphere technique [2]. In this study, the regional blood flow in liver indicates the hepatic artery blood flow.

The results of the on–off tests were assessed by the paired t-test. Statistical significance was considered at a P value < 0.05.

Results

By the administration of propranolol, aortic blood flow and cardiac output were reduced to 67% and 66% of the control value, respectivley. In test 1 (EAB only on), regional blood flows in the left and right ventricles and the brain were significantly increased. In test 2 (VAC only on), the aortic blood flow and cardiac output were significantly increased. The regional blood flows in the right ventricle, liver, kidney, and brain were significantly increased. However, there was no significant change in the regional blood flow in the left ventricle. In test 3 (both devices on), the aortic blood flow and cardiac output were significantly increased. All five regional blood flows were significantly increased (Table 1).

Discussion

This study demonstrates the useful effects of EAB and VAC on regional blood flows in vital organs. In test 1, EABC significantly increased regional blood flows in both ventricles. The regional blood flow in brain also significantly increased. In test 2, both cardiac ouput and aortic blood flow increased significantly. Consequently, the regional blood flows in liver, kidney, and

Table 1. Changes in regional blood flows and hemodynamic parameters

	Control	EAB		VAC		EAB + VAC	
		Off	On	Off	On	Off	On
LV (ml·min^{-1}·g^{-1})	1.19 ± 0.21	0.64 ± 0.16	0.80 ± 0.24**	0.56 ± 0.16	0.59 ± 0.18	0.53 ± 0.14	0.74 ± 0.21**
RV (ml·min^{-1}·g^{-1})	0.82 ± 0.14	0.41 ± 0.11	0.50 ± 0.13**	0.36 ± 0.10	0.39 ± 0.11**	0.38 ± 0.09	0.53 ± 0.12**
Liver[a] (ml·min^{-1}·g^{-1})	0.43 ± 0.14	0.15 ± 0.06	0.16 ± 0.07	0.13 ± 0.05	0.17 ± 0.06**	0.12 ± 0.06	0.18 ± 0.08**
Kidney (ml·min^{-1}·g^{-1})	2.34 ± 0.41	1.55 ± 0.53	1.53 ± 0.57	1.29 ± 0.40	1.54 ± 0.53**	1.26 ± 0.48	1.54 ± 0.55**
Brain (ml·min^{-1}·g^{-1})	0.66 ± 0.16	0.36 ± 0.16	0.43 ± 0.17*	0.31 ± 0.08	0.37 ± 0.09**	0.31 ± 0.08	0.42 ± 0.11**
AoF (l·min^{-1})	1.50 ± 0.56	1.06 ± 0.45	1.16 ± 0.45	1.00 ± 0.47	1.23 ± 0.49**	1.07 ± 0.45	1.21 ± 0.47**
CO (l·min^{-1})	1.46 ± 0.35	0.97 ± 0.25	0.98 ± 0.26	0.88 ± 0.28	1.11 ± 0.37**	0.89 ± 0.26	1.15 ± 0.35**

EAB, extra-aortic balloon; VAC, ventricular assist cup; LV, left ventricle; RV, right ventricle. AoF, aortic blood flow; CO, cardiac output.
*P < 0.05 vs off value; **P < 0.01 vs off value.
[a] Hepatic artery blood flow.

brain were significantly increased. The regional blood flow in the left ventricle did not change significantly, because the VAC has no effect during the diastolic phase, and the coronary perfusion mainly occurs during the diastolic phase [3]. On the other hand, regional blood flow in the right ventricle increased significantly, because the compressive forces exerted by the right ventricle were far less than those exerted by the left ventricle, and perfusion of the right ventricle was not interrupted during systole [4]. In test 3, the beneficial effect of using both the EAB and VAC was shown. Theoretically, the VAC supports both ventricles. However, pulmonary systolic pressure did not significantly change in test 3, though it significantly increased in test 2. This suggests that the VAC moved from the ideal position in test 3. This problem is crucial, and must be addressed before chronic use of these devices.

Methods of assisted circulation that involve no blood-contacting surface do not require any anticoagulant therapy. They can avoid the risk of embolism and hemorrhage. Among these methods, cardiomyoplasty and/or aortomyoplasty and direct mechanical ventricular actuation (DMVA) are used for mechanical circulatory support, experimentally and clinically [5,6]. Takahashi and co-workers reported that assisted circulation using both dynamic cardiomyoplasty and aortoplasty improved left ventricular function in an acute heart failure model [7]. Dynamic cardiomyoplasty and aortoplasty could be as promising as some biomechanical assist devices, because they use one's own skeletal muscles. However, enlarged heart size is a serious limitation to muscle wrapping, particularly when the size of the muscle flap is small [5].

The mechanism of DMVA is as follows: positive and negative pneumomatic forces operate on a diaphragm within the cup to actuate the ventricles into respective systolic and diastolic configurations. Our VAC was designed to have a systolic configuration like DMVA, and it assisted circulation during the systolic phase. It did not provide circulatory assistance during the diastolic phase, so we used the VAC combined with the EAB. As the VAC and EAB operate in opposite phases, a single controller could control both devices. Though further improvements are required, this device is unique for its technical simplicity, easy installation, and absence of blood contact. With this device, an electric driver such as an axillar pump, which normally generates nonpulsatile flow, can produce pulsatile flow. These characteristics are advantageous for potential use an implantable assist device (Fig. 1).

In conclusion, the combination of the EAB and VAC is applicable and effective, and is a very promising implantable device for chronic heart failure.

References

1. Odaguchi H, Yozu R, Kashima I, Mitsumaru A, Kanda K, Tsutsui N, Tsutsui Y, Kawada S (1996) Experimental study of extraaortic balloon counterpulsation as a bridge to other mechanical assists. ASAIO J 42:190–194
2. Hale SL, Alker KJ, Kloner RA (1988) Evaluation of nonradioactive, colored microspheres for measurement of regional myocardial blood flow in dogs. Circulation 78:428–434
3. Braunwald E, Soble BE (1992) Coronary blood flow and myocardial ischemia In: Braunwald E (ed) Heart disease. Saunders, Philadelphia, pp 1161–1199

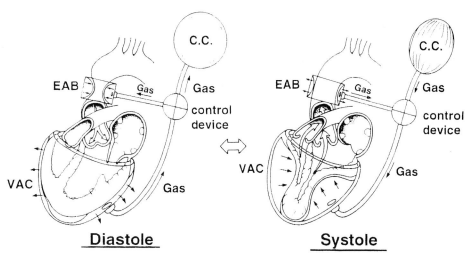

Fig. 1. A schema of the proposed application of an assist device comprising an implantable ventricular assist cup (*VAC*) and an extra-aortic balloon (*EAB*). *C.C.*, compliance chamber

4. Hutton I (1986) Physiology of myocardial perfusion. In: Wheatly DJ (ed) Surgery of coronary artery disease. Chapman and Hall, London, pp 41–49
5. Carpentier AF, Chachques JC, Grandjean PA (1995) Dynamic cardiomyoplasty at nine years. In: Lewis T, Graham TR (eds) Mechanical circulatory support. Edward Arnold, London, pp 277–284
6. Anstadt MP, Anstadt GL, Lowe JE (1991) Direct mechanical ventricular actuation: a review. Resuscitation 21:7–23
7. Takahashi R, Yozu R, Kurosaka Y, Kawada S (1993) Assisted circulation using cardiomyoplasty together with aortomyoplasty. Artif Organs 17:914–918

Implantable Rotary Blood Pump Performs as Well as Pulsatile Pneumatic Assist Device

Bart Meyns[1], Thorsten Siess[2], Yosuke Nishimura[1], Rozalia Racz[1], Ramadan Jashari[1], Helmut Reul[2], and Willem Flameng[1]

Summary. A new implantable rotary blood pump (the diagonal pump) was tested. Hemodynamic performance and organ perfusion were analyzed in a heart failure model and compared to the performance of a pulsatile assist device (Medos, Aachen, Germany). Six sheep were instrumented with a 50 Fr. left atrial inflow cannula and a 16-mm Dacron outflow graft to the descending aorta. After control measurements, left ventricular heart failure was induced by intracoronary injection of microspheres. Measurements were repeated during heart failure, during mechanical support with the Medos device, and during support with the new rotary blood pump. Organ perfusion was analyzed by injection of colored microspheres. Cardiac output, arterial blood pressure, left and right atrial pressure, and first derivative of the left ventricular pressure were all significantly changed during heart failure. These parameters were restored by both types of mechanical support to exactly the same level. Organ perfusion was significantly reduced in all organs during heart failure. There was no difference in organ perfusion with the diagonal pump compared with the pulsatile Medos device. Hemodynamic status and organ perfusion due to left ventricular failure are restored in exactly the same way by a nonpulsatile miniature rotary blood pump and a pneumatic pulsatile assist device (Medos). Rotary blood pumps can be miniaturized and are therefore more attractive than pulsatile displacement pumps for long-term mechanical support.

Key words: Rotary blood pumps — Organ perfusion — Heart failure — Diagonal pump

Introduction

Rotary blood pumps as well as pulsatile assist devices have been used in patients in heart failure to restore the circulation [1]. The success of long-term mechanical support awaiting heart transplantation has driven many investigators to the development of a device for chronic use [2–5]. Rotary blood pumps can be miniaturized and are therefore more attractive than pulsatile devices. The nonpulsatility of the rotary blood pumps is considered to be a minor disadvantage [6]. Still, many doubts remain concerning the actual in vivo performance of these new rotary blood pumps, especially in cases of heart failure. We tested the performance of a new rotary blood pump for chronic use in a series of animal experiments. Hemodynamic performance and organ perfusion were analyzed in the nonfailing and the failing heart model during support with the new pump and with a classical pulsatile assist device.

Materials and Methods

Pumps

The new blood pump used in this study is designed for prolonged heart assist. It is a single-stage rotary blood pump and is currently being developed at the Helmholtz Institute for Biomedical Engineering in Aachen, Germany. The pump itself (Fig. 1) consists of an integrated pump and d.c. motor unit, including a magnetic coupling between both units to eliminate any kind of seal. For mid- to long-term pump operation, a seal would be a disadvantage since ultimately any seal deteriorates and fails.

The pump has a maximum outer diameter of 25 mm and an overall length of the pump housing of 70 mm, which allows either thoracic or abdominal pump positioning. The single-stage pump unit consists of an impeller and a stator which combine the two basic principles of an axial pump (high flow, but low pressure rise) and of a centrifugal pump (low flow, but high pressure rise). This mixed flow design leads to a diagonal pump which appears to be well suited for an implantable assist device, since the impeller design leads to rather low rotational speeds in comparison with axial pumps and is less flow-pressure dependent than most centrifugal pumps. Hence, it is less complicated to control the pump–ventricular interaction in vivo.

Figure 2 shows the hydraulic characteristics of the pump measured in a water-glycerol solution with a viscosity similar to blood ($\mu = 3.6$ mPa.s) and with the rotational speed being measured via an integrated speedometer. According to Fig. 2 the acceptable range of rotational speeds (3000 rpm $< n <$ 8000 rpm) will cause tolerable wear and ensure long operation peri-

[1] Department of Cardiac Surgery, Gasthuisberg University Hospital, Herestraat 49, 3000 Leuven, Belgium
[2] Helmholtz Institute, Aachen, Germany

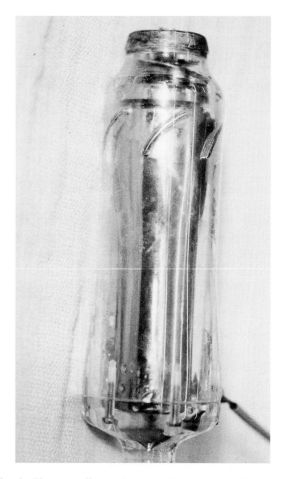

Fig. 1. The new diagonal rotary blood pump. The device measures 25×70 mm

ods, whereas the afterload stability allows the pump to be operated with an atrial-aortic cannulation, despite pressure heads which are high in comparison with an apical-aortic cannulation.

The pulsatile device used was the clinical available, pneumatically driven Medos (Medos, Aachen, Germany) device.

Experimental Protocol

Six sheep with a mean weight of 67.6 kg (± 2.73 kg) were anesthetized and instrumented. All animals received human care in compliance with the "Guide for the Care of and Use of Laboratory Animals" published by the National Institutes of Health. A 50 Fr. left atrial inflow cannula was introduced and a 16-mm Dacron outflow graft was sutured to the descending thoracic aorta. Baseline measurements included hemodynamic parameters: arterial blood pressure (ABP), cardiac output (CO), left atrial pressure (LAP), first derivative of the left ventricular pressure (dP/dt), mixed venous oxygen pressure (SvO_2) as well as peripheral organ perfusion by injection of colored microspheres [7–9].

Heart failure was induced by injection of 100-μm microspheres in the lateral branch of the left coronary artery. This produced a profound low cardiac output state (drop in cardiac output by 55% $\pm$ 6% of the baseline value), while the model remained stable, free of arrhythmia. Measurements were repeated during heart failure, with the Medos assistance, and with the

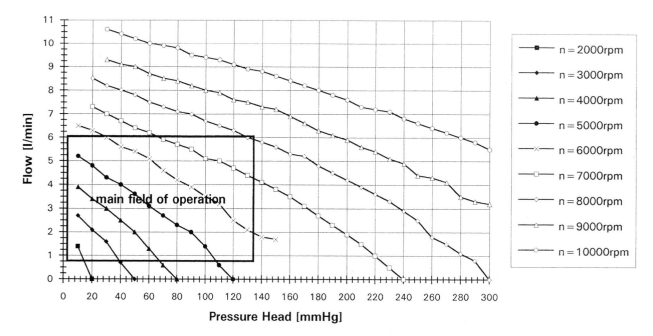

Fig. 2. The hydraulic characteristics of the pump measured in a water-glycerol solution with a viscosity similar to blood ($\mu = 3.6$ mPa.s). rpm = rotations per minute

diagonal pump assistance. During heart failure and mechanical support, no other therapeutic actions such as increasing the circulatory volume or inotropic support were undertaken. Each animal underwent pulsatile as well as nonpulsatile support. The order of support was alternated in each animal. The mechanical support was maintained for 20 min to allow stabilization of the hemodynamic parameters before the colored microspheres were injected. The change from one device to the other was immediate as they were both connected to the same cannulas.

Statistics

Continuous data are presented with their standard deviation. Data for different modes of mechanical support were compared using the two-tailed paired t-test. A probability value of less than 5% ($P < 0.05$) is considered significant.

Results

The hemodynamic state of the animals severely deteriorated after the induction of heart failure. Cardiac output, perfusion pressures, and mixed venous oxygen pressure all significantly changed (Table 1). Mechanical support by either the diagonal pump or the Medos device improved all hemodynamic parameters. The improvement by both devices was equal. Cardiac output could not be restored to baseline values as no fluid administration was allowed in the experimental protocol.

Table 1. Hemodynamic parameters

	Control	Heart failure	Medos pump	Diagonal pump
ABP systolic (mmHg)	110 (9)	60 (18)*	110 (13)	92 (19)
ABP diastolic (mmHg)	91 (8)	45 (17)*	81 (15)	87 (15)
LAP (mmHg)	14 (2)	29 (1)*	0 (1)*	0 (1)*
Cardiac output (l/min)	5 (0,7)	2.2 (0,7)*	3.6 (0.8)*	3.7 (1)*
dP/dt (mmHg/s)	1953 (390)	512 (360)*	714 (360)*	838 (580)*
SvO₂ (mmHg)	56 (22)	39 (11)*	46 (12)	46 (12)

Values are means, with standard deviations in parentheses. ABP, arterial blood pressure; LAP, left atrial pressure; dP/dt, first derivative of the left ventricular pressure; SvO_2, mixed venous oxygen pressure.
*Significantly different from control value ($P < 0.05$).

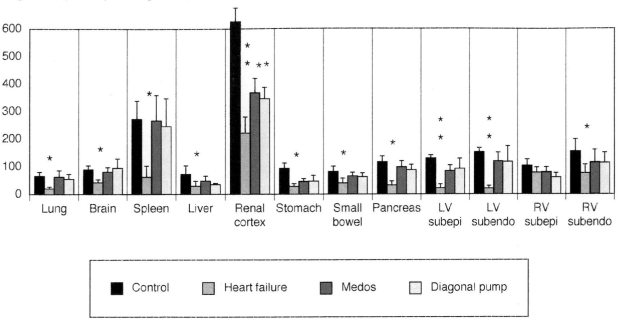

Fig. 3. Mean organ blood flow (+standard error) in various organs during control, heart failure, diagonal pump support, and Medos support. *Stars* indicate the level of significance in differences from the control values (*$P < 0.05$, **$P < 0.001$). *RV*, right ventricle; *LV*, left ventricle; *subepi*, subepicardial; *subendo*, subendocardial

Organ perfusion, measured by colored microsphere content, was significantly reduced in all organs during ischemia (Fig. 3). The pulsatile Medos pump and the diagonal pump improved organ perfusion to exactly the same extent in all organs. Myocardial perfusion, severely impaired during shock, was also improved to baseline values during assistance with the Medos or the diagonal pump.

Discussion

New technical developments in recent years have promoted the small rotary blood pumps as candidates for a chronic circulatory support device [4,5]. The advantages are obvious: the devices can be miniaturized and the pumps allow a native cardiac activity. In addition, Y. Nosé has shown in his extensive work that the body will adapt to long-term nonpulsatile flow as long as the delivered blood flow is high enough [6]. These findings triggered our group to work on this new diagonal blood pump.

However, still some physiological questions remain, First, the future recipients of these devices will be patients in chronic or acute cardiac failure. Because of the specific interaction between rotary blood pump performance and their own cardiac activity, the hemodynamic performance of these devices will be changed. As shown in this model of acute heart failure, the flow produced by both pulsatile and nonpulsatile devices is exactly the same. This is because the administration of fluids was equal (none in both cases) and the inflow cannulation was identical (the same atrial cannula).

In clinical practice it is crucial that the implanted assist device firstly succeeds in overcoming the low cardiac output state from which the patient is dying. We showed that the new diagonal pump restores both hemodynamics and organ perfusion to exactly the same level as a classical pulsatile assist device in cardiogenic shock.

Secondly, the implantation of any device for chronic support should be a low morbidity and mortality procedure. The size reduction of the rotary blood pumps allows a simplification of surgical implantation procedures. We tested the diagonal pump in an atrial inflow position because we believe that atrial inflow allows a less traumatic implantation and possible explantation. Clearly, pump performance is superior with an apical inflow for the pump but patient survival is more the issue than pump performance. Possible disadvantages of atrial inflow are (1) less pronounced unloading of the left ventricle, (2) a possible reduction in myocardial perfusion, and (3) the thrombogenicity of an atrial cannula. In order to defend atrial inflow, we had to show that myocardial perfusion was sufficient. In our series, left ventricular myocardial perfusion was significantly decreased during shock, and both pumps (diagonal and Medos) restored myocardial perfusion to baseline values with the atrial inflow. For the purpose of this acute experiment we used a 50 Fr. atrial inflow cannula. In a chronic implantation, this cannula will be replaced by suturing a graft to the left atrium to avoid thrombus formation.

These short pump runs were insufficient to judge the level of thrombus formation within the pump. Chronic animal studies are being performed to do so.

References

1. Meyns BP, Sergeant PT, Daenen WJ, Flameng WJ (1995) Left ventricular assistance with the transthoracic 24F Hemopump for recovery of the failing heart. Ann Thorac Surg 60:392–397
2. Frazier OH, Rose EA, Macmanus Q, Burton NA, Lefrak EA, Poirier VL, Dasse KA (1992) Multicenter clinical evaluation of the Heartmate 1000 IP left ventricular assist device. Ann Thorac Surg 53:1080–1090
3. Dew MA, Kormos RL, Roth LH, Armitage JM, Pristas JM, Harris RC, Capretta C, Griffith BP (1993) Life quality in the era of bridging to cardiac transplantation. ASAIO J 39:145–152
4. Ohtsubo S, Nosé Y (1996) Evolution towards the development of totally implantable rotary blood pumps. Artif Organs 20:461–462
5. Nosé Y, Kawahito K, Nakazawa T (1996) Can we develop a nonpulsatile permanent rotary blood pump? Yes, we can. Artif Organs 20:467–474
6. Nosé Y (1993) Nonpulsatile mode of blood flow required for cardiopulmonary bypass and total body perfusion. Artif Organs 17:92–102
7. Kowallik P, Schultz R, Guth BD, Schade A, Paffhausen W, Gross R, Heusch G (1991) Measurement of regional myocardial blood flow with multiple colored microspheres. Circulation 83:974–982
8. Rudolph AM, Heymann MA (1967) The circulation of the fetus in utero: Methods of studying distribution of blood flow, cardiac output and organ blood flow. Circ Res 21:163–184
9. Wieland W, Wouters PF, Van Aken H, Flameng W (1993) Measurement of organ blood flow with coloured microspheres: a first time-saving improvement using automated spectophotometry. Proc Comp Cardiol 9:691–694

Implantation of a Ventricular Assist Device in Animals: Progress and Regress

Taiji Murakami, Daiki Kikugawa, Koichi Endoh, Yoshiaki Fukuhiro, and Takashi Fujiwara

Summary. Two types of ventricular assist device (VAD) were tested in vitro and in vivo. A biventricular bypass type total artificial heart utilizing two pusher-plate pumps was implanted in 11 sheep. Following the implantation, the animal's heart was fibrillated. They survived for 2–48 days, with an average of 11.3 days. The pump flow ranged from 90 to 100 ml/min per kg. Other hemodynamic data and the hematological data were normal, except for a low hemoglobin level. We have been developing an implantable motor-driven VAD in collaboration with the Baylor College of Medicine. This pump provided 8 l/min output against a mean afterload of 120 mmHg with a filling pressure of 20 mmHg. Nine in vivo studies have been conducted. Three sheep survived for 10–12 h. The pump flow ranged from 0.8 to 2.5 l/min. From these data, left atrial cannulation may not be sufficient to drain adequate blood flow into the pump.

Key words: Pneumatic blood pump — Biventricular bypass system — Implantable motor-driven left ventricular assist device

Introduction

More than 2000 implanted devices have been reported through January 1994, and 584 ventricular assist devices (VADs) or total artificial hearts (TAHs) have been implanted as bridges to heart transplantation [1]. When these results were analyzed according to the type of support, a significantly higher proportion of those patients who received univentricular support survived, and there was a trend toward overall diminished survival with biventricular support. This may be understood in terms of the severity of the underlying pathology. To solve this difficult problem, we have developed a biventricular support system for use as a bridge to transplantation or in patients with postcardiotomy shock. This paper describes our biventricular support system using pneumatic pumps and presents data on a sheep that survived after the pump implantation.

Pneumatic VADs have been employed extensively in patients with a failing heart, but problems with pneumatic pumps have become apparent, including tethering of the patients to external drive systems and the possibility of infection through drive lines that penetrate the chest wall. To overcome these problems, we have developed an implantable motor-driven left ventricular assist device (LVAD) in collaboration with Baylor College of Medicine, Houston, TX, USA. In this report, we describe the design of the prototype console-based LVAD and the results of in vivo studies.

Materials and Methods

Description of the Biventricular Bypass System

The system consists of a pair of pneumatically powered pusher-plate type blood pumps, a pneumatic power unit, and a control system. The pumps, with a stroke volume of 60 ml for the left side and 40 ml for the right side, were used to clarity the independence of the pumping. The blood-contacting surface was coated with segmented polyurethane. Björk-Shiley monostrut valves of 25 mm and 21 mm were used in the inflow and the outflow ports, respectively. The two pumps are operated in a variable rate (VR) mode. In the VR mode, the Hall effect signal is utilized to regulate the pump stroke volume at a constant level, while its rate is allowed to vary depending on its preload and afterload [2].

Description of the Motor-Driven LVAD

The LVAD has two major components: an implantable pump/actuator unit and an external control console. The unit consists of an epoxy pump housing, a conically shaped polyolefin rubber diaphragm attached with a pusher-plate, and an actuator case housing for a high-speed direct-current brushless motor and planetary roller screw. Twenty-one mm St. Jude Medical valves were used in the inflow and outflow ports. The design stroke volume is 63 ml. The roller screw nut fixed inside the motor rotor is supported by two bearings mounted on either side of the motor stator. As the rotating unit turns, the rotational force

Department of Thoracic and Cardiovascular Surgery, Kawasaki Medical School, 577 Matsushima, Kurashiki, Okayama 701-01, Japan

445

of the motor is translated to the rectilinear motion of the roller screw through a sliding mechanism generated by three stabilizer rods with Teflon guides. The control unit can handle both the variable rate and fixed rate modes.

Biventricular Bypass In Vivo Study

Eleven sheep were used as the experimental animals. General anesthesia was induced and the chest was opened through the fifth intercostal space. The drainage cannula (12 mm in diameter) of the left bypass pump was inserted into the left atrium through the Dacron atrial cuff sutured to its appendage, while an outflow cannula (12 mm in diameter) was anastomosed to the descending aorta. For the right bypass circuit, the drainage cannula was inserted into the right atrium through the atrial cuff and a return cannula was anastomosed to the pulmonary artery. After the control data were obtained, the heart was fibrillated by an electrical shock, and the artificial hearts maintained the entire circulation. The chest was closed and the animal was placed in a special cage. Anticoagulant was not applied after the operation.

The Motor-Driven LVAD In Vivo Study

Nine sheep were used as the experimental animals. Device implantation was carried out under general endotracheal anesthesia. The inflow conduit was inserted into the left ventricular apex in three animals and into the left atrium in six. An 18-mm woven Dacron outflow graft was anastomosed to the thoracic descending aorta. The device was placed in a subcutaneous pocket in the abdominal wall. The drive and vent lines penetrated the skin. No anticoagulants were used except during surgery.

Results

Eleven animals weighing 45–60 kg with biventricular byapass survived 2 to 48 days (mean 11.3 days). Table 1 summarizes the results of in vivo experiments. The cause of termination was respiratory failure in four animals, infection in three, mechanical trouble in three, and bleeding from the arterial line in one.

The pump flow ranged from 90 to 100 ml/min per kg. The mean aortic pressure was kept around 80 mmHg. The central venous pressure was elevated on the first postoperative day and it remained at 10 mmHg thereafter. Values of venous lactate, which indicates the state of peripheral circulation, dropped significantly on the third postoperative day (Fig. 1).

The hemoglobin level had a tendency to decrease after the third postoperative day. On the 14th day, it decreased to 7.3 ± 1.0 mg/dl. The serum free hemoglobin level was maintained at less that 10 mg/dl. Antithrombin III, which is a good indicator of disseminated intravascular coagulation, decreased markedly in the first 3 days, and returned to the control level on the 10th day. Total protein decreased significantly on the first day and it was kept below 6 g/dl during the entire course (Fig. 2).

The performance of the motor-driven LVAD was tested in a mock circulatory system. The LVAD provided 8 l/min of output against a mean afterload of 120 mmHg with a filling pressure of 20 mmHg when the pump was operated in the variable rate mode. When the pump rate was 120 bpm in the fixed rate mode, the maximum flow was 6.5 l/min (Fig. 3).

Nine in vivo studies using motor-driven LVADs have been conducted. Table 2 summarizes the body weight, duration of the experiment, pump flow, and

Table 1. Summary of biventricular bypass in vivo study

Number	Body weight (kg)	Duration (days)	Cause of termination
1	52	12	Bleeding from arterial line
2	55	6	Pneumonia
3	60	3	Drive console trouble
4	50	48	Sepsis
5	60	9	Drive line occlusion
6	57	20	Respiratory failure
7	50	11	Respiratory failure
8	53	3	Sepsis
9	53	2	Sepsis
10	45	5	Respiratory failure
11	56	5	Drive console trouble
Mean ± S.D.	54 ± 4	11.3 ± 12.7	

Fig. 1. Biventricular bypass hemodynamic data. *significant compared with control ($P < 0.05$); **Significant compared with control ($P < 0.01$)

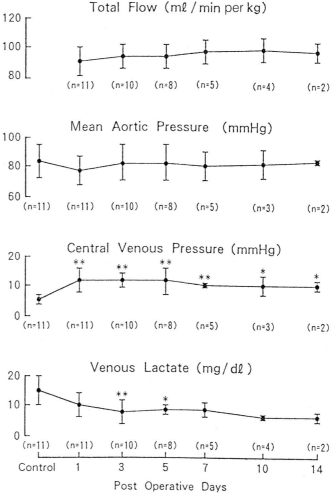

Table 2. Summary of motor-driven left ventricular assist device in vivo study

Number	Body weight (kg)	Cannulation	Pump time (h)	Pump flow (l/min)	Cause of termination
1	42	Apex	0		Bleeding
2	60	LA	12	1.5	Vent tube obstruction
3	58	LA	0		Respiratory failure
4	45	LA	10	2.5	Respiratory failure
5	50	LA	0		Respiratory failure
6	54	Apex	0		VF
7	73	Apex	0		VF
8	50	LA	0		Bleeding
9	50	LA	11	0.8	Thrombus formation within pump

LA, left atrium; VF, ventricular fibrillation.

cause of termination. The mean body weight was 53.6 kg, ranging from 42 to 73 kg. Three animals survived 12, 10, and 11 h, respectively. The mean pump flow was 1.6 l/min, ranging from 0.8 to 2.5 l/min. The cause of termination was respiratory failure in three animals, bleeding in two, ventricular fibrillation in two, vent tube obstruction in one, and thrombus formation within the pump in one.

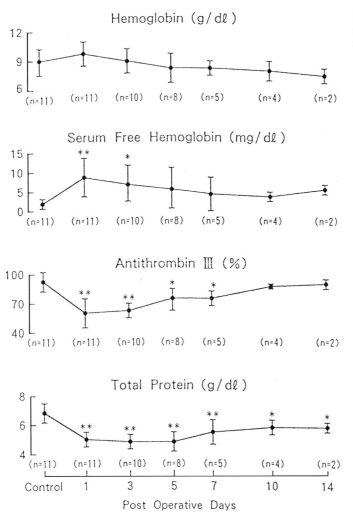

Fig. 2. Biventricular bypass hematology data. *Significant compared with control ($P < 0.05$); **significant compared with control ($P < 0.01$)

Discussion

To date, of 584 patients who have received ventricular assistance in conjunction with heart transplantation, 201 (34.4%) have received biventricular support and 191 (32.7%) have received a total artificial heart (TAH). Discharge rates were significantly lower when patients were supported with either biventricular VADs or TAHs than when they were supported with LVADs. This may be understood in terms of the severity of biventricular failure.

We have been developing a biventricular bypass system for use as a bridge to heart transplantation or for permanent use. The goal of this experiment was to establish a biventricular bypass system with total circulatory maintenance ability. In TAH experiments, the control method is an important factor in optimizing pump performance. To date, most total artificial hearts have used atrial pressure as a parameter to control the rate of filling of the ventricle. This method provides

two alternatives for pumping the heart: constant frequency with variable stroke volume and variable frequency with constant stroke volume [3]. The former control method, the fixed rate mode, operates two pumps in the fill-limited mode. Therefore, pressure measurement is required to regulate right and left pump flow. The latter control method (variable rate mode) insures complete filling and ejection of the pump, and the pumping rate is allowed to vary from beat to beat with changes in filling pressure and afterload. In this fill-empty operation, blood stagnation in the pump is eliminated and invasive measurement is no longer required. It was for these reasons that we employed the VR mode as a control method in this experiment. Although the hemodynamic performance of a TAH operated in the independent VR mode has been fully justified [4], in this experiment, a question arises concerning the pump flow sensitivity to the filling pressure due to its narrow cannulae. With this system operated in the independent VR mode, the

(L/min)

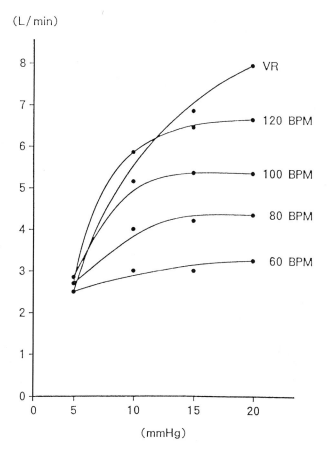

(mmHg)

Fig. 3. In vitro performance of the motor-driven left ventricular assist device. *VR*, variable rate; *BPM*, beats per minute. Afterload was 120 mmHg

hearts results in too few organs available for treatment via transplantation. Mechanical circulatory support systems for long-term use are needed to meet the demand of the growing number of patients with diagnoses of irreversible end-stage heart failure.

Our initial goal is to develop a console-based electrically powered LVAD system. This LVAD provides 8 l/min of output against a mean afterload of 120 mmHg with a filling pressure of 20 mmHg. In animal experiments, left atrial cannulation was done in six animals and apical cannulation in three. Three animals with left atrial cannulation survived 10 to 12 h (mean 11 h). The mean pump flow was 1.6 l/min, ranging from 0.8 to 2.5 l/min. Based on our in vitro study, this pump provides over 3 l/min of output with a filling pressure of 10 mmHg. However, the left atrial pressure may not be high enough to fill up the pump during diastole because of the high resistance created by the long inflow cannula. Further study is to be undertaken, and a newly designed apical cannula is being tested to enhance pump filling.

References

1. Mehta SM, Aufiero TX, Pae WE Jr, Miller CA, Pierce WS (1995) Combined registry for the clinical use of mechanical ventricular assist pumps and the total artificial heart in conjunction with heart transplantation: sixth official report — 1994. J Heart Lung Transplant 14:585–593
2. Takatani S, Nakatani T, Takano H, Tanaka T, Umezu M, Adachi S, Noda H, Fukuda S, Matsuda T, Iwata H, Nakamura T, Akutsu T (1986) Total artificial heart study in goats and calves with pusher-plate type blood pumps: progress and problems. Jpn J Artif Organs 15:654–659
3. Kwan-Gett CS, Wu Y, Collan R, Jacobson S, Kolff WJ (1969) Total replacement artificial heart and driving system with inherent regulation of cardiac output. ASAIO Trans 15:245–250
4. Takatani S, Harasaki H, Koike S, Yada I, Yozu R, Fujimoto L, Murabayashi S, Jacobs G, Kiraly R, Nosé Y (1982) Optimum control mode for a total artificial heart. ASAIO Trans 28:148–153
5. Aufiero TX, Magovern JA, Rosenberg G, Pae WE Jr, Donachy JH, Pierce WS (1987) Long-term survival with a pneumatic artificial heart. ASAIO Trans 33:157–161
6. Kunin CM, Dobbins JJ, Melo JC, Levinson MM, Love K, Joyce LD, DeVries W (1988) Infectious complications in four long-term recipients of the Jarvick-7 artificial heart. JAMA 259:860–864
7. Kung RTV, Yu LS, Ochs BD, Parnis SM, Macris MP, Frazier OH (1995) Progress in the development of the ABIOMED total artificial heart. ASAIO J 41:245–248
8. Harasaki H, Fukamachi K, Massiello A, Chen JF, Himley SC, Fukumura F, Muramoto K, Niu S, Wika K, Davies CR, McCarthy PM, Kiraly RJ, Thomas DC, Rintoul TC, Carriker JC, Maher TR, Butler KC (1994) Progress in Cleveland Clinic-Nimbus total artificial heart development. ASAIO J 40:494–498

hemodynamic parameters were kept at near normal levels, and hematological data were also normal except for a low hemoglobin level.

The major problems previously identified in experimental and clinical TAH recipients were local and general infections [5,6]. In this experiment, three animals died of sepsis and one died of pneumonia. Two intravascular catheters or four cannulae which directly penetrated the chest wound might have been a cause of infection. To prevent infection, a totally implantable electrohydraulic TAH has been developed and tested in vivo. The ABIOMED TAH and the Cleveland Clinic-Nimbus TAH have achieved an in vivo implant duration of 108 days and 120 days, respectively [7,8]. In the future, the implantation of a totally implantable TAH as a bridge to transplantation or for long-term use may enhance the quality of life and reduce the occurrence of infection.

Cardiac transplantation is an acceptable treatment for end-stage heart disease, but the shortage of donor

Ventricular Assist Device Made with Silicone Valves and Silicone Blood Chamber

Norimasa Mitsui[1], Shintaro Fukunaga[1], Masafumi Sueshiro[1], Shinji Hirai[1], Kimiko Katsuhara[1], Taijiro Sueda[1], Yuichiro Matsuura[1], and Shinsaku Koguchi[2]

Summary. A blood chamber integrated with a trileaflet valve was made with silicone rubber through a die-casting process. The valve, which was originally a short tube with three thick and thin portions, was turned inside-out to make a trileaflet valve. The diameter of the valve orifice was 17 mm. The bottom of the blood chamber, which was open after removing the core, was sealed with silicone glue. This blood chamber, with a volume of 70 ml, was placed in a casing made with aluminum alloy and acrylic resin, and it was driven by a pneumatic artificial heart driver. In an overflow-type mock circulatory system, a maximal flow of 6.3 l/min was achieved at the rate of 80 bpm. Regurgitation with the silicone valves was nearly equal to that of Björk-Shiley monostrut valves. The pressure gradient across the silicone valves was slightly greater than that across the monostrut valves. The device maintained good performance for 8 weeks in the mock circulatory system.

Key words: Ventricular assist device — Trileaflet valve — Silicone valve — Silicone blood chamber

Introduction

A pulsatile ventricular assist device (VAD) consists of a blood chamber and two valves at the inlet and outlet ports. Several materials have been used, including titanium alloy or polyurethane rubber for the blood chamber, and pyrolytic carbon, titanium alloy, biological materials, or polyurethane rubber for the valves [1,2]. The artificial valves used for clinical purposes have normally been employed as the valve in the VADs. Since we had access to a die-casting technique for silicone rubber for making industrial products, we have made a VAD which consists of a silicone blood chamber and two silicone trileaflet valves, by the die-casting process. Its structure, hemodynamic performance, and durability are described in this report.

Materials and Methods

The valves and the blood chamber were made with silicone rubber through the die-casting process. As shown in Fig. 1, the valve originally consisted of a short tube with three thick and thin portions, which was then turned inside-out to make a trileaflet valve. After removing the core, the open bottom of the blood chamber was sealed with silicone glue. This blood chamber had a volume of 70 ml; the diameters of the inlet and outlet were 22 mm, and that of the valve orifice was 17 mm. The thickness of the wall of the blood chamber was 1.5 mm and that of the valves was 0.4 mm at the thinnest portion. The blood chamber was then placed in a casing made with aluminum alloy and acrylic resin. We prepared another device with two Björk-Shiley monostrut (BS) valves of 25 mm in diameter instead of silicone valves to evaluate the performance of the silicone valves.

Hemodynamic performance studies were carried out using an overflow-type mock circulatory system. Preload and afterload were monitored by pressure transducers (NEC San-ei Instruments, Tokyo, Japan) and the flow of the VAD was measured by electromagnetic blood flow meters (Nihon Kohden, Tokyo, Japan). The devices were driven by a pneumatic artificial heart driver (Corat 104, Aisin Seiki, Kariya, Japan). Under the conditions of a 10-mmHg preload, 100-mmHg afterload, 140-mmHg driving pressure, 10-mmHg vacuum, and 40% in percent systole, the VAD flow was measured at the inlet and outlet ports while the driving rate was changed from 40 bpm to 140 bpm. The VAD flow was also measured under the same conditions except that the percent systole was changed from 15% to 70% at a driving rate of 60 bpm. The pressure gradient across the valves was measured with steady flow while the flow rate was changed. The durability test was performed with one device using the overflow-type mock circulatory system with a 10-mmHg preload, 100-mmHg afterload, 140-mmHg driving pressure, 10-mmHg vacuum, 40% in percent systole, and a driving rate of 80 bpm.

[1] The First Department of Surgery, Hiroshima University School of Medicine, 1-2-3 Kasumi, Minami-ku, Hiroshima 734, Japan
[2] Eba Machinery Works Co., Ltd. 2-11-21 Dejima, Minami-ku, Hiroshima 734, Japan

Fig. 1. Formation of the silicone trileaflet valve (*left four items*); the blood chamber containing the integrated silicon valve (*center*); and the complete ventricular assist device (*right*)

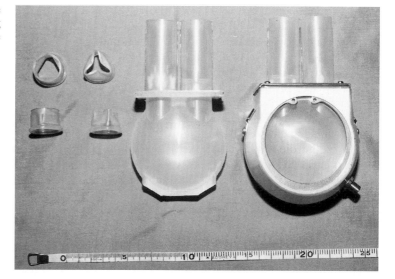

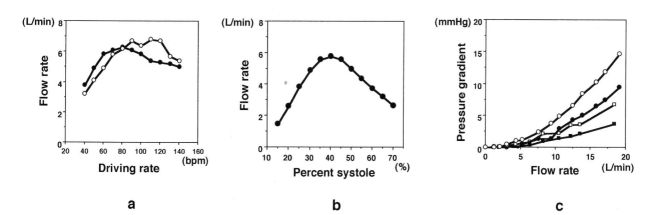

a   b   c

Fig. 2. Performance of device and valves. **a** Relationship between flow rate and driving rate. Preload 10 mmHg; afterload 100 mmHg; driving pressure 140 mmHg; vacuum 10 mmHg; percent systole 40%. *Closed circles*, with silicone valves; *open circles*, with Björk-Shiley (BS) valves. **b** Relationship between flow rate and percent systole. Preload 10 mmHg; afterload 100 mmHg; driving pressure 140 mmHg; vacuum 10 mmHg; driving rate 60 bpm. **c** Relationship between pressure gradient across the valve and flow rate. *Closed circles*, silicone valve in inlet; *open circles*, silicone valve in outlet; *closed squares*, BS valve in inlet; *open squares*, BS valve in outlet

Results

The performance of the device and valves is shown in Fig. 2. The relationship between the flow rate and driving rate is shown in Fig. 2a. When the driving rate increased, the flow rate increased up to 6.3 l/min at 80 bpm, and beyond this driving rate the flow rate began to decrease. The flow rate with the BS valves increased up to 7.2 l/min at 120 bpm and beyond 120 bpm it decreased. The relationship between the flow rate and percent systole is shown in Fig. 2b. The maximal flow rate was achieved at a percent systole of 40%. The pressure gradient across the valves is shown in Fig. 2c. The pressure gradient across the silicone valves was slightly greater than that across the BS valves at each flow rate: with the silicone valve it was around 9 mmHg at the inlet and 15 mmHg at the outlet at a flow rate of 19 l/min. From the recordings of the instantaneous flow curve at the valve, we found that the regurgitation with the silicone valves was almost the same as that with the BS valves. The device performed satisfactorily until the 55th day when the inlet valve failed, resulting in massive regurgitation.

Discussion

Silicone and polyurethane rubber are well-known antithrombogenic materials. At present, polyurethane rubber is used for the VAD because of its advantage in durability over silicone rubber. Nevertheless, we have treated silicone rubber for industrial materials, and we have applied the technique to make trileaflet valves. Then we made a silicone blood chamber for a VAD by means of the die-casting process by which trileaflet valves of silicone rubber were seamlessly built-in. The hemodynamic performance of the VAD was satisfactory on the whole. Regurgitation with the silicone valves was almost the same as that with BS valves. Although the pressure gradient across the silicone valves was slightly greater than that of the BS valves, it could in practice be tolerated. The durability of the silicone valve is not sufficient at present, and further improvement is required. Antithrombogenicity and hemolysis tests are also to be evaluated before practical application.

Acknowledgment. This work was supported by the Research Grant for Cardiovascular Disease (7A-1) from the Ministry of Health and Welfare of Japan.

References

1. Imachi K, Mabuchi K, Chinzei T, Abe Y, Imanishi K, Yonezawa T, Maeda K, Suzukawa M, Kouno A, Ono T, Fujimasa I, Atsumi K (1989) In vitro and in vivo evaluation of a jellyfish valve for practical use. ASAIO Trans 35:298–301
2. Smulders YM, Tieleman RG, Topaz SR, Bishop ND, Yu LS, Yuan B, Kolff WJ (1991) Concept of a soft, compressible artificial ventricle under evaluation. Artif Organs 15:96–102

Evaluation of Pump Performance of a Percutaneous-Type Pulsatile Left Ventricular Assist Device (MAD Type 5 and Type 6)

K. Imanishi[3], K. Imachi[1], H. Yoshito[4], T. Isoyama[1], Y. Abe[1], T. Chinzei[1], K. Mabuchi[2], N. Tsutsui[4], K. Suma[2], and I. Fujimasa[1]

Summary. We have been developing a percutaneous-type left ventricular assist device named the Modified Assist Device (MAD). The system is composed of an air-driven sac-type blood pump and cannula in which an inflow and an outflow valve have been installed. With the MAD type 5, a maximum pump flow of 2.5 l/min was obtained in a mock circulation study. For clinical application of this ventricular assist device, a new model, MAD type 6, was developed and was evaluated in in vitro and in vivo experiments. To obtain satisfactory anatomical fit and durability, a spiral was installed in the cannula of MAD type 6. In in vitro evaluation, the pressure gradients across the inflow and outflow valves were 110 mmHg and 75 mmHg at a flow rate of 2 l/min. With the MAD type 6, the index of hemolysis was almost the same as that of a centrifugal pump. The durability test was maintained for more than 30 days without deterioration of the new system. In an animal experiment, using dogs, more effective systolic unloading and diastolic augmentation were observed by the activation of the MAD type 6 than with an intra-aortic balloon pump (IABP) assist. As for the peripheral circulation, the MAD type 6 device produced greater carotid artery flow than did the the IABP assist. In conclusion, the MAD type 6, a pulsatile-flow device, appears to have a design and function suitable for clinical application.

Key words: Left ventricular assist device — Intra-aortic balloon pump — Jellyfish valve — Percutaneous access

Introduction

To obtain both pressure and flow support with a percutaneously accessible left ventricular assist device, we have been developing a circulatory assist device called the Modified Assist Device (MAD). The MAD comprises an air-driven sac-type blood pump and a cannula installed with inflow and outflow valves. With this new concept, we have designed and developed this novel circulatory assist device in prototypes from type 1 to type 5. For the clinical application of this ventricular assist device, we evaluated the pump performance of MAD type 5 from various viewpoints. On the basis of that evaluation, the newest model, MAD type 6, was designed. In this study, the pump performance of MAD types 5 and 6 was evaluated in in vivo and in vitro experiments.

Materials and Methods

Blood Pump and Cannula

The MAD type 6 consists of an air-driven blood pump and cannula.

Blood Pump. A single-port, valveless, diaphragm-type blood pump with a stroke volume of 30 ml was made of polyvinyl chloride paste. To obtain complete filling and emptying, the profile of the blood pump has been changed from ball-shaped (MAD type 5) to discoid-shaped. Moreover, the durability of the membrane of diaphragm has been increased compared with that of MAD type 5 (Figs. 1, 2).

Cannula. In MAD type 5, the outer diameter of the cannula was 7.5 mm and the inner diameter was 5.5 mm. In MAD type 6, the outer diameter was reduced to 7.0 mm, while the inner diameter was the same as that of type 5. The length of the cannula of MAd type 6 was 40 cm, which was also the same as that of type 5. To increase the flexibility and allow better anatomical fit, in type 6, the cannula was made of polyvinyl chloride paste in which a spiral of stainless steel was installed. An inflow (cone-shaped jellyfish valve: CS-JFV) and an outflow valve (lantern-shaped valve; L-V) were mounted at the apex and in the side wall 10 cm from the apex of the cannula, respectively. The valve seat of the inflow valve, which has four spokes to prevent prolapse of the valve membrane, was made of two liquid reactance polyurethane and was coated with Cardiothane (Nippon Zeon Tokyo, Japan). The total open area of the inflow valve was increased from 84 mm² (MAD type 5) to 100 mm²

[1] Institute of Medical Electronics, Faculty of Medicine, University of Tokyo, Japan
[2] Research Center for Advanced Science of Technology, University of Tokyo, Japan
[3] Department of Cardiovascular Surgery, Tokyo Women's Medical College, Daini Hospital, 2-1-10 Nishiogu, Arakawa-ku, Tokyo 116, Japan
[4] Tokai Medical Products Co. Ltd., Japan

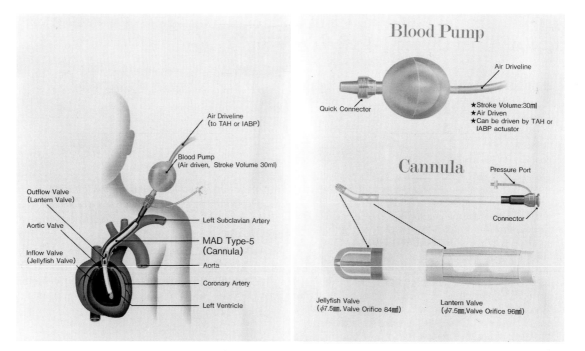

Fig. 1. A percutaneously accessible left ventricular assist device, the Modified Assist Device (MAD). Components of the MAD are shown. *TAH*, total artificial heart; *IABP*, intra-aortic balloon pump; φ, diameter

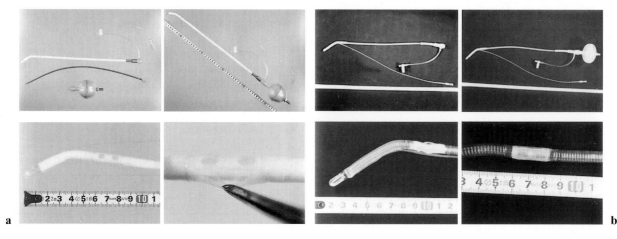

Fig. 2a,b. Cannula and blood pump of MAD type 5 (**a**) and type 6 (**b**). The *upper panels* show the cannula, which can monitor left ventricular pressure. The *lower panels* show the inflow valve (truncated conical jellyfish valve, *left*) and outflow valve (lantern valve, *right*)

(MAD type 6). The membrane of the CS-JFV is 0.1 mm thick and was made of Cardiothane by casting. For implantation of the L-V, six side holes with a total area of 96 mm² were placed 10 cm from the apex of the cannula. A valve membrane with slits was placed around the side holes (Figs. 1, 2).

Driving System

The blood pump is driven by a pneumatic driving system also used for the total artificial heart in our laboratory. The driving system can control pulse rate (beats/min), percent systolic duration (S/D ratio; %), and independent positive and negative air pressure (mmHg). The blood pump can also be driven by any kind of intra-aortic balloon pump (IABP) driver.

Control Method

During systole, the blood pump withdraws the blood from the left ventricle through the inflow valve of the cannula, and ejects to the root of the aorta through the outflow valve during diastole to increase coronary and systemic blood flow. The driver was programmed to deliver systolic pressure with a delay of 30%–45% of the R-R interval to provide diastolic augmentation.

Insertion Technique

The cannula is inserted into the subclavian artery and passed in the retrograde direction through the aortic valve into the left ventricle using the guidewire technique. Therefore, the inflow valve is placed in the left ventricle, and the outflow valve is located near the coronary orifice above the aortic valve. The blood pump is then connected to the cannula with the quick connector system (Fig. 1).

Mock Circulation Study

To assess pump performance, the relationship between the driving conditions of the MAD and the pump flow was evaluated in a mock circulation study. The pump flow was measured with afterloads of 0, 50, and 70 mmHg under the following driving conditions: positive air pressure 350 mmHg, negative air pressure 150 mmHg, S/D ratio 40%, and pulse rate 50 bpm.

A test to assess leakage through the inflow valve was performed. The relationship between leakage through the inflow valve and pressure overload was traced. To evaluate the factor limiting the maximum pump-flow, the relationship between the flow and the pressure gradients through the valves and cannula was traced.

A the durability test was performed under the following driving conditions: systolic pressure 390 mmHg, diastolic pressure 150 mmHg, S/D ratio 45%, and pulse rate 50 bpm.

Evaluation of hemolysis was performed using fresh goat blood. A hemolytic test circuit was used to compare the index of hemolysis (IH) of MAD type 5 and the centrifugal pump. The index of hemolysis was defined as grams of hemoglobin released/100 l [1]. The conditions of the hemolytic test circuit were as follows: priming volume 500 ml, pump flow 2 l/min, pressure gradient 100 mmHg, pumping time 5 h. Liberated hemoglobin and hematocrit were determined every hour, and the IH of MAD type 5 and the centrifugal pump were calculated and compared.

Animal Experiments

Mongrel dogs, weighing 15–25 kg, were operated on according to the guidelines in "Guide for the Care and Use of Laboratory Animals" of the National Institutes of Health (NIH). Anesthesia was induced with i.v. pentobarbital. The animals were incubated and maintained with a volume displacement respirator. A median sternotomy was made and the ascending aorta and right subclavian artery were exposed. Aortic flow (ml/min), carotid artery flow (ml/min), aortic pressure (mmHg), left ventricular pressure (mmHg), and pulmonary artery pressure were traced. After a dose of heparin (1.5 mg/kg) was given i.v., the MAD type 6 was inserted through the subclavian artery and passed through the aortic valve into the left ventricle. During the experiment, anticoagulation therapy, with i.v. heparin, was performed to keep the activated clotting time (ACT) at twice the control value. After confirmation of the positioning of the apex of the cannula in the left ventricle, pumping was started, using the 2:1 assist mode.

Then, the intra-aortic balloon pump (IABP) was inserted through the femoral artery. After the calculation of control hemodymamics, the effectiveness of pressure and flow support by the MAD type 6 and the IABP were compared with an on–off study. Also, the effect on the peripheral circulation of the MAD type 6 was evaluated.

After the termination of the experiment, the animals were killed with i.v. potassium chloride. The aorta was opened longitudinally from where the cannula was inserted to the aortic valve, to observe the relationship between the coronary orifice and the outflow valve. Then, the left ventricle was also opened longitudinally to the apex to observe the positioning of the inflow valve.

Results

Mock Circulation Study

In the MAD type 5, a maximum flow of 2.5 l/min was observed in the mock circulatory study under the following driving conditions: systolic pressure 350 mmHg, diastolic pressure 150 mmHg, S/D 40%, and pulse rate 50 beats/min with a preload of 10 cm H_2O and an afterload of 0 mmHg. The pump flow did not drop under 2 l/min with an increase in the afterload to 70 mmHg (2.04 l/min).

In the relationship between flow and pressure gradient at the inflow valve, outflow valve, and cannula, a maximum pressure gradient of 115 mmHg with a flow of 2 l/min was observed in the inflow valve.

The durability test was continued for 30 days without deterioration of the system.

As for the hemolysis, a linear increase in serum free hemoglobin was observed with both the MAD type 5 and the centrifugal pump. Two separate evaluations revealed that the values of the index of hemolysis (IH) were 0.0259 and 0.00853 for the MAD type 5, and 0.0134 and 0.00834 for the centrifugal pump (Fig. 3).

Animal Study

In the animal experiment, control hemodynamics were compared with those obtained with each pump. In the waveform of aortic pressure, the MAD type 6 produced stronger systolic unloading and diastolic augmentation than the IABP assist. A decrease in the systolic left ventricular pressure was observed with the activation of the MAD type 6 which was not observed during the assist with the IABP. There was a slight decrease in the pulmonary pressure with the MAD type 6. Improved aortic flow and carotid artery flow were observed with the MAD compared with the IABP assist (Fig. 4). The left ventricular work index (LVWI), a measure of the total power of the left ventricle, was also increased with the assistance by MAD type 6 (Control, 1039; IABP, 1208; MAD type 6, 1554 $g \cdot m^{-2} \cdot min^{-1}$.

At autopsy, the outflow valve was located near the coronary orifice, and no injury to the aortic valve could be observed. Proper positioning of the inflow valve and cannula were observed in the left ventricle. There was no kinking of the cannula in the subclavian artery

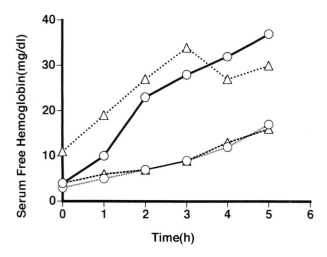

Fig. 3. Evaluation of hemolysis (liberated hemoglobin) with MAD type 5 (*circles*) and the centrifugal pump (*triangles*). Two experiments were performed: the *upper traces* represent the first experiment, and the *lower traces*, the second. The index of hemolysis (IH) was calculated. The values from experiments 1 and 2, respectively, were: MAD, 0.0259 and 0.00853; centrifugal pump, 0.0134 and 0.00834. Fresh goat blood was pumped at 2 l/min with a pressure gradient of 100 mmHg and a priming volume of 500 ml

or in the aorta because of the spiral insertion in the cannula. There was no evidence of thrombus formation in the cannula, in the inflow or outflow valves, or in the blood pump (Fig. 5).

Discussion

Several types of ventricular assist devices have been developed, mainly in the United States [2–4]. The number of patients with post-cardiotomy cardiogenic shock or heart failure for several reasons has been increasing [5]. We have been developing a percutaneously accessible, left ventricular assist device [6–9]. The number of patients who require mechanical circulation per year is consistently 220–390. The percentages of those patients able to be weaned and discharged are 40%–50% and 19%–30%, respectively [5]. Among weaned and discharged patients, there are high rates of complications such as bleeding and renal failure [5]. In such circumstances, a ventricular assist device which is easily accessible and provides strong circulatory assist is required.

In our institute, a left ventricular assist system has been developed which is percutaneously accessible and can provide pressure and flow support [8,9]. Five prototypes of the Modified Assist Device (MAD) have been developed. MAD type 5 produced stronger pressure and flow support than did the IABP, in animal experiments. Good anatomical fit in the aorta and in the left ventricle was also observed [9]. However, MAD type 5 had several problems. One of the major problems needing to be resolved was the kinking of the cannula. If kinking occurs, the pump flow decreases dramatically. To decrease the wall thickness of the cannula while maintaining the maximum pump flow, and to increase its flexibility, a spiral was installed in the cannula in MAD type 6. As observed at autopsy, anatomical fit was improved and there was almost no possibility of kinking of the cannula. The outer diameter of the cannula in MAD type 6 was decreased from 7.5 mm to 7.0 mm, but the inner diameter was the same as that of MAD type 5. Therefore, the maximum pump flow (2.5 l/min) did not decrease.

To investigate the factor limiting the maximum pump flow, a mock circulation study was performed with MAD type 5. The inflow valve was found to be the limiting factor determining the maximum pump flow. The opening area of the inflow valve was the most important factor from the viewpoints of both maximum pump flow and hemolysis.

An evaluation of hemolysis with the MAD type 5 in comparison with the centrifugal pump was performed. The index of hemolysis, defined as grams of hemoglobin released per 100 l, was calculated [1]. The comparison of hemolysis, performed twice during the

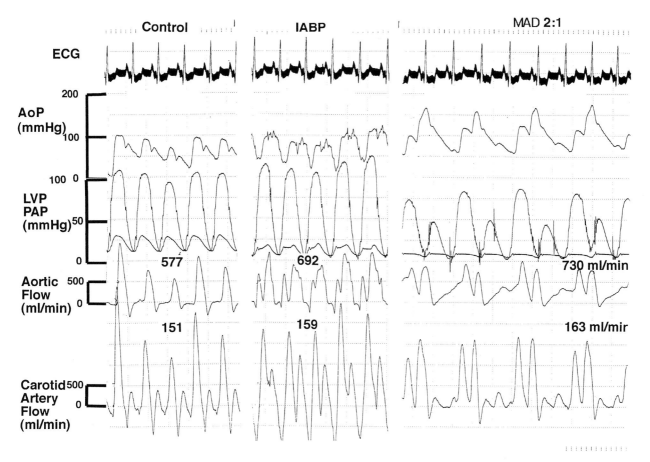

Fig. 4. Comparison of support by MAD type 6 (*right panel*) and IABP (*center panel*). Control, *left panel*, Chart speed, 25 mm/s, *AoP*, aortic pressure; *LVP*, left ventricular pressure (*higher peaks*); *PAP*, pulmonary arterial pressure (*lower peaks*). Flow data (ml/min) are shown *above the trace* for aortic flow and carotid artery flow

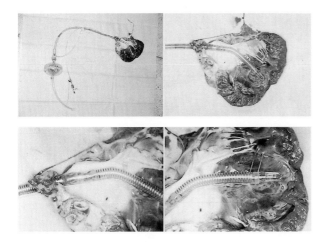

Fig. 5. MAD type 6 gave good anatomical fit in the ascending aorta and left ventricle

study, indicated almost no significant difference in the index of hemolysis. This results suggested that the design of the MAD pump was acceptable for clinical application from the viewpoint of hemolysis.

In the animal experiment, MAD type 6 provided the same circulatory assistance as obtained with type 5. With respect to pressure, MAD support gave stronger systolic unloading and diastolic augmentation than did IABP support. During assistance by MAD type 6, left ventricular pressure was always kept at a lower level than aortic pressure. The mean aortic flow was also increased compared with IABP assist. As a measure of the total power of the left ventricle under assistance by the MAD or IABP, the left ventricular work index (LVWI) was calculated. MAD type 6 produced a higher LVWI than did the IABP assist. These results suggested that left ventricle was in a resting condition during assistance by the MAD type 6.

Mean carotid artery flow, a peripheral flow, also increased with the assistance by the MAD type 6.

There was reverse flow in the waveform of the carotid artery under assistance by the IABP. However, there was no reverse flow in the waveform of carotid artery flow with the MAD type 6. Preservation of myocardium was more effective with the MAD than with the IABP assist.

Conclusions

1. The MAD type 6 has advanced closer toward an optimal design for percutaneous access and stable circulatory assist with pulsatile flow.
2. MAD types 5 and 6 produced pulsatile flow and satisfactory circulatory assistance in terms of both blood pressure and systemic blood flow.
3. There was no significant difference in hemolysis between the MAD and the centrifugal pump.
4. The design and pump performance of the MAD type 6 appear suitable for clinical application.

References

1. Oku T, Harasaki H, Smith W. Nosé Y (1988) A comparative study of four nonpulsatile pumps. ASAIO Trans 34:500–504
2. Ruzevich SA, Pennington DG, Kanter KR, Swartz MT, McBride LR, Termuhlen DF (1987) Long-term follow-up study of survivors of postcardiotomy circulatory support. ASAIO Trans 33:177–181
3. Wampler RK, Moise JC, Frazier OH, Olsen DB (1988) In vivo evaluation of a peripheral vascular access axial flow blood pump. ASAIO Trans 34:450–454
4. Whalen RK, Hurford WE, Skoskiewicz M, Wonders TR, Zapol WM (1987) A new right ventricular assist device. The extracorporeal pulsatile assist device (EPAD). ASAIO Trans 33:223–226
5. Mehta SM, Aufiero TX, Pae WE Jr, Miller CA, Pierce WS (1996) Results of mechanical ventricular assistance for the Treatment of post cardiotomy cardiogenic shock. ASAIO J 42(3):211–218
6. Imachi K, Mabuchi K, Chinzei T, Abe Y, Imanishi K, Yonezawa T, Maeda K, Suzukawa M, Kouno A, Ono T, Fujimasa I, Atsumi K (1989) In vitro and in vivo evaluation of a jellyfish valve for practical use. ASAIO Trans 35:298–301
7. Imachi K, Mabuchi K, Chinzei T, Abe Y, Imanishi K, Suzukawa M, Yonezawa T, Kouno A, Ono T, Atsumi K, Fujimasa I (1991) Blood compatibility of the jellyfish valve without anticoagulant. ASAIO Trans 37(3):220–222
8. Imanishi K, Imachi K, Abe Y, Chinzei T, Mabuchi K, Fujimasa I, Atsumi K, Suma K (1989) Development of a new circulatory assist method with the combined effects of intra-aortic balloon pumping and counter-pulsation: First report. ASAIO Trans 35(3):715–717
9. Imanishi K, Imachi K, Yoshito H, Isoyama T, Abe Y, Chinzei T, Mabuchi K, Kanda K, Tsutsui N, Suma K, Fujimasa I (1996) A percutaneously accessible pulsatile left ventricular assist device: Modified Assist Device type-5. Artif Organs 20(2):147–151

Automatic Regulation of Output of an Electrohydraulic Left Ventricular Assist Device Using the Polymer Bellows Water Pressure and Motor Current

Jae-Soon Choi[1], Yung-Ho Jo[1], Won-Woo Choi[1], Seong-Keun Park[1], Kyong-Sik Om[1], Jong-Jin Lee[1], Yong-Soon Won[2], Won-Gon Kim[3], and Byoung-Goo Min[1]

Summary. An electrohydraulically driven left ventricular assist device (LVAD) has been developed in our laboratory. Over years of in vitro and in vivo testing, a "suction" problem has been pointed out as one of the major problems related to the device mechanism. The suction problem involves collapse of the left atrium, which can be caused by excessive negative pressure generated by the active blood-filling mechanism, and can lead to damage to the atrium or an air-embolism. We have developed methods for properly controlling the assistance output, depending upon the inlet pressure conditions. Algorithms have been developed for setting an absolute limit to negative pressure and for the regulation of the diastolic velocity of the device. The regulating system is based on the estimation of left atrial pressure (LAP), using the internal pressure of the polymer bellows and the motor current as raw information indicating the status of the left atrium. The estimation is based upon direct analysis of the signal wave form, coupled with the use of fuzzy logic in determining significant parameters such as the systolic peak, diastolic peak, and diastolic integral. Results of experiments using a mock-circulation system have shown that the new control system performs satisfactorily in detecting suction. An animal experiment was conducted to verify the feasibility of the methods. In a 17-day experiment using an adult sheep with a left ventricular assist device, there was no sign of damage or suction-related problems when we used the new method for controlling the diastolic velocity depending upon the bellows water pressure. In this paper, the methods are described and the results are documented.

Key words: Ventricular assist — Atrial collapse — Motor current — Water pressure — Fuzzy logic — Flow regulation

Introduction

We have been developing an electrohydraulic left ventricular assist device (LVAD). We chose an electrohydraulic device because (1) using incompressible water can give more precise control of assist output, so we can synchronize assist pumping more precisely with the ECG; (2) an active blood-suction mechanism can induce more cardiac output than the passive mechanisms of pneumatic devices or others; and (3) the mechanism, algorithms, and various research results can readily be applied to a totally implantable device [1].

In our device however, the active blood-suction mechanism can cause excessive suction. Excessive suction can lead to damage of the myocardium or an air-embolism, because of left atrial collapse and air intrusion through the suture site. This has been pointed out as one of the major problems with our device [2], and some rotary blood pumps were reported to have a similar problem [3].

We have solved this problem through various electrical algorithms and mechanical methods. Electrical algorithms are estimation and regulation algorithms. They estimate the status of the left atrium or blood volume, and regulate the velocity of the device. For estimation, they use the motor current and the bellows pressure signal. They include a simple pressure limiter using the characteristics of these signals, and a fuzzy-logic suction detector. The simple pressure limiter limits the minimum absolute bellows pressure, so that it does not fall below a set point, and sets limits to the negative pressure gradient. The fuzzy detector makes decisions using fuzzy logic on the peaks and integrals of signals. In addition, a mechanical improvement was made. We tried an additional mechanical bellows for compliance-chamber and magnetic coupling in the pumping sac. This improvement prevented suction without a large loss of flow or energy.

Materials and Methods

Device Overview

The major components are the actuator, pumping sac, water conduit, blood chamber, and controller. The torque generated by the servo d.c. motor is converted to reciprocal force through the ball screw. It pumps the bellows-type pumping sac ("bellows"), which transmits the pressure to the blood sac in the blood chamber

[1] Department of Biomedical Engineering, Graduate School of Engineering, Seoul National University 28 Youngun-Dong, Chongno-Ku, Seoul 110-744, Korea
[2] Department of Thoracic Surgery, College of Medicine, Ehwa Women's University, 11-1 Daehyun-Dong, Seodaemun-Ku, Seoul 120-750, Korea
[3] Department of Thoracic Surgery, College of Medicine, Seoul National University, Seoul, Korea

459

through the water conduit. The water conduit (Toyox, Tokyo, Japan) is reinforced with a spring to prevent kinking, and filled with water. Its length and inner diameter are 1.2 m and 12 mm, respectively. The blood chamber can be equipped either with two mechanical valves (Medtronic Hall valve 21A, Minneapolis, MN, USA) or two polymer valves (Department of Biomedical Engineering, Seoul National University Hospital). The stroke volume of the blood sac is about 48 cm^3. The inlet from the left atrium and the outlet to the aorta are cannular and polymer tube (Tygon, Norton Performance Plastics, Arkon, OH, USA) with a $\frac{1}{2}$-in. inner diameter, respectively, and their lengths are about 40 cm (exact lengths are determined by the surgeon during the operation). Longer lengths of conduit can cause more consumption of energy, but since the amount of energy consumption is not important with our system, lengths of conduits only have to be in an appropriate range without large variance. The controller consists of a microcontroller (Intel 80C196KC, Intel Corporation, Santa Clara, CA, USA) for motor control and a PC (Intel 80486) for monitoring. It can operate in three modes — fixed rate mode, automatic flow regulation mode, and synchronized mode. In synchronized mode, the pumping can be synchronized to the heart rate at up to at least 160 bpm. In the automatic mode, it regulates assist flow according to (1) the left atrial pressure (LAP) or aortic pressure (AoP), estimated from the motor current consumed by the actuator; and (2) the measured pressure in the bellows.

Using Polymer Bellows Water Pressure

We use a pressure sensor measuring the internal water pressure of the polymer bellows. This pressure is related to LAP, which indicates the state of the left

atrium or the blood volume in the atrium. Under low LAP or low filling volume, the pressure drops below normal levels, and when suction occurs, LAP goes far negative abruptly. Therefore, adjustment of the pumping action to limit or regulate this pressure is needed to prevent suction.

We implemented two simple pressure limiters [4]. One is an absolute limiter, and the second is a local minimum limiter. The absolute pressure limiter prevents a large negative peak. It monitors the bellows pressure at 1-ms intervals, and stops the actuator when the pressure goes lower than the set point; then after some delay (800 ms) for passive filling, it restarts pumping at low speed (60 bpm). The second limiter was used because a local minimum of bellows pressure can occur when blood filling is interrupted by low blood volume or another abnormal inlet conduit state — for example, cannula kinking. The limiter monitors the moving gradient of bellows pressure during successive 20-ms intervals, and stops the actuator when the gradient goes negative twice; goes to second minimum, then after some delay (800 ms) for passive filling, it restarts pumping at a low speed (60 bpm).

Using Motor Current

In an in vitro experiment using a mock circulation system, we observed that motor current consumed by the device is related to the LAP or inflow status (Fig. 1), as some other researchers have reported [5,6]. Significant factors include the systolic maximum, diastolic maximum, systolic sum, and diastolic sum. In the case of the diastolic signal, a low filling volume induces the device to do more work to overcome the lower negative pressure in the conduit, and this is reflected by a higher maximum and larger sum. The occurrence of

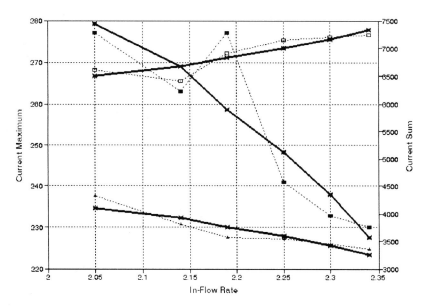

Fig. 1. Relationship between inflow rate (1/min) and motor current (not calibrated). *Triangles*, diastole current sum; *open squares*, systole current sum; *closed squares*, systole current maximum; *solid lines* are fitted curves

suction is reflected in an excessively high peak or second peak of current. Low filling affects systole also. In the early stage of systole, the motor needs low energy because the negative pressure in the bellows helps the motor, but in the middle stage, it comes up with a sudden load without the help of internal bellows pressure, so the current goes high abruptly. Therefore, using this factor, we can adequately determine the motor velocity.

Fuzzy Controller

Bellows pressure and motor current data were observed to have comparatively large deviations, and this complicates the decision on the appropriate pumping speed. Therefore, we used fuzzy logic in the controller for this decision [7]. We tested two types of fuzzy-logic controller. One uses the diastolic bellows pressure maximum, the diastolic bellows pressure sum, and the motor current maximum ratio (systolic to diastolic)

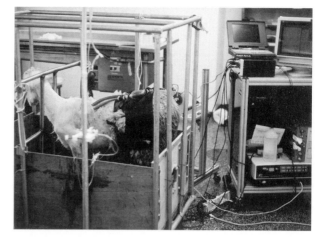

Fig. 2. In vivo test of the new control system in an adult sheep for 17 days (23 Jan 1996–8 Feb 1996)

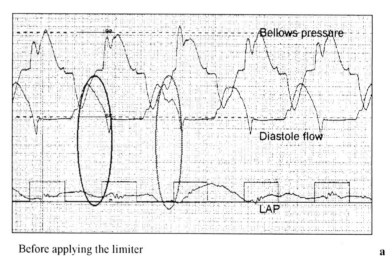

Before applying the limiter   **a**

Fig. 3a,b. In vivo test of the pressure limiter. **a** Before application of the limiter. **b** After application of the limiter; note the hiatus in bellows pressure and diastolic flow showing that the pump had stopped. *Ovals*, suction; *LAP*, left atrial pressure. Polygraph speed, 50 mm/s

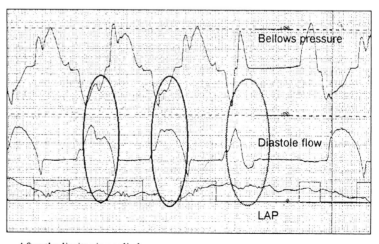

After the limiter is applied   **b**

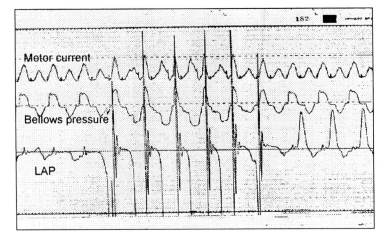

a   Before using fuzzy detector

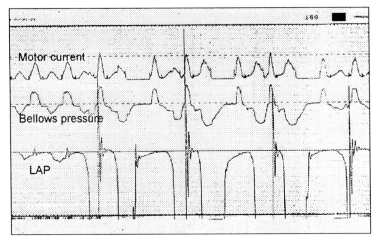

b   After using fuzzy detector

Fig. 4a,b. Suction detection using fuzzy logic controller type I in a mock-circulation experiment (polygraph chart). **a** Before using the fuzzy detector. **b** After using the fuzzy detector; note the hiatus in current and bellows pressure

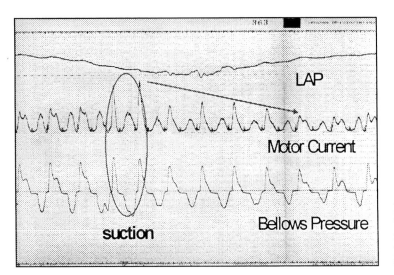

Fig. 5. Suction detection using fuzzy logic controller type II in a mock-circulation experiment. *Oval*, suction; *arrow* shows decrease of peak current indicating gradual resolution of suction event

as input, and its output regulates diastole velocity at low LAP, and determines whether to stop the device or not when suction occurs [8]. The other type of controller uses the diastolic motor current maximum, the diastolic motor current sum, and the systolic motor current sum as input, and its output controls the diastole velocity at low LAP, and determines whether to stop the device or not when suction occurs [9]. Fuzzification uses five steps of the conventional triangular member function. Fuzzy inference and defuzzification are unified into a simple weighted sum function, because output variance is not so large as the input variable combinations.

Experiments

The pressure limiter was implemented in the motor controller, while the fuzzy-logic controller was implemented in the monitoring PC to utilize the high-level language and faster calculation speed supported in the PC. For the in vitro test, we used our mock-circulation system, which has a mock left atrium. Signals were recorded by a polygraph (Fukuda Denshi MCS-5000, Tokyo, Japan) and a monitoring PC. In an in vivo test, an adult sheep was used as the experimental animal (Fig. 2). The test was done over a 17-day period from January 23 to February 8, 1996.

Results

Results are presented in Figs. 3–5. Figure 3 shows the results of the in vivo test of the pressure limiter. Low negative bellows pressure or low LAP was detected successfully, and the pump was stopped automatically. After a 17-day test of the controller in a sheep, autopsy results showed no damage or problem related to suction [10]. However, the pressure gradient detector showed some unexpected faults in operation and mistakes in coding, which were found and fixed later. Figures 4, 5 show the results of in vitro tests of fuzzy controllers types I (Fig. 4) and II (Fig. 5) using a mock circulation system. Both types of controller show good detection of suction and regulation of pump velocity. However, in both, the abrupt motor-stop function for suction prevention responded with a 1-beat delay, because the fuzzy controller is implemented in the monitoring PC and the monitoring PC cannot transmit the motor-stop command until one stroke ends. This problem can be solved by implementing the fuzzy controller in the motor controller.

Discussion

We proposed three electrical methods to prevent suction and regulate assist output with respect to inflow state automatically. We were able to verify the feasibility of all methods proposed for practical use; in particular, the pressure-limiting method proved its good performance through a 17-day in vivo test using an adult sheep. For more rigorous control of assistance flow, system modeling and further experimental analysis are in progress.

References

1. Choi J-U (1992) A study on the development of an electrohydraulic left ventricular assist device. Ph D dissertation, Seoul National University, Seoul, pp 18–19
2. Lee S-W (1995) Pump output regulation algorithm for an electrohydraulic left ventricular assist device using pressure waveform analysis. ME dissertation, Seoul National University, Seoul, pp 10–11
3. Stöcklmayer C, Dorffner G, Schmidt C, Schima H (1995) An artificial neural network-based noninvasive detector for suction and left atrium pressure in the control of rotary blood pumps: an in vitro study. Artif Organs 19:719–724
4. Choi J-S, Ahn Y-H, Lee S-W, Jung C-I, Min B-G (1995) An improvement of velocity control method for prevention of left atrium collapse in left ventricular assist device. Proceedings of KOSOMBE (Korea Society of Medical and Biological Engineering) Spring conference 1995, 71(1):251–255
5. Choi W-W, Kim H-C, Min B-G (1996) A new automatic cardiac output control algorithm for moving actuator total artificial heart by motor current waveform analysis. Int J Artif Organs 19:189–193
6. Trinkl J, Havlik P, Mesana T, Mitsui N, Morita S, Demunck JL, Tourres JL, Monties JR (1993) Control of a rotary pulsatile cardiac assist pump driven by an electric motor without a pressure sensor to avoid collapse of the pump inlet. ASAIO J 39:M237–M241
7. Yoshizawa M, Takeda H, Yambe T, Nitta S (1994) Assessing cardiovascular dynamics during ventricular assistance. IEEE J Eng Med Biology Nov/Dec:687–692
8. Choi J-S, Choi W-W, Jo Y-H, Park S-K, Min B-G (1995) Development of a stroke output control algorithm using a fuzzy logic for a left ventricular assist device. Proceedings of the 10th Korea Automatic Control conference internation program, Oct 23–25, 1995, pp 514–517
9. Choi J-S, Choi W-W, Jo Y-H, Park S-K, Min B-G (1995) Development of an algorithm for regulation of inlet blood flow in electrohydraulic left ventricular assist device using fuzzy logic. Proceedings of KFIS (Korea Fuzzy Logic and Intelligent Systems Society) Fall Conference 1995 5(2):387–392
10. Jae-Soon C, Chanil C, Won-Woo C, Seong-Keun P, Yung-Ho J, Kyoung-Sik O, Jong-Jin L, Yong-Soon W, Hee-Chan K, Won-Gon K, Byoung-Goo M (1996) Evaluation of electrohydraulic left ventricular assist device through animal experiment. Proceedings of KOSOMBE (Korea Society of Medical and Biological Engineering) Spring conference 1996 18(1):84–87

Scintigraphic Analysis of Cell Adhesion in Oxygenators and Internal Organs

Robert C. Eberhart, Jun Li, M. Kurt Sly, Parag Shastri, Rohan Bhujle, John N. Gaffke, James E. Clift, Yun-Wei Ye, Michael E. Jessen, Robert Chao, Anca Constantinescu, and Padmakar Kulkarni

Summary. We studied dynamic platelet and neutrophil adhesion on cardiopulmonary bypass (CPB) circuit surfaces and in internal organs by quantitative dual-isotope gamma scintigraphy. Microporous polypropylene oxygenators were allocated to four groups: uncoated (I) and siloxane/caprolactone coated (SMA) (II) Cobe Duo oxygenators ($n = 8$); or uncoated (III) and Carmeda heparin treated (IV) Medtronic Maxima oxygenators ($n = 4$). Pigs were subjected to 90 min of normothermic CPB. During CPB, 4%–25% of the platelet and neutrophil populations deposited on oxygenator surfaces, in correlation with circulating cell numbers. Platelet deposits increased during the first 20–30 min of CPB in all groups; deposits stabilized, then declined slightly after 60 min (I, III, IV). Deposits dropped sharply after 20 min (II). Neutrophil deposits increased continuously (I, II) or stabilized (III), or were significantly reduced (IV). Post CPB, increased sequestered cell populations were observed in liver and lung, in correlation with decreased deposits of cells on circuit surfaces. Carmeda heparin treatment reduced neutrophil adhesion, but not platelet adhesion. SMA treatment reduced platelet adhesion, but not neutrophil adhesion.

Key words: Platelet — Neutrophil — Cardiopulmonary bypass — Internal organs — Imaging

Introduction

Oxygenator membranes pose the greatest challenge to the hemostatic and inflammatory systems of the host during cardiopulmonary bypass (CPB). Data on platelet and neutrophil accumulation and/or release from the surfaces of CPB circuitry during CPB are lacking. We developed a gamma imaging system that simultaneously measures platelet and neutrophil kinetics on biosurfaces and internal organs. We report results for two oxygenators (Cobe Duo [Cobe Cardiovascular, Arvada, CO, USA] and Medtronic Maxima [Medtronic Cardiopulmonary, Irvine, CA, USA]) with separate surface treatments (siloxane/caprolactone [SMA, Thoratech Laboratories, Berkeley, CA, USA]

Joint Biomedical Engineering Program, The University of Texas Southwestern Medical Center at Dallas and The University of Texas at Arlington, 5323 Harry Hines Blvd., Dallas, TX 75235-9130, USA

and Carmeda heparin [Medtronic Cardiopulmonary]) and a common centrifugal pump (Medtronic Biomedicus, Eden Prarie, MN, USA).

Materials and Methods

Male farm pigs 35–40 kg were premedicated with ketamine (20 mg/kg IM) and anesthetized with isoflurane. A 43-ml blood sample was drawn for platelet labelling with ^{111}In-oxine [1]. A 70-ml blood sample was then drawn for neutrophil labelling with ^{99m}Tc-exametazime [2]. Platelets and neutrophils were reinfused and the pig was prepared for CPB employing a median sternotomy and standard methods, including systemic heparin (300 U/kg IV) and flow rates of 75–100 ml·kg^{-1}·min^{-1}. The activated clotting time (ACT) was maintained greater than 400 s with supplemental heparin. Oxygenator, pump, and internal organs were imaged (Fig. 1) with a two-dimensional gamma camera (GE 400T, General Electric, Milwaukee, WI, USA). Intensity distributions were corrected for energy overlap, camera-object spacing sensitivity, plastic and tissue gamma absorption, and for the blood pool. Differences from control values were analyzed by Student's t-test.

Results

Reductions of cell counts during CPB were typical for hemodilution by circuit priming and fluid infusion. There were no intergroup differences in pressure, infusion volume, heparin, or activated clotting time (ACT). Platelet adhesion was detected at all timepoints in the centrifugal pump and in the Cobe Duo oxygenators (groups I and II), with much greater deposition in the oxygenators. Platelet deposits increased over the first 30 min of CPB in group I to a maximum at 60 min, declining thereafter to about half peak value at the end of CPB. Based on a 5.3-m^2 membrane + netting surface area, the peak platelet surface concentration was 30/1000 μm^2. The mean surface deposit during CPB was 16% of the pre-CPB circulating platelet mass (Fig. 2). SMA-treated

Fig. 1. Schematic diagram of the ex vivo cardiopulmonary bypass (CPB) system setup. The field of view includes the oxygenator and blood pump during CPB, and the pig thorax and upper abdomen before and after CPB

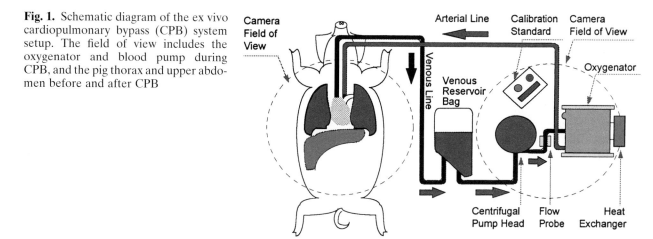

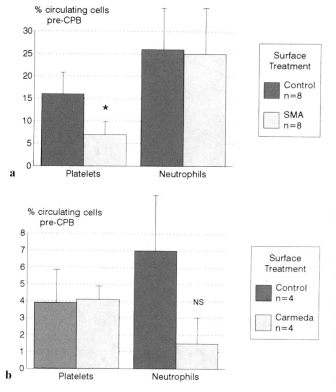

Fig. 2a,b. Platelet and neutrophil deposition. **a** Cobe Duo microporous polypropylene sheet membrane oxygenators, coated with siloxane/caprolactone (*SMA, gray bars*) or untreated (*black bars*). **b** Medtronic Maxima microporous polypropylene hollow fiber oxygenators, coated with Carmeda heparin (*gray bars*) or untreated (*black bars*). Data are averaged over 90 min of cardiopulmonary bypass (*CPB*)

oxygenators accumulated significantly fewer platelets; 7% of the pre-CPB value (Fig. 2a). Neutrophil deposits were also higher on the oxygenators than on the centrifugal pump, increasing continuously to a peak concentration at the end of CPB of $1.4/1000\,\mu m^2$,

25% of the pre-CPB neutrophil mass (Fig. 2a) and suggesting a CPB-induced demargination.

Large platelet deposits were also observed on the uncoated and Carmeda-treated Medtronic oxygenators. There were no differences in mean surface deposits for groups III and IV, both approximately 4% of the pre-CPB circulating platelet values (Fig. 2b). Platelet deposits peaked at 30 min, then stabilized and declined, earlier than in group I. Based on a 2.0-m^2 membrane surface area, platelet surface concentrations (III and IV) were the same, $41/1000\,\mu m^2$, slightly higher than in group I. Circulating platelet counts throughout CPB were lower than the theoretically predicted values from hemodilution, correlating with the higher deposits on the oxygenator membranes. Neutrophil deposition tended to be lower for Carmeda (IV) oxygenators than controls (III) (Fig. 2b); the small sample size ($n = 4$) prevented this difference from becoming statistically significant. The initial neutrophil transients were larger, and deposits peaked later, than for the corresponding platelet pattern. The group III peak surface concentration of neutrophils was $1.5/1000\,\mu m^2$.

SMA treatment (II) preserved average platelet counts in liver and lung during the post-CPB observation period. In contrast, untreated (I) Cobe oxygenators were associated with decreased platelet numbers in liver and lung, with a similar but nonsignificant tendency in heart. The preservation of organ platelets correlates with the increased group II circulating cell concentrations observed during CPB. SMA treatment (II) tended to increase neutrophil accumulations in heart, liver, and lung, relative to pre-CPB controls. No such increase was obtained in the untreated group (I). Neither uncoated (III) nor Carmeda-heparin-treated Medtronic oxygenator circuits (IV) preserved platelet counts in heart, lung, or liver. Neutrophil counts in heart and lung were significantly lower in untreated controls (Fig. 2b);

Carmeda treatment preserved neutrophils in these organs.

Discussion

Accumulation of significant numbers of platelets and neutrophils occurs on foreign surfaces during CPB, with maximal uptakes observed on the surfaces of oxygenator membranes. Flat-sheet oxygenators generally require netting to support the blood gap, while wound hollow fiber oxygenators do not. Despite the much larger blood–polymer contact surface for the flat-sheet oxygenators, cell surface densities were roughly equivalent to those for the wound hollow fiber oxygenators when the entire blood-contacting polymer surface was taken into account. Much lower levels of platelet and neutrophil accumulation were found on centrifugal pump surfaces. These are subject to much higher fluid shear, which may inhibit stable adhesion of cells. An interesting difference was observed between the two types of surface treatments in this study. The siloxane/caprolactone (SMA) treatment inhibited platelet adhesion on oxygenator membranes and preserved them for the circulation. However, SMA treatment did not alter neutrophil adhesion patterns; in fact, more neutrophils entered the circulation for perfusions with the treated surfaces than for perfusions with control surfaces. In contrast, the Carmeda surface heparinization treatment had no influence on platelet adhesion during CPB, while neutrophil adhesion was nonsignificantly reduced by the Carmeda treatment. Post-CPB, we observed decreased numbers of adherent platelets and neutrophils on the washed surfaces of both types of oxygenators subjected to both types of surface treatment. These results are consistent with published observations for Carmeda-treated oxygenators. Despite the platelet-sparing effect of Carmeda treatment inferred from studies of oxygenators post-CPB, our results suggest that platelets nevertheless are attracted to and retained on these treated surfaces during CPB. Platelet activation (whole blood impedance aggregometry) roughly tracks the platelet adhesion results. Further activation or traumatization of platelets or neutrophils cannot be inferred from these results. Nevertheless, the surface interaction is shown to be a significant one, for both types of cells, for both types of oxygenators. Those surface treatments which decreased cell deposition on pump-oxygenator surfaces, increased, in general, circulating cell counts and increased the accumulations (sequestered and blood pool) in internal organs. Our results do not permit the conclusion that cells sequestered in organs are more, or less, activated by the surface treatment than the corresponding cells from control studies. Nevertheless, it is significant that shifts, sometimes major, in cell accumulations are observed in internal organs. These results suggest that related functional imaging studies of these populations may be rewarding in regard to our understanding the fate of cells traumatized by CPB.

Acknowledgments. Kimberly Jones, Nicklett Minnella, Srinivasan Natarayan, Ashit Pandit, Satthya Raja, Parag Shastri, and Kurt Sly also contributed to this research. Supported by a grant from the Texas Advanced Technology Program, and financial assistance from Cobe Cardiovascular and Medtronic Cardiopulmonary

References

1. Thakur MI, Walsh L, Malech HL, Gottschalk A (1981) Indium-111-labeled human platelets: improved method, efficacy and evaluation. J Nucl Med 22:381–385
2. Dewanjee MK (1990) Techniques of labeling white cells with ^{99m}Tc HMPAO. Semin Nucl Med 20:21

Surface Fixation of Lumbrokinase via Photochemical Reaction of Azidophenyl Group

Hyun Jung Kim[1,2], Yasuhide Nakayama[3], Jongwon Kim[1,2], Takehisa Matsuda[3], and Byoung Goo Min[1]

Summary. A new method for the immobilization of lumbrokinase (LK) on polymer was developed. The method is based on the photochemical reaction of the azidophenyl group, which produces a highly reactive phenylnitrene upon ultraviolet (UV) light irradiation. First, an aminated polymer, partially derivatized with a photoreactive phenyl azido group in its side chains, was coated onto a polyurethane (PU) surface. Subsequently, the surface was exposed to UV light. To induce the carboxyl group on the UV-light-treated surface, poly(methyl vinyl ether-co-maleic acid) (MAcMEC) was reacted. LK was immobilized on the PU surface using 1-ethyl-3-(3-dimethylaminopropyl)carbodiimide (EDC) in aqueous solvent. Electron spectroscopy for chemical analysis (ESCA) and water contact angle measurement before and after sequential surface reactions revealed that LK was immobilized successfully. The LK immobilized on the PU surface had fibrinolytic activity. In conclusion, LK immobilization via this photochemical reaction will be useful in improving the blood compatibility of blood-contacting polymer.

Key words: Lumbrokinase — Polyurethane — Photochemical reaction — Azidophenyl functional group

Introduction

To covalently immobilize biomacromolecules onto polymer surfaces, it is necessary to have functional groups on the polymer surface such as amine, carboxyl, isocyanate, or hydroxyl groups [1]. Since most conventional polymers except for polysaccharides have no such functional groups on the surface, they must be modified by the addition of reactive groups for the covalent immobilization of biomacromolecules.

We aimed to introduce the amine group onto the surface of polyurethane (PU) by photochemical reaction of the azidophenyl group from poly(allylamine)

(AzPhPAL) [2]. Ultraviolet (UV) light irradiation has made it possible to generate an AzPhPAL layer on the PU surface without any alteration of the bulk properties of the polymer. The grafted AzPhPAL layers on the PU surface were further subjected to a condensation reaction with poly(methyl vinyl ether-co-maleic acid) (MAcMEC) and 1-ethyl-3-(3-dimethylaminopropyl)carbodiimide (EDC) to generate the carboxyl groups that were used for immobilization of Lumbrokinase (LK).

The modified surfaces were characterized by electron spectroscopy for chemical analysis (ESCA) and attenuated total internal reflection–Fourier transform infrared spectroscopy (ATR-FTIR). The amount of amino functional group was evaluated by orange II assay (dye-binding method). In addition, we evaluated the fibrinolytic activity of the immobilized LK to demonstrate the efficacy of surface derivatization without changing the biological properties of the immobilized protein.

Materials and Methods

Poly(allylamine hydrochloride) (10 mmol equivalents for each monomer unit), 4-azidobenzoic acid (3.6 mmol), and a small amount of $KHCO_3$ (2 mmol) were dissolved in deionized water (70 ml) with cooling in an ice bath. ECD (4.4 mmol) in dimethylformamide (DMF, 50 ml) was added to the mixture while stirring and cooling in an ice bath. The reaction was allowed to stand overnight under continuous stirring. The product was concentrated under reduced pressure, and extensive dialysis using a seamless cellulose tube was conducted in deionized water for one day. The dialyzed polymer was freeze-dried in vacuum to obtain a white solid. Ten microliters of AzPhPAL solution in ethanol and deionized water 2:1 v/v (0.5 g/100 ml) was spread on the PU (20 × 20 mm). The surface was UV-irradiated for 1 min using a Hamamatsu UV lamp (intensity 2.2 mW/cm²) and thoroughly washed with running water for 1 h. To generate the carboxyl group on the photoreacted PU surface, the PU was placed in 2 mmol MAcMEC solution containing 2.4 mmol EDC and 0.05 M KH_2PO_4, pH 4.5, at 25°C for 3 h. The PU

[1] Institute of Medical and Biomedical Engineering, Seoul National University Hospital, 28 Youngun-Dong, Chongno-Ku, Seoul 110-744, Korea
[2] Biomedlab Company, Dongsung Bldg., 1-49 Dongsung-Dong, Jongno-Gu, Seoul 110-510, Korea
[3] National Cardiovascular Center Research Institute, 5-7-1 Fujishirodai, Suita, Osaka 565, Japan

with the introduced carboxyl groups was placed in 0.03 M EDC solution in 0.05 M KH$_2$PO$_4$, pH 4.5, at 4°C for 1 h and then washed with PBS of pH 7.4. The resulting PU, containing the *O*-acylisourea group, was placed in 1 mg/ml bovine albumin or 1 mg/ml LK solution in PBS, pH 7.4, and the solution was kept at 4°C for 20 h [3].

Fibrinogen (0.8 g/100 ml) was dissolved in 0.2 M borate buffer, pH 7.8, containing 0.05 M NaCl. The solution was incubated in 37°C for 30 min and filtered. The fibrinogen solution (10 ml) and 10 μl of thrombin (500 U/ml) were added to a petri dish. The mixed solution was incubated for 2 h. To evaluate the fibrinolytic activity of the immobilized LK, the size of the clear zone around the PU was determined.

Results

The degree of substitution of azidophenyl groups was by amino groups in AzPhPAL 4.4%, determined from UV spectroscopic measurement (λ_{max} 266 nm).

A thin layer coating of AzPhPAL with the azidophenyl groups on a PU surface was obtained by coating with 10 μl of AzPhPAL solution (0.5 g/100 ml in ethanol:deionized water, 2:1 v/v). Ethanol was used as a hydrophobic solvent for increasing the solubility of AzPhPAL. To induce carboxyl groups on the AzPhPAL-treated PU surface, a PU having 9×10^{-8} mol/cm^2 of amino group on its surface was reacted with MAcMEC and EDC in 0.05 M KH$_2$PO$_4$ at 25°C for 3 h [3]. The carboxyl groups on the PU surface-treated with MAcMEC were used for amide bond formation between the LK and the aminated PU.

Figure 1 shows the ESCA spectra of a nontreated PU surface (a), the photochemically fixed surface (b), and the PU surface with immobilized LK (c). UV irradiation of the AzPhPAL casting surface resulted in the ESCA spectral changes shown in Fig. 1b. The N1s signal increased and the C1s subpeaks were markedly changed. Immobilization of LK on the AzPhPAL-treated PU surface caused an appreciable change in the C1s and S2p spectra. These results indicated that AzPhPAL and LK were chemically fixed on the PU (summarized in Table 1).

Static contact angles toward water of PU before and after surface grafting with AzPhPAL were measured. The water wettability measurement showed that the surface nature was drastically changed, from hydrophobic to hydrophilic, upon surface grafting by AzPhPAL (Table 2). The receding angle ($\frac{1}{2}\theta_{rec}$) was 3.40° ± 0.216° for AzPhPAL-treated PU. After LK immobilization on the AzPhPAL-treated PU, the receding angle ($\frac{1}{2}\theta_{rec}$) was reduced to 1.87° ±

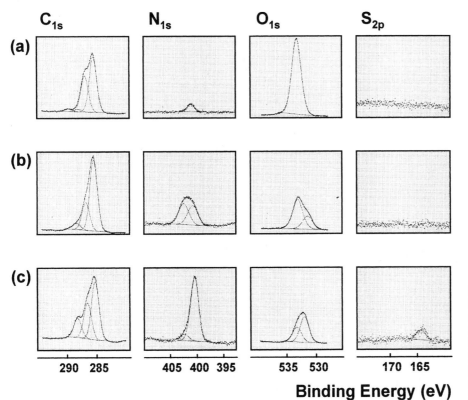

Fig. 1. Electron spectroscopy for chemical analysis (ESCA) spectra of nontreated polyurethane (PU) surface (**a**), PU surface photochemically fixed with poly(allylamine) (AzPhPAL) (**b**), and PU surface with immobilized Lumbrokinase (LK) (**c**)

Table 1. Elemental ratios of the polymer surface obtained by electron spectroscopy for chemical analysis (ESCA)

Polyurethane treatment	N/C	O/C	S/C
Nontreated	0.0247	0.6936	n.d.
CW	0.1388	0.4478	n.d.
CUW	0.1717	0.3804	n.d.
CUWL	0.2228	0.2833	0.0043

CW, coated with 10µl poly(allylamine) (AzPhPAL) and washed; CUW, coated with 10µl AzPhPAL, irradiated by UV light, and washed; CUWL, coated with 10µl AzPhPAL, irradiated with UV, washed, and reacted with Lumbrokinase; n.d., not detected.

Table 2. Contact angles of polyurethane and derivatized polyurethane, measured in water using the sessile drop technique

Polyurethane treatment	$\frac{1}{2}\theta_{adv}$	$\frac{1}{2}\theta_{rec}$
Nontreated	38.0° ± 0.000°	28.5° ± 0.368°
CUW	37.6° ± 0.873°	3.40° ± 0.216°
CUWL	32.2° ± 0.205°	1.87° ± 0.287°

θ_{adv}, advancing contact angle; θ_{rec}, receding contact angle.

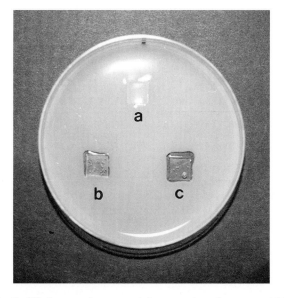

Fig. 2. Fibrin test plate containing samples of untreated PU (**a**), PU with LK physically adsorbed to its surface (**b**), and PU with LK photochemically immobilized on its surface (**c**)

0.287°. Therefore, the LK-treated PU surface is more hydrophilic than the AzPhPAL-treated surface.

To demonstrate the fibrinolytic activity of the LK photochemically immobilized on PU, we used the fibrin plate test. Figure 2 shows that the size of the clear zone around the PU with LK immobilized by photochemical reaction (c in Fig. 2) was larger than that around the PU surface with physically adsorbed LK (b in Fig. 2). These results indicate that LK retains fibrinolytic activity after immobilization on the PU surface by photochemical reaction with AzPhPAL.

Discussion

Various methods have been tried to immobilize enzymes, peptides, and phospholipids on polymer surfaces [4,5]. In this paper, a new method for protein fixation, utilizing a photoreactive azidophenyl group, was developed to fix LK chemically onto a PU surface. With this method, we can overcome the considerable limitations in the availability of surface functional groups, and it can readily be applied to complex-shaped devices. Aryl azides, including phenyl azide, are more thermally and chemically stable than alkyl or acyl azides. Therefore, we synthesized AzPhPAL using 4-azidobenzoic acid and poly(allylamine). AzPhPAL and MAcMEC can be dissolved in aqueous solvent. By virtue of their stability and solubility, we could use them for surface modification of PU without any change in the physical and morphological properties of the polymer. The condensation reaction between MAcMEC and LK in aqueous solution with EDC is one of the most conventional methods for immobilization of LK on PU surface without affecting the polymer's physical properties. This surface modification, via photochemical fixation of AzPhPAL and subsequent coupling of MAcMEC, provides the following advantages: (1) much less limitation in the choice of polymer surfaces to be modified, (2) less surface destruction, and (3) uniform grafting of a given region of complex-shaped devices.

Conclusion

Following treatment of PU with AzPhPAL by photochemical reaction, LK could be immobilized onto the surface of the PU. Under optimum conditions, 10^{-8} mol/cm^2 of amino group from AzPhPAL could be introduced onto the PU surface. The surface possessing the amino group was characterized by ESCA spectra. The carboxyl group was introduced by the reaction of MAcMEC with the aminated PU surface. This functional group, introduced onto the PU surface, proved to be useful in the covalent conjugation of LK using EDC.

References

1. Ryu GH, Han DK, Park S, Kim MR, Min BG (1995) Surface characteristics and properties of lumbrokinase-immobilized PU. J Biomed Mater Res 29:403–409

2. Sugawara T, Matsuda T (1994) Novel surface graft copolymerization method with micro-order regional precision. Macromolecules 27:7809–7814
3. Sano S, Kato K, Ikada Y (1993) Introduction of functional groups onto the surface of polyethylene for protein immobilization. Biomaterials 14(11):817–822
4. Cai SX, Wybourne MN, Keana JFW (1994) *N*-hydroxysuccinimide ester functionalized perfluorophenyl azides as novel photoreactive heterobifunctional cross-linking reagents. The covalent immobilization of biomolecules to polymer surfaces. Bioconjug Chem 5(2):151–157
5. Massia SP, Hubble JA (1990) Covalent surface immobilization of Arg-Gly-Asp and Tyr-IIe-Gly-Ser-Arg-containing peptides to obtain well-defined cell adhesion substrates. Anal Chem 187:292–301

The Effect of Lumbrokinase, a Trypsin-Like Enzyme from *Lumbricus rubellus,* on Human Blood Cells

Jae Hee Shim[1,2], Yong Doo Park[1], Won Hee Choi[1], Jongwon Kim[1,2], Seonyang Park[3], and Byoung Goo Min[1]

Summary. Lumbrokinase (LK), a trypsin-like enzyme, was efficiently purified from a crude preparation of earthworm (*Lumbricus rubellus*). The purification procedure was as follows: dissolving crude powder in saline for 3 days; 30%–60% ammonium sulfate gradient fractionation of the soluble fraction; and column chromatography on DEAE-cellulose anion exchange and then *p*-aminobenzamidine sepharose 6B. Lumbrokinase has a molecular weight of 34.2 kDa, is not dependent on metal ions, is heat-stable, and has a very broad optimal pH range. To examine whether LK hydrolyzed fibrin directly without human blood cell damage, various human blood cells were prepared for characterization of LK activity. The hemolysis of erythrocytes was assayed using a UV spectrophotometer, the degradation pattern of plasma proteins was assessed by sodium dodecyl sulfate-polyacrylamide gel electrophoresis, and the lysis of protein constituents of platelet-rich plasma and platelets (platelets were separated by Bio-gel A-50 gel filtration) was measured. To investigate whether LK causes spontaneous platelet aggregation, the effect of antiaggregation by adenosine diphosphate (ADP) was measured using an aggregometer. It was shown that, in spite of its proteolytic activity, LK did not cause lysis of erythrocytes, or excessive degradation of protein in plasma, platelets, or platelet-rich plasma. Nor did LK cause spontaneous platelet aggregation. The antiaggregation effect by ADP was not observed.

Key words: Earthworm — Lumbrokinase — Purification — Blood cell — Platelet antiaggregation effect

Introduction

The incidence of thrombotic disorders, including cerebral stroke, myocardial infarction, and venous thromboembolism, is rapidly increasing in Korea. Various therapeutic agents are used for thrombotic diseases, including anticoagulants and antiplatelet drugs, which may retard or prevent further progression of thrombotic lesions. However, they cannot actively lyse thrombotic clots. Thrombolytic agents, however, can lyse the thrombi, and currently available thrombolytic agents are used for various thrombotic disorders. In Oriental regions, a number of traditional treatment regimens have been used for thrombotic diseases. However, most natural products have not so far been evaluated in a scientific way. For the first time, a novel fibrinolytic enzyme called lumbrokinase was extracted from the earthworm (*Lumbricus rubellus*) by Mihara, 1983 [1]. Recently, we purified lumbrokinase by a simpler method than Mihara's, obtaining a trypsin-like protease from the earthworm. This study was designed to evaluate the effectiveness of lumbrokinase from the earthworm (*L. rubellus*), a component of traditional Oriental antithrombotic drugs [2], and to assess the antithrombotic activity of lumbrokinase immobilized on an artificial heart surface [3]. In this study, we present a simple purification procedure for the fibrinolytic enzyme, its biochemical characteristics, and the effect of lumbrokinase on human blood cells.

Materials and Methods

Materials

Sodium dodecyl sulfate polyacrylamide gel electrophoresis and Bio-gel A-50 were from Bio-Rad (Richmond, CA, USA), earthworm powder (species: *L. rubellus*) was purchased from Cisam Guin Compost in Kiheoung, Korea, dialysis membrane (cutoff size: 10 kDa) was from Spectrum (Laguna Hills, CA, USA), diethylaminoethyl (DEAE) sephadex A-25, *p*-aminobenzamidine insolubilized on sepharose 6B, bovine fibrinogen, aprotinin, soybean trypsin inhibitor, ε-aminocaproic acid, and ethylene diamine tetraacetic acid (EDTA) were from Sigma (St. Louis, MO, USA), and the ultra-filtration (membrane cutoff size: 10 kDa) was from Amicon (Beverly, MA, USA).

Methods

Purification and Biochemistry of LK

Purification of fibrinolytic enzyme (LK) from earthworm (*L. rubellus*) was carried out by pretreatment

[1] Institute of Biomedical Engineering, College of Medicine, Seoul National University, 28 Youngun-Dong, Chongno-Ku, Seoul 110-744, Korea
[2] Biomedlab Co., Dongsung Bldg., 1-49 Dongsung-Dong, Jongno-Gu, Seoul 110-510, Korea
[3] Department of Internal Medicine, College of Medicine, Seoul National University, Seoul, Korea

and two-step column chromatography comprising DEAE-anion exchange and benzamidine affinity column chromatography [2]. Sodium dodecyl sulfate polyacrylamide gel electrophoresis (SDS-PAGE) was carried out to prove that the purified protein formed a single band. Proteins were quantitated by using the Bradford method [4]. LK was dissolved in each buffer with different pH values and incubated at various temperatures for 2h (Fig. 1). Fibrinolytic activity was examined by the fibrin plate method [6]. LK was incubated with various protein inhibitors. In separate incubations, aprotinin, soybean trypsin inhibitor, ε-aminocaproic acid, and EDTA were added to final concentrations of 100 kIU/mℓ, 0.8 mg/mℓ, 0.8 mg/mℓ, and 1 mM, respectively.

Plasma Degradation Studies

First, plasma was diluted with phosphate buffered saline (PBS) to give 10mg protein per ml. LK (0.1mg) was then added (to give a weight ratio of 100:1). The reaction mixture was incubated at 37°C for various time intervals. The reaction mixture containing sample buffer under denaturing conditions was added for SDS-PAGE (Fig. 2).

The Effect of LK on Blood Cells

Red blood cells and platelet-rich plasma (PRP) were separated by centrifugation, and platelets were further purified by gel filtration (Bio-gel A-50). An absorption spectrum peak around 415 nm is characteristic of free hemoglobin. The release of proteins in PRP and platelets was observed by monitoring absorbance at 280 nm. These samples, treated by LK at protein ratios of 100:1 and 10:1 (w/w) were incubated at 37°C for vari-

ous time intervals. The absorbance was recorded at 25°C after the indicated time intervals (Figs. 3–5). Blood from healthy volunteers was collected in 3.8% sodium citrate (9 vol blood/1 vol citrate) and immediately centrifuged at 25°C for 10 min at 250 × g to obtain PRP and then centrifuged at 1500 × g for 10 min to obtain platelets and platelet-poor plasma. Platelet aggregation was recorded with a platelet aggregometer at 37°C using siliconized glass tubes. Changes in light transmission of the platelet suspensions were recorded under continuous stirring (900 rpm). The reaction mixture consisted of 450 μℓ of PRP preincubated for 1.5 min and added prior to 50 μℓ of 2 mg/mℓ LK at 37°C, and then after 1.5 min, 0.2 mM adenosine diphosphate (ADP) in LK was added (line II) (Fig. 6) [5]. Line I is the control that was treated with ADP only after 3 min. The maximum aggregation response obtained from the addition of ADP, an aggregation agonist, was given a value of 90% aggregation (Fig. 6) [5]. Line I of Fig. 7 is PRP that was treated with ADP only after 3 min and line II is treated with LK only after 1.5 min [5].

Results

It has been reported that there are six kinds of fibrinolytic enzymes with different fibrinolytic activity in the earthworm [1]. The enzyme with the highest fibrinolytic activity, lumbrokinase (LK), was eluted from DEAE-Sephadex at between 300 and 400 mM sodium chloride. The pooled fraction was further purified by *p*-aminobenzamidine column chromatography. The enzyme appears to be homogeneous by SDS-

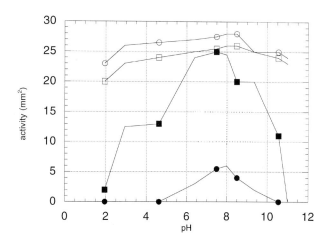

Fig. 1. Stability of purified lumbrokinase to temperature and pH. *Open circles*, 25°C; *open squares*, 45°C; *closed squares*, 66°C; *closed circles*, 78°C. Activity was assayed by the fibrin plate method, and the *ordinate* shows the area of fibrinolysis

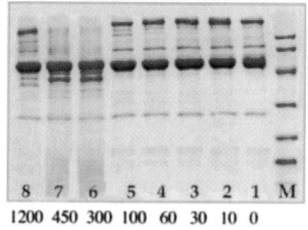

Fig. 2. Degradation of platelet-poor plasma protein by lumbrokinase (LK), assessed by sodium dodecylsulfate-polyacrylamide gel electrophoresis (SDS-PAGE). *Numbers on gel*, well numbers; *M*, molecular weight marker proteins; numbers below gel, incubation time (min)

Fig. 3. Release of hemoglobin from erythrocytes treated with LK at an LK: total hemoglobin of 10:1 (*closed circles*) and 100:1 (*open circles*). *O.D.*, optical density. The O.D. at 415 nm reflects free hemoglobin

Fig. 4. Release of protein from platelets treated with LK for various time intervals at an LK: platelet protein of 10:1 (*closed circles*) and 100:1 (*open circles*)

Fig. 5. Release of protein from platelet-rich plasma (PRP) treated with LK for various times at an LK: PRP protein of 10:1 (*closed circles*) and 100:1 (*open circles*)

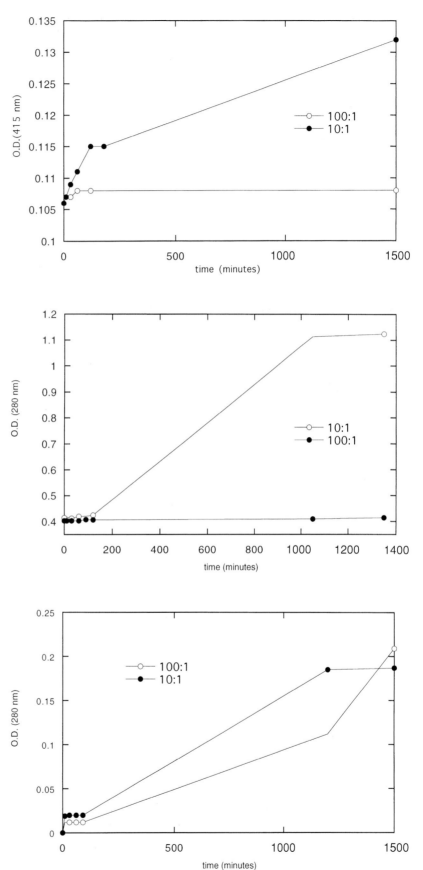

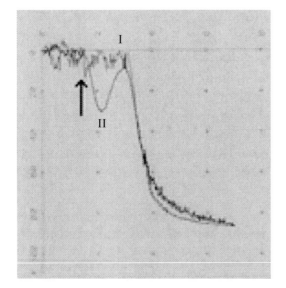

Fig. 6. Antiaggregation effect of ADP-induced platelets when platelets were treated with LK. Line *II* is the reaction mixture that consisted of 450 μℓ of platelet-rich plasma (PRP) preincubated for 1.5 min and added prior to 50 μℓ of 2 mg/mℓ LK at 37°C (*arrow*). After 1.5 min, 0.2 mM adenosine diphosphate (ADP) in LK was added. Line *I* is the control, treated with ADP only after 3 min

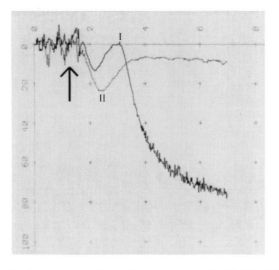

Fig. 7. Aggregation effect of platelets treated with LK. Line *I* is PRP that was treated with ADP only after 3 min and the line *II* is PRP treated with LK only after 1.5 min (*arrow*)

PAGE. This enzyme showed almost constant fibrinolytic activity throughout the range pH 2–11 and retained activity at up to 70°C (Fig. 1). When the enzyme was treated with aprotinin or soybean trypsin inhibitor, LK activity was not detected at all. LK activity did not require the addition of metal ions, and the chelator EDTA had no effect. Therefore, this enzyme

is a trypsin-like protease, not dependent on metal ions, heat-stable, and active over a very wide pH range. LK did not cause excessive degradation of proteins in plasma, release of erythrocyte hemoglobin, or release of protein from platelets (Figs. 2–5). Furthermore, LK had no effect on platelet antiaggregation induced by ADP, and did not itself cause platelet aggregation (Figs. 6, 7). In this study, LK was found to be an effective fibrinolytic agent rather than an antiplatelet drug. This enzyme was also suitable for immobilization on artificial heart surfaces.

Discussion

The biochemical characteristics of LK and its effects on human blood cells may be summarized as follows:

1. The enzyme (34.2 kDa) was purified to near homogeneity following the benzamidine affinity chromatography.
2. The enzyme displayed almost constant fibrinolytic activity at pH 2–11 and retained activity at up to 70°C.
3. Using several protease inhibitors, the enzyme has been shown to be a trypsin-like enzyme.
4. LK did not cause excessive degradation of human plasma protein.
5. The release of hemoglobin from erythrocytes treated by LK was not excessive.
6. Damage to PRP in human blood caused by LK was not apparent.
7. Lysis of platelets in human blood treated by LK was not excessive.
8. LK did not cause platelet aggregation, nor prevent ADP-induced aggregation.

The pathway of LK to fibrinolysis is different from that of the conventional antithrombotic agents such urokinase and tissue plasminogen activator (tPA). We observed that LK hydrolyzes fibrin directly, without plasminogen activation (data not shown). Most enzymes are unstable at high temperature and extreme pH, but under these conditions LK was very stable. Also, in spite of its proteolytic activity, LK did not cause much damage to blood cells. The artificial heart has problems of thrombosis and infection. If LK were to be immobilized by covalent bonding to the surfaces of an artificial heart, we expect that the immobilized LK would be able to prevent thrombosis.

References

1. Mihara H, Sumi H, Akazawa K, Yoneta T, Mizunoto H (1983) Fibrinolytic enzymes extracted from the earthworm. Thromb Haemost 50:258

2. Mihara H, Sumi II, Yoneta T, Mizumoto H, Ikeda R, Seiki M, Maruyama M (1991) A novel fibrinolytic enzyme extracted from the earthworm, *Lumbricus rubellus*. Jpn J Phys 41:461–472

3. Ryu GH, Park S, Han DK, Kim YH, Min B (1993) Antithrombotic activity of a lumbrokinase immobilized polyurethane surface. ASAIO J 39(3):M314–M318

4. Bradford MM (1976) A rapid sensitive method for the quantitation of microgram quantities of protein utilizing the principle of protein-dye binding. Annal Biochem 72:246–254

5. Ahmed NK, Tennant KD, Markland FS, Lacz JP (1990) Biochemical characteristics of fibrolase, a fibrinolytic protease from snake venom. Hemostasis 20(3):147–154

6. Astrup T, Mullertz S (1952) The fibrin plate method for estimating fibrinolytic activity. Arch Biochem Biophys 40:346–351

Multivariate Analysis of Key Factors in Clinical Results of Postcardiotomy Circulatory Support

Masaya Kitamura, Shigeyuki Aomi, Mitsuhiro Hachida, Hiroshi Nishida, Masahiro Endo, and Hitoshi Koyanagi

Summary. To examine key factors contributing to the clinical results of postcardiotomy circulatory support, we evaluated 53 patients (33 men, 20 women) who underwent the circulatory support in our institution. Their ages ranged from 22 to 74 (mean 51) years. Of 53 patients, 32 had valvular, 19 had ischemic, and 2 had congenital heart disease. After operation, 21 patients underwent venoarterial bypass (VAB), 20 had biventricular bypass (BVB), and 8 had left ventricular bypass (LVB). The remaining 4 patients received a pulsatile left ventricular assist device (LVAD). The weaning and discharge rates of the patients by support types were 52.4% and 28.6% with VAB, 75.0% and 55.0% with BVB, 87.5% and 37.5% with LVB, and 75.0% and 50.0% with LVAD, respectively. Overall, the weaning rate was 67.9% and the discharge rate was 41.5%. As a multivariate analysis, the logistic regression method was applied to perioperative variables before and during postcardiotomy circulatory support. Selected independent key factors (odds ratio) of significant difference ($P < 0.05$) were: support type (7.547) for unsuccessful weaning; and presupport cardiogenic shock (17.246), support type (8.780), and support duration (1.487) for nonsurvival. These results indicate that the early application of support before cardiogenic shock and the appropriate selection of support type are key factors in successful postcardiotomy circulatory support.

Key words: Circulatory support — Multivariate analysis — Postcardiotomy heart failure — Mortality — Morbidity

Introduction

Many perioperative factors are supposed to affect the final outcome of postcardiotomy circulatory support. This investigation was undertaken to evaluate key factors contributing to the clinical results of postcardiotomy circulatory support.

Patients and Methods

Between 1984 and October 1995, 53 patients underwent postcardiotomy circulatory support for perioperative ventricular failure in our institution. There

Department of Cardiovascular Surgery, The Heart Institute of Japan, Tokyo Women's Medical College, 8-1 Kawada-cho, Shinjuku-ku, Tokyo 162, Japan

were 33 men and 20 women, and their ages ranged from 22 to 74 (mean 51) years. Of the 53 patients, 32 patients had valvular, 19 had ischemic, and 2 had congenital heart disease.

Venoarterial bypass (VAB) with oxygenation was used for biventricular failure with respiratory insufficiency, and recently, biventricular bypass (BVB) has been applied by preference for left-dominant biventricular failure. Left ventricular bypass (LVB) or a left ventricular assist device (LVAD) [1] was employed for isolated left ventricular failure. As a new technique of emergency VAB, percutaneous cardiopulmonary support (PCPS) [2] was mainly used for acute cardiogenic shock after weaning from standard cardiopulmonary bypass, and it was converted to BVB or LVB if necessary.

In this study, we assessed the clinical results of circulatory support in association with perioperative variables, and key factors contributing to the outcome were analyzed by the logistic regression method. For this multivariate analysis, the age and gender of patients, the functional class according to the New York Heart Association classification, the category of heart disease, the left ventricular ejection fraction, the history of previous cardiac surgery, dysfunction of other organs, and so forth were selected as preoperative variables. The surgical procedure, operation duration, aortic cross-clamp time, presupport cardiogenic shock, ventricular fibrillation, type of circulatory support, support duration, and so on were evaluated as operative variables.

Results

Of the 53 patients after cardiovascular surgery, 21 patients underwent VAB, 20 patients had BVB, 8 patients had LVB, and the remaining 4 patients underwent LVAD support. The duration of support ranged from 3 to 312h (mean 34.9h).

With respect to support duration, in 34 patients with circulatory support of less than 24h, 24 (70.6%) were weaned from the support and 18 (52.9%) were discharged from the hospital. In contrast, 3 of 14 patients (21.4%) with circulatory support between 24 and 96h and only 1 of 5 patients (20%) with support of over 96h remained alive and were discharged from the hospital.

Concerning hemodynamic condition at the introduction of circulatory support, the clinical outcome for patients with or without presupport cardiogenic shock was compared. Severe hypotension, less than 70mmHg, or ventricular fibrillation which required cardiac resuscitation was defined as presupport cardiogenic shock. Eleven of 19 patients (57.9%) who received circulatory support after cardiogenic shock could be weaned from the support, but only 2 patients (10.5%) were discharged from the hospital. Of 34 patients in whom circulatory support was initiated without cardiogenic shock, 25 (73.5%) were weaned and 20 (58.8%) survived.

Regarding the type of circulatory support, the weaning and discharge rates of the patients were 52.4% and 28.6% with VAB, 75.0% and 55.0% with BVB, 87.5% and 37.5% with LVB, and 75.0% and 50.0% with LVAD, respectively. Overall, a 67.9% weaning rate and a 41.5% discharge rate were achieved in this series of patients.

The results of the logistic regression analysis are presented in Table 1. The type of support (odds ratio: 7.547) was a key factor correlating with continued dependence on support, and for patients who did not survive to be discharged, presupport cardiogenic shock (17.246), support type (8.780), and support duration (1.487) were identified as independent key factors of significant difference ($P < 0.05$).

Discussion

In the present study, 53 patients (1.1%) of about 5000 who underwent cardiac operations received various circulatory supports for postcardiotomy ventricular failure. According to the combined registry (ASAIO-ISHLT) [3], 1279 patients had undergone postcardiotomy circulatory support as of December 1993 and

584 patients (45.7%) had been weaned from the support; 323 patients (25.3%) were discharged from hospital.

Our current strategy of circulatory support for postcardiotomy heart failure consists of the combined usage of VAB, BVB, LVB, and LVAD. If the patients are unable to be weaned from cardiopulmonary bypass, VAB with oxygenation is maintained for the evaluation of left and right ventricular performance and respiratory function. In the case of left-dominant biventricular failure, BVB is applied for balanced support of both ventricles. Short-term LVB or intermediate-term LVAD is selected for isolated left ventricular failure. In an emergency, such as the sudden onset of cardiogenic shock in an intensive care unit after operation, PCPS is the support of choice for saving the brain, heart, and other organs. After achieving hemodynamic stabilization, an appropriate type of circulatory support will be selected to obtain sufficient recovery of the left and/or right ventricle. Although this strategy has been reasonably successful, with a 67.9% weaning rate and a 41.5% discharge percentage, some patients with intractable biventricular failure needed a more long-term biventricular assist system [4]. A more precise evaluation of the emergency grade, the severity of biventricular failure, and other organ functions would be necessary to obtain a more appropriate indication for circulatory support for postcardiotomy ventricular failure.

From the result of the logistic regression analysis in this investigation, selected independent determinants of significant difference were support type for nonweaning, and presupport cardiogenic shock, support type, and duration for mortality. For the practical treatment of patients with postcardiotomy cardiogenic shock, PCPS is the quickest method of support for saving the brain, heart, and major organs, and stepwise conversion to advanced circulatory support is important for effective recovery of the failing heart.

With the retrospective review of the 53 patients in this series, we suggest that the patients who died during or after the circulatory support might have been saved by earlier or more appropriate conversion to another type of circulatory support. In terms of postcardiotomy circulatory support, our method of BVB appeared to be very useful for evaluation of the type of heart failure, with or without pulmonary failure. Therefore, all 20 patients with VAB could be candidates for BVB. Concerning the type of heart failure in each patient, the types readily varied during the early postoperative period, and appropriate conversion might be necessary for effective recovery of left and/or right ventricles and lungs.

Overall, the results of this investigation suggest that early application of support before profound cardiogenic shock and the appropriate selection of support

Table 1. Key factors contributing to the clinical results of postcardiotomy circulatory support

Event	Variable	Odds ratio	P value
Support dependence	Support type	7.547[a]	0.0462
Nondischarge	Cardiogenic shock	17.246	0.0146
	Support type	8.780[a]	0.0458
	Support duration	1.487[b]	0.0368

[a] Venoarterial bypass (VAB) versus non-VAB.
[b] Ratio increase per 10h.

type might be key factors in successful circulatory support for postcardiotomy heart failure.

References

1. Pae WE, Miller CA, Matthews Y, Pierce WS (1992) Ventricular assist devices for postcardiotomy cardiogenic shock. J Thorac Cardiovasc Surg 104:541–553
2. Phillips SJ, Ballenteine B, Slonine D, Hall J, Vandehaar J, Kongtahworn C, Zeff RH, Skinner JR, Reckmo K, Gray D (1983) Percutaneous initiation of cardiopulmonary bypass. Ann Thorac Surg 36:223–225
3. Aufiero TX (1994) Combined registry (ASAIO-ISHLT) for the clinical use of mechanical ventricular assist pumps and the total artificial heart. In: 40th annual meeting of American Society for Artificial Internal Organs, San Francisco, CA, April 14–16, 1994
4. Guyton RA, Schonberger JPAM, Everts PAM, Jett GK, Gray LA, Gielchinsky I, Raess DH, Vlahakes GJ, Woolley SR, Gangahar DM, Soltanzadeh H, Piccione WJ, Vaughn CC, Boonstra PW, Buckley MJ (1993) Postcardiotomy shock: clinical evaluation of the BVS 5000 biventricular support system. Ann Thorac Surg 56:346–356

Clinical Experience with Percutaneous Cardiopulmonary in Postcardiotomy Cardiogenic Shock

Yukihiko Orime, Motomi Shiono, Hiroaki Hata, Shinya Yagi, Saeki Tsukamoto, Haruhiko Okumura, Kin-ichi Nakata, and Yukiyasu Sezai

Summary. From April 1990 to June 1996, 14 patients who had been suffering from post-cardiotomy cardiogenic shock were supported by a heparin-coated percutaneous cardiopulmonary support (PCPS) system. Of these patients, 8 (57%) (group I) could be weaned from PCPS, and 6 (group II) could not. Of the group I patients, 7 were discharged from our hospital (long-term survival rate 50%). One patient died from cardiac rupture due to severe myocardial infarction. In group II, cerebral vascular damage was recognized in two cases and renal failure in three. As for aortic cross-clamp time and cardiopulmonary bypass (CPB) time, there were no significant differences between the groups. However, the time delay from initiation of CPB to that of PCPS in group I (212 min) was significantly shorter than that in group II (390 min). This heparin-coated PCPS system was very simple and easy to control. It demonstrated long-term biocompatibility without systemic heparinization. Quicker application of this system is expected to play an important role in preventing severe complications, such as multisystem organ failure, and to obtain better clinical results.

Key words: Percutaneous cardiopulmonary support (PCPS) — Heparin-bonded materials — Postcardiotomy cardiogenic shock — Multisystem organ failure

Introduction

Currently several types of mechanical assist device and oxygenator are clinically available for postcardiotomy cardiogenic shock cases [1,2]. Appropriate device selection is the most important factor in obtaining a better clinical result. In this paper, we introduce our experience with the percutaneous cardiopulmonary support system (PCPS), and also compare factors involved in the outcomes of wean-able and nonweanable cases.

Second Department of Surgery, Nihon University School of Medicine, 30-1 Oyaguchi Kamimachi, Itabashi-ku, Tokyo 173, Japan

Materials and Methods

Percutaneous Cardiopulmonary Support System

Our percutaneous cardiopulmonary support (PCPS) system [3] consists of a centrifugal pump, a membrane oxygenator, and a reservoir. For a centrifugal pump, we used the BioMedicus BP-80 (Medtronic, Minneapolis, MN, USA) and its console. The entire blood-contacting surface of our PCPS system was coated by heparin-bonded materials. For example, the centrifugal pump and percutaneous cannulae were coated by Carmeda (Medtronic). The oxygenator, reservoir, and tube were coated by Duraflo-II (Baxter Bentley Division, Irvine, CA, USA) [4]. Due to this new technology, it can be used long-term with low-dose systemic heparinization.

Patients

From April 1990 to June 1996, we introduced the heparin-coated PCPS system in 14 patients with an average age of 66 years: 11 men and 3 women. Their diagnoses were ischemic disease in 7, valvular in 3, and aortic in 4. The indication for use of this system was cardiopulmonary bypass (CPB) weaning in 6 and postoperative low-output syndrome (LOS) in 8.

We divided those patients into two groups: eight (57%) patients could be weaned from PCPS (group I); their average age was 64; five were men and three women. Their original diseases were: three ischemic heart, one valvular, and four aortic. Five of these patients were supported because of CPB weaning, and three because of postoperative LOS. Group II comprised six patients who could not be weaned from CPB. Their average age was 66. All patients were men; four had ischemic heart disease and two had valvular disease. PCPS was introduced for CPB weaning in one patient and LOS in five (Table 1).

Clinical results and complications in the two groups were reviewed. In addition, comparative study was done on those parameters involving time: cardiopulmonary bypass time (CPBT), aortic cross-clamp time (ACCT), time delay from initiation of CPB to that of PCPS, and support time.

Table 1. Characteristics of patients in groups I and II

	Group I	Group II
Number	8	6
Age (years)	64 ± 20	66 ± 8
Gender (male/female)	5/3	6/0
Preoperative diagnosis		
Ischemic heart disease	3	4
Valvular disease	1	2
Aortic disease	4	0
Indications		
CPB wean	5	1
Postoperative LOS	3	5

CPB, cardiopulmonary bypass; LOS, low output syndrome.

Table 2. Comparisons of groups I and II

	Group I	Group II	P value
ACCT (min)	80 ± 33	74 ± 28	NS
CPBT (min)	236 ± 94	203 ± 80	NS
Time delay (min)	212 ± 74	309 ± 201	<0.05
Support time (h)	22 ± 10	72 ± 48	<0.05

ACCT, aortic cross-clamp time; CPBT, cardiopulmonary bypass time; Time delay, from initiation of cardiopulmonary bypass to that of percutaneous cardiopulmonary support; NS, not significant.

Results

In group I, six patients were discharged from our hospital without any complications. One suffered from renal dysfunction; however, he recovered and was discharged. The other one died from cardiac rupture because of massive myocardial infarction. The long-term survival of patients from both groups was seven (50%). In group II, the complications included central nervous system disturbance in two patients, renal failure in three, and lower extremity ischemia in two.

The ACCT was 80 ± 33 min in group I and 74 ± 28 min in group II, showing no significant difference. The CPBT was 236 ± 94 min in group I and 203 ± 80 min in group II, indicating no significant difference. However, the time delay between CPB and PCPS in group II (390 ± 201 min) was significantly ($P < 0.05$) longer than that in group I (212 ± 74 min). Similarly, the duration of support in group II (72 ± 48 h) was significantly ($P < 0.05$) longer than that in group I (22 ± 10 min) (Table 2).

Discussion

Recently, several types of centrifugal pumps have been developed and they are clinically available, not only as a main pump for CPB, but also for postcardiotomy cardiac support, because of their simple, easy, and reliable controllability and low cost [5,6]. The PCPS system with a centrifugal pump and an oxygenator is also widely used for postcardiotomy cardiogenic shock cases. As a strategy for these cases of severe heart failure, suitable selection of the device and support system and appropriate postoperative management play a significant role in the survival rate of these patients.

Our PCPS system can be operated simply and easily, and set up very quickly with simple surgical techniques. It was very effective for recovery from severe cardiac failure, indicating a satisfactory clinical result (weaning rate, 57%; long-term survival rate, 50%).

This heparin-coated PCPS system demonstrated excellent biocompatibility, and it could be used for an extended period (more than 48 h) with low-dose, or no, systemic heparinization. As an anticoagulant therapy, nafamostat mesilate (Futhan; Torii Pharmacy, Tokyo, Japan) was administered intravenously at a dose of $1 \text{mg} \cdot \text{kg}^{-1} \cdot \text{h}^{-1}$. In fact, we never used heparin during PCPS. In spite of the absence of systemic heparinization, the activated clotting time could be maintained within the range 180–230 s.

However, there are several limitations when using PCPS. We had some thromboembolic complications, such as ischemic injuries in cannulated legs. Because of the limited duration of support, we had to change the oxygenator, the pump, or the whole system frequently [7]. We experienced left heart failure in spite of support in some patients. Nevertheless, we consider that appropriate usage of the device will improve its clinical results.

It is pertinent to note that the effect of "time delay" may be caused by a different etiology. Of the six patients in group II, who could not be weaned from PCPS, five were supported by PCPS because of postoperative low-output syndrome (LOS), which means that all these cases could be weaned from cardiopulmonary bypass. Thus, the time interval between the initiation of CPB to the start of PCPS (i.e., the time delay) was longer than that of group I (in which of eight patients, three were assisted due to LOS). That is why the time delay of group II was significantly longer than that of group I, as discussed earlier.

Conclusion

A total of 14 patients were supported by a heparin-coated PCPS system, resulting in a 57% weaning rate and a 50% survival rate. Owing to this new heparin coating technology, it can be used for an extended period without systemic heparinization, demonstrating excellent biocompatibility. Quicker application of this system will play an important role in preventing severe complications, such as multisystem organ failure, and obtaining better clinical results.

References

1. Frazier OH, Rose EA, Macmanus Q, Burton NA, Lefrak EA, Poirier VL, Dasse K (1992) Multicenter clinical evaluation of the Heartmate 1000 IP left ventricular assist device. Ann Thorac Surg 53:1080–1090
2. McCarthy PM, Portner PM, Tobler HG, Starnes VA, Ramasamy N, Oyer PE (1991) Clinical experience with the Novacor ventricular assist device system: bridge to transplantation and the transition to permanent application. J Thorac Cardiovasc Surg 102:578–587
3. Orime Y, Shindo S, Shiono M, Hata H, Yagi S, Tsukamoto S, Okumura H, Sezai Y (1996) Experiences of postcardiotomy assist: Pneumatic ventricular assist device or venoarterial bypass with percutaneous cardiopulmonary support. Artif Organs 20:721–723
4. Belboul A, Al-khaja N, Gudmundsson M, Karlsson H, Uchino T, Liu B, El-Gatit A, Bjell A, Roberts D, William-Olsson G (1993) The influence of heparin-coated and uncoated extracorporeal circuits on blood rheology during cardiac surgery. J Extra-corporeal Technol 25:40–46
5. Noom GP, Sekela ME, Glueck J, Coleman CL, Feldman L (1990) Comparison of Delphin and BioMedicus pumps. ASAIO Trans 36:616–619
6. Noon GP (1991) BioMedicus ventricular assistance. Ann Thorac Surg 52:180–181
7. Shiono M, Sezai Y (1995) Pneumatic ventricular assist device: Its problems and future trends. Ann Thorac Cardiovasc Surg 1:85–91

Feasibility of Ferromagnetic Artificial Cells for Artificial Circulation

Yoshinori Mitamura[1], Tatsuhiko Wada[2], and Eiji Okamoto[1]

Summary. The feasibility of assisting artificial circulation by the use of ferromagnetic artificial cells was studied experimentally and theoretically. The results indicated that artificial circulation with ferromagnetic artificial cells could become feasible if artificial cells with a magnetization of 113 kA/m (at 0.28 T) become available.

Key words: Artificial heart — Artificial blood cells — Ferrofluids

Introduction

It is known that oxyhemoglobin is diamagnetic while deoxyhemoglobin is paramagnetic. The successful direct magnetic separation of red cells from blood has been reported [1]. Antibody-conjugated magnetoliposomes for targeting cancer cells and their application in hyperthermia have been reported [2]. A ferrofluidic actuator for an implantable artificial heart has been studied by the authors [3]. These studies have led us to investigate the possibility of artificial circulation using biocompatible ferromagnetic artificial cells in the blood.

Materials and Methods

A ferrofluid and a combination of a ferrofluid and an iron cylinder (6.67 mm in outer diameter and 28.7 mm in length) were used as substitutes for ferromagnetic artificial cells. The pressure–flow characteristics were measured using the apparatus shown in Fig. 1. An array of two poles of ring solenoids with an air gap of 10 mm was mounted near the glass tube (7.60 mm in inner diameter). The flux density was 0.236 Tesla (T). The solenoids were alternately activated. Two experiments were conducted: (1) a magnetic fluid consisting of magnetite particles (Ferricolloid HC-50 Taiho, To-

kyo, Japan) was used in the glass tube; (2) the magnetic fluid and an iron cylinder were used. The iron cylinder was immersed in the ferrofluid.

Results

A flow of 38–8 ml/min was obtained against a pressure of 12.5–16.3 mmHg in experiment 1, and 80–24 ml/min against a pressure of 53–240 mmHg in experiment 2 (Fig. 2).

Discussion

The pressure applied to the ferrofluid was calculated. The magnetic flux density (B) at the center line of the gap was measured with a flux meter (Gaussmeter, 9640. F. W. Bell, Orlando, FL, USA). The magnetic field strength (H) was calculated by $H = B/\mu_0$ where μ_0 is the magnetic permeability of free space. The pressure was calculated by the following equation

$$P = \mu_0 \int M \cdot dH$$

where M was magnetization. With the use of the ferrofluid, pressures of 12.5–16.3 mmHg were obtained experimentally (Fig. 2). Extrapolating the results, we obtained a maximum pressure of about 20 mmHg for zero flow. The calculated maximum pressure was 21.7 mmHg. The pressure, therefore, can be reasonably estimated by the calculation.

Calculation showed that magnetic substances could move against a pressure of 100 mmHg if they had a magnetization of 113 kA/m (at a magnetic flux of 0.28 T). The magnetic fluid had a saturation magnetization of 35.6 kA/m, while that of magnetite was 479 kA/m.

As for the size of the particles, the ferrofluid utilized in this study consists of magnetite particles of about 10 nm in diameter. The magnetite particles are coated with surfactant. The antibody-conjugated magnetoliposomes have a diameter of 80 nm [2]. In the capillary membrane there are pores with a width of 8–9 nm. Therefore, the artificial cells should have a diameter larger than 9 nm. If the magnetite particles are coated

[1] Department of Electronic and Information Engineering, School of Engineering, Hokkaido Tokai University, 5-1-1-1 Minamisawa, Minami-ku, Sapporo, Hokkaido 006, Japan
[2] Department of Physics, College of Medical Technology, Hokkaido University Kika-12, Nishi-5, Kita-ku, Sapporo, Hokkaido 060, Japan

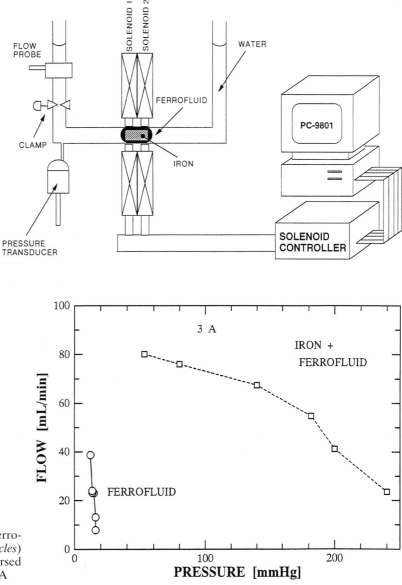

Fig. 1. Apparatus used for measuring the pressure–flow characteristics of a ferrofluid with and without an immersed iron cylinder

Fig. 2. Pressure–flow characteristics of a ferrofluid containing magnetite particles (*circles*) and of the ferrofluid containing an immersed iron cylinder (*squares*). Coil current was 3A

or encapsulated with biocompatible proteins or phospholipids, the artificial cells can flow within a capillary without leaking out of the membrane.

The flow obtained in this study was mainly limited by the size of the device utilized. The inner diameter of the glass tube was 7.6 mm and the maximum stroke of the magnetic plug was limited to 23.4 mm. The theoretical maximum stroke volume, therefore, was 1.06 ml. Experimentally, a maximum stroke volume of 0.8 ml (80 ml at 100 bpm) was obtained. The difference from the calculated value was due to leakage through the gap between the glass wall and the iron cylinder. Higher flow could be obtained with a device of a larger scale. Further studies are required for clinical application of this method, but the prospect of using it to

assist artificial circulation in a particular organ or tissue is interesting.

References

1. Melville D, Paul F, Roath S (1975) High gradient magnetic separation of red cells from whole blood. IEEE Trans Magnetics MAG-11:1701–1704
2. Shinkai M, Suzuki M, Iijima S, Kobayashi T (1994) Antibody-conjugated magnetoliposomes for targeting cancer cells and their application in hyperthermia. Biotechnol Appl Biochem 21:125–137
3. Mitamura Y, Okamoto E (1993) Study of a ferrofluidic actuator for an implantable artificial heart. Jpn J Artif Organs 22:748–753

Arterial Resonance Inferred from Analysis of Arterial Impedance

Shinichi Kobayashi[1], Shinichi Nitta[1], Tomoyuki Yambe[1], Taro Sonobe[1], and Hiroyuki Hashimoto[2]

Summary. At an irregular point in an artery, a pulse wave is reflected, generating a characteristic impedance. An arterial branch is a major origin of such reflection waves. It may be possible to make an artery resonate by using an artificial heart which is carefully controlled to generate the appropriate frequency for the target point. In this report, arterial impedance was studied in animal experiments. Total cardiopulmonary bypasses were performed using a vibrating flow pump generating a 10–40-Hz oscillating blood flow. It was found that the value of arterial impedance at around 30 Hz was increased compared with that at other driving frequencies. Blood flow distribution was also changed at 30 Hz; the left common carotid arterial blood flow rate underwent a relative increase with a 30-Hz oscillating blood flow. These results indicate that 30 Hz is a point of significance in determining the frequency characteristics of this artery. It is postulated that resonance of the artery caused a reflection wave from the aortic arch at 30 Hz. The power generated by pulsatile flow is the product of mean flow and amplitude. It may be important to study the hemodynamics from the viewpoint of alternating current theory, i.e., considering arterial impedance, as well as direct current theory. Arterial resonance may become an important factor in the management of the artificial circulation of blood.

Key words: Vibrating flow pump — Oscillating blood flow — Arterial resonance — Reflection wave — Arterial impedance

Introduction

Arterial impedance has previously been studied within a beat frequency range of 0–12 Hz, based on the natural heartbeat [1]. It was shown in some reports that arterial impedance was influenced by the reflection wave from an arterial branch [2]. In the present study, high-frequency oscillating blood flow (10–40 Hz) was used for extracorporeal circulation, and the arterial impedance at these high frequencies was estimated. Arterial impedance fluctuated with frequency, and the blood flow distribution was also changed by the blood flow frequency. This fluctuation may be the result of a reflection wave from the arterial branch causing arterial resonance.

Materials and Methods

Total cardiopulmonary bypass circulation was performed on eight adult goats (45–65 kg). A roller pump (RP) and a vibrating flow pump (VFP) were used as blood pumps for comparison [3]. The aortic pressure (AOP), systemic blood flow rate (SF), central venous pressure (CVP), and left common carotid arterial blood flow rate (CAF) were measured to study the arterial impedance and blood flow distribution. (Cobe disposable pressure manometer; Cobe, USA; Nihon Koden MFV-3100; Nihon Koden, Tokyo, Japan; Camino DPM-420; Camino, USA; Transonic Systems T101; Transonic Systems, Ithaca, NY USA). The extracorporeal circuit was primed with lactated Ringer solution, D-mannitol, $NaHCO_3$, dextran $(C_6H_{12}O_6)_n$, antihemolytic agent, and heparin (20000 IU). The priming volume was approximately 1.5 l.

Results

Figure 1a shows the blood flow distribution ratio for the carotid artery (CAF/SF) at various frequencies of oscillation. The CAF/SF was significantly increased when driven by the VFP at 30 Hz compared with RP driving. This result indicates a change in blood flow distribution at 30 Hz. Figure 1b shows the arterial impedance during oscillating blood flow at various frequencies. The absolute magnitude of the arterial impedance increased at 20–30 Hz. This fluctuation may have some relationship with the observed change in carotid arterial blood flow relative to systemic blood flow at 30 Hz.

Discussion

Arterial impedance study of natural heartbeats is shown in Fig. 1c. Fluctuation at 5–12 Hz has previously been postulated to be formed by a reflection wave

[1] Department of Medical Engineering and Cardiology, Institute of Development, Aging, and Cancer, and [2] Institute of Fluid Science, Tohoku University, 4-1 Seiryo-machi, Aoba, Sendai, Miyagi 980, Japan

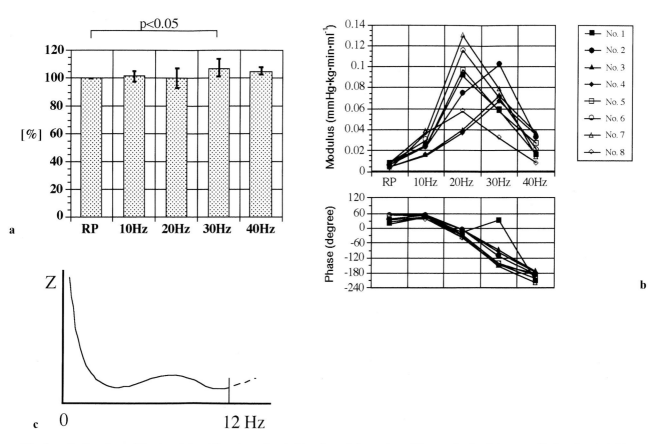

Fig. 1. a Ratio of carotid artery blood flow to systemic blood flow (CAF/SF) at various frequencies of oscillation. At 30 Hz, the blood flow ratio of the carotid artery was significantly higher. **b** Arterial impedance at various frequencies of oscillation. *Key* shows experiment number. Aortic impedance was calculated to estimate the frequency characteristics of the artery. The peak absolute magnitude of arterial impedance was at 20–30 Hz. **c** Aortic impedance (Z) during natural pulsatile blood flow at various frequencies of oscillation. Aortic impedance during natural heartbeats is shown. The fluctuation of impedance in the higher frequency region may be caused by a reflection wave from the arterial branch

from the femoral arterial branch [4]. Generally speaking, resonance occurs when there is an interaction between the progressive wave and a reflection wave. An arterial branch is a good source of reflection waves. The aortic arch and the carotid arterial branch may be the major points of reflection. An appropriate frequency of the progressive wave is postulated to exist for generating the enhanced reflection from the arterial branch. Arterial impedance is a good index for describing the frequency characteristics of artery. Rapid change of input impedance must be observed at the stated frequency of resonance. In this study, significant changes in both arterial input impedance and CAF/SF were observed at 30 Hz in animal experiments [5]. These results may indicate that the carotid arterial blood flow rate was changed by the control of blood flow frequency, though the total blood flow rate did not change. At 30 Hz, the oscillating blood flow might generate arterial resonance by producing a reflection wave from the carotid arterial branch [6]. The

carotid arterial blood flow rate might have changed as a result.

Conclusion

The carotid arterial blood flow rate was increased when the vibrating flow pump provided oscillating blood flow at 30 Hz, even though the total blood flow rate was unchanged compared with that at other frequencies. Arterial input impedance was also significantly changed at 30 Hz. The blood flow distribution may be influenced by the blood flow frequency because the arterial circulatory system is composed of elastic vessels. Arterial resonance may be the reason for the change in CAF/SF.

Acknowledgment. This work is partly supported by Grants-in-Aid for Developmental Scientific Research from the

Japanese government (06558118, 06555052, 07557309, 055570639).

References

1. Attinger EO (1996) Use of Fourier series for the analysis of biological systems. Biophys J 6:291
2. Bertram CD, Greenwald SE (1992) A general method of determining the frequency dependent propagation coefficient and characteristic impedance of an artery in the presence of reflections. J Biomech Eng 114:2–9
3. Nitta S, Hashimoto H, Sonobe T, Katahira Y, Yambe T, Naganuma S, Tanaka M, Satoh N, Miura M, Mouri H, Hiyama H, Matsuki H (1991) The newly designed uni-valved artificial heart. ASAIO Trans 37(3):M240–M241
4. Milnor RW (1989) Hemodynamics, vol 2. Williams and Wilkins, Baltimore
5. Kobayashi S, Nitta S, Yambe T, Naganuma S, Tanaka M, Kasai T, Hashimoto H (1994) Carotid arterial impedance during oscillated blood flow. Artif Organs 18:627–632
6. Kobayashi S, Nitta S, Yambe T, Naganuma S, Hashimoto H, Fukuju T, Mouri H, Kouichi T (1995) Experimental study of physiological advantages of assist circulation using oscillated blood flow. Artif Organs 19(7):704–707

Artificial Heart Flow Visualization Tests — A Comparative Study of Different Valves, Ventricle Geometries, and Control Parameters

Z. Nawrat, Z. Malota, and Z. Religa

Summary. Flow visualization tests were performed for Polvad and Poltah ventricles. The purpose of our investigation was the optimalization of flow pattern inside the chamber, depending on the valve type and driving mode. To evaluate sectional flow patterns, a He-Ne laser planar light was applied and the ventricle was scanned segmentally in different directions. The motion of tracing silicon particles was observed and video recorded. Analysis of pictures saved by computer was performed by an original, simple functional method, which provided information about local washing and about the tendency of particles to move to the inflow and outflow channels of the ventricle during all phases of the cycle. Recirculation and stagnation zones for different types of valves and control parameters were identified, and the optimal orientation for valves in ventricles was determined. The flow distribution characteristics of a pulsatile blood pump depend on the type and orientation of valves mounted in it. The ventricle geometry and control parameters influence flow phenomena inside the chamber.

Key words: Total artificial heart — Ventricular assist device — Artificial heart tests — Flow visualization tests

Introduction

The time- and spatial-flow pattern inside the artificial heart chamber is one of the basic factors determining the efficiency and biological safety of pumping. Local areas of the chamber may experience dangerous shear velocities (critical values of shear stress for morphotic (red cells, white cells, platelets etc.) blood elements reached during a given time), dependent on directions of local flow velocities and chamber's wall geometry (collision with the wall), and fluctuations of local flow velocities with respect to their values and directions. The simplest method for the observation of flow stagnation zones, recirculation zones, or areas where the shear stress and flow velocity values reach their peaks, is laser flow visualization (Fig. 1).

The purpose of these investigations is the determination of the influence of driving mode and valve type on flow–pressure biophysical phenomena in the chamber, knowledge deemed essential for the safety of clinical application of artificial heart chambers and heart assist device chambers.

Devices

The pneumatically drive, membrane-type Polish ventricular assist device, Polvad (U-shaped), and the Polish artificial heart, Poltah (of spherical geometry), were developed in the Artificial Heart Laboratory, Silesian Medical Academy (Zabrze, Poland) and manufactured by Plastmed (Żywiec, Poland). The chambers, along with the electropneumatic driving units JSN 201 and JSN 301 built by the Research and Development Centre for Electronic Medical Equipment (Zabrze, Poland), valves constitute the pump system.

The original Polish valves, Polbio (porcine valves sewn on delrin stent, and fixed according to our own, original method, designed and manufactured in FCSD Zabrze, Poland, specially mede for the artificial heart) and the commercial Sorin (SO) tilting disc valve (Biomedica, Italy) were tested.

Methods

Laser flow visualization tests, providing qualitative flow pictures, velocity fields, and detection of flow recirculation and stagnation areas, were performed. To evaluate sectional flow patterns, a He-Ne 25-mW laser planar light was applied and the ventricle was scanned segmentally in different directions. The motion of tracing silicon particles was observed and video recorded. The valve affects the flow pattern, creating, for a given phase (opening), a characteristic spatial flow distribution. We performed visualization of valves mounted in the chambers, looking for their optimal orientations and configurations for both chambers.

One problem not yet satisfactorily solved is the interpretation of laser flow visualization pictures. We therefore developed our own method: the functional analysis of flow character. The method is based on the observation that the quality of a flow system should be

Foundation for Development of Cardiac Surgery and Silesian Medical Academy, Zabrze, Wolności 345a, Poland

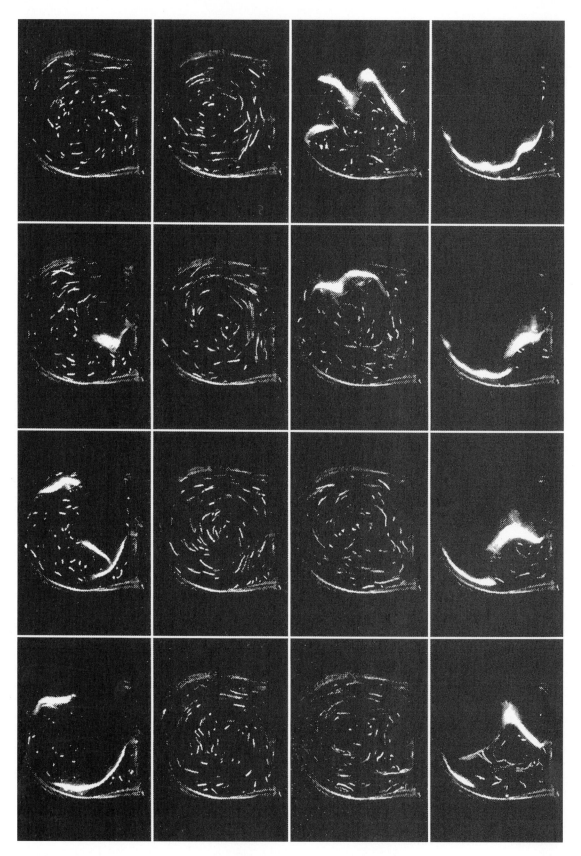

Fig. 1. Polish ventricular assist device (Polvad) equipped with Polbio valves: flow visualization tests during one cycle of pumping. Test conditions: heart rate = 70 bpm, % systole (%sys) = 50%, average pressure at outlet (P_{out}) = 13.3 kPa, average pressure at inlet (P_{in}) = 1 kPa

Fig. 2. Scheme of functional division of measurement visualization areas in the Polvad and the Polish artificial heart (Poltah). *A,B,1,2,3,4* represent predetermined divisions on the planes of visualization; *out*, outlet; *in*, inlet

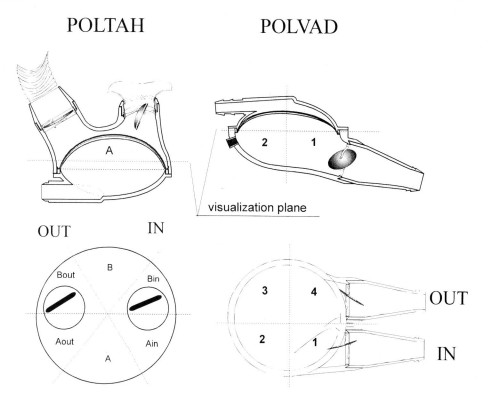

judged from the point of view of the function that the flow has to fulfill. The artificial heart is a pump that should cause fluid flow from the inlet (atrial) to the outlet channel and provide blood with a pre-determined amount of energy to overcome the load, in order to create the clinically desired pressure–flow state in the circulatory system. For long-term pumping of blood, both goals must be reached while preventing deleterious effects on blood elements. Therefore, it is essential to minimize undesired phenomena occurring at a blood–artificial surface interface.

That is why, for functional analysis, the chamber was divided into areas where, for a given section, every local flow velocity vector was assigned its components in the outlet and inlet directions as well as the component tangential to the chamber wall. The analysis of time changes of the first two components allows us to track down the dynamics of flow patterns during the entire cycle, and to detect inertial effects and determine passage time. The tangential component is responsible for effective washing of areas in the vicinity of the wall. The full analysis makes possible the classification of the pictures obtained so that, since digital picture recording is suitable for computer analysis and gives results that are easy to interpret, the conclusions regarding the causes of phenomena and their regulation may be drawn easily.

The Functional Method of Flow Pattern Examination

1. We divide the chamber into areas of predetermined geometrical and functional character: the wall vicinity area, the valve neighborhood area, the central area, etc.
2. Every trace of a particle suspended in a fluid, whose length is proportional to the flow velocity (the path covered during the exposure time) is characterized by three numbers:

   V_r — the component of the velocity vector (a line tangent to the trajectory) in the direction tangential to the chamber wall

   V_{in} — the component of the velocity vector in the direction tangential to the shortest path to the inlet channel

   V_{out} — the component of the velocity vector in the direction tangential to the shortest path to the outlet channel

3. The analysis concerns the constant or pulsatile flow visualization; it is important to analyze consecutive pictures (a change in flow direction may indicate disordered flow, flow traps, and recirculation).

This method allows us to describe flow velocity dynamics (value and direction) during the cycle, and spatial dependencies on the geometry of the chamber.

Results and Analysis

We analyzed the pictures of flow in a plane 0.5 cm offset from the membrane–chamber junction plane. Figure 2 shows the easiest way of dividing the observation plane. The aim of our analysis is to determine the average, maximum, and minimum values of the velocity in a cycle for a particular section, as well as the change of direction of velocity during one cycle.

In Fig. 3 we analyzed a set of pictures taken during one cycle of work of the right Poltah chamber. The pictures were taken simulating the parameters of pul-

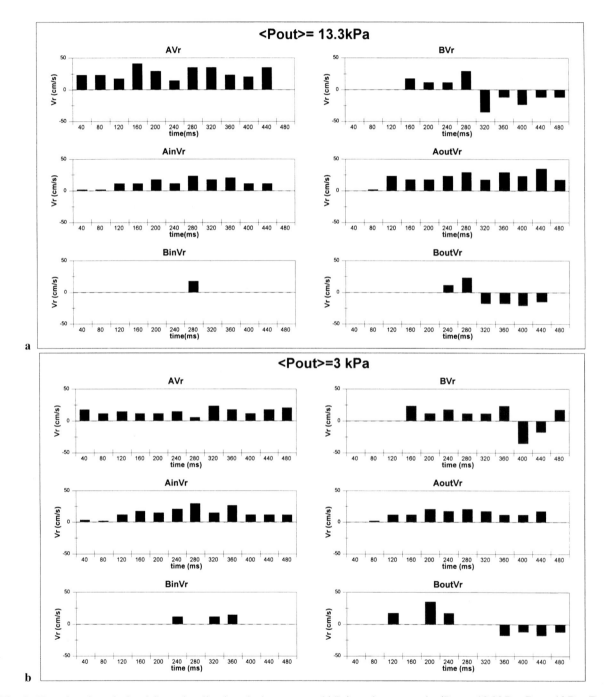

Fig. 3. Functional analysis of flow visualization during one pumping cycle of the Poltah equipped with a Sorin disc valve (heart rate = 70 bpm) under **b** pulmonary (P_{out} = 3 kPa, P_{in} = 1 kPa, systolic/diastolic driving pressure (DP) DP = 10 kPa/ −2 kPa) and **a** systemic (P_{out} = 13.3 kPa, P_{in} = 1 kPa, Dp = 30 kPa/−5 kPa) work conditions. A,B, areas (see Fig. 2); V_r, component of velocity vector tangential to chamber wall

monary circulation [afterload (P_{pa}) = 3 kPa, preload (P_{atr}) = 1 kPa, and systolic/diastolic driving pressure (DP) DP = 10 kPa/−2 kPa)] and systemic circulation [(P_{ao}) = 13.3 kPa, P_{atr} = 1 kPa, and DP = 30 kPa/−5 kPa)] to assess the influence of pressure conditions on the washing of the chamber. For a chamber working in a low-pressure system, washing of a wall vicinity area was less effective in the central area, A, and in the outlet area, A_{out} (up to 60% reduction of maximum velocity value and average velocity value for one cycle, during the exposure). Nevertheless, there was a 125% improvement of the washing of the inlet area, A_{in}. In conditions of pulmonary circulation we obtained smaller (83%) maximum velocity values in the B_{in} area, while for the B_{out} area maximum velocities were even greater (150%) than those appearing in the conditions of systemic circulation. From the functional point of view, the flow conditions in B_{out} were worse

because of its positive average velocity value. This means that the average velocity vector in this outlet region was directed toward the inlet channel. In conclusion, the velocities of washing in the wall vicinity in all regions were around half the velocities obtained during tests under systemic condition, except the area A_{in}.

We also assessed the influence of the shape of the chamber on the flow organization inside it by measuring (Fig. 4) the total trace area for every picture in a cycle taken at 40-ms intervals. This simple method demonstrates also that the use of a biological valve having a central flow pattern decreases the washing of the wall vicinity area near the inlet valve (Fig. 5). For the chamber section parallel to the plane of membrane assembly, vortex flow with an axis in the center of the chamber (cyclone type) lasts for a shorter time for valves of axial flow than for properly oriented, tilting-

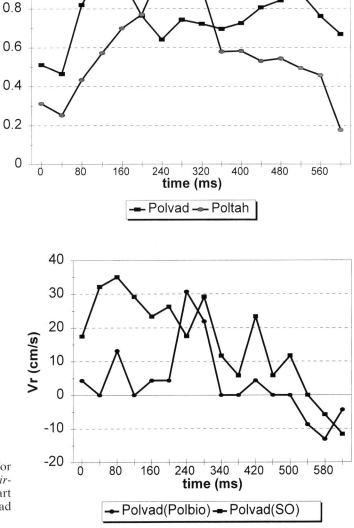

Fig. 4. Comparison of velocity fields obtained with trace area method for the Polvad (*rectangles*) and the Poltah (*ovals*) for the same work conditions

Fig. 5. Comparison of flow velocity (VA_r) in area 1 for the Polvad equipped with different valves: Polbio (*circles*) or Sorin So (*rectangles*). Tests conditions: heart rate = 70 bpm, aortic pressure (P_{ao}) = 13.3 kPa; preload (P_{atr}) = 1 kPa; 50% systole

disc valves, remains longer when driving parameters are properly chosen, and is most significantly developed in U-shaped chambers (where connectors are located at a small angle to the membrane assembly plane).

In these U-shaped chambers, we observed a strong dependence of the flow pattern picture on the orientation of the inlet disc valve. Figure 6 shows the analysis of one cycle of work of the ventricular assist device (VAD) chamber for two inlet disc valve orientations differing by 180°. We observe a halved average wall vicinity flow in area 1, a tenfold decrease in area 2, and a threefold decrease in area 3. In the wall vicinity area

of the outlet region there is a 25% improvement. For a valve orientation such that the main portion of the flow is directed toward the central part of the chamber, we observe stagnation and reticulation areas near the walls. There are two neighboring, dynamic vortex structures inside the chamber.

The washing conditions are also dependent on time-dependent driving parameters — % systole (%sys) and frequency. In Fig. 7 we show results obtained when the frequency was changed from 70 to 90 bpm for a %sys value of 40% (at which the cycle time is used most effectively). The increase of frequency resulted in significant increase of flow velocity inside the

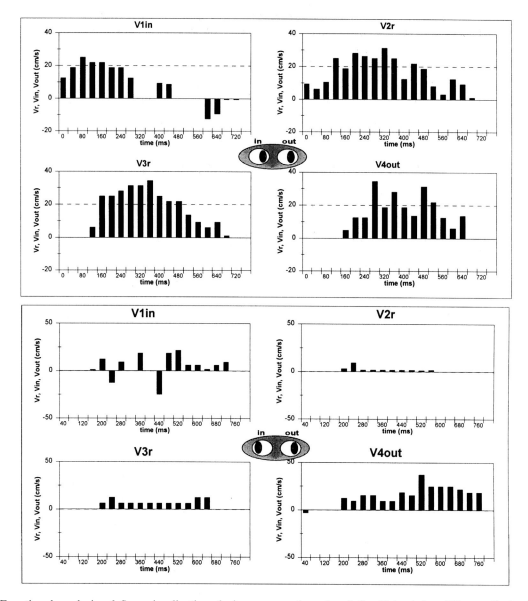

Fig. 6. Functional analysis of flow visualization during one work cycle of the Polvad for different Sorin disc valve orientations. Test conditions: heart rate = 70 bpm, $P_{ao} = 13.3$ kPa, $P_{atr} = 1$ kPa, 50% systole. *V1–4*, velocities in areas 1–4, respectively, of Fig. 2

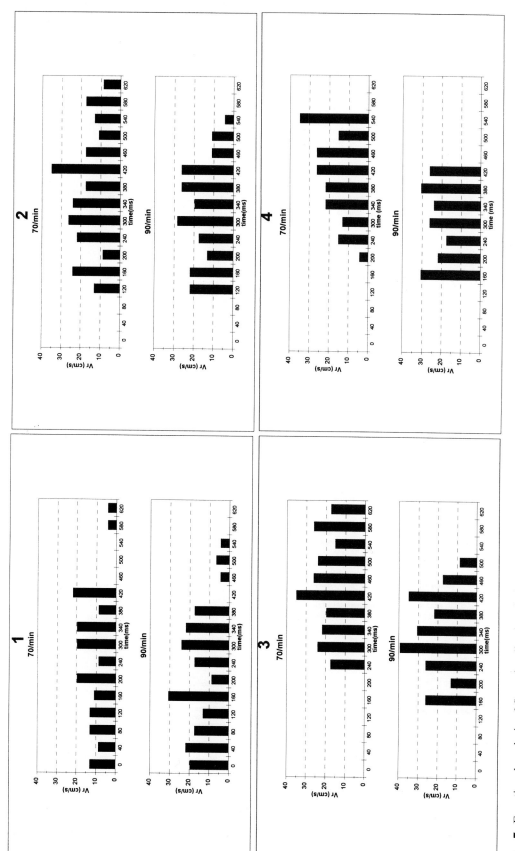

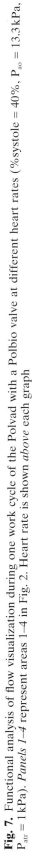

Fig. 7. Functional analysis of flow visualization during one work cycle of the Polvad with a Polbio valve at different heart rates (%systole = 40%, P_{ao} = 13.3 kPa, P_{atr} = 1 kPa). *Panels 1–4* represent areas 1–4 in Fig. 2. Heart rate is shown *above* each graph

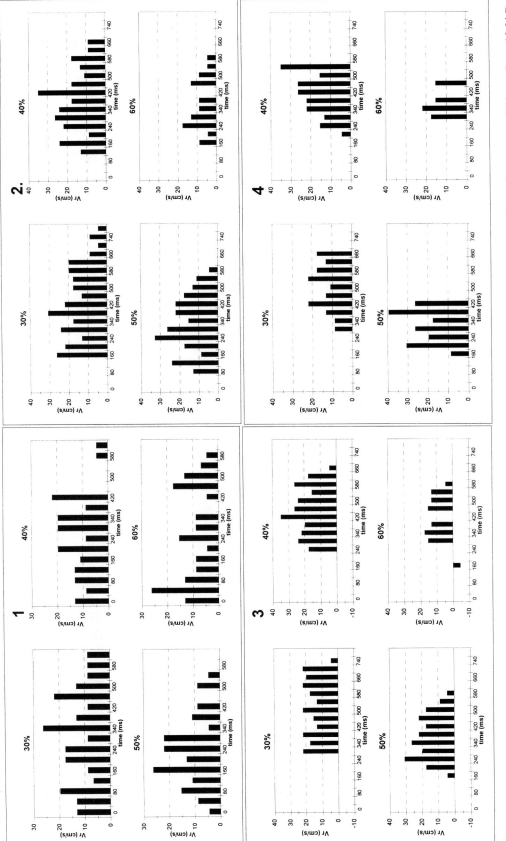
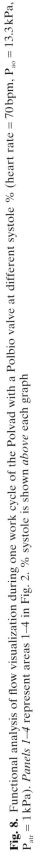

Fig. 8. Functional analysis of flow visualization during one work cycle of the Polvad with a Polbio valve at different systole % (heart rate = 70bpm, P_{ao} = 13.3 kPa, P_{atr} = 1kPa). *Panels 1–4* represent areas 1–4 in Fig. 2. % systole is shown *above* each graph

chamber, mostly in the early diastolic phase. The average velocity value in areas 1 and 2 increased by 20% but did not change significantly in areas 3 and 4. Generally, when the increase of frequency decreases ejection or filling we observe worse washing of areas distant from the inlet and outlet channels.

Changing the percent of systole, we observed a decrease in the average washing velocity value when the chamber filling time was lowered. It was almost halved at 60% systole (when the volume flowing into the chamber in one cycle was 60 ml) compared with the value at 30% systole (when the volume flowing into the chamber was 70 ml) (Fig. 8). The most interesting thing is the difference in this influence for different areas. We observed a clear decrease of washing up to a %sys value of 60% mostly for areas 2 and 3 inside the chamber. For a %sys of 30% a central, cyclone-type vortex lasted for 360 ms while for the %sys value of 60% the vortex lasted for 200 ms during one cycle.

A full picture of flow conditions in the chamber may be obtained by analyzing the pictures obtained for all interesting sections, and the components of velocity, V_r, V_{in}, and V_{out}.

Conclusion

Global and local flow characteristics depend on the chamber geometry. The valves and driving method influence flow organization both in the global sense (e.g., the duration of a cyclone-type structure during the heart cycle) and the local sense (affects proper washing). Disc valves are better for controlling washing processes. The proposed functional method for flow pattern analysis is significant for the comparison of test data.

Successful Dynamic Cardiomyoplasty with Pharmaceutical Support

Victor V. Nikolaychik, Valeri S. Chekanov, Matthew D. Silverman, Mark M. Samet, Donald H. Schmidt, and Peter I. Lelkes

Summary. Dynamic cardiomyoplasty is an attractive alternative to heart transplantation. We used fibrin sealant to facilitate the intraoperative bonding of skeletal muscle to the myocardial wall, focusing on prevention of ischemia-reperfusion injuries in the skeletal muscle flap, and enhancement of angiogenesis in the "repaired" heart. In a sheep model, we used autologous fibrin sealant to join the tissues, to create a provisional matrix for angiogenesis, and to act as a depot for the delivery of agents aimed at minimizing ischemia-reperfusion lesion formation. Coadministered with the fibrin sealant were the following pharmaceuticals: deferoxamine (an iron chelator), pyrrolostatin (a free radical scavenger), and aprotinin (a protease inhibitor). Five days after cardiomyoplasty, the skeletal muscle was stimulated with a progressive electrical regimen. After two months, the skeletal muscle showed none of the signs of necrosis or ischemia-reperfusion damage seen in the controls. The layer of fibrin sealant rapidly (<2 weeks) became densely vascularized with capillaries. The expedited angiogenesis provided an organic bridge between skeletal muscle and myocardium. By contrast, in controls there was poor contact between the tissues, with evidence of fiber deterioration and loss of vascular network integrity in the transposed muscle flap. Even greater angiogenic stimulation was seen when pharmaceuticals were included into the fibrin meshwork, which minimized the formation of ischemia-reperfusion lesions. Over time, these agents promoted much more extensive vascularization than did fibrin sealant alone. This therapeutic strategy, using a pharmacologically-enhanced fibrin sealant, is clearly beneficial for countering muscle flap postoperative injury, and may open promising pathways for the design of other biomechanical assist devices.

Key words: Cardiomyoplasty — Angiogenesis — Muscle damage — Ischemia-reperfusion prevention — Fibrin sealant

Introduction

More than a decade ago, dynamic cardiomyoplasty (CMP) was introduced as a biological assist to the failing heart; i.e., wrapping skeletal muscle, usually latissimus dorsi muscle (LDM), around the heart, and pacing it in synchrony with the ventricle. To date, the number of long-term survival studies are few, and reported early benefits are controversial [1–3]. Unlike total artificial heart replacement or left ventricle assist devices, the full potential of CMP is not realized immediately after surgery. Termination of myocardial dilatation, augmentation of ventricular contraction, and provision of an additional blood supply from the muscle flap require time to become established.

During CMP, the mobilized LDM remains perfused by its primary blood source (i.e., the thoracodorsalis artery), but is separated from substantial secondary arterial sources. It was hoped that, eventually, natural revascularization of the LDM would occur. Unfortunately, no such natural angiogenic response follows, resulting in minimal revascularization and poor bonding of the traumatized, ischemic skeletal muscle to the mobile myocardial wall.

Surgical trauma, ischemia, and readmission of oxygen causes a burst of free radical production, platelet aggregation, and leukocyte adherence to the endothelium. Iron ions in extravasate cause added damage to both the vessel wall and surrounding muscle tissue by further elevating local free radical concentrations. Endothelial cells are particularly susceptible to ischemia-reperfusion injury. Lasting postischemia pathological sequelae render these cells chronically dysfunctional, and they do not undergo angiogenesis.

A therapeutic strategy must be devised to minimize damage in the LDM flap if we are to fully enjoy the expected benefits of CMP. In this study, we analyzed the ability of a pharmaceutically enhanced fibrin sealant to prevent ischemia-reperfusion injury, and to promote angiogenesis, in isolated muscle flaps and in the complete CMP.

Materials and Methods

Skeletal Muscle Pockets. In eight sheep under general anesthesia, the anterior border of the right LDM was completely mobilized, leaving undisturbed the vessels entering the LDM from the posterior border [4]. An-

University of Wisconsin Medical School and Milwaukee Heart Project, Milwaukee Clinical Campus, Sinai Samaritan Medical Center, Laboratory of Cell Biology, P.O. Box 342, Milwaukee, WI 53201-0342, USA

497

terior and posterior regions of the LDM were super-
imposed and sutured together, forming three 3 × 5-cm
pockets (Fig. 1a). The pockets contained fibrin sealant
(FS) alone, or FS supplemented with either aprotinin,
deferoxamine, or pyrrolostatin; empty pockets served
as controls.

Dynamic Cardiomyoplasty. Dynamic cardiomyoplasty was performed through a left anterolateral
thoracotomy, by established protocols [4]. Briefly, the
left LDM was dissected from the distal attachments,
with the neurovascular pedicle intact, and was
wrapped around the heart and sutured to the pericardium. Five days postoperatively, a progressive regimen of electrical stimulation was started, increasing
every ten days in both pace and duration. The final set
consisted of 6 impulses per burst, with a 1:2
cardiosynchronization ratio. In four sheep, autologous
FS alone, or FS supplemented with aprotinin, was inserted in the pockets between the LDM flap and the
myocardium (Fig. 1b). In four other sheep, the pockets
were left untreated and served as controls.

Autologous Fibrin Sealant. Concentrated fibrinogen
was prepared from citrated sheep blood, using standard procedures for plasma cryoprecipitation [5]. Two
different syringes were filled with thrombin (USP) and
autologous cryoprecipitate, which were simultaneously applied to the intermuscular space. Aprotinin
(10,000 U/ml), pyrrolostatin (10 µM), or deferoxamine
(20 mg/ml) were added to the fibrinogen solution just
before application.

Total Capillary Cross-Sectional Area. The total capillary cross-sectional area in tissue samples was assessed
after conventional indirect immunoperoxidase staining of endothelial cells for von Willebrand factor.

Results

Mobilization of LDM results in reduction of the functional vasculature and presents a constant threat of
flap necrosis, mostly to its distal part. Indeed, 12 weeks
postoperatively, the LDM is largely atrophic, and
contains many regions of adipose degeneration and
fibrotic tissue formation. In our LDM pocket model
(Fig. 1), the initial pathologic events were discernable
within three hours after surgery, with margination of
leukocytes obvious throughout the LDM vasculature.
This phenomenon was maximal on day 7, and per-
sisted until day 16 (Fig. 2a). These observations
suggest that leukocyte–endothelium interactions,
probably resulting in the localized elevation of both
free radical and protease concentrations, are primary
early initiators of LDM degeneration.

When FS was introduced between the ischemic and
normal LDM in the muscle pocket model (Fig. 2b),
and between the LDM and myocardium during CMP,
it served as a scaffold for the construction of a new
pseudolayer, which was clearly well-vascularized after
16 days. Eight weeks after either procedure, the LDM
flaps in the FS-treated groups appeared nonischemic,
and of a similar thickness to normal LDM. In addition,
adipose degeneration was significantly reduced, and
blood vessels of various diameters were abundant
at the interface (Table 1). By contrast, the non-FS-
treated controls displayed obvious ischemic damage.
These findings demonstrate that FS can be instrumen-
tal in promoting tight bonding of an initially ischemic

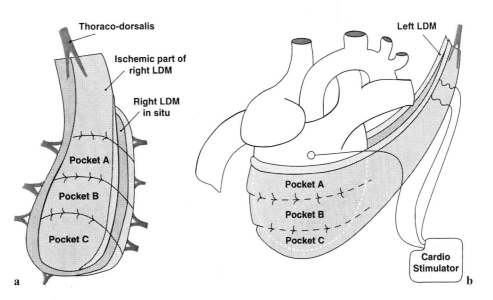

Fig. 1. Schematic of experimental setup: latissimus dorsi muscle (*LDM*) pocket model and dynamic cardiomyoplasty. **a** Overview of a right skeletal muscle flap and experimentally introduced pockets. **b** Outline of cardiomyoplasty performed with the contralateral LDM; experimentally introduced pockets between the ailing myocardium and electrically stimulated LDM are indicated

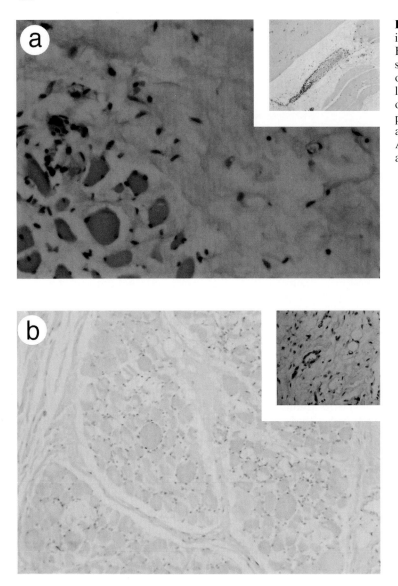

Fig. 2. Histological section of the contact interlayer between LDM/LDM pockets. **a** Hematoxylin and eosin (H&E) stained biopsy sample taken from an ischemic control pocket on day 16. *Inset* indicates margination of leukocytes. **b** H&E stained histological section of ischemic pocket taken 16 days after FS application. The LDM appears nonischemic and adipose degeneration is significantly reduced. As shown in the *inset*, well-vascularized areas are present in the fibrin meshwork interlayer

Table 1. Comparison of total capillary cross-sectional areas in skeletal muscle–myocardium interlayer

Biopsy localization and fibrin sealant composition	LDM/LDM interface (%)		
	Day 16	Day 30	Day 56
Control, empty pocket	3.0 ± 0.97	2.9 ± 0.93	3.6 ± 0.69
FS without additives	4.1 ± 0.38	5.1 ± 0.19	5.5 ± 0.18[a]
FS + aprotinin	5.2 ± 1.11	7.8 ± 1.38[a,b,c]	8.5 ± 1.10[a,b]
FS + pyrrolostatin	7.9 ± 1.78	8.1 ± 1.46[a,b]	9.4 ± 1.76[a,b]
FS + deferoxamine	5.1 ± 1.23	6.3 ± 0.67[a]	7.4 ± 1.03[a,b]

	CMP interface (%)		
	Day 16	Day 30	Day 56
Control, classic CMP	—	—	3.9 ± 0.24
FS without additives	—	—	5.3 ± 0.33[a]
FS + aprotinin	—	—	9.2 ± 0.91[a,b]

Value: mean ± SD (% total area).
FS, fibrin sealant; LDM, latissimus dorsi muscle; CMP, cardiomyoplasty.
[a] $P < 0.05$ vs control; [b] $P < 0.05$ vs FS; [c] $P < 0.05$ vs day 56.

LDM flap to other muscle tissues, including the moving, complex contours of the heart.

The introduction of fibrin meshwork onto a damaged area does not completely protect the tissue from leukocyte-mediated injury. Although there are many experimental agents that can be used to effectively minimize further injury to the surgically traumatized tissue, we focused on pharmacological protectors that were co-administered with FS. Specifically, we tested whether FS, which had been spiked with deferoxamine, an iron chelator, could inhibit free radical damage in LDM pockets. Local reduction of free iron enhanced angiogenesis (Table 1), but the pocket periphery still contained zones of visible degeneration.

We also explored whether local availability of pyrrolostatin, a free radical scavenger [6], would be effective in reducing the effects of ischemic insult. We found that, within one month, the combination of FS and pyrrolostatin enhanced angiogenesis and reduced injury in the LDM flap (Table 1), with even greater efficacy than did deferoxamine. This confirms the important role of free radicals in mediating postoperative vascular damage, and provides a new approach for its control.

Protease release from leukocytes is a key event in ischemic muscle damage, and might inhibit active angiogenesis. In agreement with this hypothesis, inclusion of the serine protease inhibitor aprotinin into the fibrin meshwork enhanced revascularization in both the LDM pocket model and in CMP (Table 1), as compared with FS alone. Moreover, eight weeks post-CMP, in addition to supporting a dense capillary network, aprotinin, in combination with fibrin meshwork, caused the ingrowth of massive vessels from the LDM flap to the myocardium (Fig. 3).

Discussion

For CMP to be successful, ischemic damage to the cardiac-assisting skeletal muscle must be restricted. Following surgical transposition, the traumatized LDM requires an adequate blood supply to efficiently provide nutrients and remove toxic metabolites. Thus, the patency of its vasculature, initially compromised, must be rapidly regenerated. The angiogenic potential of healthy muscle is extremely high, and it is much more densely vascularized, with larger bore capillaries than most other tissues [7]. Ideally, it would recover quickly following CMP, and might even serve as an important supplemental blood supply for the failing heart. In practice, however, classical CMP results in negligible establishment of vascular connections between these tissues. In addition, many of the microvessels that are severed during surgery continue leaking blood into the intermuscular site. Traditionally, such microbleeding has been arrested by surface application of thrombin alone or in combination with fibrinogen, forming local fibrin clots in the treated area.

Previously, the combination of fibrinogen and thrombin has also been used in surgical procedures as a passive tissue adhesive, to prevent postsurgical leaks, to fill voids, and to ensure good attachment after tissue grafting [8]. We envisioned employing fibrin meshwork in a more active role in the restoration of vascular integrity after CMP, with encouraging results. By inserting FS between closely apposed muscles, we were able to create a provisional matrix, within which extensive angiogenesis occurred, resulting in the evolution of a complex vascular network which acted as a functional bridge between the two tissues. With time,

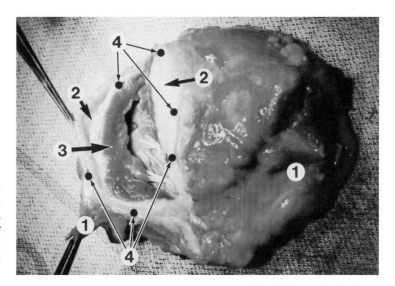

Fig. 3. Gross appearance of the "repaired" heart 56 days after cardiomyoplasty (CMP) with pharmaceutical support: *1*, LDM flap wrapped around the heart; *2*, pseudolayer of intensified fibrin sealant; *3*, myocardium; *4*, newly formed blood vessels of significant diameter within pseudolayer

this interlayer became enriched with collagen bundles and elastin fibers, giving it both strength and distensibility. These characteristics allow the LDM and the myocardium to remain closely juxtaposed, without interfering with cardiac contractile dynamics. Additionally, this arrangement might limit future cardiac dilatation, the so-called Girdling effect [1–3].

Elevated free iron in tissues, owing to erythrocyte extravasation and lysis which follows operational trauma, is a known mediator of inflammatory reactions and ischemia-reperfusion damage [9]. Redox active metal ions, particularly iron, catalyze the Harber-Weiss reaction, dramatically increasing the local concentration of free radicals. Fibrin mesh-work alone acts as a physical barrier to erythrocyte extravasation and subsequent lysis. Deferoxamine binds ferric iron with high affinity, and prevents iron-catalyzed hydroxyl radical formation. By using deferoxamine as an intrinsic component of FS, we are able to provide to the regenerating tissues an additional measure of protection from free radical damage.

Proteases that are released from activated leukocytes and from damaged and ischemic muscle are likely to inhibit vascular regeneration following CMP. Indeed, incorporation of the serine protease inhibitor aprotinin into FS reduced protease-mediated tissue damage, and resulted in a more rapid reestablishment of the microvascular network. We intend in the future to test the efficacy of other protease inhibitors, and combinations of protease inhibitors, in maximizing this protective effect.

The present study demonstrates diverse pharmacological approaches which can successfully enhance FS-based vascularization of intermuscular layers following CMP. Despite the inevitable presence of inflammatory infiltrates after surgery, the endothelial cells surrounding the operative site are fully capable, provided the proper physical and chemical environment, of elaborate vessel repair in the LDM flap. Localized delivery of select bioactive agents can shift the chemical milieu to one which promotes rapid and extensive vascular regeneration. Furthermore, the infiltration of large vessels into the FS matrix suggests that development of anastomoses between branches of LDM and myocardial arteries is possible, and these could act as an important alternative blood source.

The use of transposed LDM in cardiac assist designs promises significant clinical merit. By combining the adhesive and structural properties of FS with its ability to store and deliver various pharmacologic agents, we are able to enhance the activity of physiological repair mechanisms in ischemic muscle, resulting in rapid and lasting vascular regeneration. This approach appears to be a feasible means for effecting dramatic improvements in tissue functional integrity after dynamic cardiomyoplasty, and, as a result, the successful outcome of this operation. We are currently evaluating whether increasing local concentrations of known angiogenic factors, by inclusion of either purified agents or the cells which produce them into the FS, can further potentiate these promising observations.

Acknowledgments. This work was supported in part by the Milwaukee Heart Research Foundation. We are grateful to Ms. Michelle Rieder, Mrs. Dawn M. Wankowski, and Dr. Gennady Tchekanov for their participation and assistance in the project.

References

1. Magovern GJ, Simpson KA (1996) Clinical cardiomyoplasty: review of the ten-year United States experience. Ann Thorac Surg 61:413–419
2. Moreira LFP, Stolf NAG, Braile DM, Jatene AD (1996) Dynamic cardiomyoplasty in South America. Ann Thorac Surg 61:408–412
3. Chekanov VS, Krakovsky AA, Buslenko NS, Riabinina LG, Andreev DB, Shatalov KV, Dubrovsky IA, Shetty K (1994) Cardiomyoplasty: review of early and late results. Vasc Surg 28(7):482–488
4. Chekanov VS, Tchekanov GV, Rieder MA, Eisenstein R, Wankowski DM, Schmidt DH, Nikolaychik VV, Lelkes PI (1996) Biological glue increases capillary ingrowth after cardiomyoplasty in an ischemic cardiomyopathy model. ASAIO J 42(5):M480–M487
5. DePalma L, Criss VR, Luban NLC (1993) The preparation of fibrinogen concentrate for use as fibrin glue by four different methods. Transfusion 33:717–720
6. Kato S (1993) Pyrrolostatin, a novel lipid peroxidation inhibitor from *Streptomyces chrestomyceticus*. J Antibiotics 46(6):892–899
7. Hudlicka O, Brown M, Eggington S (1992) Angiogenesis in skeletal and cardiac muscle. Physiol Rev 72:369–417
8. Silver FM, Wang MC, Pins GD (1995) Preparation and use of fibrin glue in surgery. Biomaterials 16(12):892–903
9. Muntane J, Puig-Parellada P, Mitjavila M (1995) Iron metabolism and oxidative stress during acute and chronic phases of experimental inflammation: effect of iron-dextran and deferoxamine. J Lab Clin Med 126:435–443

Scientific Exhibitions

Exhibition Address List

1. **Pneumatic Driving Unit for Ventricular Assist and Intra-Aortic Balloon Pump (IABP)**
   Aisin Human Systems Co. Ltd.
   2–3 Showa-cho, Kariya, Aichi 448, Japan
2. **Baxter Novacor Wearable Electrical Left Ventricular Assist System (LVAS)**
   Baxter Limited
   Novacor Project, Product Development, Cardiovascular Group
   4 Rokuban-cho, Chiyoda-ku, Tokyo 102, Japan
3. **DeBakey Ventricular Assist Device (VAD)**
   Eiki Tayama
   Department of Surgery, Baylor College of Medicine, One Baylor Plaza, Houston, TX 77030, USA
4. **The Chang Heart Assist Device — An Inexpensive "Bridge" System**
   CHAD Research Laboratories
   PO Box 264, Surry Hills, NSW 2010, Australia
5. **Eccentric Roller Type Artificial Heart**
   Shintaro Fukunaga
   The First Department of Surgery, Hiroshima University School of Medicine, 1-2-3 Kasumi, Minami-ku, Hiroshima 734, Japan
6. **Totally Implantable Motor-Driven Assist Pump System**
   Eiji Okamoto
   Department of Electronic and Information Engineering, Hokkaido Tokai University, 5-1-1-1 Minamisawa, Minami-ku, Sapporo, Hokkaido 005, Japan
7. **Centrifugal Pump with a Magnetically Suspended Impeller: Kyoto — NTN Pump**
   Kazunobu Nishimura
   Department of Cardiovascular Surgery, Kyoto University Faculty of Medicine, 54 Kawahara-cho, Shogoin, Sakyo-ku, Kyoto 606, Japan
8. **Artificial Hearts Developed at the National Cardiovascular Center, Osaka, Japan**
   Yoshiyuki Taenaka, Toru Masuzawa, and Eisuke Tatsumi
   Director, Department of Artificial Organs Research Institute, National Cardiovascular Center, 5-7-1 Fujishiro-dai, Suita, Osaka 565, Japan
9. **Intraventricular Artificial Heart (Iva-Heart)**
   Sun Medical Technology Research Corp.
   1-3-11 Suwa, Suwa, Nagano 392, Japan
10. **New Developments of the Moving-Actuator Type Total Artificial Heart**
    Byoung Goo Min
    Chairman and Professor, Department of Biomedical Engineering, Seoul National University Hospital, 28 Youngun-Dong, Chongno-Ku, Seoul 110-744, Korea
11. **Linear Pulse Motor-Driven Total Artificial Heart System: Kuniko III**
    Hajime Yamada
    Professor, Department of Electrical and Electronic Engineering, Faculty of Engineering, Shinshu University, 500 Wakasato, Nagano 380, Japan
12. **The HeartMate Vented Electric Left Ventricular Assist System**
    Thermo Cardiosystems
    Seidler Bernstein Inc.
    215 First Street, Cambridge, MA 02142, USA
13. **Tohoku University Pneumatically Driven Total Artificial Heart (TAH) and Totally Implantable Ventricular Assist System Using a Vibrating Flow Pump (VFP)**
    Tomoyuki Yambe
    Institute of Development, Aging and Cancer, Tohoku University, 4-1 Seiryo-cho, Aoba-ku, Sendai, Miyagi 980-77, Japan

14. TOW NOK Component System III Heart Lung System, AVECOR AFFINITY Oxygenation Systems
Tonokura Ika Kogyo Co. Ltd.
5-1-13 Hongo, Bunkyo-ku, Tokyo 113, Japan

15. New Concept of the Artificial Heart
Kou Imachi

Department of Biomedical Engineering, Graduate School of Medicine, The University of Tokyo, 7-3-1 Hongo, Bunkyo-ku, Tokyo 113, Japan

1. Pneumatic Driving Unit for Ventricular Assist and Intra-Aortic Balloon Pump (IABP) (Aisin Human Systems Co. Ltd.)

The CORART 104 is a multipurpose pulsation-type driving unit which can be applied to left and right ventricular assistance simultaneously and also to intra-aortic balloon pumping. The driving unit has a compressor, vacuum pump, and battery built in, and, furthermore, provides a remote controller and a back-up unit against an emergency. As a distinctive feature, air pressure is accurately controlled with a high-speed electromagnetic valve developed by Aisin Seiki Co. Ltd.

The CORART BP1, a new generation IABP, provides beat-to-beat optimization and automatic control for timing and volume of balloon inflation/deflation even in patients with severe tachyarrhythmias. With the sensored AISIN balloon catheter, the system is automatically driven by one-switch operation, and provides the potential for enhanced circulatory support to the sickest patients, reducing IABP staffing requirements in the coronary care unit.

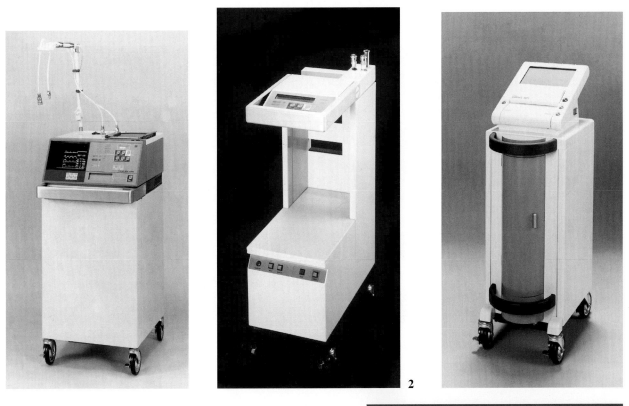

1   2   3

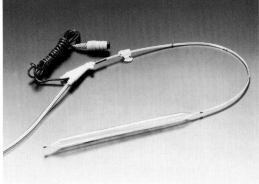

Fig. 1. CORART 104
Fig. 2. Back-up unit
Fig. 3. CORART BP1 (IABP drive unit)
Fig. 4. Sensored IABP catheter   4

2. Baxter Novacor Wearable Electrical Left Ventricular Assist System (LVAS) (Baxter Limited)

Following its first successful clinical application as a bridge to heart transplantation at Stanford University Medical Center in 1984, the Baxter Novacor LVAS has been used widely at more than 52 medical institutions throughout the United States, Europe, South America, and Japan. A total of 491 patients have received implantation of the device, and as of October 1996, the cumulative supporting period has exceeded 88 years. The longest supporting period (797 days) with the Novacor LVAS has been reported at Berlin German Heart Center in Germany, following which the patient was discharged. In 1992, conversion from the conventional console-type control system to the battery-powered wearable compact controller made it possible for the patients to move around freely, and thus has remarkably improved their quality of life. In 1994, the CE Mark for Europe was granted, which made sales of the device in Europe possible. In 1996, clinical investigation was started in Japan also.

The operating principle of the Baxter Novacor LVAS is simple. The pump sack is pressed by a pair of electromagnetic solenoids, and as the result the blood is ejected. Blood enters the pump freely by de-energizing, and thereby neutralizing, the solenoid. Ejection timing is achieved by synchronized counterpulsation to the natural heart.

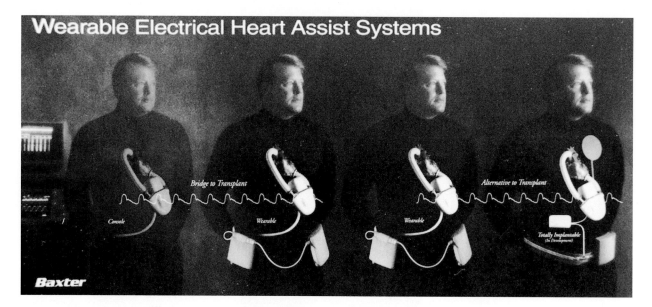

Fig. 1. Evolution of Novacor Left Ventricular Assist System (LVAS)

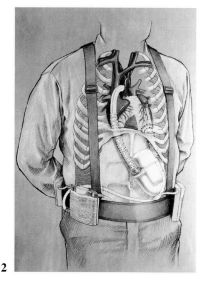

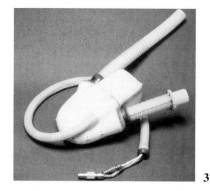

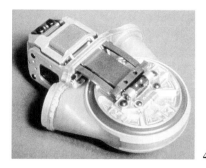

Fig. 2. Novacor wearable LVAS
Fig. 3. Implantable blood pump
Fig. 4. Uncovered blood pump

3. DeBakey Ventricular Assist Device (VAD)
(Baylor College of Medicine)

An implantable axial flow ventricular assist device has been under development as a joint project between the Baylor College of Medicine and NASA/Johnson Space Center. The components of the pump consist of a spinning inducer/impeller with a fixed flow straightener and diffuser residing within a flow tube. Magnets are installed in the impeller, and this impeller is rotated by the brushless motor stator. Computer Aided Design (CAD), Computer Aided Manufacturing (CAM), and Computer Aided Engineering (CAE) were aggressively applied for prototype fabrication and optimization. More than 50 configurations have been fabricated and tested. To date, the pump has been optimized in terms of hydraulic efficiency, hemolysis, and thrombosis. The pump requires less than 10 watts to deliver 5l/min against 100mmHg at 10000–11000rpm. A Normalized Index of Hemolysis of less than 0.003mg/100l has been achieved. Several models have accomplished completely thrombus-free performance after 2 weeks' ex vivo implantation. Following the success of the ex vivo experiments, a series of in vivo experiments has been initiated aiming for 6 months' thrombus-free implantation.

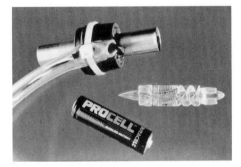

Fig. 1. DeBakey ventricular assist device (VAD). The small size (25mm × 25mm × 35mm) enables the device to be implanted in either a child's or an adult's chest cavity. The pump can provide 5l/min against 100mmHg with less than 10 watts of electrical power

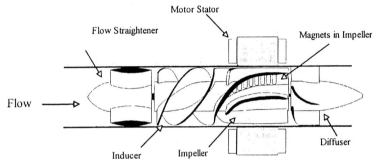

Fig. 2. The schematic drawing of the DeBakey VAD. The flow is created by rotation of the impeller, which is supported by the flow straightener and flow diffuser. The magnets are installed in the inducer/impeller

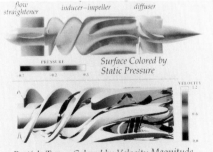

Fig. 3. For the prototype, Computer Aided Design (CAD), Computer Aided Manufacturing (CAM), and Computer Aided Engineering (CAE) were aggressively applied. These technologies shortened the design cycle time and resulted in an optimized device. More than 50 configurations have been fabricated and tested

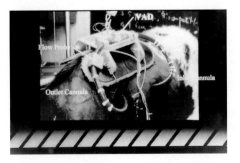

Fig. 4. Ex vivo implantation in calves. Several models have already achieved 2 weeks' implantation without thrombus formation in the pump. Following this success, a series of in vivo experiments have been initiated with the goal of 6-month, thrombus-free implantation

4. The Chang Heart Assist Device — An Inexpensive "Bridge" System (CHAD Research Laboratories)

Ventricular assist devices (VADs) for "bridge to other therapy" are good candidates for lower-cost technologies, particularly in the areas of pump fabrication and valve and driver design. With the advent of less-expensive VADs should come increasing willingness of clinicians to use these devices in cases where pharmacologic or intra-aortic balloon support is currently employed.

The Chang Heart Assist Device (CHAD) has been designed for ease of manufacture, and uses injection moulding for the rigid case and valve housings, and vacuum forming methods to produce the flexing diaphragm. All blood-contacting surfaces are solution-coated with a biocompatible polyurethane following assembly, to provide a continuous smooth layer. The blood pump incorporates integral valved conduits with ball occluders which provide good central flow characteristics to enhance the formation of a persistent "spiral vortex" within the pumping chamber.

A self-contained pneumatic driver has been designed which features a colour touch-screen interface. Multiple parameters are monitored by both main and backup microprocessors allowing fuzzy logic control of driving parameters and fault detection. This driver is made from stock components and is assembled onto a rigid chassis, which allows easy assembly and keeps all the components in tight and precise alignment whilst taking up all reaction forces.

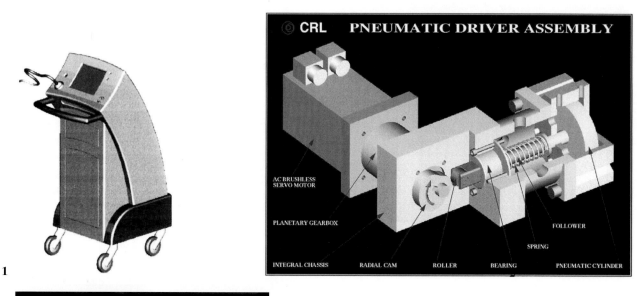

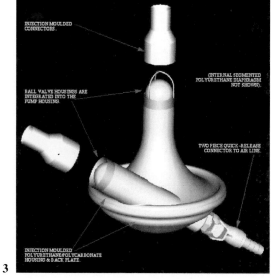

1

3

Fig. 1. Self-contained driver unit with touch-screen user interface
Fig. 2. Mechanical driver assembly featuring integral chassis
Fig. 3. "Spiral vortex" ventricular assist device (VAD) concept with integral ball valves

5. Eccentric Roller Type Artificial Heart (Hiroshima University)

Toward a completely implantable total artificial heart system, we have designed an eccentric roller type artificial heart. Blood chambers are made of silicone rubber and are toroidal in shape, and the actuator of the artificial heart is a drum-type eccentric roller, as shown in Fig. 1. The main characteristics of the artificial heart are that it discharges blood in pulsatile mode and that it requires no reversing of the motor. We tested the actuator with an overflow-type circulatory system of 100 mmHg afterload. It worked at the roller speeds of 50, 100, and 150 rpm producing outputs of 1.7, 3.7, and 5.4 l/min, respectively, as shown in Fig. 2.

Silicone Trileaflet Valve for Artificial Hearts.

Silicone trileaflet valves were developed for use in the artificial heart. The valves and the blood chamber are made en bloc using a die caster. The blood chamber is placed in a casing and is driven by a pneumatic artificial heart driver, as shown in Fig. 3. In an overflow-type circulatory system, the maximal flow of 6.3 l/min was achieved at a rate of 80 bpm, as shown in Fig. 4. The pressure gradient across the silicone valves was slightly greater than that across the existing valves for clinical use. The device has worked well for eight weeks in the circulatory system.

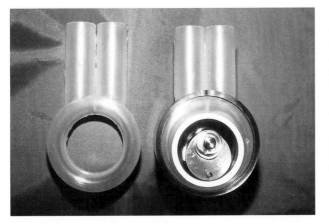

Fig. 1. Toroidal silicone blood chamber (*left*) and the eccentric roller squeezing the blood chamber (*right*)

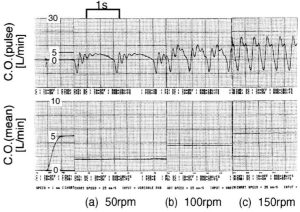

Fig. 2. Cardiac output (*C.O.*) of the eccentric roller type artificial heart: *upper*, instantaneous flow rate; *lower*, mean flow rate

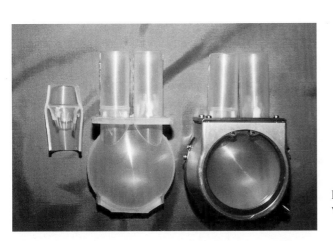

Fig. 3. Cross-section of the silicone trileaflet valve (*left*), valve-integrated blood chamber (*center*), and external view of the ventricular assist device (*right*)

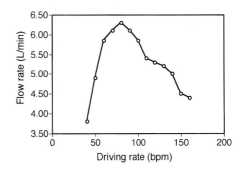

Fig. 4. Relationship of flow rate and driving rate of the ventricular assist device

6. Totally Implantable Motor-Driven Assist Pump System (Hokkaido Tokai University)

We have been developing a totally implantable motor-driven assist pump system that consists of a transcutaneous energy transmission system, a motor-driven assist pump, and a bidirectional optical telemetry system. The motor-driven assist pump consists of a brushless direct current motor driving a ball-screw and a pusher-plate-type blood pump. The ball screw converts high-speed bidirectional rotational motion of the motor into recti-linear movement of the pusher-plate.

Concurrently, we have also been developing polytetrafluoroethylene (PTFE)-coated ball-bearings to increase the endurance of the motor-driven assist pump. The goal of the PTFE-coated ball-bearings is two years' life in a humidity of 100% without any lubricant. The PTFE-coated ball-bearing system consists of stainless steel inner and outer rings, a stainless steel cage, and stainless steel balls. The raceways on both the rights and the cage are coated with PTFE (5 μm) as a solid lubricant. For verification of its endurance, the PTFE-coated ball-bearing prototype has been tested in a bearing test system for 551 days (as of November 18, 1996). By monitoring results of the power of particular frequencies in sound and vibration signals from the ball-bearings, we have not detected any sign of deterioration of the bearings.

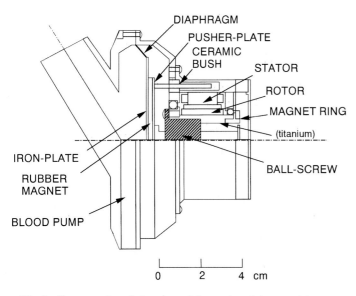

Fig. 1. Cross-sectional drawing of the motor-driven assist pump

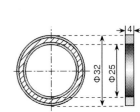

Fig. 2. Motor-driven assist pump, implantable controller, and its compliance chamber. The motor-driven assist pump displaces a volume of 350 ml and weighs 790 g. The pump stroke volume is 65 ml

Fig. 3. Polytetrafluoroethylene (PTFE)-coated ball-bearing system

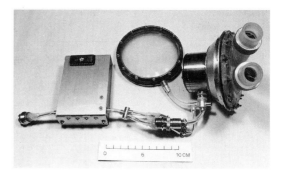

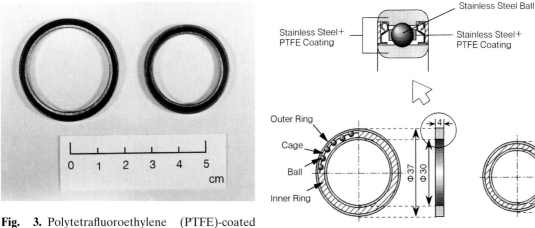

Basic Dynamic Load Capacity 77kgf
Basic Static Load Rating 100kgf
Number of Balls 24

Basic Dynamic Load Capacity 68kgf
Basic Static Load Rating 94kgf
Number of Balls 21

Fig. 4. Constitution of PTFE-coated ball-bearing system. The raceways are coated with PTFE as a solid lubricant. Units are mm

7. Centrifugal Pump with a Magnetically Suspended Impeller: Kyoto — NTN Pump (Kyoto University and NTN Corporation)

A centrifugal pump with a magnetically suspended impeller has been developed in Kyoto University in collaboration with NTN Corporation. The pump is composed of three parts: a motor unit, a pump housing, and a magnetic bearing. The pump housing has an impeller inside that pumps blood flow in and out. The rotor of the motor and the corresponding impeller have 24 pairs of permanent magnets that produce magnetic attraction. On the opposite side of the impeller, electromagnets produce contrary magnetic force against the permanent magnets so as to float the impeller inside the casing. The magnetic bearing contains three electromagnets and gap sensors which detect the distance between the impeller and the electromagnets so that any instability of the impeller can be actively controlled. The hemolysis test showed that this pump was better than the Biomedicus pump with respect to destruction of blood components. Chronic animal experiments are in progress using sheep in which the pumps have been extracorporeally placed. To date, seven sheep have undergone implantation of the pumps and the longest survival was 46 days. The pump flow rates during the experiment were 2.5–5.0 l/min under a pressure head of 100–140 mmHg. The implantable version of the Kyoto-NTN pump is a promising device for long-term clinical use.

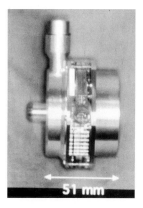

Fig. 1. Overview of a current version of the Kyoto-NTN pump. The pump is designed as an implantable left ventricular assist system

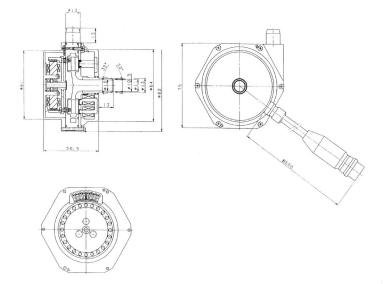

Fig. 3. Cross-sectional view and blueprint of the pump

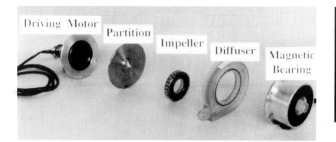

Fig. 2. Components of the Kyoto-NTN pump

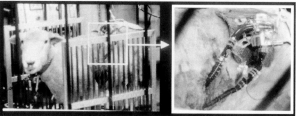

Fig. 4. Chronic animal experiment using sheep

8. Artificial Hearts Developed at the National Cardiovascular Center, Osaka, Japan (National Cardiovascular Center)

Two types of electric artificial heart have been developed for long-term use at the National Cardiovascular Center, Osaka, Japan. One is a centrifugal pump (NCVC-2) with a unique structure for chronic support. The pump is driven by magnetic coupling and has no shaft for rotation, no seal around the rotating part, and a balancing hole at the center of the impeller and the thrust bearing. The pump ran for more than a year as a left heart bypass in a chronic animal experiment.

The second device is a totally implantable electrohydraulic (EH) artificial heart. The components of the system are diaphragm-type ventricles, an intracorporeal and separately placed regenerative pump as an EH actuator, flexible stainless steel tubes to connect these two parts, an externally coupled transcutaneous energy transfer system, a transcutaneous optical telemetry system, an internal battery, and an internal control-drive unit. This device is now being tested in a chronic animal experiment.

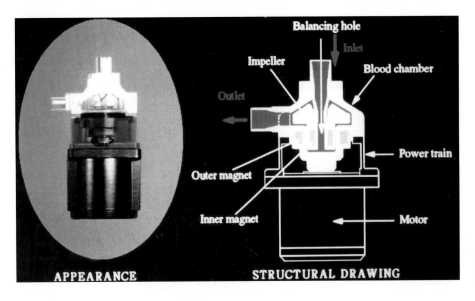

Fig. 1. NCVC-2 type centrifugal pump for long-term use

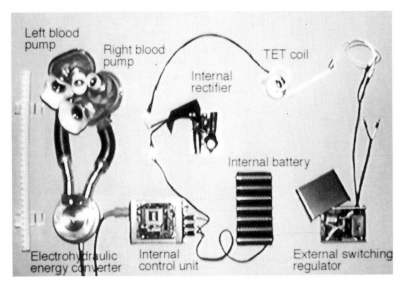

Fig. 2. A totally implantable electrohydraulic (EH) artificial heart system
1. EH blood pumps: implantable in 50–70 kg animals
   — Pump output performance: up to 8 l/min driven with transcutaneous energy transfer (TET) system
   — Efficiency: 10% at 6 l/min of cardiac output (within 4°C temperature rise)
2. TET system: 80% d.c.–d.c. efficiency in a chronic animal experiment
   — Internal rectifier: $74 \times 55 \times 20$ mm
   — External switching circuit: $59 \times 80 \times 31$ mm
3. Transcutaneous optical telemetry (TOT) system: stable positioning and generous allowance of sensor displacement
4. Internal battery: 120 ml and 280 g (Li ion battery)
5. Internal control drive unit: $70 \times 70 \times 20$ mm

9. Intraventricular Artificial Heart (Iva-Heart)
(Tokyo Women's Medical College, University of Pittsburgh, Waseda University, and Sun Medical Technology Research Corp.)

We have developed an intraventricular artificial heart. This device is an axial flow blood pump for use as an implantable left ventricular assist device (LVAD). The blood pump has a recirculating purge system with a mechanical seal. This is a breakthrough system, where purge fluid circulates within the pump and motor to minimize blood clotting and heat generation in the seal area of the pump rotary shaft. This purge system results in little leakage or clotting of blood during long-term use. Diamond-like carbon (DLC) coating is an original surface treatment method which has excellent antithrombogenicity.

The pump was implanted in a calf (168 days of support). It was inserted into the left ventricular (LV) cavity via the LV apex and the outlet cannula was passed antegrade across the aortic valve without any difficulty. Blood was withdrawn from the LV cavity through the inlet ports at the pump base, and discharged into the ascending aorta.

Pump function and hemodynamics remained stable throughout the experiment. No cardiac arrhythmias were detected, even during treadmill exercise tests. The plasma free hemoglobin level remained in an acceptable range (<10mg/dl). Post mortem examination did not reveal any interference between the pump and the mitral apparatus. No major thromboembolism was detected in the vital organs.

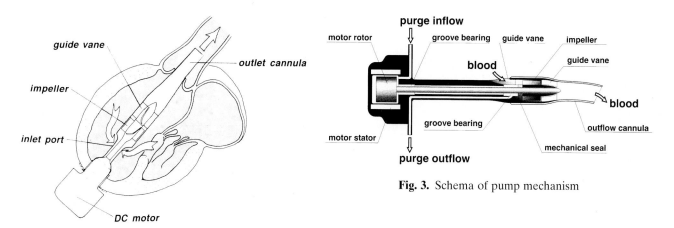

Fig. 1. Schema of blood flow

Fig. 3. Schema of pump mechanism

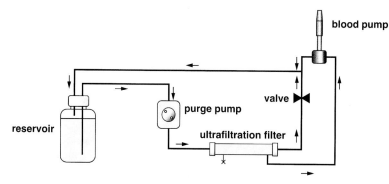

Fig. 2. Schema of recirculating purge system

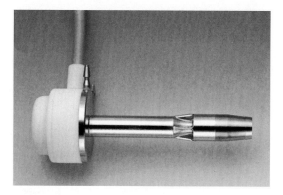

Fig. 4. Iva-Heart (prototype no.9)
Materials
Pump body, impeller, pump casing: titanium alloy
Outlet cannula: silicon
Motor casing: polytetrafluoroethylene (PTFE)
Surface treatment: diamond-like carbon (DLC) coating
Pump weight: 170g
Impeller diameter: 13.9mm
Shaft sealing: mechanical seal
Purge consumption <10cm³/day

10. New Developments of the Moving-Actuator Type Total Artificial Heart
   (Seoul National University)

The electromechanical total artificial heart (TAH) developed in Seoul National University Hospital was verified as acceptable for human implantation through several successful animal experiments.

In the last two years (1994–1996), the TAH has been re-designed to be small (600–650cm³ total volume), and lightweight (approximately 950g), as well as improved to overcome the three practical problems that faced the animal experiments. First, we implemented modifications to the blood pump housing to resolve the problem of anatomical compatibility through the construction of a 3-dimensional model of the TAH, the human thoracic cavity, and the large vessels, from magnetic resonance imaging (MRI) and computed tomography studies. Secondly, the intraventricular surface of the blood sacs was modified with fibrinolytic and anti-infective surface treatments. Thirdly, the regulation mechanism of cardiac output (CO) was improved by analyzing the measured pressure of the interventricular volume space (IVP). This was very beneficial, to achieve CO regulation in response to the physiological demand as well as the prevention of atrial collapse due to suction. As an accurate indicator hemodynamic status, the IVP was used to predict the preload condition.

The three improvements will assist in the application of the newly developed implantable electromechanical artificial heart for long-term implantation.

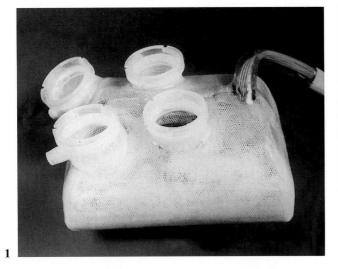

1

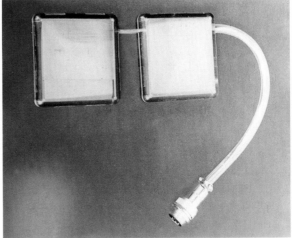

2

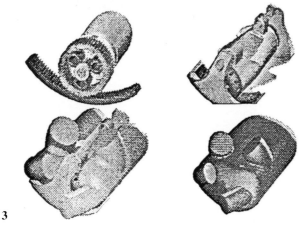

3

Fig. 1. The moving-actuator type total artificial heart (TAH)
Fig. 2. The redesigned electronics assembly for an implantable total artificial heart
Fig. 3. The new blood pump. Solid model of the energy convertor and rack gear of the Korean TAH (*upper left*); outer case assembled to this model (*upper right*); two blood sacs for the left ventricle and right ventricle assembled in the correct position (*lower left*); and solid model of assembled Korean TAH (*lower right*)

For the relationship between the imbalanced pump output and interrentricular space pressure, refer to Fig. 3 in the chapter by Jo, this volume.

11. Linear Pulse Motor-Driven Total Artificial Heart System: Kuniko III
(Shinshu University)

A human body model equipped with a linear pulse motor-driven total artificial heart (linear TAH) system has been developed and dubbed "Kuniko III." She has a linear TAH, a mock circulatory system, a drive control unit, and a transcutaneous energy transmission (TET) system. The systemic and pulmonary circulation have been improved in this new system. The linear TAH consists of a linear pulse motor, two pusher plates, two sac-type blood pumps, and four Jellyfish valves. The volume of the linear TAH is 580 ml. The linear TAH pumps out the blood by expanding and compressing the blood pumps according to the reciprocating motion of the pusher plates attached at the mover of the linear pulse motor. The TET system is made up of a d.c.–a.c. inverter, a transcutaneous transformer utilizing amorphous magnetic fiber, and an a.c.–d.c. converter. The TET system transmits the electric energy from a d.c. power supply outside of her body to the linear TAH within her body without piercing the skin. The excitation frequency to the transformer is 120 kHz. The pumping rate of the linear TAH is displayed on an outside pumping rate meter through a photocoupler.

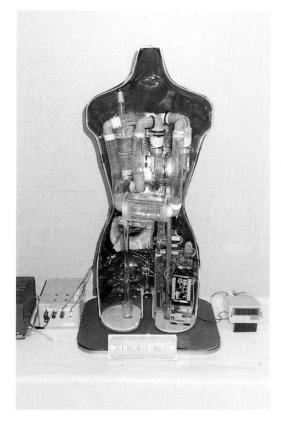

Fig. 1. External view of Kuniko III

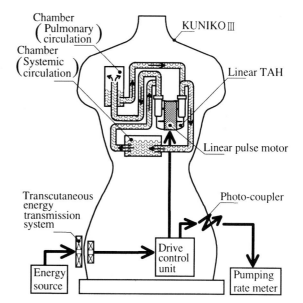

Fig. 2. Constitution of Kuniko III. *TAH*, total artificial heart

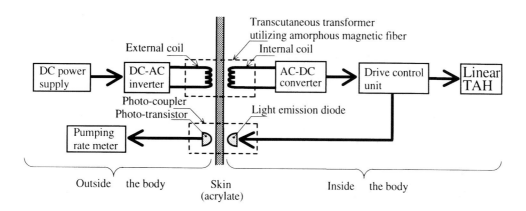

Fig. 3. Block diagram of the transcutaneous energy transmission system in Kuniko III

12. The HeartMate Vented Electric Left Ventricular Assist System (Thermo Cardiosystems)

The HeartMate vented electric blood pump is an implantable device that takes over the pumping function of seriously damaged or diseased hearts. The system comprises an implantable left ventricular assist device (LVAD), along with external power and control electronics. In addition, the system's lightweight, belt-mounted controller gives patients complete mobility. The LVAD features a blood pump and an integrally coupled, high-efficiency electric motor. This motor produces one eject cycle during a single revolution. When the eject is complete, the motor halts, permitting the pump to be refilled by the left ventricle.

The pump's unique textured blood-contacting surfaces encourage the deposition of a tightly adhered fibrin/cellular matrix, rich in a variety of cells, including endothelial cells. The resulting pseudo-neointima reduces the need for anticoagulation and may reduce the risk of thromboembolic complications.

Thermo Cardiosystems is a leader in the research and development of implantable left ventricular assist systems. Our air-driven HeartMate is the only implantable heart-assist device approved in the United States for commercial sale, and our electric system is under clinical evaluation to sustain patients awaiting transplant, and as an alternative to medical therapy for nontransplant candidates.

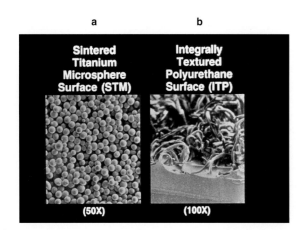

Fig. 1. The HeartMate vented electric blood pump in situ. *LVAD*, left ventricular assist device

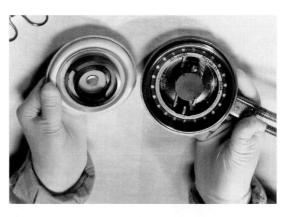

Fig. 2. The LVAD's high-efficiency electric motor

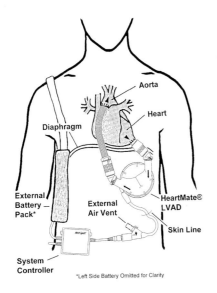

Fig. 3. a Sintered titanium microspheres and **b** Cardioflex polyurethane

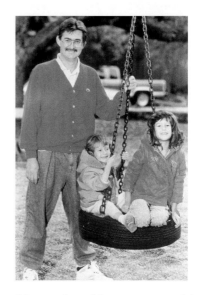

Fig. 4. HeartMate patient able to resume activities of daily living

13. Tohoku University Pneumatically Driven Total Artificial Heart (TAH) and Totally Implantable Ventricular Assist System Using a Vibrating Flow Pump (VFP) (Tohoku University)

A pneumatically driven TAH system was developed using a silicone ball valve in a sac-type artificial blood pump. It can be mounted into the thoracic cavity of the healthy adult goat and may be able to produce enough blood flow for the systemic circulation. The blood sac was improved to generate round shaped blood streamline on the basis of fluid science studies. An electromagnetic rotating ball pump was shown in one exhibition (Fig. 1). The rotating ball pump was for the extracorporeal circulation. A model totally implantable ventricular assist system using a vibrating flow pump (VFP) was shown in the other exhibition (Fig. 2). The VFP may be built as a small-sized artificial heart, because of its short stroke volume with high-frequency driving. This system was totally implantable and was driven by a transcutaneous energy transmission system (TETS). The TETS, developed at Tohoku University, was made from copper line with spokewise-placed cobalt amorphous fibers. Electromagnetic radiation from outside was shut out and energy transfer efficiency was increased by using this seal with amorphous fibers.

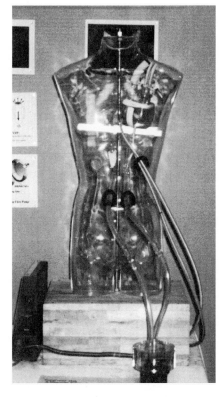

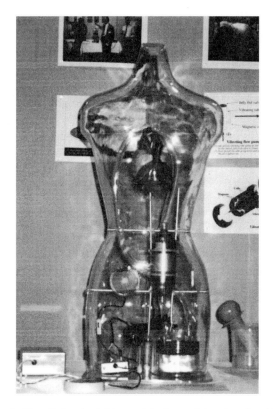

Fig. 1. Pneumatically driven total artificial heart (TAH) and rotary ball pump

Fig. 2. Totally implantable ventricular assist system in which a vibrating flow pump (VFP) is used

14. TOW NOK Component System III Heart Lung System, AVECOR AFFINITY Oxygenation Systems (Tonokura Ika Kogyo Co. Ltd.)

The latest version of our heart lung system, Compo, has made another step further to meet today and tomorrow's high demands of the operation room. Compo has been developed to be user-friendly as well as being friendly to the patient. Various messages can be displayed during the operation on a large screen liquid crystal display (LCD) monitor (option). With this monitor, the user can easily observe the necessary information. We have used our unique Ω-shaped casing on the pump head. Our in-house experiment has confirmed that the Ω-shaped casing has a far lower hemolysis level than the conventional U-shaped head casing.

AVECOR Membrane Oxygenator AFFINITY

The AFFINITY has been developed to meet all the demands for an oxygenator in today's cardiopulmonary bypass. A very high gas exchange performance with a small profile, a blood flow path with minimum blood shear and shunts, low pressure drop within the blood flow path; all of these features were made possible by using a highly sophisticated computational fluid dynamics program. The completely transparent housing employed for the product allows very high visibility of the blood flowing throughout the oxygenator. This high quality oxygenation system has an optional reservoir, both hardshell and a reservoir bag.

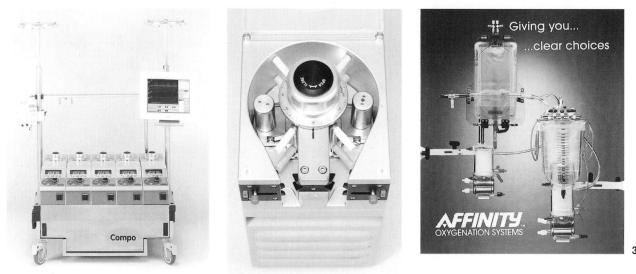

1,2

Fig. 1. Heart Lung System Compo III
Fig. 2. Ω-Shaped pump casing
Fig. 3. AFFINITY Oxygenation System

15. New Concept of the Artificial Heart
(The University of Tokyo)

The University of Tokyo has been developing an artificial heart (AH) since 1959. To date, many significant outcomes have been generated by out laboratory with new concepts in hardware and software. Typical new conceptual AH work includes development of the jellyfish valve, a polymer membrane valve, and the study of the 1/R control method of the total artificial heart (TAH) in which the TAH goat itself controls cardiac output by changes in the total peripheral resistance. Using these technologies, we achieved the survival of a goat for 532 days with a pneumatically driven TAH in 1995. TAH research is now moving to ward a totally implantable TAH.

We exhibited two new conceptual AH systems, the undulation pump-TAH (UP-TAH) and the modified assist device (MAD). The UP-TAH is a very compact (75 mm in diameter and 80 mm long) TAH composed of two undulation pumps and two brushless DC motors. It could be implanted into the chest cavity of a goat weighing 42 kg. The MAD is a percutaneously accessible ventricular assist device composed of a valveless single-port diaphragm-type pump and a cannula 6.5 mm in diameter with a small inflow and outflow valve. It is driven pneumatically and can pump 2 to 3 L/min of pulsatile flow.

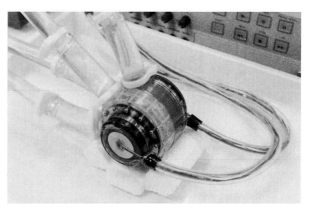

Fig. 2. The UP-TAH, the world's most compact TAH

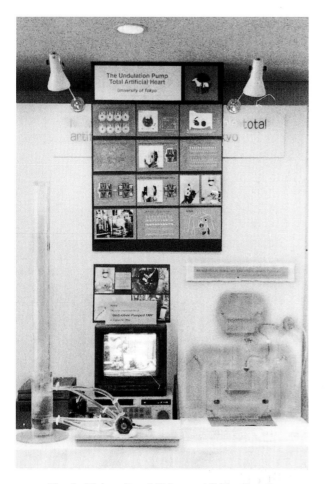

Fig. 1. University of Tokyo exhibition booth

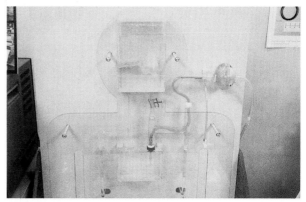

Fig. 3. The MAD exhibited in a mock circulatory system

Key Word Index